Blood Cells

Blood Cells
A Practical Guide

Barbara J. Bain MBBS, FRACP, FRCPath

Professor of Diagnostic Haematology
St Mary's Hospital Campus of Imperial College
Faculty of Medicine, London
and Honorary Consultant Haematologist,
St Mary's Hospital, London

Fourth Edition

Blackwell
Publishing

First published 1989 (Published by Gower Medical Publishing)
Second edition 1995
Third edition 2002
Fourth edition 2006

2   2007

Library of Congress Cataloging-in-Publication Data

Bain, Barbara J.
     Blood cells : a practical guide / Barbara J. Bain. — 4th ed.
        p. ; cm.
     Includes bibliographical references and index.
     ISBN: 978-1-4051-4265-6 (alk. paper)
     1. Blood cells.   2. Blood cell count.
     [DNLM: 1. Blood Cell Count.   2. Blood Cells—physiology.   3. Hematologic Tests—methods.
QY 402 B162b 2006]   I. Title.

     RB45.B27 2006
     612.1′1—dc22

                                                                                            2005031759

ISBN: 978-1-4051-4265-6

A catalogue record for this title is available from the British Library

Set in 9/12pt Palatino by Graphicraft Limited, Hong Kong
Printed and bound in Singapore by Fabulous Printers Pte Ltd

Commissioning Editor: Maria Khan
Editorial Assistant: Saskia Van der Linden
Development Editor: Rob Blundell
Production Controller: Kate Charman

For further information on Blackwell Publishing, visit our website:
http://www.blackwellpublishing.com

The publisher's policy is to use permanent paper from mills that operate a sustainable forestry policy,
and which has been manufactured from pulp processed using acid-free and elementary chlorine-free
practices. Furthermore, the publisher ensures that the text paper and cover board used have met
acceptable environmental accreditation standards.

Contents

Preface

Blood Cells has been written with both the practising haematologist and the trainee in mind. My aim has been to provide a guide for use in the diagnostic haematology laboratory, covering methods of collection of blood specimens, blood film preparation and staining, the principles of manual and automated blood counts and the assessment of the morphological features of blood cells. My objective has been that the practising haematologist should find this book sufficiently comprehensive to be a reference source while, at the same time, the trainee haematologist and biomedical scientist should find it a straightforward and practical bench manual. I hope that the medically trained haematologist will gain a fuller understanding of the scientific basis of an important segment of laboratory haematology while the laboratory scientist will understand more of the purpose and clinical relevance of laboratory tests. I trust it is not too ambitious to hope to be 'all things to all men'. This edition has been expanded to keep it as comprehensive and up-to-date as possible and includes more guidance on the further tests that should be performed for any given provisional diagnosis. The chapter on supplementary tests now includes more details on the role of immunophenotyping. In addition, cytogenetic and molecular genetic techniques are discussed briefly. However, microscopy and the automated full blood count remain the core of the book. My overriding purpose has been to show that microscopy not only provides the essential basis of our haematological practice but can also lead to the excitement of discovery. The decline in the number of blood films made and the increasingly heavy clinical commitments of any haematologist who is not purely a laboratory haematologist make this book more than ever necessary. If I succeed in sending the reader back to the microscope with renewed interest and enthusiasm I shall be well satisfied.

Barbara J. Bain
London, 2006

Acknowledgements

I remain grateful to thank Dr John Matthews, Mr Alan Dean, the late Dr Kate Ozanne and Dr Ketan Patel who between them critically read the manuscripts for the first, second and third editions of this book. The specialist registrars of St Mary's Hospital kindly shared the task of reviewing the fourth edition. I should like to thank also the many other colleagues who provided blood films for photography and those others, numbering in their hundreds, with whom I have discussed interesting and difficult diagnostic problems over the last 35 years. I should like to acknowledge Dr Helen Dodsworth without whose comment to an editor this book might not have happened. Finally, in this latest and, possibly, last edition, I should like to remember and acknowledge those who taught me to examine blood films, particularly but not only the late Professor Sir John Dacie, Professor David Galton, Professor Sunitha Wickramasinghe and Professor Daniel Catovsky.

List of abbreviations

aCML atypical chronic myeloid leukaemia
ACTH adrenocorticotropic hormone
AIDS acquired immune deficiency syndrome
ALL acute lymphoblastic leukaemia
AML acute myeloid leukaemia
ANAE α-naphthyl acetate esterase
ANBE α-naphthyl butyrate esterase
ATLL adult T-cell leukaemia/lymphoma
ATP adenosine triphosphate
B-PLL B-lineage prolymphocytic leukaemia
CAE chloroacetate esterase
CD cluster of differentiation
CDA congenital dyserythropoietic anaemia
CDC Centers for Disease Control
CGL chronic granulocytic leukaemia
CHCM cellular haemoglobin concentration mean
   (Technicon H.1 series counters)
CLL chronic lymphocytic leukaemia
CLL/PL CLL, mixed cell type
CML chronic myeloid leukaemia
CMML chronic myelomonocytic leukaemia
CMV cytomegalovirus
CV coefficient of variation
DDAVP 1-deamino-8-D-arginine vasopressin
DNA deoxyribonucleic acid
EBV Epstein–Barr virus
EDTA ethylenediaminetetra-acetic acid
ESR erythrocyte sedimentation rate
FAB French–American–British (classifications of
   haematological neoplasms)
FBC full blood count
FDA Food and Drug Administration
FISH fluorescence *in situ* hybridization
FITC fluorescein isothiocyanate
G6PD glucose-6-phosphate dehydrogenase
G-CSF granulocyte colony-stimulating factor
GM-CSF granulocyte macrophage colony-
   stimulating factor
GPI glycosylphosphatidylinositol

Hb haemoglobin concentration
Hct haematocrit
HDW haemoglobin distribution width
HELLP haemolysis, elevated liver enzymes and
   low platelet (syndrome)
HEMPAS hereditary erythroid multinuclearity
   with positive acidified serum test
HES hypereosinophilic syndrome
HHV6 human herpesvirus 6
HIV human immunodeficiency virus
HLA histocompatibility locus antigen
HPFH hereditary persistence of fetal haemoglobin
HPLC high performance liquid chromatography
HTLV-I human T-cell lymphotropic virus I
HTLV-II human T-cell lymphotropic virus II
ICSH International Committee (now Council) for
   Standardization in Haematology
IL interleukin
ITP idiopathic (autoimmune) thrombocytopenic
   purpura
JMML juvenile myelomonocytic leukaemia
LCAT lecithin-cholesterol acyl transferase
LDH lactate dehydrogenase
LI lobularity index (H.1 series counters)
LUC large unstained cells (H.1 series counters)
MALT mucosa-associated lymphoid tissue
MCH mean cell haemoglobin
MCHC mean cell haemoglobin concentration
M-CSF macrophage colony-stimulating factor
MCV mean cell volume
MDS myelodysplastic syndrome/s
MGG May-Grünwald–Giemsa (stain)
MIRL membrane inhibitor of reactive lysis
MPC mean platelet component concentration
MPM mean platelet mass
MPO myeloperoxidase
MPV mean platelet volume
MPXI mean peroxidase index (H.1 series counters)
NAP neutrophil alkaline phosphatase

NASA naphthol AS acetate esterase
NASDA naphthol AS-D acetate esterase
NCCLS National/Committee for Clinical Laboratory Standards
NK natural killer (cell)
NRBC nucleated red blood cell
PAS periodic acid–Schiff (reaction)
PCDW platelet component distribution width
PCH paroxysmal cold haemoglobinuria
PCR polymerase chain reaction
Pct plateletcrit
PCV packed cell volume
PDW platelet distribution width
Peg-rHuMGDF polyethylene glycol recombination human megakaryocyte growth and development factor
PHA phytohaemagglutinin
PLL prolymphocytic leukaemia
PMDW platelet mass distribution width
PNH paroxysmal nocturnal haemoglobinuria
POEMS polyneuropathy, organomegaly, endocrinopathy, M protein, skin changes (syndrome)
PRV polycythaemia rubra vera
RBC red blood cell count

RDW red cell distribution width
RNA ribonucleic acid
RT-PCR reverse transcriptase polymerase chain reaction
SBB Sudan black B
SD standard deviation
SI Système International
SLVL splenic lymphoma with villous lymphocytes
TNCC total nucleated cell count
T-PLL T-lineage prolymphocytic leukaemia
TRAP tartrate-resistant acid phosphatase
TTP thrombotic thrombocytopenic purpura
WBC white blood cell count
WHO World Health Organization
WIC WBC in the impedance channel (Cell-Dyn instruments)
WOC WBC in the optical channel (Cell-Dyn instruments)

Note to the reader

Unless otherwise stated, all photomicrographs have been stained with a May-Grünwald–Giemsa stain and have a final magnification of approximately 912.

1 Blood sampling and blood film preparation and examination

Obtaining a blood specimen

Performing an accurate blood count and correctly interpreting a blood film require that an appropriate sample from the patient, mixed with the correct amount of a suitable anticoagulant, is delivered to the laboratory without undue delay. No artefacts should be introduced during these procedures.

The identity of the patient requiring blood sampling should be carefully checked before performing a venepuncture. This is usually done by requesting the patient to state surname, given name and date of birth and, for hospital inpatients, by checking a wristband to verify these details and, in addition, the hospital number. To reduce the chance of human error, bottles should not be labelled in advance. The person performing the phlebotomy must conform to local guidelines, including those for patient identification. Although traditionally more attention has been given to patient identification in relation to blood transfusion it should be noted that wrong treatment has also followed misidentification of patients from whom samples are taken for a blood count and identification must also be taken seriously in this field. More secure identification of inpatients can be achieved by the use of electronic devices in which the patient's identity is scanned in from a barcoded wristband by means of a hand-held device.

Patients should either sit or lie comfortably and should be reassured that the procedure causes only minimal discomfort; they should not be told that venepuncture is painless, since this is not so. It is preferable for apprehensive patients to lie down. Chairs used for venepuncture should preferably have adjustable armrests so that the arm can be carefully positioned. Armrests also help to ensure patient safety, since they make it harder for a fainting patient to fall from the chair. I have personally observed one patient who sustained a skull fracture when he fainted at the end of a venepuncture and fell forward onto a hard floor, and two other patients, neither previously known to be epileptic, who suffered epileptiform convulsions during venepuncture. Such seizures may not be true epilepsy, but consequent on hypoxia following brief vagal-induced cessation of heart beat [1]. If venepunctures are being performed on children or on patients unable to cooperate fully then the arm for venepuncture should be gently but firmly immobilized by an assistant. Gloves should be worn during venepuncture, for the protection of the person carrying out the procedure. Non-latex gloves must be available if either the phlebotomist or the patient is allergic to latex. The needle to enter the patient must not be touched, so that it remains sterile.

Peripheral venous blood

In an adult, peripheral venous blood is most easily obtained from a vein in the antecubital fossa (Fig. 1.1) using a needle and either a syringe or an evacuated tube. Of the veins in the antecubital region the median cubital vein is preferred, since it is usually large and well anchored in tissues, but the cephalic and basilic veins are also often satisfactory. Other forearm veins can be used, but they are often more mobile and therefore more difficult to penetrate. Veins on the dorsum of the wrist and hand often have a poorer flow and performing venepuncture at these sites is more likely to lead to bruising. This is also true of the anterior surface of the wrist where, in addition, venepuncture tends to be more painful and where there is more risk of damaging vital structures. Foot veins are not an ideal site for venepuncture and it is rarely necessary to use them. Injuries that have been associated with obtaining a blood sample from the antecubital fossa include damage to the lateral antebrachial cutaneous nerve [2] and inadvertent

Basilic vein

Median cubital vein

Cephalic vein

Accessory cephalic vein

Fig. 1.1 Anterior surface of the left arm showing veins most suitable for venepuncture.

arterial puncture. Complications are more likely with the less accessible basilic vein than with the median antecubital or the cephalic vein. If anterior wrist veins have to be used there is a risk of damage to the radial or ulnar nerve or artery. Use of foot veins is more likely to lead to complications, e.g. thrombosis, infection or poor healing.

When a vein is identified it is palpated to ensure it is patent. A patent vein is soft and can be compressed easily. A thrombosed vein feels cord-like and is not compressible. An artery has a thicker wall and is pulsatile. If a vein is not visible (in some dark-skinned or overweight people) it is identified by palpation after applying a tourniquet to achieve venous distension. If veins appear very small, warming of the arm to produce vasodilatation helps, as does tapping the vein and asking the patient to clench and unclench the fist several times.

It should be noted that pathogenic bacteria can be cultured from reusable tourniquets and it is prudent practice to use disposable tourniquets at least for patients at particular risk of infection [3].

The arm should be positioned on the armrest so that the vein identified is under some tension and its mobility is reduced. The skin should be cleaned with 70% ethanol or 0.5% chlorhexidine and allowed to dry, to avoid stinging when the skin is penetrated. A tourniquet is applied to the arm, sufficiently tightly to distend the vein, but not so tightly that discomfort is caused. Alternatively, a sphygmomanometer cuff can be applied and inflated to diastolic pressure, but the use of a tourniquet is usually quicker and simpler. If it is particularly important to obtain a specimen without causing haemoconcentration, e.g. in a patient with suspected polycythaemia, the tourniquet should be left on the arm only long enough to allow penetration of the vein. Otherwise it can be left applied while blood is being obtained, to ensure a continuing adequate flow of blood. It is preferable that the tourniquet is applied for no more than a minute, but the degree of haemoconcentration is not great, even after 10 minutes application. The increase of haemoglobin concentration and of red cell count is about 2% at 2 and at 10 minutes [4].

Fig. 1.2 Venepuncture technique using needle and syringe.

Blood specimens can be obtained with a needle and an evacuated tube (see below) or with either a needle or a winged blood collection cannula (a 'butterfly') and a syringe. A winged cannula is preferable for small veins and difficult sites. A 19 or 20 gauge needle is suitable for an adult and a 21 or 23 gauge for a child or an adult with small veins. When using a syringe, the plunger should first be moved within the barrel of the syringe to ensure that it will move freely. Next the needle is attached to the syringe, which, unless small, should have a side port rather than a central port. The guard is then removed. The needle is now inserted into the vein with the bevel facing upwards (Fig. 1.2). This may be done in a single movement or in two separate movements for the skin and the vein, depending on personal preference and on how superficial the vein is. With one hand steadying the barrel of the syringe so that the needle is not accidentally withdrawn from the vein, blood is withdrawn into the syringe using minimal negative pressure. Care should be taken not to aspirate more rapidly than blood is entering the vein, or the wall of the vein may be drawn against the bevel of the needle and cut off the flow of blood. If the tourniquet has not already been released this must be done before withdrawing the needle. Following removal of the needle, direct pressure is applied to the puncture site with cotton wool or a sterile gauze square, the arm being kept straight and, if preferred, somewhat elevated. Adhesive plaster should not be applied until pressure has been sustained for long enough for bleeding from the puncture site to have stopped.

The needle should be removed from the syringe before expelling the blood into the specimen container, great care being taken to avoid self-injury with the needle. The needle should be put directly into a special receptacle for sharp objects without resheathing it. The blood specimen is expelled gently into a bottle containing anticoagulant and is mixed gently by inverting the container four or five times. Forceful ejection of the blood can cause lysis. Shaking should also be avoided. The specimen container is then labelled with the patient's name and identifying details and, depending on hospital standard operating procedure, possibly also with a bar-code label, which is also applied to the request form and subsequently to the blood film. The time of venepuncture should also be recorded on the bottle. Bottles should not be labelled in advance away from the patient's bedside as this increases the chances of putting a blood sample into a mislabelled bottle. Recording the time of venepuncture is important both to allow the clinician to relate the laboratory result to the condition of the patient at the time and also to allow the laboratory to check that there has been no undue delay between venepuncture and performing the test.

When blood is taken into an evacuated tube the technique of venepuncture is basically similar. A double-ended needle is screwed into a holder, which allows it to be manipulated for venepuncture (Fig. 1.3). Alternatively, a winged cannula can be attached to an evacuated tube, using a plastic holder into which an adaptor is screwed. Once the vein has been entered an evacuated tube is inserted into the holder and is pushed firmly so that its rubber cap is penetrated by the needle, breaking the vacuum and causing blood to be aspirated into the tube (Fig. 1.4).

Fig. 1.3 Venepuncture technique using an evacuated container; the distal end of the needle has been screwed into the holder and the proximal needle has then been unsheathed and inserted into a suitable vein.

Fig. 1.4 Venepuncture technique using an evacuated container; the evacuated container has been inserted into the holder and forced onto the sharp end of the needle.

Evacuated tubes are very convenient if multiple specimens are to be taken, since several evacuated tubes can be applied in turn. Only sterile vacuum tubes should be used for obtaining blood specimens. In children and others with very small veins an appropriately small vacuum tube should be used so that excessive pressure does not cause the vein to collapse. Once all necessary specimen tubes have been filled, the needle is withdrawn from the vein, still attached to the holder. To reduce the possibility of a needle-prick injury it is necessary to either: (i) use a specially designed device that permits the needle to be discarded with a single-hand technique; (ii) remove the needle from the holder with a specially designed safe device; or (iii) throw away the holder with the needle. When blood samples are obtained with an evacuated tube system the anticoagulant from one tube may contaminate another. Heparin may interfere with coagulation tests, ethylenediaminetetra-acetic acid (EDTA) with calcium measurements and fluoride with haematological investigations. It is therefore advised, by the NCCLS (National Committee for Clinical Laboratory Standards, now renamed Clinical and Laboratory Standards Institute) that samples be taken in the order shown in Table 1.1 [5].

Table 1.1 Recommended order for taking blood samples.

Blood culture tubes
Plain glass tubes for serum samples
Sodium citrate tubes
Gel separator tubes/plain plastic tubes for serum
Heparin tubes/heparin gel separator tubes
EDTA tubes
Fluoride tubes for glucose

EDTA, ethylenediaminetetra-acetic acid.

If there is a need for a large specimen or a large number of specimens either an evacuated tube system or a syringe and winged cannula should be used. In the latter case the tubing is pinched off to allow several syringes in turn to be attached. This technique is also useful in children and when small veins make venepuncture difficult.

A blood specimen should not be taken from a vein above the site of an intravenous infusion, since dilution can occur. However, venepuncture below the site of an infusion is not associated with clinically significant inaccuracy.

'Capillary blood'

It is often necessary to obtain blood by skin puncture in babies and infants and in adults with poor veins. 'Capillary' or, more probably, arteriolar blood may be obtained from a freely flowing stab wound made with a sterile lancet on the plantar surface of a warmed and cleansed heel (babies less than 3 months of age and infants), the plantar aspect of the big toe (infants) or a finger, thumb or ear lobe (older children and adults). The correct site for puncture of the heel is shown in Fig. 1.5. The lateral or posterior aspect of the heel should not be used in a baby, as the underlying bone is much closer to the skin surface than it is on the plantar aspect. In older patients a finger (excluding the fifth finger) or the thumb is preferred to an ear lobe, since bleeding from the ear lobe may be prolonged in a patient with a haemostatic defect, and pressure is difficult to apply. The palmar surface of the distal phalanx is the preferred site on a digit, since the underlying bone is closer to the skin surface on other aspects. The middle or ring finger of the non-dominant hand is preferred; these digits are less painful than the index finger. In adults, skin

Yes No Yes

Fig. 1.5 The areas of the foot of a baby or infant that are suitable for obtaining capillary blood.

punctures should ideally be more than 1.5 mm deep in order that the lancet passes through the dermal–subcutaneous junction where the concentration of blood vessels is greatest, permitting a free flow of blood. Lancets used for heel puncture in full-term babies must not exceed 2.4 mm in length, since this is the depth below the skin of the calcaneal bone. Much shorter lancets are available and should be selected for use in premature babies. Osteomyelitis of the calcaneal bone has resulted from inadvertent puncture of the bone [6]. Previous puncture sites should be avoided, to reduce the risk of infection. Safety lancets, with a blade that retracts permanently after first use, have been developed in order to reduce the risk of accidental injury to phlebotomy staff. They are available in sizes appropriate for adults and children, infants and premature neonates.

Capillary samples should be obtained from warm tissues so that a free flow of blood is more readily obtained. If the area is cool then it should be warmed with a wet cloth, no hotter than 42°C. The skin should then be cleansed with 70% isopropanol and dried with a sterile gauze square (since traces of alcohol may lead to haemolysis of the specimen). The first drop of blood may be diluted with tissue fluid and should be wiped away with a sterile gauze square. Flow of blood may be promoted by gentle pressure, but a massaging or pumping action should not be employed, since this may lead to tissue fluid being mixed with blood.

Capillary blood can be collected into reusable glass pipettes or into glass capillary tubes. Reusable pipettes are not recommended, since they require cleaning. Capillary tubes coated with EDTA can be used, but tubes containing heparin are not suitable for full blood count (FBC) specimens since cellular morphology and staining characteristics are altered. Disposable pipettes complete with diluent, suitable for both automated and manual counts, are commercially available. Caution is necessary if glass capillary tubes are used, because of the risk of injury to the person obtaining the blood sample [7]. Caution should also be employed in the use of spring-loaded skin-prick devices, since transmission of hepatitis B from one patient to another has occurred when there has been failure to change the platform as well as the lancet between patients [8]. However, automated lancets do ensure a standardized depth of penetration. Use of one proprietary automated incision device (Tenderfoot) has been reported to cause less bruising and to be associated with less haemolysis of capillary samples than when the device is not used [9,10].

Platelet counts performed on capillary blood are often lower than are those on venous blood [11] and other parameters may also vary (see Chapter 5). The precision of measurement of haemoglobin concentration (Hb) on a single drop of capillary blood is poor and it is therefore recommended that several drops be put into an EDTA-containing tube [12].

Cord blood

Blood samples can be obtained from the umbilical cord immediately after birth. Cord blood is best obtained with a syringe and needle after removing any blood from the surface of the cord with a gauze square. Expressing blood from the cut end of the cord can introduce Wharton's jelly into the blood sample, with subsequent red cell agglutination. Haematological parameters on cord blood are not necessarily the same as those obtained from capillary or venous specimens from the neonate.

Obtaining a blood specimen from other sites

It may sometimes be necessary to obtain blood from the femoral vein or from indwelling cannulae in various sites. When blood is obtained from a cannula the first blood obtained may be diluted by infusion fluid or contaminated with heparin and should be discarded. In infants, blood can be obtained from scalp veins or jugular veins.

Anticoagulant and specimen container

The anticoagulant of choice for blood count specimens is one of the salts of EDTA. K_2EDTA, K_3EDTA and Na_2EDTA have all been used. The preferred anticoagulant, recommended by the International Committee (now Council) for Standardization in Haematology (ICSH), is K_2EDTA in a final concentration of 1.5–2.2 mg/ml [13]. Both dry EDTA and EDTA in solution are in use. If screw-capped tubes are being used, a solution has the advantage that mixing of blood specimens is easier so clotted specimens are less common. However, if a dry evacuated tube system is used, in which the inside of the tube is coated with the anticoagulant, poor mixing is not a problem. It should also be noted that some parameters are altered by dilution, and if too little blood is taken into a tube, dilution may be appreciable. Excess EDTA also has deleterious effects on cell morphology in stained blood films. Na_2EDTA is less soluble than the potassium salts. K_3EDTA causes undesirable cell shrinkage, which is reflected in a lower microhaematocrit (see p. 24).

Many laboratories use automated blood counting instruments with a sampling device, which is able to perforate the rubber cap of a blood specimen container and thus reduces unnecessary handling of blood. To take advantage of this it is necessary that not only evacuated tubes but also all blood containers have rubber caps that can be penetrated and resealed without permitting leakage.

Guidelines

Guidelines for the procedure of venepuncture [5] and for the protection of phlebotomists and laboratory workers from biological hazards [14] have been published by the NCCLS. It is recommended that 'standard precautions' proposed by the Centers for Disease Control (CDC), previously referred to as 'universal precautions', should be applied to phlebotomy. This policy means that all blood specimens are regarded as potentially infectious. The following specific recommendations are made [14]:

1 Gloves should preferably be worn for all phlebotomy; their use is particularly important if the phlebotomist has any breaks in the skin, if the patient is likely to be uncooperative, if the phlebotomist is inexperienced or if blood is being obtained by skin puncture.

2 Gloves should be changed between patients.

3 An evacuated tube system should be used in preference to a needle and syringe.

4 If a needle and syringe has to be used and it is then necessary to transfer blood to an evacuated tube the rubber stopper should not be removed. The stopper should be pierced by the needle and blood should be allowed to flow into the tube under the influence of the vacuum. To avoid the possibility of a self-inflicted wound the evacuated tube **must not be held in the hand** during this procedure, but instead should be placed in a rack.

Needle-prick injury

Precautions should be taken to avoid needle-prick (needle-stick) injuries. Hepatitis B can be readily transmitted by such injury, particularly when the patient is HBe antigen positive. Overall transmission rates of 7–30% have been reported following needle-prick injuries involving infected patients. If the patient is HBe antigen positive, the rate of transmission is of the order of 20% if hepatitis B immunoglobulin is given after the injury and about 30–40% if it is not given [15,16]. Reported rates of transmission of hepatitis C have varied from zero to 7%, with a mean of 1.8% [17] but, when sensitive techniques are used, the rate of transmission has been found to be about 10% [18]. Transmission occurs only from patients who are positive for hepatitis C viral RNA [17]. Human immunodeficiency virus (HIV) is much less readily transmitted than hepatitis B or C but a risk does exist. In 3430 needle-prick injuries reported up to 1993 the overall transmission rate was 0.46% [19]. Other infections that have been transmitted occasionally by needle-prick injury include malaria, cryptococcosis, tuberculosis, viral haemorrhagic fever and dengue fever [20–24].

A risk of injury and viral transmission also exists if glass capillary tubes are used for blood collection,

and alternative blood collection devices have therefore been advised by the USA's Food and Drug Administration (FDA) [7].

Because it has proved impossible to eliminate needle-stick injuries totally, all hospitals should have agreed policies for meeting this eventuality. Both laboratory managers and occupational health services have a responsibility in this regard. Staff who are performing venepunctures should be offered vaccination against hepatitis B and the adequacy of their antibody response should be verified; if a needle-prick injury from a known hepatitis B-positive source occurs, the antibody titre should be checked and a booster vaccination should be given if necessary [14]. Phlebotomists with an inadequate antibody response to vaccination should, in the event of a needle-prick injury from an infected source, be offered hepatitis B immunoglobulin. Phlebotomists who have chosen not to be vaccinated should be offered hepatitis B immunoglobulin and vaccination should again be offered. Antiretroviral prophylaxis should be offered to those exposed to a risk of HIV exposure through needle-stick injury and ideally should be administered within a few hours of exposure; the risk of infection becoming established is reduced but not eliminated [25]. Prophylaxis offered may be zidovudine alone but double or triple agent antiretroviral therapy (e.g. zidovudine plus lamivudine with or without indinavir or nelfinavir) is likely to be more effective. Current CDC recommendations can be found on the CDC's web site (http://www.cdc.gov). The use of nevirapine is not recommended because of the possibility of serious toxicity [26]. There appears to be no effective post-exposure prophylaxis for hepatitis C infection [17] but the consensus view is that interferon therapy is indicated in acute infection including that acquired by needle-stick injury. Interferon alpha-2b in a dose of 5 million units daily for 4 weeks followed by the same dose three times a week for a further 20 weeks has been found to be efficacious [27]. Unless all new staff are routinely tested for HIV, occupational health services should consider at least offering storage of serum samples so that baseline HIV testing is possible in the event of a subsequent needle-prick injury. If this policy is not followed, serum storage should be offered in the event of a needle-prick injury from a seropositive source or from a source of unknown HIV-status.

Making a blood film

A blood film may be made from non-anticoagulated (native) blood, obtained either from a vein or a capillary, or from EDTA-anticoagulated blood. Chelation of calcium by EDTA hinders platelet aggregation so that platelets are evenly spread and their numbers can be assessed more easily (Fig. 1.6). Films prepared from capillary blood usually show prominent platelet aggregation (Fig. 1.7) and films from native venous blood often show small aggregates (Fig. 1.8). Films prepared from native venous or capillary blood are free of artefacts due to storage or the effects of the anticoagulant. A few laboratories still use such films as a matter of routine, but otherwise their use is obligatory for investigating abnormalities such as red cell crenation or white cell or platelet aggregation that may be induced by storage or EDTA. Conversely, making a blood film from EDTA-anticoagulated blood after arrival of the blood specimen in the laboratory has the advantage that some of the artefacts that may influence the validity of results obtained from automated instruments are more likely to be detected, e.g. the formation of fibrin strands, aggregation of platelets or agglutination of red cells induced by

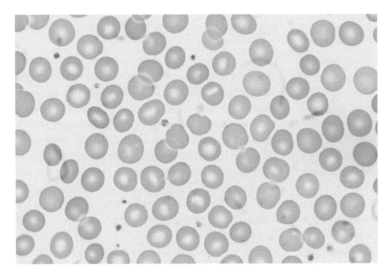

Fig. 1.6 A blood film from EDTA-anticoagulated blood showing an even distribution of platelets.

Fig. 1.7 A blood film from non-anticoagulated capillary blood showing the aggregation of platelets that usually occurs.

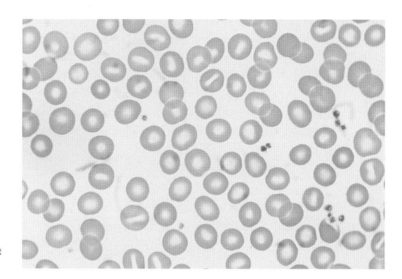

Fig. 1.8 A blood film from non-anticoagulated venous blood showing the minor degree of platelet aggregation that usually occurs.

cold agglutinins. Good laboratory practice includes recording the date and time the specimen is received in the laboratory and making a film shortly after receipt of the specimen. In this way the length of any delay in transit is known and attribution of morphological changes to prolonged storage of EDTA-anticoagulated blood ('storage artefact', see p. 63) can be confirmed.

Manual spreading of a blood film on a glass slide (wedge-spread film)

Glass slides must be clean and free of grease. They should not be too porous or background staining is increased [28]. A spreader is required and must be narrower than the slide. If a coverslip is to be applied the spreader must also be narrower than the coverslip so that cells at the edge of the blood film are covered by the coverslip and can be easily examined microscopically. A spreader can be readily prepared by breaking the corner off a glass slide after incising it with a diamond pen; this provides a smooth-edged spreader that is large enough to be manipulated easily. Spreaders made by cutting transverse pieces from a slide are inferior since they are more difficult to handle and have at least one rough edge that may damage gloves or fingers.

The laboratory worker spreading blood films should wear gloves. A drop of blood (either native or anticoagulated) is placed near one end of the slide.

Anticoagulated blood from screw-top containers can be applied to the slide using a capillary tube, which is then discarded. A drop of blood from specimen containers with penetrable lids can be applied to the slide by means of a special device that perforates the lid. The spreader is applied at an angle of 25–30°, in front of the drop of blood, and is drawn back into it (Fig. 1.9). Once the blood has run along its back edge, the spreader is advanced with a smooth steady motion so that a thin film of blood is spread over the slide. If the angle of the spreader is too obtuse or the speed of spreading is too fast, the film will be too short. An experienced operator learns to recognize blood with a higher than normal haematocrit (Hct), which is more viscous and requires a more acute angle to make a satisfactory film and, conversely, blood with a lower than normal Hct, which requires a more obtuse angle. The spreading technique should produce a film of blood with a fairly straight tail. A film of the shape of a thumbprint means that, when observing the film microscopically and moving across the film, the observer moves from an area that is optimal for identification of cells to an area that is too thick. It is important that the spreader is wiped clean with a dry tissue or gauze square after each use since it is otherwise possible to transfer abnormal cells from one blood film to another (Fig. 1.10).

As soon as slides are made they should be labelled with the patient's name and the date or with an

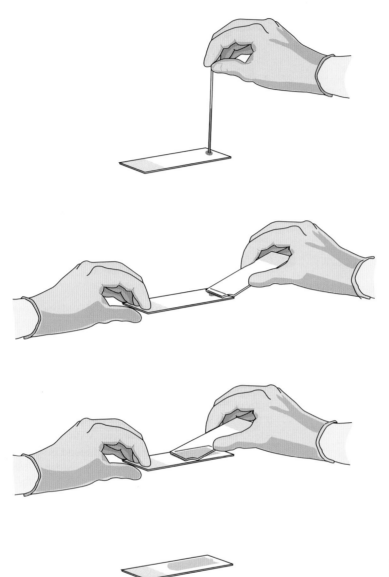

Fig. 1.9 The method of spreading a blood film.

identifying number. Small numbers of slides can be labelled with a diamond marker or by writing details on the thick part of the film. The fastest way to label large numbers of slides is with a methanol-resistant pen or by writing in pencil on the frosted end of a slide. Slides that are frosted at one end on **both** sides are useful because they avoid waste of staff time ensuring that the slide is the right way up. Blood films should be dried rapidly. A hot-air blower or a fan to increase air circulation can be useful. If films are dried slowly, there is shrinkage of cells that can lead to the appearance of cytoplasmic blebs and villi, bipolar lymphocytes, hyperchromatic nuclei and inapparent nucleoli [28]; these changes can occur not only in normal cells but also in neoplastic cells so that their characteristic features are less apparent.

Fig. 1.11 shows a well-spread film in comparison with examples of poor films resulting from faulty technique.

Unless otherwise stated, this book deals with morphology as observed in wedge-spread films.

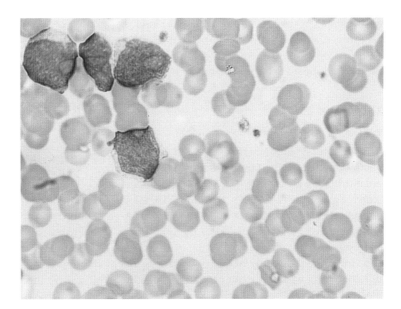

Fig. 1.10 Blast cells from a patient with acute leukaemia that have been inadvertently transferred to the blood film of another patient by the use of an inadequately cleaned spreader.

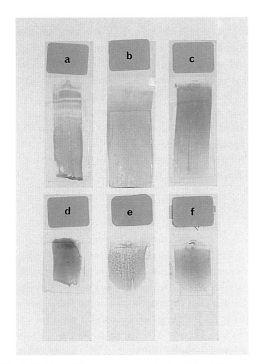

Fig. 1.11 Unsatisfactory and satisfactory blood films: (a) uneven pressure has produced ridges; (b) too broad and too long—the edges and the tail of the film cannot be examined adequately; (c) too long and streaked by an uneven spreader; (d) too thick and short due to the wrong angle or speed of spreading; (e) even distribution of blood cells has been interrupted because the slide was greasy; (f) satisfactory.

Most of the photographs are of manually spread films, which were prepared from recently collected EDTA-anticoagulated blood.

Other methods of spreading thin films

Automated spreading of blood films

Wedge-spread films can be prepared by mechanical spreaders, which can be integrated into a staining machine or an automated full blood counter. A film of blood one cell thick can also be spread on a glass slide by centrifugation in a specially designed centrifuge, but this method is little used.

Films from blood with a very high Hct

If blood has a very high Hct, e.g. Hct > 0.60, Hb > 20 g/dl, it can be impossible to make a good blood film, even if the angle and the speed of spreading are adjusted. Mixing a drop of blood and a drop of either saline or blood group AB plasma reduces viscosity so that a film can be made in which details of red cell morphology can be appreciated.

Buffy coat films

Buffy coat films are useful to concentrate nucleated cells, e.g. to look for low-frequency abnormal cells or bacteria. A tube of anticoagulated blood is centrifuged and a drop of the buffy coat is mixed with a drop of autologous EDTA-anticoagulated plasma and spread in the normal manner.

Thick films

Thick films are required for examination for malarial parasites and certain other parasites, the red cells being lysed before the film is examined. Parasites are much more concentrated in a thick film, so that searching for them requires less time. To make a thick film, several drops of native or EDTA-anticoagulated blood are placed in the centre of a slide and stirred with a capillary tube or an orange stick into a pool of blood of such a thickness that typescript or a watch face can be read through the blood (Fig. 1.12). The blood film is not fixed but, after drying, is placed directly into an aqueous Giemsa stain so that lysis of red cells occurs; this allows the organisms to be seen more clearly.

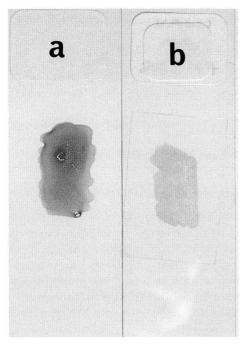

Fig. 1.12 Thick films for examination for malarial parasites: (a) unstained film showing the correct thickness of the film of blood; and (b) film stained without fixation, causing lysis of red cells.

Unstained wet preparations

Unstained wet preparations are useful for searching for motile parasites such as microfilariae, which can be seen agitating the red cells. A drop of anticoagulated blood is placed on a slide and covered with a coverslip.

Fixation, staining and mounting

Fixation

Following air drying, thin films are fixed in absolute methanol for 10–20 minutes. Poor fixation and characteristic artefactual changes occur if there is more than a few per cent of water in the methanol (Fig. 1.13); this renders interpretation of morphology, particularly red cell morphology, impossible and, if the film is not examined carefully, can give a mistaken impression of hypochromia. In warm, humid climates it may be necessary to change methanol solutions several times a day. Similar artefactual changes can be produced by condensation on slides. In humid climates, slides should be fixed as soon as they are thoroughly dry. A hot-air blower can be used to accelerate drying. In any circumstances, prolonged delay in fixation should be avoided as this can lead to alteration in the staining characteristics of the film, which can acquire a turquoise tint.

Staining

There is little consistency between laboratories in the precise stain used to prepare a blood film for microscopic examination, but the multiple stains in use are based on the Romanowsky stain, developed by the Russian protozoologist in the late nineteenth century [29]. Romanowsky used a mixture of old methylene blue and eosin to stain the nucleus of a malarial parasite purple and the cytoplasm blue. Subsequently, Giemsa modified the stain, combining methylene azure and eosin. The stain most commonly used in the UK is a combination of Giemsa's stain with May-Grünwald stain; it is therefore designated the May-Grünwald–Giemsa (MGG) stain. The stain most commonly used in North America is Wright's stain, which contains methylene blue and

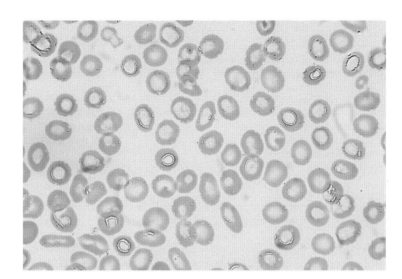

Fig. 1.13 Artefactual changes produced by 5% water in the methanol used for fixation.

eosin; the methylene blue has been heated, or 'polychromed', to produce analogues of methylene blue. Sometimes this is combined with Giemsa's stain to give a Wright–Giemsa stain, which is generally held to give superior results. It has been demonstrated by chromatography that dyes prepared by traditional organic chemistry methods are not pure, dyes sold under the same designation containing a variable mixture of five to ten dyes [30]. Variation between different batches prepared by the same manufacturer also occurs.

The essential components of a Romanowsky-type stain are: (i) a basic or cationic dye, such as azure B, which conveys a blue-violet or blue colour to nucleic acids (binding to the phosphate groups of DNA and RNA) and to nucleoprotein, to the granules of basophils and, weakly, to the granules of neutrophils; and (ii) an acidic or anionic dye, such as eosin, which conveys a red or orange colour to haemoglobin and the eosinophil granules and also binds to cationic nuclear protein, thus contributing to the colour of the stained nucleus. A stain containing azure B and eosin provides a satisfactory Romanowsky stain [29], as does a mixture of azure B, methylene blue and eosin [30]. The ICSH reference method for the Romanowsky stain [31], which uses pure azure B and eosin Y, gives very satisfactory results but such pure dyes are expensive for routine use. Satisfactory and reasonably consistent staining can be achieved using good quality commercial stains and an automated staining machine. This method has been used for staining the majority of blood films photographed for this book.

Traditionally, cytoplasm that stains blue and granules that stain purple have both been designated 'basophilic', and granules that stain violet or pinkish-purple have been designated 'azurophilic'. In fact all these hues are achieved by the uptake of a single basic dye such as azure B or A. 'Acidophilic' and 'eosinophilic' both refer to uptake of the acidic dye, eosin, although 'acidophilic' has often been used to describe cell components staining pink, and 'eosinophilic' to describe cell components staining orange. The range of colours that a Romanowsky stain should produce is shown in Table 1.2.

Staining must be performed at the correct pH. If the pH is too low, basophilic components do not stain well. Leucocytes are generally pale, with eosinophil granules a brilliant vermilion. If the pH is too high, uptake of the basic dye may be excessive leading to general overstaining, it becomes difficult to distinguish between normal and polychromatic red cells, eosinophil granules are deep blue or dark grey, and the granules of normal neutrophils are heavily stained, simulating toxic granulation.

Stain solutions may need to be filtered shortly before use, to avoid stain deposit on the blood film, which can be confused with red cell inclusions. If an automated staining machine is used, superior results are usually achieved with a dipping technique, in

Cell component staining	Colour
Chromatin (including Howell–Jolly bodies)	Purple
Promyelocyte granules and Auer rods	Purplish-red
Cytoplasm of lymphocytes	Blue
Cytoplasm of monocytes	Blue-grey
Cytoplasm rich in RNA (i.e. 'basophilic cytoplasm')	Deep blue
Döhle bodies	Blue-grey
Specific granules of neutrophils, granules of lymphocytes, granulomere of platelets	Light purple or pink
Specific granules of basophils	Deep purple
Specific granules of eosinophils	Orange
Red cells	Pink

Table 1.2 Characteristic staining of different cell components with a Romanowsky stain.

which the entire slide is immersed in the stain, than with a flat-bed stainer, in which staining solution is applied to a horizontal slide. The latter type of staining machine is more prone to leave stain deposits on the slides and, if the blood film is too long or badly positioned, some parts of it may escape staining.

Destaining an MGG-stained blood film can be done by flooding the slide with methanol, washing in water and then repeating the sequence until all the stain has gone. This can be useful if only a single blood film is available and a further stain, e.g. an iron stain, is required.

Staining for malarial parasites

The detection and identification of malarial parasites is facilitated if blood films are stained with a Giemsa (or Leishman) stain at pH 7.2. At this pH, cells that have been parasitized by either *Plasmodium vivax* or *Plasmodium ovale* have different tinctorial qualities from non-parasitized cells and are easily identified. The inclusions in parasitized cells are also evident (see p. 145).

Mounting

If films are to be stored, mounting gives them protection against scratching and gathering of dust. As stated above, the coverslip should be sufficiently wide to cover the edges of the blood film. A neutral mountant that is miscible with xylene is required.

As an alternative to mounting, blood films can be sprayed with a polystyrene or acrylic resin.

If films are not to be stored, a thin film of oil can be smeared on the stained slide to permit microscopic examination at low power before adding a drop of oil to permit examination with the oil immersion lens.

Storage of slides

Ideal patient care and continuing education of haematology staff dictate that blood films should be stored as long as possible, preferably for some years. Unfortunately, the very large numbers of blood specimens now being processed daily by most haematology laboratories means that this is often difficult. The most economical way to store slides is in metal racks in stacking drawers. Labels showing the patient's name, the date and the laboratory number should be applied in such a way that they can be read when the slides are in storage. Slides that have been freshly mounted should be stored in cardboard trays or stacked in racks, separated from each other by wire loops until the mountant has hardened and dried. When the mountant is no longer sticky, slides can be stacked closely together for maximum economy of space. Glass slides are heavy and if large numbers are to be stored the floor of the room may need to be strengthened.

When a patient has a bone marrow aspiration performed, a blood film should always be stored permanently with bone marrow films so that when it is necessary to throw out old peripheral blood films to make room for new ones, at least this film is available for review. A laboratory should also maintain a separate file of teaching slides. These

Ring to adjust left ocular

Ocular

Rotating nosepiece

Arm

Objective

Slide retainer

Stage

Coarse focus

Condensor lens

Lever to open iris diaphragm

Fine focus

Centering knobs

Knob to move stage

Condensor focus knob

Field diaphragm ring

Lamp housing (may also, preferably, be located at back of microscope)

Fig. 1.14 A drawing of a microscope showing the names of the individual parts.

should include examples of rare conditions and typical examples of common conditions.

Setting up and using a microscope

All laboratory workers should learn to set up a microscope correctly early in the course of their training. The following is the correct procedure for setting up a binocular microscope.

1 If you need to move or lift the microscope do so using only the arm (Fig. 1.14). Sit at the microscope and make sure that the height is correct for comfortable viewing. Adjust the chair or the height of the microscope above the bench, as necessary.

2 Plug in the electric lead and switch on the mains power supply.

3 Turn on the microscope.

4 Turn up the rheostat until there is a comfortable amount of light.

5 Lower the stage and rotate the × 10 objective into place; it will click when it engages.

6 Select a slide and place it on the stage, being careful to place it with the blood film and cover slip uppermost. Handle the slide only by its edges. Secure the slide with the levers provided for this purpose.

7 Raise the condenser as high as it will go.

8 Open the field diaphragm and the condenser aperture diaphragm fully.

9 Move the stage until the film of blood is beneath the objective, in the beam of light.

10 Raise the stage, looking at the slide from the side or the front rather that using the oculars (eyepieces), until the slide almost touches the objective.

11 Adjust the position of the oculars so that they match your interpupillary distance and look at the slide through the oculars, making sure that the light is at a comfortable level.

12 Lower the slide slowly using the coarse focus knob until the slide comes into focus.

13 Using the coarse and then the fine focus, focus on the slide with your right eye to the right ocular then, without moving the slide, rotate the ring on the left ocular so that the image recorded by your left eye is also sharp. (With some microscopes it is possible to adjust both oculars.)

14 Close the field iris diaphragm fully. The field iris diaphragm is near the lamp and controls the area of illumination.

15 Lower the condenser until the edge of the field iris diaphragm comes into focus. Adjust the focus by moving the condenser so that the edges of the diaphragm appear faintly blue rather than faintly red (Köhler illumination). Check that the aperture in the field iris diaphragm is centred and, if it is not, centre it using the two centring screws on the condenser.

16 Open the field iris aperture so that the whole field of view is illuminated but no wider. If it is opened too wide, stray light will enter the field of view (particularly important for photography, for which purpose the diaphragm can be closed further till only the photographic frame is illuminated).

17 Using the appropriate lever or ring, close the condenser aperture diaphragm to about 70–80% of the numerical aperture marked on the objective. A condenser scale near the lever or ring permits this to be done. This aperture controls the angular aperture of the cone of light that reaches the condenser lens. The more you close this aperture the less light there is and the lower the resolution but the greater the contrast and depth of focus. For optimal optics, the condenser aperture iris should be reset for each objective.

18 Examine the slide with the $\times 10$ objective*, then rotate in a $\times 40$ objective. Readjust the focus and the condenser aperture iris and adjust the field iris diaphragm so that only the field of view is illuminated. Re-examine the slide.

19 Before using an oil immersion lens, rotate out the non-oil objective and put a drop of immersion oil in the centre of the slide. Rotate in an oil immersion objective, e.g. $\times 60$ or $\times 100$, and focus, using the coarse and then the fine focus and adjust the condenser aperture iris. Be careful not to rotate in any objective other than an oil immersion objective while there is a drop of oil on the slide. If you are not sure if an objective is for oil immersion or not, read its label. Do not use excess oil and do not mix two different types of oil. Do not overfill a bottle of oil or oil will get on your fingers.

20 After examining a slide with an oil immersion objective, gently wipe the oil from the objective and from the slide. If the slide has been freshly mounted, remove the oil gently so that the cover slip is not accidentally removed, removing enough of the oil that a non-oil lens will not be contaminated if the slide is again placed on a microscope stage. Removing oil from slides does not require lens tissues; ordinary tissues are satisfactory. Non-mounted blood films are not advised but, if they are used, be careful to minimize scratching of the blood film when removing oil.

21 When you have finished working, rotate back in the lowest power objective and lower the stage. Remove traces of oil from any oil immersion lens using methanol and lens tissues. Turn down the rheostat before turning off the microscope. Do not leave the microscope turned on when you are away from your workstation; in some poorly designed microscopes the lamp is very close to the field diaphragm and prolonged heat will damage the leaves of the diaphragm.

22 Keep the microscope clean. Dust can be removed with a small brush. Lenses should be cleaned only with lens tissues. These can be moistened with methanol (or a mixture of 3 parts methanol to 7 parts ether).

23 Cover the microscope with a dust cover when not in use.

* Note: microscopes used by haematology laboratories do not usually have a $\times 4$ objective fitted, unless histological sections are also being examined. If a $\times 4$ objective is to be used, e.g. for examining a trephine biopsy section, swing out the condenser before viewing the slide.

Identifying the source of a problem and preventing problems

1 If there is no light, check that the light beam has not been deflected to a camera.

2 If you cannot focus on a blood film check if the slide is upside down and make sure that there are not two coverslips instead of one. Some microscopes have a 'stop' on the coarse focus; if necessary, release it. Rarely, very thick slides may make it impossible to focus with a high power lens if a coverslip is mounted. Unsuitably thick coverslips can have the same effect.

3 If you cannot see the image clearly, clean the slide using tissues and methanol. Sealed methanol-soaked squares of tissue used to prepare the arm for venepuncture are convenient for cleaning slides and avoid the need to have a bottle of methanol in the microscopy laboratory. If cleaning the slide does not help, clean the objective gently using a lens tissue and methanol. Do not use xylene unless you are unable to get the lens clean with methanol.

4 If you wear spectacles you will find that it is impossible to use a microscope with bifocal or varifocal lenses. Modern plastic spectacle lenses are easily scratched and if there is an antiglare coating to the lenses this can also be scratched. Be sure that the oculars have a protective rubber guard if you are using spectacles with this type of lens or lens coating.

Examining a blood film

1 Check the label of the slide (patient identity and date).

2 Examine the film macroscopically for unusual characteristics.

3 Adjust the microscope as above and examine the film microscopically, examining the edges and the tail and then the whole film under low power, e.g. × 10 objective.

4 Next examine the whole film with a × 40 or × 50 objective. This is the most important part of the film examination as it is possible to scan the entire film to note any rare abnormal cells. Be systematic: look specifically at red cells, white cells and platelets.

5 Examine with an oil immersion lens only if there is some particular reason to do so.

Test your knowledge

Multiple choice questions (MCQ)

(1–5 answers may be correct)

MCQ 1.1 Blood for a full blood count should normally be anticoagulated with
(a) Heparin   T/F
(b) Citrate   T/F
(c) Calcium   T/F
(d) Fluoride   T/F
(e) A sodium or potassium salt of EDTA   T/F

MCQ 1.2 A needle-prick injury can lead to transmission of
(a) Hepatitis B   T/F
(b) Hepatitis C   T/F
(c) Human immunodeficiency virus (HIV)   T/F
(d) Malaria   T/F
(e) Dengue fever   T/F

MCQ 1.3 Good phlebotomy practice includes
(a) Labelling the necessary tubes carefully before going to the patient's bedside   T/F
(b) Shaking the blood sample vigorously to ensure that the anticoagulant is dissolved   T/F
(c) Holding a specimen container firmly in the non-dominant hand if it is necessary to transfer blood from a syringe and needle to an evacuated container   T/F
(d) Recording family name, given name and date and time of sampling on the specimen container   T/F
(e) Wearing gloves for the procedure   T/F

MCQ 1.4 Skin puncture 'capillary' blood samples
(a) Often have a higher platelet count than venous samples   T/F
(b) Ideally are obtained from the posterior or lateral aspect of the heel   T/F
(c) If obtained from an ear lobe, sometimes result in persistent bleeding   T/F
(d) Should be obtained by a puncture at least 1.5 mm deep   T/F
(e) Should exclude the first drop of blood   T/F

Extended matching question (EMQ)

Only one answer is correct

EMQ 1.1
Theme: Romanowsky-stained blood film

Options
A Blue-grey
B Deep blue
C Deep purple
D Orange
E Pink
F Red
G Black
H Bluish-green

For each structure choose the most accurate term from the options listed above to describe the colour in a correctly stained blood film. Each option may be used once, more than once or not at all.

Cellular structure	Matching option
1 Howell–Jolly body	
2 Döhle body	
3 Pappenheimer body	
4 Cytoplasm of atypical lymphocyte	
5 Basophil granules	

References

1 Roddy SM, Ashwal S and Schneider S (1983) Venipuncture fits: a form of reflex anoxic seizure. *Pediatrics*, **72**, 715–717.

2 Sander HWE, Conigliari MF and Masdeu JC (1998) Antecubital phlebotomy complicated by lateral antebrachial cutaneous neuropathy. *N Engl J Med*, **339**, 2024.

3 Golder M, Chan CL, O'Shea S, Corbett K, Chrystie IL and French G (2000) Potential risk of cross-infection during peripheral-venous access by contamination of tourniquets. *Lancet*, **355**, 44.

4 Mull JD and Murphy WR (1993) Effects of tourniquet-induced stasis on blood determinations. *Am J Clin Pathol*, **39**, 134–136.

5 NCCLS. *H3-A4—Procedure for the collection of diagnostic blood specimens by venipuncture; approved standard*, 4th edn. NCCLS, Wayne, PA, 1998.

6 Hammond KB (1980) Blood specimen collection from infants by skin puncture. *Lab Med*, **11**, 9–12.

7 Anonymous (1999) Glass capillary tubes: joint safety advisory about potential risks. *Lab Med*, **30**, 299.

8 Polish LB, Shapiro CN, Bauer F, Klotz P, Ginier P, Roberto RR *et al.* (1992) Nosocomial transmission of hepatitis B virus associated with the use of a spring-loaded finger-stick device. *N Engl J Med*, **326**, 721–725.

9 Vertanen H, Laipio ML, Fellman V, Brommels M and Viinikka L (2000) Hemolysis in skin puncture samples obtained by using two different sampling devices from preterm infants. Paper presented at 24th World Congress of Medical Technology, Vancouver, Canada.

10 Vertanen H, Fellman V, Brommels M and Viinikka L (2000) An automatic incision device causes less damages to the heels of preterm infants. Paper presented at 24th World Congress of Medical Technology, Vancouver, Canada.

11 Brecher G, Schneiderman M and Cronkite EP (1953) The reproducibility and constancy of the platelet count. *Am J Clin Pathol*, **23**, 15–26.

12 Conway AM, Hinchliffe RF and Anderson LM (1998) Measurement of haemoglobin using single drop of skin puncture blood: is precision acceptable? *J Clin Pathol*, **51**, 248–250.

13 ICSH Expert Panel on Cytometry (1993) Recommendations of the International Council for Standardization in Haematology for ethylenediaminetetraacetic acid anticoagulation of blood for blood cell counting and sizing. *Am J Clin Pathol*, **100**, 371–372.

14 NCCLS. *M29-A—Protection of laboratory workers from instrument biohazards and infectious disease transmitted by blood, body fluids, and tissue: approved guideline*. NCCLS, Wayne, PA, 1997.

15 Masuko K, Mitsui T, Iwano K, Yamazaki C, Aikara S, Baba K *et al.* (1985) Factors influencing postexposure immunoprophylaxis of hepatitis B viral infection with hepatitis B immune globulin. High deoxyribonucleic acid polymerase activity in the inocula of unsuccessful cases. *Gastroenterology*, **88**, 151–155.

16 Seeff LB, Wright EC, Zimmerman HJ, Alter HJ, Dietz AA, Felsher BF *et al.* (1978) Type B hepatitis after needle-stick exposure: prevention with hepatitis B immune globulin. A final report of the Veterans Administration Cooperative study. *Ann Intern Med*, **88**, 285–293.

17 Ramsay ME (1999) Guidance on the investigation and management of occupational exposure to hepatitis C. *Commun Dis Public Health*, **4**, 258–262.

18 Mitsui T, Iwano K, Masuko K, Yamazaki C, Okamoto H, Tsuda F *et al.* (1992) Hepatitis C virus infection in medical personnel after needlestick accident. *Hepatology*, **126**, 1109–1114.

19 Heptonstall J, Gill ON, Porter K, Black MB and

Gilbart VL (1993) Health care workers and HIV: surveillance of occupationally acquired infection in the United Kingdom. *Commun Disease Rep*, **3**, 147–153.

20 Bending MR and Maurice PD (1980) Malaria: a laboratory risk. *Postgrad Med J*, **56**, 344–345.

21 Glaser JB and Garden A (1985) Inoculation of cryptococcosis without transmission of the acquired immunodeficiency syndrome. *N Engl J Med*, **312**, 266.

22 Kramer F, Sasse SA, Simms JC and Leedom JM (1993) Primary cutaneous tuberculosis after a needlestick injury from a patient with AIDS and undiagnosed tuberculosis. *Ann Intern Med*, **119**, 594–595.

23 Advisory Committee on Dangerous Pathogens. *Management and control of viral haemorrhagic fevers*. The Stationery Office, London, 1996.

24 De Wazières B, Gil H, Vuitton DA and Dupond JL (1998) Nosocomial transmission of dengue from a needlestick injury. *Lancet*, **351**, 498.

25 Katz MH and Gerberding JL (1997) Postexposure treatment of people exposed to the human immunodeficiency virus through sexual contact or injection drug use. *N Engl J Med*, **336**, 1097–1100.

26 Gottlieb S (2001) Nevirapine should not be prescribed for needlestick injuries. *BMJ*, **322**, 126.

27 Jaeckel E, Cornberg M, Wedemeyer H, Sanantonio T, Mayer J, Zankel M *et al*. (2001) Treatment of acute hepatitis C with interferon alfa-2b. *N Engl J Med*, **345**, 1452–1457.

28 Nguyen D and Diamond L. *Diagnostic Hematology: a Pattern Approach*. Butterworth-Heinemann, Oxford, 2000.

29 Wittekind D (1979) On the nature of the Romanowsky dyes and the Romanowsky–Giemsa effect. *Clin Lab Haematol*, **1**, 247–262.

30 Marshall PN, Bentley SA and Lewis SM (1975) A standardized Romanowsky stain prepared from purified dyes. *J Clin Pathol*, **28**, 920–923.

31 ICSH (1984) ICSH reference method for staining blood and bone marrow films by azure B and eosin Y (Romanowsky stain). *Br J Haematol*, **57**, 707–710.

Answers to test questions

Multiple choice questions

MCQ 1.1	FFFFT
MCQ 1.2	TTTTT
MCQ 1.3	FFFTT
MCQ 1.4	FFTTT

Extended matching questions

EMQ 1.1

1 C

2 A

3 B

4 B

5 C

2 Performing a blood count

In the past, blood counts were performed by slow and labour-intensive manual techniques using counting chambers, microscopes, glass tubes, colorimeters, centrifuges and a few simple reagents. The only tests done with any frequency were estimations of haemoglobin concentration (Hb), packed cell volume (PCV) and white blood cell count (WBC). Hb was estimated by a method depending on optical density and was expressed as mass/volume, or even as a percentage in relation to a rather arbitrary 'normal' that represented 100%. PCV was a measurement of the proportion of a column of centrifuged blood that was occupied by red cells. Now expressed as a decimal fraction representing volume/volume, it was initially expressed as a percentage. White cells were counted microscopically in a diluted blood sample in a haemocytometer, a counting chamber of known volume. All cell counts were expressed as the number of cells in a unit volume. The red blood cell count (RBC) was performed occasionally, mainly when there was a need to make an estimate of red cell size. Platelets were counted, by light or phase-contrast microscopy, only when there was a clear clinical need. From the primary measurements relating to red cells other values were derived: the mean cell volume (MCV), mean cell haemoglobin (MCH) and mean cell haemoglobin concentration (MCHC). The formulae for these derived measurements are as follows:

$$MCV \, (fl) = \frac{PCV \, (l/l) \times 1000}{RBC \, (cells/l) \times 10^{-12}}$$

$$MCH \, (pg) = \frac{Hb \, (g/dl) \times 10}{RBC \, (cells/l) \times 10^{-12}}$$

$$MCHC \, (g/dl) = \frac{Hb \, (g/dl)}{PCV \, (l/l)}$$

These and many other measurements are now made on automated and semi-automated instruments within minutes using either modifications of the manual techniques or totally new technologies. Measurements are precise, i.e. repeated measurements on the same sample give very similar results. As long as the instruments are carefully calibrated and the blood has no unusual characteristics, measurements are also accurate, i.e. they give results that are very close to 'truth'. However, despite the widespread use of automated instruments, the manual techniques remain important both as reference methods and in the investigation of blood samples that appear to give anomalous test results on automated instruments. They also illustrate the principles that underlie various measurements.

Basic techniques

Haemoglobin concentration

To measure haemoglobin concentration (Hb), a known volume of carefully mixed whole blood is added to a diluent which lyses red cells to produce a haemoglobin solution; lysis occurs because of the hypotonicity of the diluent, but may be accelerated by the inclusion in the diluent of a non-ionic detergent to act as a lytic agent. The Hb is then determined from the light absorbance (optical density) of the solution of haemoglobin or its derivative at a selected wavelength.

Cyanmethaemoglobin method

The International Committee (now Council) for Standardization in Haematology (ICSH) has recommended a reference method in which haemoglobin is converted to cyanmethaemoglobin (haemiglobin-cyanide) [1]. This method has three significant advantages:

1 Haemoglobin, methaemoglobin and carboxyhaemoglobin are all converted to cyanmethaemoglobin

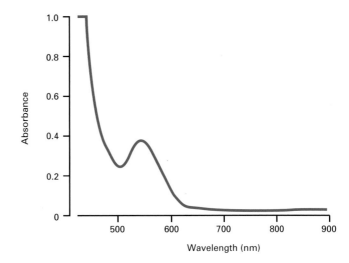

Fig. 2.1 Absorbance spectrum of cyanmethaemoglobin.

and are therefore included in the measurement. Of the forms of haemoglobin likely to be present in blood, only sulphaemoglobin—usually present in negligible amounts—is not converted to cyanmethaemoglobin, although carboxyhaemoglobin is more slowly converted than the other forms.

2 Stable secondary standards that have been compared with the World Health Organization (WHO) international standard are readily available for calibration.

3 Cyanmethaemoglobin has an absorbance band at 540 nm, which is broad and relatively flat (Fig. 2.1) and thus measurements can be made either on a narrow-band spectrophotometer or on a filter photometer or colorimeter that reads over a wide band of wavelengths.

The reference method requires the addition of a diluent that contains: (i) potassium cyanide and potassium ferricyanide, to effect the conversion to methaemoglobin; (ii) dihydrogen potassium phosphate to lower the pH, accelerate the reaction, and allow the reading of light absorbance at 3 minutes rather than 10–15 minutes; and (iii) a non-ionic detergent, to accelerate cell lysis and reduce the turbidity due to precipitation of lipoproteins (and to a lesser extent red cell stroma), which is otherwise a consequence of the lower pH achieved by the dihydrogen potassium phosphate [2]. The absorbance of light by the solution is measured at 540 nm in a spectrophotometer. At this wavelength, the light absorbance of the diluent is zero; either water or,

preferably, the diluent can be used as the blank. No standard is required, since the haemoglobin concentration can be calculated from the absorbance, given that the molecular weight and the millimolar extinction coefficient of haemoglobin are known. However, the wavelength of light produced by the instrument must be verified and the absorbance scale calibrated. A reference solution of cyanmethaemoglobin can be used for calibration.

In routine practice, Hb is usually measured by means of a photometer or colorimeter in which light of approximately 540 nm is produced by use of a yellow-green filter such as the Ilford 625. The light passing through the solution is detected by a photoelectric cell and the instrument scale shows either light absorbance or transmittance. Comparison of the instrument reading with that for a reference solution allows calculation of the Hb; this is most conveniently performed using a standard curve or a conversion table. Alternatively, the photometer can be calibrated to produce a direct readout of Hb; a reference cyanmethaemoglobin solution is suitable for verifying the accuracy of instruments of this type.

Certain characteristics of pathological blood samples may lead to inaccuracy in a cyanmethaemoglobin estimation of Hb. The presence of sulphaemoglobin will lead to slight underestimation of total haemoglobin: a concentration of 15 g/dl will be measured as 14.8 g/dl if 5% of haemoglobin is present as sulphaemoglobin [2]. The slow conversion of carboxyhaemoglobin to methaemoglobin leads to overestimation of the Hb if the test is read at 3 minutes, since carboxyhaemoglobin absorbs more light at 540 nm than does cyanmethaemoglobin. The maximum possible error that could be caused if 20% of the haemoglobin were in the form of carboxy-haemoglobin, a degree of abnormality that may be found in heavy smokers, would be 6% [2].

Spectrophotometers and photometers are both sensitive to the effect of turbidity, which may be caused by a high WBC, high concentrations of lipids or plasma proteins, or non-lysed red cells. Increased turbidity causes a factitiously elevated estimate of Hb. When the WBC is high, turbidity effects are circumvented by centrifugation or filtration of the solution prior to reading the absorbance. When turbidity is due to a high level of plasma protein (either when a paraprotein is present or when there is polyclonal hypergammaglobulinaemia resulting from severe chronic infection or inflammation), it can be cleared by the addition of either potassium carbonate or a drop of 25% ammonia solution. When turbidity is due to hyperlipidaemia, a blank can be prepared from the diluent and the patient's plasma or the lipid can be removed by diethyl ether extraction and centrifugation. The target cells of liver disease or red cells containing haemoglobin S or C may fail to lyse in the diluent and, again, increased turbidity produces a factitiously high reading of Hb. Occasionally, this phenomenon is observed without any identifiable abnormality in the red cells to account for it. Making a 1 : 1 dilution in distilled water ensures complete lysis of osmotic-ally resistant cells.

The cyanmethaemoglobin method has been modified for application in automated instruments by the use of various lytic agents and by reading absorbance after a shorter time or at a different wavelength.

Other methods

Alternative methods of measuring Hb are not widely used except when they have been incorpor-ated into haemoglobinometers. Such methods usu-ally require standardization by reference back to a cyanmethaemoglobin standard, but they otherwise avoid the use of cyanide, which is potentially toxic if released into the environment in large quantities.

Haemoglobin can be converted into a sulphated derivative with maximum absorbance at 534 nm by addition of sodium lauryl sulphate [3]. Conversion is almost instantaneous and methaemoglobin, but not sulphaemoglobin, is converted. This method correlates well with the reference method that is employed for calibration. This method is suitable for use with a spectrophotometer and has also been incorporated into several automated instruments.

Hb can also be measured following conversion to azidmethaemoglobin by the addition of sodium nitrate and sodium azide. This is the method employed by one portable haemoglobinometer (HemoCue, Clandon Scientific Ltd.), which employs measurements at two wavelengths, 570 and 880 nm, to permit compensation for turbidity. A modification of this instrument permits accurate measurements down to 0.1 g/l, so that it is also suitable for measurement of dilute solutions of haemoglobin, e.g. haemoglobin in fluid salvaged during surgery or haemoglobin in plasma or urine [4].

Hb can be measured as oxyhaemoglobin, in which case concentration of carboxyhaemoglobin, sulphaemoglobin and methaemoglobin will not be measured accurately. An artificial or secondary standard is needed. This method has been incor-porated into directly reading haemoglobinometers, which are standardized to give the same result as a cyanmethaemoglobin method.

Hb can be measured as haematin produced under alkaline conditions. The alkaline–haematin method measures carboxyhaemoglobin, sulphaemoglobin and methaemoglobin, although it does not adequately measure haemoglobin F or haemoglobin Bart's, which are resistant to alkaline denaturation. An artificial standard is required. The acid–haematin method is less reliable and is not recommended.

Hb can be estimated without chemical con-version by measuring absorbance at 548.5 nm, at which wavelength deoxyhaemoglobin and oxyhae-moglobin both have the same optical density and that of carboxyhaemoglobin is not much less. Hb is calculated by comparison of absorbance with that of an artificial standard. Absorbance can also be integrated between 500 and 600 nm, the integral absorbance of oxyhaemoglobin, deoxyhaemoglobin and carboxyhaemoglobin being similar over this waveband.

New methods for the estimation of haemoglobin concentration have been introduced specifically for near-patient testing (see p. 54).

(see p. 54)

Recommended units

The ICSH has recommended that Hb be expressed as g/l (mass concentration), or as mmol/l (molar concentration) in terms of concentration of the haemoglobin monomer. The conversion factor, if Hb is expressed in g/l, is 0.06206, i.e. an Hb of 120 g/l = 120 × 0.06206 mmol/l = 7.45 mmol/l. If Hb is expressed in molar concentration, then MCH and MCHC should also be expressed in this manner. An MCH of 27 pg is equivalent to 1.70 fmol. Similarly, an MCHC of 330 g/l (33 g/dl) is equivalent to 20 mmol/l. There are no clear practical advantages in expressing Hb as molar concentration and the potential for confusion and risk to patients if conversion to these units were to be attempted might be considerable. Despite the advice of the ICSH, many laboratories, preferring familiarity to correctness, continue to express Hb as g/dl.

Packed cell volume

The packed cell volume (PCV) is the proportion of a column of centrifuged blood that is occupied by red cells. Some of the measured column of red cells represents plasma that is trapped between red cells. The PCV is expressed as a decimal fraction representing l/l (litres/litre). The terms 'packed cell volume' and 'haematocrit' (Hct) were initially synonymous and were used interchangeably, but the ICSH has now recommended that PCV be reserved for estimates made by the traditional technique of centrifugation and Hct for estimates derived by other methods on automated instruments. The original method of measuring the PCV, as devised by Maxwell Wintrobe, required 1 ml of blood and prolonged (30 minutes to 1 hour) centrifugation in graduated glass tubes with a constant internal bore. This method, sometimes referred to as the macrohaematocrit, is the basis of the reference method [5], but for routine use it is cumbersome and slow. Since, for these reasons, it is no longer used in the diagnostic laboratory, it will not be discussed further. It has been replaced by the microhaematocrit, which has

clinical usefulness by itself, can be combined with the Hb to derive an estimate of the MCHC, and can be used to calibrate automated counters.

Microhaematocrit

A small volume of blood is taken by capillarity into an ungraduated capillary tube (usually 75 mm long with an internal diameter of 1.2 mm) leaving about 15 mm unfilled. The end of the tube distant from the column of blood is sealed by heat, or by modelling clay or a similar product. It is then centrifuged for 5 or 10 minutes, at a high *g* value (for example 10 000–15 000 *g*) in a small, specially designed centrifuge, to separate the column of blood into red cells, buffy coat and plasma (Fig. 2.2). The PCV is read visually on a scale, the buffy coat of white cells and platelets being excluded from the measurement. The ICSH has published a selected method that employs 5 minutes centrifugation [6]. A further 3 minutes centrifugation is advisable if the sample is polycythaemic, in order to reduce the abnormal plasma trapping [7]. The microhaematocrit is usually measured on ethylenediaminetetra-acetic acid (EDTA)-anticoagulated venous blood but it can also be performed on capillary blood if the sample is taken into a microhaematocrit tube the interior of which is coated with heparin (2 iu). Plastic (polycarbonate) tubes are available and are safer than glass tubes.

A microhaematocrit can also be measured automatically by an instrument that is suitable for

Fig. 2.2 Measurements of packed cell volume (PCV) by the microhaematocrit technique; paired tests from three patients are shown.

Table 2.1 Some factors affecting the microhaematocrit.

	Factors decreasing the microhaematocrit	Factors increasing the microhaematocrit
Consequent on dilution	Use of EDTA solution rather than dry EDTA (0.5% lower)	
Consequent on an alteration in the amount of trapped plasma	Longer period of centrifugation Increased centrifugal force (e.g. increased radius of centrifuge or increased speed of centrifugation)	Shorter period of centrifugation Decreased centrifugal force
	Elevated ESR	Microcytosis (e.g. iron deficiency or thalassaemia trait) Sickle cell trait or sickle cell disease Spherocytosis Reduced flexibility of red cells on prolonged storage at room temperature
Consequent on red cell shrinkage	Excess EDTA [12,13] K_3EDTA rather than K_2EDTA or Na_2EDTA [11] (about 2% lower) Narrower tubes than recommended [14] Soda lime tubes [14] Fully oxygenated blood [15]	K_2EDTA or Na_2EDTA Borosilicate tubes Deoxygenated blood [15]

EDTA, ethylenediaminetetra-acetic acid; ESR, erythrocyte sedimentation rate.

near-patient testing, which incorporates a centrifuge and an infrared analyser [8].

It should be noted that there are hazards associated with determining the microhaematocrit. Glass capillary tubes may break during insertion of modelling clay, leading to a penetrating injury and blood inoculation to the user. In one case human immunodeficiency virus (HIV) was transmitted and the house officer concerned subsequently developed the acquired immune deficiency syndrome (AIDS) [9,10]. Glass capillary tubes can also break during centrifugation, leading to a risk of injury and viral transmission [10].

The microhaematocrit has several sources of imprecision and inaccuracy. Because of the smallness of the tube, reading the level correctly can be difficult. Tubes may taper or be of an uneven bore. The seal is not flat, tending to be convex if modelling clay is used and concave if heat sealing is employed, although the error introduced by the type of seal is usually minor [11]. The amount of plasma trapping is usually around 1–3%, but is variable. It is less with longer periods of centrifugation and higher *g* values, but is also affected by other technical factors and by

the characteristics of the blood sample (Table 2.1). It should be noted that in the USA blood is usually taken into K_3EDTA, and in the UK it is more usually taken into K_2EDTA; because of the cell shrinkage that occurs, the microhaematocrit with K_3EDTA is about 2% lower than with K_2EDTA [16]. The precision of the microhaematocrit can be improved by making at least three replicate measurements and taking the average; this is necessary when a manual PCV is used to calibrate an automated instrument. It has been recommended that, because of the increase in microhaematocrit that occurs with deoxygenation, blood should be fully oxygenated when a microhaematocrit is used for calibration of an automated instrument [15].

Plasma trapping

Attempts have been made to make the microhaematocrit more accurate by 'correcting' the PCV for plasma trapping. A more accurate PCV means that an estimated MCV is also more accurate. In experimental conditions this can be done by labelling plasma proteins with ^{131}I and determining the amount of radioactive isotope that is trapped in the red cell column. The correction may itself be inaccurate, since estimates of plasma trapping are lower when ^{131}I-labelled fibrinogen is used than when ^{131}I-labelled albumin is used [11]. Such correction is clearly impracticable in routine diagnostic practice and it has been suggested that an arbitrary plasma trapping correction should be applied instead, particularly when the estimated PCV is to be used for calibration. This procedure is not recommended since, although the correction to be applied is based on experimental evidence, it is nevertheless arbitrary when applied to an individual blood sample and there is no agreement as to what percentage correction is appropriate. Different studies have produced estimates varying from 1.3% to 3.2% for mean plasma trapping. The ICSH Committee on Cytometry reference method does allow for the effect of plasma trapping [17] (see below). It is important that a standard procedure be used and that if a laboratory chooses to use a plasma trapping correction in calibrating an instrument it applies this correction when determining the reference range and continues to apply it when testing patient or blood donor samples.

Minor alterations in technique such as using or not using a plasma trapping correction can alter the percentage of blood donors whose donations are deferred, or the clinician's assessment of whether or not a polycythaemic patient requires venesection. A similar variation of a few per cent in the MCV can be diagnostically important in screening for thalassaemia trait and can render nomograms devised for this purpose invalid. There is a similar effect on the use of MCV as a screening tool unless precisely the same technique is used in calibrating the instrument when the reference range is devised and when the patient samples are studied.

One circumstance in which a plasma trapping correction is considered appropriate is when a microhaematocrit is being used for estimation of total red cell mass. Allowance should be made for the greater degree of plasma trapping of polycythaemic blood. It is suggested that if the PCV is less than 0.50 after centrifugation for 5 minutes, 2% correction should be applied; if it is greater than 0.50, a further 5 minutes centrifugation should be carried out and the correction should be 3% [18].

Reference method

The ICSH reference method for the PCV [17] is based on determination of the Hb on whole blood and packed red cells, following centrifugation in a microhaematocrit centrifuge. The measurement on packed red cells is performed on cells obtained from the middle of the column of red cells where there is little trapping of plasma or white cell contamination. It therefore produces a measurement that does not include trapped plasma. The reference PCV is

$$\frac{\text{Standard whole blood haemoglobin concentration}}{\text{Packed red cell haemoglobin concentration}}$$

For blood with a normal haematocrit, a spun microhaematocrit is usually within 0.01 l/l of the reference PCV.

A 'surrogate reference method' using a microhaematocrit determined in borosilicate capillary tubes has also been proposed, this method being more applicable to diagnostic haematology laboratories [19]. It also produces a measurement that is free of the effect of trapped plasma.

Other haematocrit methods

With automated instruments in current use, Hct is computed from the number and size of electrical impulses generated by red cells passing through a sensor (see pp. 36 and 39).

The red cell count

The red cell count (RBC) was initially performed by counting red cells microscopically in a carefully diluted sample of blood contained in a counting chamber (haemocytometer) with chambers of known volume [20]. Although this method was capable of producing satisfactory results if great care was exercised, it proved very unreliable in routine use because of a high degree of imprecision, and it was also very time-consuming. For this reason the RBC and the parameters derived from it were measured or calculated on only a minority of blood specimens.

More precise and therefore more clinically useful RBCs can be performed on single-channel semi-automated impedance counters (see p. 35), such as the Coulter Counter model ZM, which count cells in an accurately fixed and known volume of diluted blood as they pass through an aperture. Although accurate setting of thresholds is needed, the instruments do not require calibration. The raw instrument cell counts produced are non-linear with increasing cell concentration because of the greater likelihood of two cells passing through the aperture simultaneously (coincidence); depending on the instrument, coincidence correction may be an automatic function of the instrument or may be carried out by the user by reference to a table. White cells are also included in the RBC. Because red cells are normally at least 100-fold more numerous than white cells the inaccuracy introduced by this is usually not great. RBCs determined on single-channel impedance counters are much more precise than those produced in counting chambers and they can also be produced with much less labour. They are therefore more clinically useful. They can be used with a manual Hb and PCV to calculate MCV and MCH, which are also much more precise than those derived from manual RBCs.

RBCs from single-channel semi-automated impedance counters can also be used to calibrate fully automated blood cell counters that count electrical impulses generated by red cells passing through a sensor (see p. 35). Automated instruments count of the order of 20 000–50 000 cells, so that the precision is again much greater than that of a haemocytometer count based on 500–1000 cells.

The reference method for the RBC employs a semi-automated single-channel aperture-impedance method with accurate coincidence correction being achieved by extrapolation from counts on serial dilutions [21].

Derived red cell variables—red cell indices

Given the three measured variables (Hb, PCV and RBC), it is possible to derive the MCV, MCH and MCHC. When no plasma trapping correction is used, the MCV derived from a microhaematocrit will be an overestimate of the true value and the MCHC will be an underestimate. This is of no clinical consequence, since reference ranges will be derived in the same manner. The measured and derived variables that describe the characteristics of red cells are often referred to collectively as the red cell indices.

The white cell count

A manual white cell count (WBC) is performed after diluting an aliquot of blood in a diluent that lyses red cells and stains the nuclei of the white cells [20]. White cells are counted microscopically in a haemocytometer with chambers of known volume. Nucleated red blood cells (NRBC) cannot be readily distinguished from white cells in a counting chamber. If NRBC are present their percentage can be counted on a stained blood film and the total nucleated cell count (TNCC) can be corrected. The manual WBC is imprecise, but this is of less practical importance than the imprecision of the RBC since clinically important changes in WBC are usually of sufficient magnitude to be detected even with an imprecise method.

White cells can also be counted in diluted whole blood following red cell lysis, using a single-channel semi-automated impedance counter. In fully automated counters, white cells are counted by impedance technology or light scattering. Automated counters are inadequate for counting very low numbers of white cells, e.g. for ensuring that units of blood products for transfusion have fewer than 5×10^8 white cells. In this circumstance, flow cytometry following staining of white cell nuclei with a DNA stain is required [22].

The reference method for the WBC employs a semi-automated single-channel aperture-impedance method with accurate coincidence correction being achieved by extrapolation from counts on serial dilutions [21]. The lower threshold is set between the noise produced by red cell stroma and the signals from leucocytes.

The platelet count

Platelets can be counted in a haemocytometer using either diluted whole blood (in which red cells can be either left intact or lysed) or platelet-rich plasma (prepared by sedimentation or centrifugation). If very large platelets are present, a whole-blood method is preferred to the use of platelet-rich plasma to avoid the risk of large heavy platelets being lost during preparative procedures. The use of platelet-rich plasma may be preferred if the platelet count is low. When the method leaves platelets intact, large platelets can be distinguished from small red cells by the platelet's shape, which may be oval rather than round, and by its irregular outline, with fine projections sometimes being visible. Use of ammonium oxalate, which lyses red cells, as a diluent produces a higher and more accurate count than use of formol-citrate, which leaves red cells intact [23]. Platelet counts are best performed on anticoagulated venous blood obtained by a clean venepuncture. Counts on blood obtained by finger-prick tend to be lower.

Platelets can be visualized in the counting chamber by light or phase-contrast microscopy. When using light microscopy, brilliant cresyl blue can be added to the diluent. This stains platelets light blue and facilitates their identification. On light microscopy, platelet identification is aided by their refractivity. It is easier to identify platelets by phase-contrast microscopy and such counts are therefore generally more precise.

Manual platelet counts are generally imprecise, particularly when the count is low. They are also very laborious, so that when this was the only technique available, counts were performed only when there was a clear clinical indication.

Platelets can be counted by semi-automated methods using impedance counters following the preparation of platelet-rich plasma. Coincidence correction and the use of two thresholds, to exclude both debris and contaminating red cells and white cells, are necessary. These techniques are also laborious and the several steps involved make them prone to error.

Laboratories with instrumentation suitable for an automated RBC but not an automated platelet count can estimate the platelet count indirectly by measuring the RBC and calculating the platelet count on the basis of the red cell : platelet ratio in a stained blood film.

However, the only satisfactory way to perform the number of platelet counts required by modern medical practice is with fully automated blood cell counters. Such instruments count platelets by impedance, light-scattering or optical fluorescence technology. In a further refinement of the method, a monoclonal antibody to a platelet glycoprotein can be incorporated so that platelets are reliably distinguished from other small particles. Counts are generally precise, even at low levels, but unusual characteristics of the blood sample can cause inaccuracy (see p. 184). Manual haemocytometer counts remain necessary in some patients with giant platelets which, with many automated counters, cannot be distinguished from red cells.

Various proposals have been made for a reference method for the platelet count. The platelet count can be determined indirectly, using the reference method for the RBC and determining the red cell : platelet ratio on an automated instrument that is capable of distinguishing reliably between these two cell types. Alternatively, the platelet count can be determined by flow cytometry using a fluorochrome-labelled monoclonal antibody, such as CD41, CD42a or CD61, that binds specifically to platelets. Either a known amount of fluorescent beads can be used as a calibrant, or the ratio of red cells to fluorescent platelets can be determined and the platelet count can be calculated from a reference RBC [24–26]. The latter procedure is preferred, and is now the proposed international reference method [27], since dilution errors do not affect the count; a mixture of CD41 and CD61 directly labelled antibodies is employed. It should be noted that, when there is an inherited platelet membrane defect with absence of one of the platelet glycoproteins, the relevant monoclonal antibody will not bind to platelets, hence the use of two antibodies. A similar flow cytometry technique has been recommended for routine platelet counts in severely thrombocytopenic patients, when an accurate platelet count is particularly important for determining whether or not a platelet transfusion is needed [28].

The differential white cell count

A differential white cell count is the assigning of leucocytes to their individual categories, this categorization being expressed as a percentage or, when the WBC is available, as an absolute count. The ICSH recommends that the differential leucocyte count be expressed in absolute numbers [29]. A differential count carried out by a human observer using a microscope is referred to as a manual differential count. It is usually performed on a wedge-spread film, prepared either manually or with a mechanical film spreader. Automated differential counts are now generally performed by flow cytometry as part of a full blood count (FBC), differentiation between categories being based on the physical characteristics of the cells and sometimes on their biochemical characteristics.

Cells that are normally present in the peripheral blood can be assigned to five or six categories, depending on whether non-segmented or band forms of neutrophils (see p. 91) are separated from segmented neutrophils or are counted with them. The differential count also includes any abnormal cells that may be present. NRBC can be included as a separate category in the differential count or, alternatively, their number can be expressed per 100 white cells. In the former case the uncorrected count is designated the TNCC rather than the WBC, and this is used for calculating absolute cell numbers. In the latter case, the TNCC is corrected to a WBC by subtracting the number of NRBC. Laboratories should consistently follow one or other convention of expressing counts. In my opinion, it is probably better **not** to correct the TNCC to a WBC, but to calculate absolute counts from the TNCC and the percentage of each cell type, NRBC being included in the differential count. The advantage of this policy is that the TNCC is likely to be a precise measurement, whereas the ratio of NRBC to WBC, calculated by counting NRBC/100 WBC, is likely to be imprecise; it is better not to replace a precise measurement of the TNCC with an imprecise estimate of the WBC. The USA's National Committee of Clinical Laboratory Standards (NCCLS), however, recommends that NRBC be expressed per 100 WBC [30].

Differential white cell counts, like all laboratory tests, are subject to both inaccuracy and imprecision. Manual differential counts are generally fairly accurate, but their precision is poor, whereas automated counts are generally fairly precise but are sometimes inaccurate.

Inaccuracy

With a manual differential count, inaccuracy or deviation from the true count results both from maldistribution and from misidentification of cells.

Maldistribution of cells

The different types of white cell are not distributed evenly over a slide. The tail of the film contains more neutrophils and fewer lymphocytes, whereas monocytes are fairly evenly distributed along the length of the film [31]. When large immature cells (blasts, promyelocytes and myelocytes) are present they are preferentially distributed at the edges of the film rather than in the centre and distally rather than proximally, in relation to lymphocytes, basophils, neutrophils and metamyelocytes [32]. The maldistribution of cells is aggravated if a film is too thin or if a spreader with a rough edge has been used. Various methods of tracking over a slide have been proposed to attempt to overcome errors due to maldistribution (Fig. 2.3). The method shown in Fig. 2.3a compensates for maldistribution between the body and the tail, but not for maldistribution between the centre and the edge, whereas the 'battlement' method shown in Fig. 2.3b tends to do the reverse, since the customary 100-cell differential count will not cover a very large proportion of the length of the blood film. A modified battlement track (Fig. 2.3c) is a compromise between the two methods. In practice, the imprecision of a manual

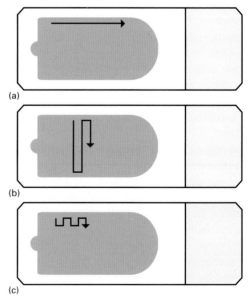

(a)

(b)

(c)

Fig. 2.3 Diagrams of blood films showing tracking patterns employed in differential white blood cell count: (a) tracking along the length of the film; (b) battlement method; and (c) modified battlement method—two fields are counted close to the edge parallel to the edge of the film, then four fields at right angles, then two fields parallel to the edge and so on.

count is so great that a small degree of inaccuracy caused by maldistribution of cells is not of any great consequence. If there is white cell aggregation, the maldistribution of cells is so great that an accurate differential count is impossible.

Misidentification of cells

Inaccuracy due to misidentification of cells is usually not great when differential counts are performed by experienced laboratory workers on high quality blood films. An exception to this is the differentiation between band forms and segmented neutrophils. Criteria for making this distinction differ between laboratories, and there is also inconsistency in the application of the criteria within a laboratory because of an element of subjectivity. Occasionally it is also difficult to distinguish a monocyte from a large lymphocyte or a degranulated basophil from a neutrophil. Marked storage artefact renders a differential count very inaccurate; specifically, degenerating neutrophils may be misclassified as NRBC and preferential disintegration of neutrophils can cause a factitious elevation of the lymphocyte count. Inaccuracy can also be introduced into a count if many smear cells (see p. 124) are present and are not included in the count. If the smear cells are, for example, lymphocytes, then the percentage and absolute number of lymphocytes will be falsely low and the percentage and absolute number of all other cell types will be falsely high. Smear cells whose nature can be determined should be counted with the category to which they belong. Smear cells, the nature of which is not clear, should be counted as a separate category or the percentage and absolute number of cells of most categories will be falsely elevated.

Imprecision

The imprecision or lack of reproducibility of a count can be expressed as either the standard deviation (SD) or the coefficient of variation (CV) of replicate counts. The small number of cells conventionally counted in a manual differential count leads to poor precision [33]. When replicate counts are made of the percentage of cells of a given type among randomly distributed cells, the SD of the count is related to the square root of the number of cells counted. Specifically, the SD of the proportion of a given cell type, θ, is equal to [34]:

$$\sqrt{\frac{\theta(1-\theta)}{n}}$$

The 95% confidence limits of the proportion, i.e. the limits within which 95% of replicate counts would be expected to fall, are equal to $\theta \pm 1.96$ SD. The confidence limits of a given percentage of cells when 100 or more cells are counted are shown in Table 2.2. It will be seen that the confidence limits are wide. For example, the confidence limits of a 10% eosinophil count on a 100-cell differential count are 4–18%. The precision of the absolute count of any given cell count cannot be any better than the precision of the percentage but, if it is calculated from an automated WBC which itself is quite a precise measurement, it is not a great deal worse. The imprecision of a manual differential count is greatest for those cells that are present in the smallest numbers, particularly the basophils. If it is diagnostically important to know whether or not there is basophilia then it is necessary to improve precision, either by performing an absolute basophil count in a haemocytometer or by counting many more than the usual 100 cells (e.g. at least 200–500 cells). Similarly, if neutrophils constitute only a small proportion of cells (e.g. in chronic lymphocytic leukaemia), it is again necessary to count a larger number of cells to improve precision and determine whether there is neutropenia. Although the precision of a manual count could be improved by routinely counting more cells, it is not feasible in a diagnostic laboratory to routinely count more than 100 or, at the most, 200 cells. The poor precision of the count of cells present in the smallest numbers means that the reference limits for manual basophil and eosinophil counts include zero. It is therefore impossible on the basis of a manual count to say that a patient has basopenia or eosinopenia. It should also be noted that the precision of the band count is so poor that it is not generally very useful to count band cells separately from segmented neutrophils. A comment such as 'left shift' or 'increased band cells' can be made when such cells are clearly increased.

There is no internationally agreed reference method for the manual differential count, though

Observed percentage of cells	Total number of cells counted (n)				
	100	200	500	1000	10 000
0	0–4	0–2	0–1	0–1	0–0.04
1	0–6	0–4	0–3	0–2	0.8–1.2
2	0–8	0–6	0–4	1–4	1.7–2.3
3	0–9	1–7	1–5	2–5	2.7–3.3
4	1–10	1–8	2–7	2–6	3.6–4.4
5	1–12	2–10	3–8	3–7	4.6–5.4
6	2–13	3–11	4–9	4–8	5.5–6.5
7	2–14	3–12	4–10	5–9	6.5–7.5
8	3–16	4–13	5–11	6–10	7.4–8.6
9	4–17	5–15	6–12	7–11	8.4–9.6
10	4–18	6–16	7–14	8–13	9.4–10.6
15	8–24	10–21	12–19	12–18	14.6–15.4
20	12–30	14–27	16–24	17–23	19.6–20.4
25	16–35	19–32	21–30	22–28	24.6–25.4
30	21–40	23–37	26–35	27–33	29.5–30.5
35	25–46	28–43	30–40	32–39	34.5–35.5
40	30–51	33–48	35–45	36–44	39.5–40.5
45	35–56	38–53	40–50	41–49	44.5–45.5
50	39–61	42–58	45–55	46–54	49.5–50.5

Table 2.2 Precision achieved with differential counts of various numbers of leucocytes.

Ninety-five per cent confidence limits of the observed percentage of cells when the total number of cells counted (n) varies from 100 to 10 000. Ranges for n = 100 to n = 1000 are derived from reference [33].

the NCCLS has established a reference method [30]. It uses a manually wedge-spread, Romanowsky-stained film. Two hundred cells are counted by each of two trained observers using a 'battlement' track (see Fig. 2.3b). The results are averaged to produce a 400-cell differential count, which is then divided by four.

The reticulocyte count

Reticulocytes are young red cells, newly released from the bone marrow, that still contain ribosomal RNA. On exposure of unfixed cells to certain dyes, such as brilliant cresyl blue or 'new methylene blue', the ribosomes are precipitated and stained by the dye, to appear as a reticular network; as the cells are still living when exposed to the dye, this is referred to as supravital staining. With new methylene blue, red cells stain a pale greenish-blue while the reticulum stains bluish-purple.

The amount of reticulum in a reticulocyte varies from a large clump in the most immature cells (group I reticulocytes) to a few granules in the most

mature forms (group IV reticulocytes) (Fig. 2.4). The difficulty in determining whether one or two dots of appropriately stained material represent RNA has led to various definitions of a reticulocyte being proposed. The minimum requirement varies from a single dot, through two or three dots to a minimum network. Since the majority of reticulocytes in the peripheral blood are group IV, the precise definition of a reticulocyte that is employed will have an appreciable effect on the reticulocyte count. The NCCLS classifies as a reticulocyte 'any non-nucleated red cell containing two or more particles of blue-stained material corresponding to ribosomal RNA' [35]. This definition is also accepted by the ICSH [36].

The RNA, which is responsible for forming the reticulum following supravital staining, gives rise, on Romanowsky-stained films, to diffuse cytoplasmic basophilia. The combination of cytoplasmic basophilia with the acidophilia of haemoglobin produces staining characteristics known as polychromasia. Not all reticulocytes contain enough RNA to cause polychromasia on a Romanowsky-stained film, but whether polychromatic cells correspond

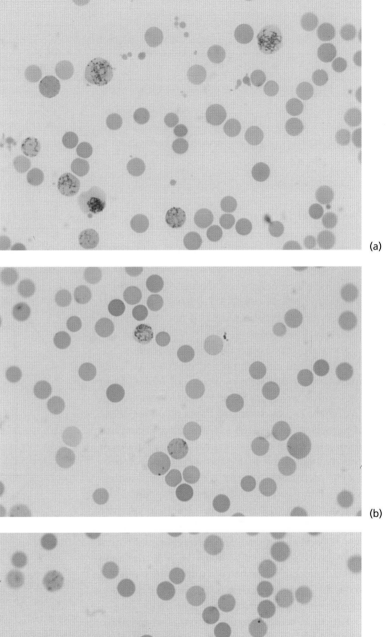

Fig. 2.4 Reticulocytes stained with new methylene blue. (a) A group I reticulocyte with a dense clump of reticulum, several group II reticulocytes with a wreath or network of reticulum and several group III reticulocytes with a disintegrated wreath of reticulum. (b) Group II, III and IV reticulocytes: the group IV reticulocyte has two granules of reticulum. There is also a cell with a single dot of reticulum. By some criteria this would also be classified as a reticulocyte. (c) Three reticulocytes and a Howell–Jolly body.

Table 2.3 The characteristic appearance of various red cell inclusions on a new methylene blue reticulocyte preparation.

Name	Nature	Appearance
Reticulum	Ribosomal RNA	Reticulofilamentous material or scanty small granules
Pappenheimer bodies	Iron-containing inclusions	One or more granules towards the periphery of the cell, may stain a deeper blue than reticulum
Heinz bodies	Denatured haemoglobin	Larger than Pappenheimer bodies, irregular in shape, usually attached to the cell membrane and may protrude through it, pale blue
Howell–Jolly bodies	DNA	Larger than Pappenheimer bodies, regular in shape, distant from the cell membrane, pale blue
Haemoglobin H inclusions	Denatured haemoglobin H	Usually do not form with short incubation periods; if present they are multiple and spherical giving a 'golf-ball' appearance, pale greenish-blue

only to the least mature reticulocytes (equivalent to the group I reticulocytes) [37] or to all but the most mature reticulocytes (group I, II and III reticulocytes) [38] is not certain.

There are certain other inclusions that can be confused with the reticulum of reticulocytes. Methods of making the distinction are given in Table 2.3 and these other inclusions are discussed in more detail in Chapter 7. Cells containing Pappenheimer bodies, in particular, can sometimes be difficult to distinguish from late reticulocytes with only a few granules of reticulofilamentous material. If necessary, a reticulocyte preparation can be counterstained with a Perls' stain (see p. 266), to identify Pappenheimer bodies, or by a Romanowsky stain, to identify Howell–Jolly bodies. When a reticulocyte preparation is fixed in methanol and counterstained with a Romanowsky stain, the vital dye, e.g. the new methylene blue, is washed out during the methanol fixation. The reticulum is then stained by the basic component of the Romanowsky stain [39].

Reticulocytes are usually counted as a percentage of red blood cells. The use of an eyepiece containing a Miller ocular micrometer disc (Fig. 2.5) facilitates counting; reticulocytes are counted in the large squares and the total red cells in the small squares, which are one-ninth of the size of the large cells. If 20 fields are counted, the reticulocytes among about 2000 cells are counted and the reticulocyte percentage is equal to:

$$\frac{\text{Reticulocytes in 20 large squares} \times 100}{\text{Erythrocytes in 20 small squares} \times 9}$$

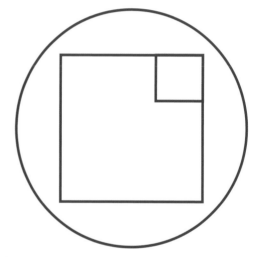

Fig. 2.5 The appearance of a Miller ocular micrometer for use in counting reticulocytes.

This method gives superior precision to counting the proportion of reticulocytes without an ocular insert [40]. Consecutive rather than random fields should be counted, since there is otherwise a tendency to subconsciously select fields with more reticulocytes [40]. It is also essential that the same principles of counting cells as are used in manual counting chamber counts are followed, i.e. the cells overlapping two of the four borders are not counted. Failure to follow this practice is thought to be the explanation of a bias towards lower counts that has been observed if a Miller disc is used [41]. The number of cells to be counted to achieve an acceptable degree of reproducibility increases as the percentage

Table 2.4 Cells to be counted to achieve a reasonably precise reticulocyte count.

Reticulocyte count (%)	Approximate number of cells to be counted in small squares for CV of 10%	Equivalent to total count of
1–2	1000	9000
3–5	500	4500
6–10	200	1800
20–25	100	900

The number of cells to be counted in the small square of a Miller graticule to achieve an acceptable degree of precision for the reticulocyte count, from reference [36].
CV, coefficient of variation.

of reticulocytes falls. If a Miller graticule is used, the number of cells that should be counted to achieve a CV of about 10% is shown in Table 2.4 [36].

Reticulocyte counts have traditionally been expressed as a percentage. If an RBC is available an absolute reticulocyte count, which gives a more accurate impression of bone marrow output, can be calculated. As an alternative, a result that is more meaningful than a percentage can be produced by correcting for the degree of anaemia as follows:

$$\text{Reticulocyte index} = \frac{\text{reticulocyte percentage} \times \text{observed PCV}}{\text{normal PCV}}$$

for example,

$$\text{Reticulocyte index} = \frac{1.2 \times 0.29}{0.45} = 0.77$$

This example shows that an apparently normal reticulocyte count can be demonstrated to be low if allowance is made for the presence of anaemia. This procedure and the use of an absolute reticulocyte count give similar information. A more complex correction [42] can be made that allows for the fact that in anaemic persons, under the influence of an increased concentration of erythropoietin, reticulocytes are released prematurely from the bone marrow and spend longer in the blood before becoming mature red cells. The reticulocyte index and the absolute reticulocyte count both give a somewhat false impression of bone marrow output in this circumstance. The reticulocyte production index [42] is calculated by dividing the reticulocyte index by the average maturation time of a reticulocyte in the peripheral blood at any degree of anaemia. Although the reticulocyte index and the reticulocyte production index have not found general acceptance, the concepts embodied in them should be borne in mind when reticulocyte counts are being interpreted.

Although the absolute reticulocyte count or one of the reticulocyte indices is to be preferred as an indicator of bone marrow output, the reticulocyte percentage has the advantage that it gives an indication of red cell lifespan. If a patient with a stable haemolytic anaemia has a reticulocyte count of 10% it is apparent that one cell in 10 is no more than 1–3 days old.

The reticulocyte count is stable with storage of EDTA-anticoagulated blood at room temperature for up to 24 hours [43] and at 4°C for several days [36]. The NCCLS reference method for the reticulocyte count is based on new methylene blue [44].

Units and approved abbreviations

The ICSH have recommended standardized abbreviations for peripheral blood variables. These are shown together with the approved units of the Système International (SI) and their abbreviations in Table 2.5.

Automated blood cell counters

Principles of operation of automated haematology counters

The latest fully automated blood cell counters aspirate and dilute a blood sample and determine 8–46 variables relating to red cells, white cells and platelets. Many counters are also capable of identifying a blood specimen (e.g. by bar-code reading), mixing it, transporting it to the sampling tube and checking it for adequacy of volume and absence of clots. Some are also linked to an automated film spreader. To avoid any unnecessary handling of blood specimens by instrument operators, sampling is usually by piercing a cap. Apart from the measurement of Hb, all variables depend on counting and sizing of particles, whether red cells, white cells or platelets. Particles can be counted and sized

Table 2.5 Units, abbreviations and symbols used for describing haematological variables*.

Variable	Abbreviation	Unit	Symbol
White blood cell count	WBC	number $\times 10^9$/l	
Red blood cell count	RBC	number $\times 10^{12}$/l	
Haemoglobin concentration	Hb	grams/litre OR	g/l
		grams/decilitre OR	g/dl
		millimoles per litre	mmol/l
Haematocrit	Hct	litre/litre	l/l
Packed cell volume	PCV	litre/litre	l/l
Mean cell volume	MCV	femtolitre	fl
Mean cell haemoglobin	MCH	picograms OR	pg
		femtomoles	fm
Mean cell haemoglobin concentration	MCHC	grams/litre OR	g/l
		grams/decilitre OR	g/dl
		millimoles per litre	mmol/l
Platelet count	Plt	number $\times 10^9$/l	
Mean platelet volume	MPV	femtolitre	fl
Plateletcrit	Pct	litre/litre	l/l
Reticulocyte count	Retic	number $\times 10^9$/l	
Erythrocyte sedimentation rate (Westergren, 1 hour)	ESR	millimitres	mm

* In addition, it should be noted that the approved abbreviation for 'international units' is iu.

either by electrical impedance or by light scattering. Automated instruments have at least two channels. In one channel a diluent is added and red cells are counted and sized. In another channel a lytic agent is added, together with diluent, to reduce red cells to stroma, leaving the white cells intact for counting and also producing a solution in which Hb can be measured. Further channels are required for a differential WBC, which is often dependent on study of cells by a number of modalities, e.g. impedance technology with current of various frequencies, light scattering and light absorbance. A separate channel or an independent instrument may be required for a reticulocyte count.

Automated instruments cannot recognize all the significant abnormalities that can be recognized by a human observer. They are therefore designed to produce accurate and precise blood counts on specimens which are either normal or show only numerical abnormalities, and to alert the instrument operator when the specimen has unusual characteristics that could either lead to an inaccurate measurement or require review of a blood film. This is often referred to as 'flagging'. Results should be flagged: (i) when the blood sample contains blast cells, immature granulocytes, NRBC or atypical lymphocytes; (ii) when there are giant or aggregated platelets or for any reason red cell and platelet populations cannot be separated; and (iii) when there is an abnormality likely to be associated with factitious results.

A new challenge to automated instruments is the production of accurate red cell indices, as well as total haemoglobin concentration, in patients who are infused with haemoglobin-based blood substitutes. This can be achieved with Bayer instruments (see below), which measure size and haemoglobin concentration of individual red cells [45].

Beckman–Coulter instruments

Blood cells are extremely poor conductors of electricity. When a stream of cells in a conducting medium flows through a small aperture across which an electric current is applied (Fig. 2.6) there is a measurable increase in the electrical impedance across the aperture as each cell passes through, this increase being proportional to the volume of conducting material displaced. The change in impedance is therefore proportional to the cell

Stopcock

Wire from internal electrode

Internal electrode

Wire from external electrode

External electrode

Aperture through which cells in suspension are drawn

Mercury-containing manometer for controlling and metering flow through the aperture

Wires from electrodes which stop and start particle counting

Fig. 2.6 Semi-diagrammatic representation of part of Coulter Counter, model FN, showing the aperture tube and the manometer used for metering the volume of cell suspension counted. Right: diagrammatic representation of the cross-section of the aperture tube of an impedance counter.

volume. Cells can thus be both counted and sized from the electrical impulses that they generate. This is the principle of impedance counting, which was devised and developed by Wallace Coulter in the late 1940s and 1950s and which ushered in the modern era of automated blood cell counting.

Aperture impedance is determined by capacitance and inductance as well as by resistance. Various factors apart from cell volume influence the amplitude, duration and form of the pulse, these being related to the disturbance of electrical lines of force as well as to the displacement of the conducting medium. Cell shape is relevant, as well as cell volume, so that cells of increased deformability, which can elongate in response to shear forces as they pass through the aperture, appear smaller than their actual size and rigid cells appear larger [46]. Furthermore, cells that pass through the aperture off centre produce aberrant impulses and appear larger than their actual

size. Cells that recirculate through the edge of an electrical field produce an aberrant impulse, which is smaller than that produced by a similar cell passing through the aperture; a recirculating red cell can produce an impulse similar to that of a platelet passing through the aperture. Cells that pass through the aperture simultaneously, or almost so, are counted and sized as a single cell; the inaccuracy introduced requires correction, known as coincidence correction. Aberrant impulses can be edited out electronically. Sheathed flow or hydrodynamic focusing can direct cells to the centre of the aperture to reduce the problems caused both by coincidence and by aberrant impulses. Both sheathed flow and sweep flow behind an aperture can prevent recirculation of cells.

Impedance counters generally produce very precise measurements of cell volume and haemoglobin content and concentration. However, there are some inaccuracies inherent in the method, which are greater when cells are abnormal. The voltage pulse produced by a cell passing through the sensing zone can be regarded as the cell's electrical shadow, which suggests a particle of a certain size and shape. A normal red cell probably passes through the aperture in a fusiform or cigar shape [46], producing an electrical shadow similar to its actual volume, whereas a sphere produces an electrical shadow 1.5 times its actual volume [46]. A fixed rigid cell will appear larger than its actual volume. Furthermore, cell deformability is a function of haemoglobin concentration within an individual cell. The effect of cell shape is not the same with all impedance counters. In one study the inaccuracy was greater with a Coulter STKR and a Cell-Dyn 3000 than with a Sysmex K-1000 and was not seen with a Sysmex NE-8000 [47].

Beckman–Coulter instruments (previously Coulter counters) initially measured Hb by a modified cyanmethaemoglobin method. For example, with the Coulter Counter S Plus IV, Hb was derived from the optical density at approximately 525 nm after a reaction time of 20–25 seconds. A cyanide-free reagent for Hb determination was subsequently introduced. Coulter instruments count and size red cells, white cells and platelets by impedance technology. Platelets and red cells are counted and sized in the same channel. The measurement of MCV and RBC allow the Hct to be derived, and the measurement of mean platelet volume (MPV) and the platelet count allow

the derivation of an equivalent platelet variable, the plateletcrit (Pct). The MCH is derived from the Hb and the RBC. The MCHC is derived from the Hb, RBC and MCV. The variation in size of red cells is indicated by the red cell distribution width (RDW), which is the SD of individual measurements of red cell volume. The equivalent platelet variable is the platelet distribution width (PDW). There is often some overlap in size between small red cells and large platelets. Depending on the model of instrument, platelets and red cells may be separated from each other by a fixed threshold, e.g. at 20 fl, or by a moving threshold, or the data from counts between two thresholds, e.g. 2 and 20 fl, may be used to fit a curve, which is extrapolated so that platelets falling beyond these thresholds, e.g. between 0 and 70 fl, are also included in the count. White cells are counted in a separate channel, the Hb channel, following red cell lysis. NRBC present are mainly included in the 'WBC'. Histograms of volume distribution of white cells, red cells and platelets are provided (Fig. 2.7).

The fully automated Coulter instruments— Coulter STKS, MAXM, HmX, Gen S and LH750— produce a five-part differential white cell count, which is based on various physical characteristics of white cells, following partial stripping of cytoplasm (Fig. 2.8; Table 2.6). Three simultaneous measurements are made on each cell: (i) impedance measurements with low-frequency electromagnetic current, dependent mainly on cell volume; (ii) conductivity

Fig. 2.7 Histograms produced by a Coulter S Plus IV automated counter showing volume distribution of white cells, red cells and platelets.

Fig. 2.8 Printouts of Coulter STKS automated counter. (a) Scatter plot of white cell volume against discriminant function 1. There are four white cell populations: NEUT, neutrophils; EOS, eosinophils; MONO, monocytes; and LYMPH, lymphocytes. (b) Scatter plots of white cell volume against discriminant function 2 showing three white cell populations: GRAN, neutrophils, eosinophils and basophils; MONO, monocytes; and LYMPH, lymphocytes. (c) Scatter plots of white cell volume against discriminant function 3 showing three white cell populations; BASO, basophils; MONO, monocytes; and LYMPH, lymphocytes. (d) Histogram showing size distribution of red cells and platelets.

measurements with high-frequency (radiofrequency) electromagnetic current, which alters the bipolar lipid layer of the cell membrane allowing the current to penetrate the cells and is therefore dependent mainly on the internal structure of the cell, including nucleocytoplasmic ratio, nuclear density and granularity; (iii) forward light scattering at 10–70° when cells pass through a laser beam, determined by the structure, shape and reflectivity of the cell. In recent instruments (e.g. the Gen S and LH750), the software permits further analysis of this data: conductivity measurements are corrected for the effect of cell volume so that they more accurately reflect internal cell structure and nucleocytoplasmic

Table 2.6 Technology employed in automated full blood counters performing 5–7 part differential counts.

Instrument	Technology
Coulter STKS, Gen S and LH750 (Beckman–Coulter)	(i) Impedance with low frequency electromagnetic current (ii) Conductivity with high frequency electromagnetic current (iii) Laser light scattering
A^cT 5diff counter (Beckman–Coulter)	(i) Impedance measurements following differential lysis (ii) Impedance technology and absorbance cytochemistry (after interaction with chlorazole black)
Sysmex SE-9000 (Sysmex Corporation)	(i) Impedance with low frequency electromagnetic current (ii) Impedance with high frequency electromagnetic current (iii) Impedance with low frequency electromagnetic current at low and high pH
Sysmex XE-2100 (Sysmex Corporation)	(i) Impedance with low frequency electromagnetic current (ii) Impedance with radiofrequency electromagnetic current (iii) Forward light scatter (iv) Sideways light scatter (v) Fluorescence intensity following interaction with a polymethine fluorescent dye
H.1, H.2 and H.3 and Advia 120 (Bayer)	(i) Light scattering following peroxidase reaction (ii) Light absorbance following peroxidase reaction (iii) Light scattering following stripping of cytoplasm from cells other than basophils by a lytic agent at low pH
Cell-Dyn 3500 (Abbott Diagnostics)	(i) Forward light scatter (ii) Narrow angle light scatter (iii) Orthogonal light scatter (iv) Polarized orthogonal light scatter
Cell-Dyn 4000 (Abbott Diagnostics)	As above plus: (v) NRBC count following binding to fluorescent dye
ABX Pentra 60 and ABX Pentra 120 Retic (ABX Diagnostics)	(i) Impedance (ii) Light absorbance following staining of granules with chlorazol black E (iii) Impedance following preferential stripping of cytoplasm from basophils at low pH

ratio—designated 'opacity'; light-scatter measurements are corrected for the effect of cell volume so that separation of different cell types is improved—designated 'rotated light scatter'. The abbreviation VCS (volume, conductivity, scatter) is used. Five cell populations are discriminated by three-dimensional cluster analysis based on cell volume, 'opacity' and rotated light scatter; clusters are separated by moving curvilinear thresholds. Clusters are represented graphically by plots of cell volume against three discriminant functions derived from the data. Plots of size against discriminant function 1 (mainly derived from light scatter) separate cells into four clusters: neutrophils, eosinophils, monocytes and lymphocytes plus basophils (Fig. 2.8a). Basophils are located in the upper right-hand quadrant of the lymphocyte box. Plots of size against discriminant function 2 (mainly based on conductivity measure-ments with high-frequency electromagnetic current) separate cells into three clusters—lymphocytes, monocytes and granulocytes (Fig. 2.8b). A plot of size against discriminant function 3, obtained by gating out neutrophils and eosinophils, shows basophils as a cluster separate from lymphocytes and monocytes (Fig. 2.8c). In addition, there is a multicolour three-dimensional scatter plot.

With the latest Beckman–Coulter instrument, the LH750, precision is improved by counting white cells, red cells and platelets in triplicate and by extending the counting time if the WBC or platelet count is low. Particles greater than 35 fl after red cell lysis are counted as white cells. The instrument is able to count NRBC and corrects the WBC for NRBC interference [48]. Platelets are counted between 2 and 20 fl but the curve is extrapolated to 70 fl to include large platelets. Reticulocytes can be counted

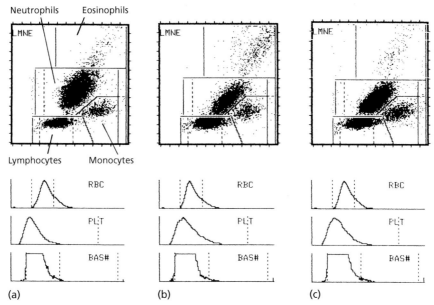

Fig. 2.9 Scatterplot and histograms produced by Beckman–Coulter A^{c}T 5diff counter: (a) normal; (b) sample with eosinophilia; (c) sample with monocytosis.

in a separate mode (see p. 49). A new red cell variable, the mean sphered cell volume (MSCV), represents the average volume of sphered red cells, measured in the reticulocyte channel [49]. Normally the MSCV is greater than the MCV (of non-sphered cells) and an inversion of this relationship suggests the presence of spherocytosis or a similar shape change [49]. The Coulter Gen S and LH750 VCS differential white cell data can be used as an 'alarm' for samples that are likely to contain malaria parasites [50].

Earlier Coulter instruments (the S Plus series and the STKR) produce a three-part differential count based solely on impedance sizing following partial stripping of cytoplasm, the categories of white cell being granulocyte, lymphocyte and mononuclear cell.

Another current instrument marketed by Beckman–Coulter instrument, the A^{c}T 5diff counter, performs a five-part differential count by means of measurements in two channels (Fig. 2.9; Table 2.6). The WBC and the basophil count are determined by impedance measurements following differential lysis, basophils being more resistant to stripping of cytoplasm in acid conditions. Other cell types are determined in a second channel using a combination of measurements of volume (by impedance technology) and absorbance cytochemistry (after

interaction with chlorazole black). Chlorazol black binds to the granules of eosinophils (most strongly), neutrophils (intermediate) and monocytes (least strongly); lymphocytes are unstained. The principles underlying the differential count on this instrument have much in common with those employed in Bayer instruments (see below). The instrument has a very small sample volume requirement so is suitable for use with paediatric samples.

Information on Beckman–Coulter instruments is available on the company website, www. beckman.com.

Sysmex and other instruments incorporating impedance measurements

After the expiry of the initial patent of Coulter Electronics, impedance counters were introduced by a number of other manufacturers, among whom Sysmex Corporation are prominent. These instruments operate according to similar principles to those of Coulter instruments. Some instruments integrate the pulse heights from the red cell channel to produce Hct and derive the MCV from the RBC and Hct while others do the reverse. Variables measured are similar to those of Coulter analysers, often including a three-part (Fig. 2.10)—or with added

3/ 6/94   NO. ✦   593341

```
WBC                          WBC       31 -
                             W-SCR     290
                             W-MCR     153
                             W-LCR     557
                             W-SCC     09 -
                             W-MCC     05
                             W-LCC     17 -
    36  72 108                   300 [fl]
RBC
                             RBC       319
                             HGB       101 -
                             HCT     0309 -
                             MCV       969
                             MCH       317
                             MCHC      327
                             RDW-SD  641 +
    25                          250 [fl]
PLT
                             PLT       38 -
                             PDW       94
                             MPV       79
                             P-LCR     131

    2      18              40  [fl]
```

Fig. 2.10 Numerical printout and histograms of white blood cell (WBC), red blood cell (RBC) and platelet (PLT) volume produced by a Sysmex NE 5000 automated haematology analyser. White cells are classified into small cells (W-SC), which are mainly lymphocytes, intermediate sized cells (W-MC), which are mainly monocytes and large cells (W-LC), which are mainly neutrophils.

technology, five-part or six-part—differential count. Platelets may be separated from red cells by fixed thresholds or moving thresholds. The RDW on most instruments represents the SD of cell size measurements. Sysmex instruments give the option of CV as an index of RDW. Most impedance counters initially measure Hb by a modified cyanmethaemoglobin method but this is now often replaced by cyanide-free methodology. For example, Sysmex instruments use a lauryl sulphate method.

Sysmex SE-9000

The Sysmex SE-9000 and later instruments have an Hb channel that is separate from the WBC channel. This permits the use of a strong lytic agent so that high WBCs are unlikely to interfere with Hb estimates. Hb estimation is by a lauryl sulphate method. There are moving thresholds for both red cells and platelets, which are counted by impedance technology. As with earlier instruments, histograms of red cell, white cell and platelet volume distribution are provided (Fig. 2.11a). The MCV on this and certain other Sysmex instruments (K-1000, NE-8000 and SE-9000) has been noted to increase on deoxygenation and decrease on oxygenation [15]. The MCHC shows inverse changes. It is likely that the same effect would be observed with other automated counters, since the same phenomenon is observed with a microhaematocrit. The NE-8000 does not show the same inaccuracy in MCV and MCHC estimates with hypochromic cells as is seen with the Coulter STKR; for the K-1000, inaccuracy is intermediate [47].

The SE-9000 produces a five-part differential count by combining data from three channels (see Table 2.6). In the granulocyte–lymphocyte–monocyte channel leucocytes are separated from red cell ghosts and platelet clumps and are divided into three major clusters (Fig. 2.11b) by a plot of radio-frequency capacitance measurements against direct current impedance measurements. Radio-frequency measurements depend on internal cellular structure—nucleocytoplasmic ratio, chromatin structure and cytoplasmic granularity—while direct current measurements depend on cell size. Eosinophils are detected by direct current measurements of cell size following exposure to a lytic agent at alkaline pH. Basophils are detected by direct current measurements of cell size following exposure to a lytic agent at acid pH. The neutrophil count is determined by subtracting basophil and eosinophil counts from the granulocyte count. Immature granulocytes can be separated from erythrocytes and the residues of other leucocytes in the immature myeloid information (IMI) channel (Fig. 2.11b, right). Any abnormalities can thus be flagged as: '? left shift', '? immature granulocytes' or '? blasts'.

The immature myeloid index has been found to be useful as a predictor of a rise in CD34-positive stem cell numbers in patients being prepared for a peripheral blood stem cell harvest, and can serve as a trigger to start monitoring the number of CD34-positive cells [51].

Fig. 2.11 Graphic output of Sysmex SE-9000 automated haematology analyser. (a) White cell scatter plots and red cell, platelet, eosinophil and basophil volume histograms on a normal sample. (b) White cell scatter plots—radiofrequency (RF) against direct current (DC)—of an abnormal sample with an increase of immature granulocytes. White cell populations shown are: GRAN, granulocytes; LYMPH, lymphocytes; MONO, monocytes (left); and immature granulocytes in a separate cluster from erythrocytes and residues of other leucocytes (right).

Sysmex XE-2100

The Sysmex XE-2100 [52] incorporates fluorescence flow cytometry into a multichannel instrument that also utilizes laser light, direct current (for impedance measurements) and radiofrequency current (for determining the internal structure of a cell) to perform a differential count (Fig. 2.12). A polymethine fluorescent dye combines with nucleic acids (nuclear DNA and RNA in cytoplasmic organelles)

Negative

WBC	7.51	[10^9/L]
RBC	4.01	[10^12/L]
HGB	13.2	[g/dL]
HCT	39.6	[%]
MCV	98.8	[fL]
MCH	32.9	[pg]
MCHC	33.3	[g/dL]
PLT	178	[10^9/L]
RDW-SD	51.9	[fL]
RDW-CV	14.4	[%]
PDW	15.8	[fL]
MPV	12.9	[fL]
P-LCR	49.3 +	[%]
PCT	0.23	[%]
NEUT	4.61	[10^9/L]	61.5	[%]
LYMPH	1.76	[10^9/L]	23.4	[%]
MONO	0.55	[10^9/L]	7.3	[%]
EO	0.55 +	[10^9/L]	7.3 +	[%]
BASO	0.04	[10^9/L]	0.5	[%]
NRBC	0.00	[10^9/L]	0.0	[/100WBC]
RET	1.28	[%]	0.0513	[10^12/L]
IRF	7.5	[%]
LFR	92.5	[%]
MFR	7.1	[%]
HFR	0.4	[%]

WBC IP Message(s)   RBC/RET IP Message(s)   PLT IP Message(s)

Fig. 2.12 Scatterplots and histograms of the Sysmex XE-2100 showing the leucocyte clusters (DIFF), the white cell count/basophil channel (WBC/BASO), immature granulocytes (IMI), nucleated red cell (NRBC), the reticulocyte channel (RET), the optical (fluorescent) platelet count (PLT-O) and red cell and platelet histograms (RBC and PLT).

of 'permeabilized' cells. This instrument has the capacity to count reticulocytes, recognize and count RNA-containing platelets and recognize and count NRBC, cells with the characteristics of immature granulocytes (promyelocytes, myelocytes and metamyelocytes, IG) and haemopoietic progenitor cells (HPC). Recognition of the latter depends on the greater lipid content of cytoplasmic membranes of more mature cells, so that differential lysis can be used to lyse mature cells and leave haemopoietic progenitor cells less damaged; this variable was also included in the SE-9500 instrument. Blast cells can be differentiated from less immature cells. The XE-2100 can operated in CBC/DIFF mode, in which TNCC are counted and the presence of NRBC is flagged, or in NRBC mode, in which NRBC are counted and the WBC is computed by subtraction of NRBC from TNCC. This instrument also has the capacity to determine a platelet count by both impedance technology and an optical method, following interaction with a fluorescent dye—the latter in the reticulocyte channel. At low counts the optical-fluorescence platelet count is usually more

accurate [53] whereas at high counts the linearity of the impedance count is better. Which count is more accurate depends on the cause of the thrombocytopenia. Patients on chemotherapy may have WBC fragments, leading to the optical count being an overestimate of the platelet count, whereas in patients with low platelet counts and large platelets, e.g. due to autoimmune thrombocytopenic purpura or thrombotic thrombocytopenic purpura, the optical count is more accurate. If the analyser is left to use the switching algorithm it will report the more accurate count.

The XE-2100 is a multichannel instrument, the channels being as follows.

1 A haemoglobin channel using a strong lytic agent and a cyanide-free reagent (lauryl sulphate) for the measurement of Hb.

2 A red cell channel/platelet channel with which red cells and platelets are counted and sized by impedance technology, following hydrodynamic focusing; in addition to the usual red cell variables, mean platelet size, platelet distribution width (the width of the platelet size histogram at 20% of the peak height) and the percentage of large platelets (platelet large cell ratio, P-LCR, platelets larger than 12 fl expressed as a percentage) are provided. An increased percentage of large platelets has been observed in patients with hyperlipidaemia and this has been suggested as a possible risk factor for thrombosis [54]. An increase in MPV, PDW and P-LCR has been observed in autoimmune thrombocytopenic purpura in comparison with aplastic anaemia [55].

3 A white cell differential channel in which neutrophils plus basophils, eosinophils, lymphocytes and monocytes are differentiated from each other, by cluster analysis, following interaction with a fluorescent dye; measurements made are of sideways light scatter (indicative of the internal structure of cells), forward light scatter (indicative of cell size) and fluorescence intensity (indicative of the size of the nucleus). Immature granulocytes are counted in this channel. An increased percentage of immature granulocytes has been found predictive of infection; however, although more predictive than the WBC it was no better than the absolute neutrophil count [56].

4 A white cell/basophil channel in which all cells except basophils are lysed so that basophils can be differentiated from other leucocytes by cluster analysis, using forward light scatter and sideways light scatter.

5 A NRBC channel in which NRBC are differentiated from white cells and from red cell ghosts by cluster analysis based on fluorescence intensity and forward light scatter, following lysis of NRBC and interaction of cells with a fluorescent dye. NRBC are less fluorescent and scatter less light than leucocytes. Persisting NRBC in the peripheral blood following stem cell transplantation have been found to correlate with a significantly worse prognosis [57].

6 An immature myeloid channel in which granulocyte precursors and putative haemopoietic stem cells can be differentiated from mature leucocytes by cluster analysis based on impedance and radiofrequency current analysis following differential lysis. The absolute count of HPC has been found to be a clinically useful measurement in determining the optimal timing for harvesting peripheral blood stem cells. Since the HPC count is quick and economical it can be used to predict when it is worthwhile performing the more slow and expensive measurement of CD34-positive cells [58].

7 A reticulocyte channel (used only when the instrument is run in reticulocyte mode) in which platelets are also enumerated optically with an immature platelet count ('reticulated platelets') being determined by a fluorescence/optical method; the fluorescent dye is a proprietary mixture of polymethine and oxazine. The immature platelet fraction has been found to be increased in conditions of increased platelet turnover, e.g. autoimmune thrombocytopenic purpura, thrombotic thrombocytopenic purpura and pregnancy-associated hypertension [59]. The instrument has a switching algorithm to select the most accurate platelet count and this should not be over-ridden [60]. Inaccurate impedance counts can occur in the presence of red cell fragments or giant platelets. Inaccurate optical/fluorescence counts can occur when white cell fragments are present, e.g. in leukaemia. The reticulocyte channel can also be used to enumerate and monitor red cell fragments in patients with microangiopathic haemolytic anaemia [61]. For further information on the reticulocyte count, see p. 49.

Information about Sysmex instruments is available on the company website www.sysmex.com.

Bayer instruments

A cell passing through a focused beam of light scatters the light, which may then be detected by photo-optical detectors placed lateral to the light beam. The degree of scatter is related to the cell size so that the cell can be both counted and sized. By placing a detector in the line of the light beam it is also possible to measure light absorbance. The light beam can be either white light or a high-intensity, coherent laser, which has superior optical qualities. The light detector can be either a photomultiplier or a photodiode both of which convert light to electrical impulses that can be accumulated and counted.

H.1 series

The H.1 series of Bayer (previously Technicon) instruments (Bayer Diagnostics)—the H.1, H.2 and H.3—count and size cells by light scattering, using

Fig. 2.13 Histograms and scatter plots of red cell volume and red cell haemoglobin concentration and white cell scatter plots produced by a Technicon H.2 counter. In the peroxidase channel forward light scatter, largely determined by cell volume is plotted against light absorbance, largely determined by the intensity of the peroxidase reaction. There are five white cell populations: NEUT, neutrophils; MONO, monocytes; LYMPH, lymphocytes; EOS, eosinophils; and LUC, large unstained cells, which are large, peroxidase-negative cells. In the basophil/lobularity channel forward light scatter, representing cell volume following differential cytoplasmic stripping, is plotted against high-angle light scatter, which is determined largely by cellular structure. There are three cell clusters, two of which overlap: BASO, basophils; MONONUC, mononuclear cells (lymphocytes and monocytes); and GRAN, granulocytes (neutrophils and eosinophils).

white light for counting and sizing leucocytes and a laser for counting and sizing red cells and platelets. The red cells are isovolumetrically sphered, so that light scatter is not dependent on cell shape and can be predicted from the laws of physics. Cells move through a laser beam, and light scattered forward is measured at a narrow (2–3°) and a wider (5–15°) angle. A comparison of the two allows the computation of the size and haemoglobin concentration of individual red cells. Histograms showing the distribution of red cell volume and haemoglobin concentration are provided, together with a plot of volume against haemoglobin concentration (Fig. 2.13). The histogram of the cell volumes permits the derivation of the MCV, RDW and Hct.

Similarly, the histogram of haemoglobin concentrations permits the derivation of the cellular haemoglobin concentration mean (CHCM) and the haemoglobin distribution width (HDW), the latter being indicative of the variation in haemoglobin concentration between individual cells. Bayer instruments measure Hb by a modification of conventional cyanmethaemoglobin methodology, and the MCH and MCHC are computed from the Hb, RBC and MCV. An optional lauryl sulphate method for Hb estimation is also available. The MCHC and CHCM are independently derived measurements, both representing the average haemoglobin concentration in a cell. They should give essentially the same result. This acts as an internal quality control mechanism since errors in the estimation of Hb, e.g. consequent on a very high WBC, cause a discrepancy between these two measurements. It would be theoretically possible to omit the haemoglobin channel and compute Hb from the CHCM, RBC and MCV derived from light-scattering measurements.

The technology of the H.1 series of instruments appears to produce accurate estimations of MCV, PCV and MCHC, which agree well with reference methods [62,63]. It has been possible to avoid the inaccuracies of earlier light-scattering instruments (in which light scattering was influenced by cellular haemoglobin concentration as well as cell size) and the inaccuracies inherent in some impedance counters (in which the electrical shadow is influenced by cellular deformability as well as cell size). Cells that cannot be isovolumetrically sphered, e.g. irreversibly sickled cells, will not be sized accurately. Similar measurements of two-angle light scatter permit platelets to be counted and sized (platelet count and MPV). A plateletcrit and PDW are also computed. Platelet counts using this technology appear to be superior, particularly when the count is low, to counts using impedance technology (Coulter or Sysmex) [26].

Hypochromic cells, as detected by these instruments, correlate with the observation of hypochromic cells on a blood film. The percentage is increased in iron deficiency and the anaemia of chronic disease. The percentage of hypochromic cells has been found to be very sensitive in the detection of functional iron deficiency in patients given erythropoietin, e.g. haemodialysis patients. Similar changes have been observed in iron-replete healthy volunteers and it has been suggested that this measurement might be useful in detecting illicit erythropoietin use by athletes [64]. However, in hospitalized patients, an increased percentage of hypochromic cells shows poor specificity for iron deficiency [65]. Hypochromic macrocytes have a different significance, being indicative of either dyserythropoiesis or an increased percentage of reticulocytes.

The differential count of the H.1 series is derived from two channels (see Table 2.6). The peroxidase channel uses white light and incorporates a cytochemical reaction in which the peroxidase of neutrophils, eosinophils and monocytes acts on a substrate, 4-chloro-1-naphthol, to produce a black reaction product, which absorbs light. Light scatter, which is proportional to cell size, is then plotted against light absorbance, which is proportional to the intensity of the peroxidase reaction (see Fig. 2.13). Neutrophils, eosinophils, monocytes and lymphocytes fall into four clusters, which are separated from each other and from cellular debris by a mixture of moving and fixed thresholds. A further cluster represents cells that are peroxidase-negative and larger than most lymphocytes, these being designated large unstained cells (LUC). In healthy subjects, LUC are mainly large lymphocytes but abnormal cells such as blast cells and atypical lymphocytes can fall into this category. In the peroxidase channel, basophils fall in the lymphocyte category. They are separated from all other leucocytes in an independent basophil/lobularity channel, on the basis of their resistance to stripping of cytoplasm by a lytic agent in acid conditions. Basophils, sized by forward light scatter, are larger than the stripped residues of other cells (see Fig. 2.13). The basophil/lobularity channel is also used to detect the presence of blasts. Forward light scatter, which is proportional to cell size, is plotted against high-angle light scatter, which is a measure of increasing nuclear density and lobulation. Blasts are detected as a population with an abnormally low nuclear density. In addition, the 'lobularity index' (LI) is a measure of the ratio of the number of cells producing a lot of high-angle light scatter (lobulated neutrophils) to cells producing less high-angle light scatter (mononuclear cells, immature granulocytes and blasts).

Instruments of the H.1 series, in addition to 'flagging' the presence of blasts, atypical lymphocytes, immature granulocytes and NRBC, produce two new white cell parameters—LI (described above) and the mean peroxidase index (MPXI). The latter is a measure of average peroxidase activity and is decreased in inherited peroxidase deficiency and also in acquired deficiency, as occurs in some myelodysplastic syndromes and myeloid leukaemias. A fall occurs during pregnancy, with a nadir at 20 weeks [66]. MPXI is increased in infection, in some myeloid leukaemias and myelodysplastic syndromes, in AIDS and in megaloblastic anaemia.

The later Bayer instrument, the Advia 120 operates on similar principles to the H.1 series instruments. The primary TNCC is provided by the basophil/lobularity channel rather than the peroxidase channel. There is improved cluster analysis in the basophil/lobularity channel permitting more accurate flagging of the presence of NRBC (Fig. 2.14). The platelet count is determined by two-dimensional analysis of size and refractive index,

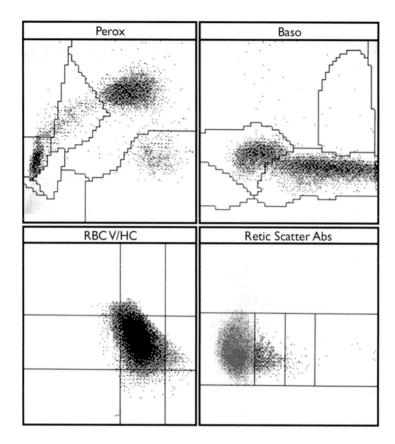

Fig. 2.14 Scatter plots produced by the Bayer Advia 120, showing the peroxidase channel (top left, Perox), the basophil channel (top right, Baso), a plot of red cell size versus haemoglobin concentration (bottom left, RBC V/HC) and the reticulocyte channel scatter plot (bottom right, Retic Scatter Abs).

using laser light scatter at two angles; this has been found to produce a more accurate platelet count than that of the H.3 [67]. There is an expanded range of platelet parameters—mean platelet component concentration (MPC), platelet component distribution width (PCDW), mean platelet mass (MPM) and platelet mass distribution width (PMDW). Reference ranges have been published and it has been suggested that the MPC may be a useful indicator of platelet activation [68].

The latest instrument in this series is the Advia 2120, which incorporates a cyanide-free haemoglobin method, enumeration of NRBC, correction of the TNCC to a WBC, and a reflex slide-spreader that adjusts for haematocrit and white cell count. The NRBC count is based on data from both the unstained area of the peroxidase channel and from a combination of data from the peroxidase channel and the basophil/lobularity channel.

Information on Bayer instruments is available on the company website www.bayer.com.

Abbott (Cell-Dyn) instruments

Cell-Dyn 3500

The Cell-Dyn 3500 (Abbott Diagnostics) is a multichannel, automated instrument incorporating both laser light-scattering and impedance technology. Hb is measured as cyanmethaemoglobin. Red cells, white cells and platelets are counted and sized by impedance technology following cytoplasmic stripping of white cells. Histograms of size distribution are provided (Fig. 2.15).

The WBC is also estimated in a light-scattering (laser) channel, which provides, in addition, an automated five-part differential count [69] (see Table 2.6). White cells mainly maintain their integrity and are hydrodynamically focused to pass in single file through the laser beam. In this channel, red cells are rendered transparent because their refractive index is the same as that of the sheath reagent. Four light-scattering parameters are measured:

Fig. 2.15 Graphic output of Cell-Dyn 3500 automated counter, showing histograms of volume distribution of RBC, platelets (PLT) and white cells (WIC) derived from the impedance channel.

1 Forward light scatter at 1–3° (referred to as 0° scatter), which is mainly dependent on cell size
2 Narrow-angle light scatter at 7–11° (referred to as 10° scatter), which is dependent on cell structure and complexity
3 Total polarized orthogonal light scatter at 70–100° (referred to as 90° scatter)
4 Depolarized orthogonal light scatter at 70–100° (referred to as 90°D scatter).

Scatter plots of white cell populations are provided (Fig. 2.16). Cells are first separated into granulocytes and mononuclear cells (Fig. 2.16a) on the basis of their lobularity and complexity. Next, granulocytes are separated into eosinophils and neutrophils on the basis of the unique ability of eosinophils to depolarize light (Fig. 2.16b). Next, the mononuclear cells are separated into monocytes, lymphocytes and degranulated basophils (basophil granules being soluble in the sheath reagent) on the basis of cell size and complexity (Fig. 2.16c). Finally, all five populations are indicated (colour coded) on a plot of lobularity against size (Fig. 2.16d). The identification of cell clusters with anomalous characteristics permits blasts, atypical lymphocytes, NRBC and immature granulocytes to be flagged.

The measurement of WBC by two technologies provides an internal quality control mechanism.

The WBC in the impedance channel (WIC) is falsely elevated if NRBC are present, whereas the WBC in the optical channel (WOC) excludes NRBC by means of a moving threshold. However, since the optical channel employs a less potent lytic agent, WOC may be falsely elevated when there are

osmotically resistant red cells, as occurs with some neonatal blood samples. The likelihood of NRBC or osmotically resistant red cells is flagged and an algorithm selects the preferred result. If a suspicion of both NRBC and osmotically resistant cells is flagged, an extended period of lysis can be used to produce an accurate WOC.

Cell-Dyn 4000

The Cell-Dyn 4000 incorporates, in addition to the variables measured by the Cell-Dyn 3500, an automated reticulocyte count and an erythroblast count [70,71]. Reticulocytes are recognized by analysis of both low-angle light scatter and green fluorescence following interaction with the DNA–RNA dye, CD4K530. They can be distinguished from platelets, leucocyte nuclei and Howell–Jolly bodies. Erythroblasts are recognized after interaction of permeabilized cells with a fluorescent DNA–RNA dye, propidium iodide, using three measurements— two light-scattering measurements relating to cell size and a measurement of red-fluorescence signals derived from erythroblast nuclei and damaged white cells. NRBC are distinguished from platelets, Howell–Jolly bodies and basophilic stippling. Since NRBC are enumerated separately from WBC, the Cell-Dyn is able to produce a WBC rather than a TNCC. The Cell-Dyn 4000 also gives a confidence estimate for the blast flag, which has been found to be clinically useful [72]. It also incorporates a 'flag' for non-viable white cells, which can alert the instrument operator to an aged sample [71] or a pathological

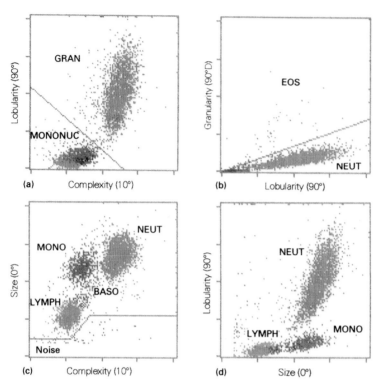

Fig. 2.16 Graphic output of a Cell-Dyn 3500 counter, showing white cell scatter plots derived from the white cell optical channel. (a) A plot of 90° scatter (indicating lobularity) against 10° scatter (indicating complexity) separates a granulocyte cluster from a mononuclear cluster. (b) 90°D (depolarized) scatter against 90° scatter separates the granulocyte cluster into eosinophils (which depolarize light) and neutrophils (which do not). (c) 0° scatter (related to size) against 10° scatter (related to complexity) separates the mononuclear cell cluster into lymphocytes, monocytes and degranulated basophils. (d) The five populations thus identified are shown on a plot of 90° scatter (related to lobularity) against 0° scatter (related to size). GRAN, granulocytes; MONONUC, mononuclear cells; NEUT, neutrophils; MONO, monocytes; LYMPH, lymphocytes; and EOS, eosinophils.

sample with an increase in apoptotic cells. There is a 'flag' for atypical lymphocytes, which has been found to be sensitive although not very specific [73]. The Cell-Dyn 4000 can be used for an immunological platelet count, employing a fluorescent-labelled CD61 monoclonal antibody [74]. This is a more expensive method, which is indicated for verifying low counts rather than being a routine method. It is indicated whenever the platelet count approaches a level that might trigger platelet transfusion (e.g. less than 20 or less than $10 \times 10^9/l$) and whenever there are giant platelets or significant numbers of red cell fragments or markedly microcytic cells [75]. This instrument has the possibility of an extended lyse period when red cells are incompletely lysed and an extended count mode for cytopenic samples. The Cell-Dyn 4000 can also be used to quantitate T cells, B cells and natural killer cells [76] and to quantitate fetal Rh D-positive cells in the circulation of an Rh D-negative mother, maternal blood being incubated with a monoclonal anti-D antibody conjugated to fluorescein isothiocyanate (FITC) [77].

Cell-Dyn instruments have been observed to given abnormal patterns in some patients with *Plasmodium falciparum* or *P. vivax* malaria, as a result of the depolarization of light by malarial pigment (haemozoin) [78]. This can serve to alert laboratory staff to this diagnosis.

Cell-Dyn Sapphire

The latest Abbott Cell-Dyn instrument is the Cell-Dyn Sapphire. It incorporates four optical detectors for polarized and depolarized light and three fluorescence detectors. The type of laser and the reagents differ from those of earlier instruments but the principles are the same. NRBC are enumerated following staining with the fluorochrome, propidium iodide; this also permits the provision of a viability index for white cells. Optional tests are a reticulocyte count, an immuno-platelet count (using a CD61 monoclonal antibody) and a measurement of CD3-positive/CD4-positive and CD3-positive/CD8-positive T cells (using fluorochrome-labelled monoclonal antibodies). The RBC can be measured by an optical as well as an impedance method. Hb is measured by imidazole ligand chemistry. As with several earlier instruments, the Cell-Dyn Sapphire may show atypical polarization events in patients with malaria, since the malarial pigment haemozoin shares with eosinophil granules the ability to depolarize light. The atypical signals appear on the neutrophil–eosinophil scatter plot in a different position from signals generated by eosinophil granules.

Information on Abbott instruments is available on the company website www.abbottdiagnostics.com.

Horiba ABX instruments

ABX instruments such as the ABX Pentra 60 and ABX Pentra DX 120 (Horiba ABX Diagnostics) are haematology analysers that have evolved from Helios Argos instruments. Red cells, white cells and platelets are counted and sized by impedance technology and histograms of size distribution are provided. The Hct is determined by summing the amplitudes of electrical signals generated by red cells and providing a coincidence correction. Platelets are separated from red cells by a floating threshold between 18 and 25 fl. Haemoglobin is measured by one of two methods, either by a cyanmethaemoglobin method or by oxidation of haem iron followed by stabilization to produce chromogenic substances that can be quantified. A five-part differential count is based on two channels (see Table 2.6). In one channel, light absorbance and impedance measurements are made, after interaction of cells with chlorazol black E, the active principle of Sudan black B (Fig. 2.17). This dye stains eosinophil granules most strongly, neutrophil granules somewhat less and monocyte granules more weakly; light absorbance of stained cells is determined both by the strength of staining of granules and the degree of complexity of the nucleus. In a second channel, basophils are differentiated from other white cells by impedance measurements following differential cytoplasmic stripping. Different white cell populations are displayed on a plot of light absorbance against impedance and are enumerated by cluster analysis (with moving thresholds). Two further abnormal white cell populations are enumerated, when present. 'Atypical lymphocytes' are both counted separately and included in the total lymphocyte count (in contrast to the Bayer instruments, where 'large unstained cells' are counted separately but excluded from the lymphocyte count). 'Large immature cells'

are counted separately but are also assigned to either the neutrophil category or the monocyte category, depending on their light absorbance. The 'atypical lymphocyte' category may include not only atypical lymphocytes in conditions such as infectious mononucleosis, but also lymphoma cells, cells of chronic lymphocytic leukaemia, small blast cells and plasma cells. The 'large immature cell' category may include myeloblasts, monoblasts, promyelocytes (including those present in promyelocytic leukaemia), myelocytes, metamyelocytes, lymphoblasts and lymphoma cells. The Pentra DX 120 also includes a reticulocyte count (see below).

Information on Pentra instruments can be found on the company website www.horiba-abx.com.

Automated differential counters

Pattern-recognition automated differential counters

CellaVision AB has produced a pattern-recognition automated differential counter, the Diffmaster Octavia, based on microscopy of an MGG or Wright–Giemsa stained blood film interpreted by a computer program employing neural networks. The identification of cells can be confirmed visually and, if necessary, altered. Information is available at www.cellavision.com.

Automated reticulocyte counts and reticulated platelet counts

Automated reticulocyte count

Most automated reticulocyte counts depend on the ability of various fluorochromes to combine with the RNA of reticulocytes. Fluorescent cells can then be counted in a flow cytometer. The fluorochromes also combine with DNA so that nucleated cells fluoresce. An alternative technology is based on staining of RNA by a non-fluorescent nucleic acid stain such as new methylene blue or oxazine 750. Reticulocytes are then detected by light scattering or light absorbance or by analysis of three different cell properties (Coulter instruments). White cells, nucleated red cells and platelets can usually be separated from reticulocytes on the basis of gating for size and

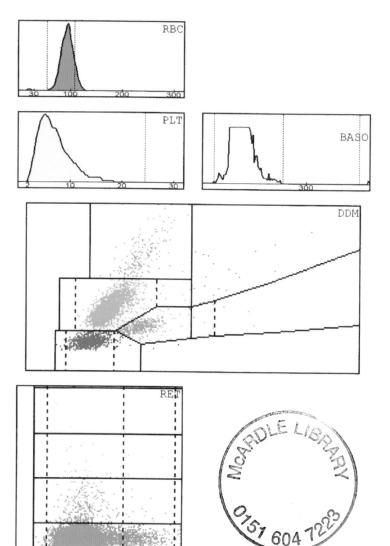

Fig. 2.17 Histograms of red cell (RBC) and platelet (PLT) size distribution and scatter plots of the differential white cell channel (DDM) and the reticulocyte channel (RET) of the Horiba ABX Pentra 120 analyser.

either their light scattering/absorbance or the intensity of their fluorescence. Reticulocyte counts can be expressed as an absolute count or as a percentage of total red cells.

Because of the large number of cells counted, automated reticulocyte counts are much more precise than manual counts. It was hoped that they might also be more accurate, since the subjective element in recognizing late reticulocytes with only one or two granules of positively staining material is eliminated. However, the automated count is altered by: (i) the choice of fluorochrome; (ii) the duration of exposure of the blood to the fluorochrome; (iii) the temperature at which the sample is kept after mixing; and (iv) the setting of thresholds—the upper threshold to exclude fluorescing nucleated cells and the lower threshold to exclude background autofluorescence.

Similar considerations apply to automated reticulocyte counts using non-fluorescent nucleic acid stains. A reference range for an automated reticulocyte count is therefore specific to an instrument and method. Reference ranges that have been established show considerable variation. It is still necessary to consider the manual count to decide whether a range represents 'truth'. Ideally, automated and manual counts should show a close correlation; mean counts should be similar, and the intercept on the y-axis of the regression line of automated counts on manual counts should be small.

Automated reticulocyte counts fall as the blood ages *in vitro*. This is likely to reflect reticulocyte maturation. It also occurs with manual counts but because of the imprecision of the manual count it is less likely to be noticed. If blood is stored at 4°C the reticulocyte count is stable for 72 hours but if it is left at room temperature a 5% fall is noted by 24 hours and a 10% fall by 48 hours [79]. Ideally counts should be performed within 6 hours of venepuncture.

Automated reticulocyte counts can be performed on general purpose flow cytometers, such as the Becton Dickinson FACScan or the Coulter EPICS XL, or on a dedicated reticulocyte counter, such as the Sysmex R-1000, R-2000 or R-3000 (Fig. 2.18). Increasingly an automated reticulocyte counting capacity is incorporated into an automated full blood counter, as in the Sysmex XE-2100 (see Fig. 2.12), the Bayer H.3 and Advia 120 (Figs 2.19 & 2.20), the Cell-Dyn 3500 and 4000, the later versions of the Coulter STKS (Fig. 2.21), the Coulter MAXM, HmX, Gen S and LH750 and the ABX Pentra 120 and Pentra Retic. Technologies employed are summarized in Table 2.7 [41,79].

Automated reticulocyte counts can also be performed by image analysis of a blood film stained with new methylene blue [80].

The automated reticulocyte count, like the manual count, is useful in determining whether anaemia is caused by failure of bone marrow output or increased red cell destruction. Because of its greater precision, the automated reticulocyte count is also useful in

monitoring the response to erythropoietin therapy in chronic renal failure and in detecting bone marrow recovery following therapy for aplastic anaemia or following chemotherapy for malignant disease.

Automated reticulocyte counters can also provide various indices of reticulocyte immaturity, since intensity of fluorescence or uptake of another nucleic acid stain is proportional to the amount of RNA in the cell. Instruments may divide reticulocytes into low, intermediate and high (or low and high) fluorescence/absorbance/light scatter, higher values indicating an increasing degree of immaturity. They may also give a mean measurement. The count of immature reticulocytes varies greatly between instruments but, nevertheless, such measurements may be of clinical significance when considered in relation to the reference range for the instrument in question. In anaemia consequent on haemolysis or blood loss, the percentage of immature reticulocytes rises as the total reticulocyte count rises [81]. However, when there is dyserythropoiesis the percentage of immature reticulocytes may be elevated despite a normal or reduced total reticulocyte count. This has been observed, for example, in acute myeloid leukaemia, the myelodysplastic syndromes, megaloblastic anaemia and aplastic anaemia [81–83]. A disproportionate increase in immature reticulocytes indicates abnormal maturation of reticulocytes [82]. In other anaemias with little dyserythropoiesis but with a poor reticulocyte response, e.g. iron deficiency anaemia or the anaemia of chronic renal failure, the absolute reticulocyte count is reduced, but the percentage of immature reticulocytes is normal. The percentage of immature reticulocytes is increased, without anaemia or any increase in the reticulocyte percentage, in

Fig. 2.18 Scatter plot of the reticulocyte count of the Sysmex R.3000. Cell volume is plotted against fluorescence intensity. A threshold separates red cells from platelets. Reticulocytes are divided into high fluorescence (HFR) representing the most immature reticulocytes, intermediate fluorescence (MFR) and low fluorescence (LFR) representing late reticulocytes.

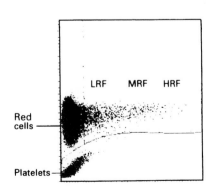

```
                                    15 : 46
NO.    596925

+RET %      11.52 [%]
+RET ♯      299.5 [×10⁹/ℓ]
−RBC         2.60 [×10¹²/ℓ]

−LFR        66.0 [%]
+MFR        25.7 [%]
+HFR         8.3 [%]

PLT DISCRIMINATION ERROR
```

RETICULOCYTE	%
RETIC	1.8

Red cells

RETICULOCYTE		
CELLS	%	#
NEG RBC	98.2	19169
RETIC	1.8	351
L RETIC	67.0	235
M RETIC	23.4	82
H RETIC	9.7	34
CELLS ACQUIRED		19693
CELLS ANALYZED		19582
GATED CELLS		19520
MEAN ABSORPTION		10.70
CAL FACT USED		1.00

RETICULOCYTE INDICES		
	RETIC CELLS	GATED CELLS
MCVr	106.3	74.4 fL
CHCMr	17.4	25.1 g/dL
RDWr	24.1	21.4 %
HDWr	3.38	4.65 g/dL
CHr	17.8	17.9 pg
CHDWr	4.5	3.7 pg

Fig. 2.19 Printout of a Bayer H.3 counter showing the scatter plot of the reticulocyte counting channel. The volume and haemoglobin content of reticulocytes and other red cells is determined by high- and low-angle light-scattering and light absorbance is measured following uptake of a nucleic acid dye, oxazine 750. Six variables of potential clinical usefulness are measured for reticulocytes as well as for total red cells: MCV, CHCM (= MCHC), RDW, HDW (in g/dl), CH (= MCH) and CHDW (HDW in pg). Cell volume is plotted against light absorbance. Reticulocytes are divided into high absorbance (H RETIC) representing early reticulocytes, intermediate absorbance (M RETIC) and low absorbance (L RETIC) representing late reticulocytes.

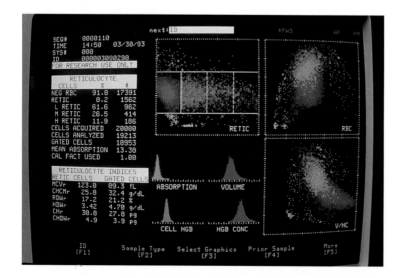

Fig. 2.20 Photograph of the colour monitor of a Bayer H.3 automated counter. The scattergram shows volume and haemoglobin content of reticulocytes (blue) in relation to size and haemoglobin content of other red cells (red) on both a Mie map and a red cell cytogram. This sample had a greatly increased reticulocyte count as a consequence of a haemolytic transfusion reaction.

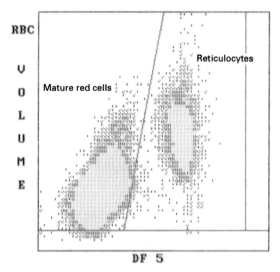

RBC

V
O
L
U
M
E

Mature red cells

Reticulocytes

DF 5

Fig. 2.21 Scatter plot of the reticulocyte channel of the Coulter Counter STKS showing clusters of mature red cells (left) and reticulocytes (right) following vital staining of reticulocytes by new methylene blue.

a significant proportion of patients with cardiac and pulmonary disease [84]. It has been suggested that this results from erythropoietin release as a response to hypoxia.

When effective erythropoiesis is restored after a period of reduced output of red cells—e.g. following bone marrow transplantation or during recovery from chemotherapy—there is a rise in the percent-

age and absolute count of immature reticulocytes in advance of any rise in the total reticulocyte percentage, neutrophil count or platelet count [85]. Similarly, an increase in the percentage of immature reticulocytes predicts haemopoietic recovery when severe aplastic anaemia is treated with immunosuppressive therapy, occurring in advance of a rise in the neutrophil count or the total reticulocyte count [86]. Immature reticulocyte counts have been found to be useful in predicting the optimal time for a peripheral blood stem cells harvest in some, but not all, studies [47].

As for the reticulocyte count, the immature reticulocyte fraction is an instrument-dependent measurement and instrument-specific reference ranges are therefore required. For example, the Pentra 120 Retic immature reticulocyte fraction is higher than that of either the Sysmex XE-2100 or the Sysmex R-2000 [87].

The most recent Bayer instruments provide other reticulocyte indices such as the haemoglobin content and concentration; haemoglobin content (CHr) provides an early sensitive index of iron deficiency but this measurement is lacking in specificity [65]. The Sysmex XE-2100 produces a measurement known as the Ret-y, which is the mean value of forward light scatter by reticulocytes. It can be converted to a reticulocyte haemoglobin equivalent, Ret-H$_e$, which gives similar information to Bayer instruments CHr in early iron deficiency [88].

Table 2.7 Technologies employed for automated reticulocyte counting in current instruments [41,79].

Instrument	Fluorochrome or stain
Fluorescence-based methods	
R-1000, R-2000, R-3000, R-3500, SE-9000 and SE-9500 (Sysmex)	Auramine O
XE-2100 (Sysmex)	A proprietary polymethine dye
Cell-Dyn 4000 (Abbott)	CD4K530 (light scatter and fluorescence intensity measurements)
XL (Beckman–Coulter)	Coriphosphine O
FACScan (Becton Dickinson)	Thiazole orange
Pentra 120 Retic (Horiba ABX Diagnostics) [79]	Thiazole orange
Non-fluorescent RNA-binding agents	
H.3 and Advia 120 (Bayer)	Oxazine 750 (absorbance measurement)
Cell-Dyn 3500 (Abbott)	New methylene blue (light scattering measurement)
STKS/MAXM/Gen S (Beckman–Coulter)	New methylene blue (VCS—volume, conductivity and scatter measurements on ghosts of sphered cells)

Reticulated platelets

Young platelets, newly released from the bone marrow, contain significant amounts of RNA; they can be identified on a blood film after exposure of the blood to methylene blue. By analogy with reticulocytes, they have been called 'reticulated platelets'. Automated reticulocyte counters can be modified to measure reticulated platelets. The Sysmex R-3000 has been modified to measure both reticulated platelets and large platelets. Reticulated platelets can also be enumerated on a flow cytometer after exposure to a fluorescent dye, such as thiazole orange, capable of binding to nucleic acids. The concentration of the fluorescent dye must be carefully judged to avoid binding to platelet components other than RNA [89]. It is also possible to use two-colour fluorescence, combining a nucleic acid stain with a fluorochrome-labelled platelet monoclonal antibody such as CD61 [90].

In most studies, an increased percentage of reticulated platelets has been found to indicate that thrombocytopenia results from increased platelet destruction rather than bone marrow failure but there is some overlapping of results and conflicting data have also been published [89,91,92]. Following bone marrow transplantation [93] and during treatment of thrombotic thrombocytopenic purpura [90], an increase in reticulated platelets heralds a rise in the platelet count.

Near-patient testing

Various small instruments are simple enough in their operation that they can be used for near-patient testing by individuals who are not fully trained biomedical scientists, but have been specifically trained for this more limited role. Some instruments measure a number of variables whereas others—e.g. the HemoCue portable haemoglobinometer (see p. 22)—measure only Hb. There are also certain methods that have been specifically developed for this setting.

An estimate of Hb can also be made by comparing the intensity of colour of a drop of blood on filter paper with a colour scale [94]. This method is suitable for screening in peripheral clinics with no ready access to laboratories. It is likely to be used particularly in developing countries, but also has potential as a test for screening blood donors prior to blood donation. The colour of a drop of blood can similarly be compared with coloured discs, as in the Lovibond Tintometer (www.tintometer.com).

A novel method for estimating Hb is employed by a portable haemoglobinometer, the HB-SCAN (Haemo Wave AB, Sweden). The unopened tube of blood is exposed to oscillating electric fields. The amount of energy absorbed at the specific (radio) frequencies used is influenced in a predictable way by the concentration of haemoglobin. The results are said by the manufacturer to be linear between 5 and 18 g/dl with a CV of 3% or less. The apparatus requires no reagents or consumables.

Another novel instrument, the Hemoscan, is a portable instrument with a hand-held probe, which is placed beneath the tongue [95]. The probe emits light that reflects from the target tissue to a tiny camera. The instrument is said to produce an estimate of Hb, PCV and WBC. A similar principle underlies the Hemo-Monitor and the Astrim, which measure Hb non-invasively on the basis of light absorbance in the near-infrared range when the fingers are inserted into the instrument [96,97]; estimates have been found to be comparable to laboratory measurements in most patients but not in those with a paraprotein [97]. However, the correlation with standard methods and the accuracy do not appear to be sufficient at present for this to be a useful advance [98].

An instrument capable of measuring haematocrit and bilirubin concentration on 25 µl of blood (Bilirubin Plus, Hematechnologies, Inc.) is potentially of value for near-patient testing on babies. The same company manufactures a near-patient instrument (ESR PLUS) that performs a modified erythrocyte sedimentation rate (which correlates well with standard methods), a Hct, Hb and total protein and bilirubin concentrations on a 25 µl EDTA-anticoagulated capillary sample. The Hct is measured optically, after centrifugation, and the Hb by photometry.

Storage of blood specimens prior to testing

If there is to be any delay in performing a blood count, the specimen should be stored at 4°C. Storage at room temperature increases the number of 'flags' and introduces inaccuracies. For example, with the H.1 series of instruments a left shift flag becomes very frequent, the MCV rises and the MCHC falls. Similarly, room temperature storage of samples for counts on a Cell-Dyn 3500 instrument was observed to cause an increased number of 'flags', a fall of the WBC as measured by the optical system (but not by the impedance system), a fall in the neutrophil percentage, a rise in the lymphocyte percentage, a rise in the MCV and a fall in the MCHC [99]. Platelet characteristics vary on storage. For example, with the Advia 120 there is a rise in the MPV and a fall in the MPC [68].

Test your knowledge

Multiple choice questions (MCQs)

(1–5 answers may be correct)

MCQ 2.1 The measurement most likely to correlate with hypochromia observed on a blood film is
(a) The RBC
(b) The PCV/Hct
(c) The MCV
(d) The MCH
(e) The MCHC

MCQ 2.2 Erroneous measurements of haemoglobin concentration by the cyanmethaemoglobin method may result from the presence of a significant proportion of
(a) Oxyhaemoglobin
(b) Deoxyhaemoglobin
(c) Carboxyhaemoglobin
(d) Sulphaemoglobin
(e) Methaemoglobin

MCQ 2.3 The platelet count may be estimated by
(a) Microscopy, using a counting chamber
(b) Impedance measurements
(c) Light-scattering measurements
(d) Estimation of their ratio to red cells, in combination with an RBC
(e) Turbidity measurements

MCQ 2.4 The International Council for Standardization in Haematology (ICSH) accepts as suitable units for the measurement of haemoglobin concentration
(a) fl
(b) g/dl
(c) g/l
(d) mmol/l
(e) %

MCQ 2.5 Fluorescence measurements are used in various automated instruments to
(a) Count platelets
(b) Measure the MCV
(c) Detect young platelets
(d) Detect and count NRBC
(e) Count reticulocytes

MCQ 2.6 An automated differential white cell count may be inaccurate because of
(a) The presence of NRBC
(b) Inherited peroxidase deficiency
(c) An increased reticulocyte count
(d) The presence of microcytic red cells
(e) Non-lysis of erythrocytes

Extended matching questions (EMQs)

Only one answer is correct.

EMQ 2.1
Theme: Red cell inclusions
Options
A An iron-containing granule on a Perls' stain
B Denatured haemoglobin
C A nuclear fragment in the cytoplasm
D An iron-containing granule on a Romanowsky stain
E A network of precipitated ribosomes
F Small granules representing ribosomes

Which option from the above list best describes the nature of the red cell inclusion?

Inclusion	Matching option
1 Heinz body	
2 Pappenheimer body	
3 Siderotic granule	
4 Howell–Jolly body	
5 Basophilic stippling	

EMQ 2.2
Theme: statistical terms
Options

A Count per unit volume
B Deviation from the true value
C The range within which a stated percentage of measurements are expected to fall
D Lack of reproducibility
E An estimate of imprecision
F An estimate of inaccuracy

Which option from the above list best explains the statistical term?

Term	Matching option
1 Imprecision	
2 Inaccuracy	
3 Confidence limit	
4 Standard deviation	
5 Coefficient of variation	

EMQ 2.3
Theme: Automated differential count
Options
A Basophil
B Eosinophil
C Erythrocyte
D Leucocyte
E Neutrophil
F Nucleated red blood cell
G Platelet
H Reticulocyte

Which option from the above list describes the cell or other particle identified by the following characteristics?

Measurement	Matching option
1 Particle size between 2 and 20 fl	
2 Intense peroxidase activity	
3 In comparison with other leucocytes, resistant to lysis	
4 Depolarized orthogonal light scatter	
5 Interaction with CD61	

References

1 International Committee for Standardization in Haematology (1978) Recommendations for reference method for haemoglobinometry in human blood (ICSH Standard EP 6/2: 1977) and specifications for international haemiglobincyanide reference preparation (ICSH Standard EP 6/3: 1977). *J Clin Pathol*, **31**, 139–143.

2 van Kampen EJ and Zijlstra WG (1983) Spectrophotometry of hemoglobin and hemoglobin derivatives. *Adv Clin Chem*, **23**, 199–257.

3 Lewis SM, Garvey B, Manning R, Sharp SA and Wardle J (1991) Lauryl sulphate haemoglobin: a non-hazardous substitute for HiCN in haemoglobinometry. *Clin Lab Haematol*, **13**, 279–290.

4 Morris LD, Pont A and Lewis SM (2001) Use of a new HemoCue system for measuring haemoglobin at low concentrations. *Clin Lab Haematol*, **23**, 91–96.

5 International Committee for Standardization in Haematology Expert Panel on Blood Cell Sizing (1980) Recommendation for reference method for determination by centrifugation of packed cell volume of blood. *J Clin Pathol*, **33**, 1–2.

6 ICSH. Selected methods for the determination of the packed cell volume. In: van Assendelft OW & England JM (eds.) *Advances in Hematological Methods: the blood count*. CRC Press, Boca Raton, 1982: 93–98.

7 Guthrie DL and Pearson TC (1982) PCV measurement in the management of polycythaemic patients. *Clin Lab Haematol*, **4**, 257–265.

8 Weatherall MS and Sherry KM (1997) An evaluation of the Spuncrit™ infra-red analyser for measurement of haematocrit. *Clin Lab Haematol*, **19**, 183–186.

9 Aoun H (1989) When a house officer gets AIDS. *N Engl J Med*, **321**, 693–696.

10 Anonymous (1999) Glass capillary tubes: joint safety advisory about potential risks. *Lab Med*, **30**, 299.

11 Crosland-Taylor PJ. The micro PCV. In: van Assendelft OW & England JM (eds.) *Advances in Hematological Methods: the blood count*. CRC Press, Boca Raton, 1982: 85–92.

12 Lampasso JA (1965) Error in hematocrit value produced by excessive ethylenediaminetetraacetate. *Am J Clin Pathol*, **44**, 109–110.

13 Pennock CA and Jones KW (1966) Effects of ethylene-diaminetetra-acetic acid (dipotassium salt) and heparin on the estimation of packed cell volume. *J Clin Pathol*, **19**, 196–199.

14 Karlow MA, Westengard JC, and Bull BS (1989) Does tube diameter influence the packed cell volume? *Clin Lab Haematol*, **11**, 375–383.

15 Bryner MA, Houwen B, Westengard J and Klein O (1997) The spun micro-haematocrit and mean cell

volume are affected by changes in the oxygenation state of red blood cells. *Clin Lab Haematol*, **19**, 99–103.

16 Lines RW and Grace E (1984) Choice of anticoagulants for packed cell volume and mean cell volume determination. *Clin Lab Haematol*, **6**, 305–306.

17 Expert Panel on Cytometry of the International Council for Standardization in Haematology (2000) ICSH recommendation for the measurement of a reference packed cell volume. *Lab Haematol*, **7**, 148–170.

18 International Committee for Standardization in Haematology (1980) Recommended methods for measurement of red cell and plasma volume. *J Nucl Med*, **21**, 793–800.

19 Bull BS, Fujimoto K, Houwen B, Klee G, van Hove L and van Assendelft OW on behalf of the ICSH Expert Panel on Cytometry (2003) International Council for Standardization in Haematology (ICSH) Recommendations for "Surrogate Reference" Method for the Packed Cell Volume. *Lab Hematol*, **9**, 1–9.

20 Bain BJ, Lewis M and Bates I. Basic haematological techniques. In: Lewis SM, Bain BJ & Bates I (eds.) *Practical Haematology*, 10th Edn. Churchill Livingstone, Philadelphia, 2006.

21 International Council for Standardization in Haematology: Expert Panel on Cytometry (1994) Reference method for the enumeration of erythrocytes and leucocytes. *Clin Lab Haematol*, **16**, 131–138.

22 Barnett D, Goodfellow K, Ginnever J, Granger V, Whitby L and Reilly JT (2001) Low level leucocyte counting: a critical variable in the validation of leucodepleted blood transfusion components as highlighted by an external quality assessment study. *Clin Lab Haematol*, **23**, 43–51.

23 Lewis SM. Visual haemocytometry. In: van Assendelft OW & England JM (eds.) *Advances in Hematological Methods: the blood count.* CRC Press, Boca Raton, 1982: 39–47.

24 Dickerhoff R and van Ruecker A (1995) Enumeration of platelets by multiparameter flow cytometry using platelet specific antibodies and fluorescent reference particles. *Clin Lab Haematol*, **17**, 163–172.

25 Tanaka C, Ishii T and Fujimoto K (1996) Flow cytometric platelet enumeration utilizing monoclonal antibody CD42a. *Clin Lab Haematol*, **18**, 265–269.

26 Harrison P, Horton A, Grant D, Briggs C and Machin S (2000) Immunoplatelet counting: a proposed new reference procedure. *Br J Haematol*, **108**, 228–235.

27 International Council for Standardization in Haematology: Expert Panel on Cytometry and International Society of Laboratory Haematology Task Force on Platelet counting (2001) Platelet counting by the RBC/platelet method: a reference method. *Am J Clin Pathol*, **115**, 460–464.

28 Norris S, Pantelidou D, Smith D and Murphy MF (2003) Immunoplatelet counting: potential for reducing the use of platelet transfusions through more accurate platelet counting. *Br J Haematol*, **121**, 605–613.

29 International Council for Standardization in Haematology: Expert Panel on Cytometry (1995) Recommendation of the International Council for Standardization in Haematology on reporting differential leucocyte counts. *Clin Lab Haematol*, **17**, 113.

30 National Committee for Clinical Laboratory Standards. *Approved Standard H20-A. Reference leukocyte count (proportional) and evaluation of instrumental methods.* USA National Committee for Clinical Laboratory Standards, Villanova, PA, 1992.

31 Talstad I (1981) Problems in microscopic and automatic cell differentiation of blood and cell suspensions. *Scand J Haematol*, **26**, 398–406.

32 Davidson E (1958) The distribution of cells in peripheral blood smears. *J Clin Pathol*, **11**, 410–411.

33 Rümke CL (1960) Variability of results in differential cell counts on blood smears. *Triangle*, **4**, 154–157.

34 England JM and Bain BJ (1976) Total and differential leucocyte count. *Br J Haematol*, **33**, 1–7.

35 Koepke IF and Koepke JA (1986) Reticulocytes. *Clin Lab Haematol*, **8**, 169–179.

36 The Expert Panel on Cytometry of the International Council for Standardization in Haematology. *ICSH Guidelines for Reticulocyte Counting by Microscopy of Supravitally Stained Preparations.* World Health Organization, Geneva, 1992.

37 Perrotta AL and Finch CA (1972) The polychromatophilic erythrocyte. *Am J Clin Pathol*, **57**, 471–477.

38 Crouch JY and Kaplow LS (1985) Relationship of reticulocyte age to polychromasia, shift cells, and shift reticulocytes. *Arch Pathol Lab Med*, **109**, 325–329.

39 Lowenstein ML (1959) The mammalian reticulocyte. *Int Rev Cytol*, **9**, 135–174.

40 Brecher G and Schneiderman MR (1950) A time-saving device for counting of reticulocytes. *Am J Clin Pathol*, **20**, 1079–1083.

41 Koepke JA (1999) Update on reticulocyte counting. *Lab Med*, **30**, 339–343.

42 Hillman RS and Finch CA (1969) The misused reticulocyte. *Br J Haematol*, **17**, 313–315.

43 Fannon M, Thomas R and Sawyer L (1982) Effect of staining and storage times on reticulocyte counts. *Lab Med*, **13**, 431–433.

44 NCCLS. *Methods for reticulocyte counting (Flow cytometry and supravital dyes); Approved guideline H44-A*, NCCLS, Wayne, PA, 1997.

45 Kunicka J, Malin M, Zelmanovic D, Katzenberg M, Canfield W, Shapiro P and Mohandas N (2001) Automated quantification of hemoglobin-based blood substitutes in whole blood samples. *Am J Clin Pathol*, **116**, 913–919.

46 Rowan RM. *Blood Cell Volume Analysis.* Albert Clark, London, 1983.

47 Paterakis GS, Laoutaris NP, Alexia SV, Siourounis PV. Stamulakatou AK, Premitis EE *et al.* (1993) The effect of red cell shape on the measurement of red cell volume. A proposed method for the comparative assessment of this effect among various haematology analysers. *Clin Lab Haematol*, **16**, 235–245.

48 Igout J, Fretigny M, Vasse M, Callat MP, Silva M, Willemont L, Gelle M and Lenormand B (2004) Evaluation of the Coulter LH750 haematology analyser compared with flow cytometry as the reference method for WBC, platelet and nucleated RBC count. *Clin Lab Haematol*, **26**, 1–7.

49 Zini G, d'Onofrio G, Garzia M and di Mario A. *Citologia Ematologica in Automazione.* Verduci Editore, Rome, 2005.

50 Fourcade C, Casbas MJ, Belaouni H, Gonzalez JJ, Garcia PJ and Pepio MA (2004) Automated detection of malaria by means of the haematology analyser Coulter GEN.S. *Clin Lab Haematol*, **26**, 367–372.

51 Gowans ID, Hepburn MD, Clark DM, Patterson G, Rawlinson PSM and Bowen DT (1999) The role of the Sysmex SE9000 immature myeloid index and Sysmex R2000 reticulocyte parameters in optimizing the timing of peripheral blood stem cell harvesting in patients with lymphoma and myeloma. *Clin Lab Haematol*, **21**, 331–336.

52 Ruzicka K, Veitl M, Thalhammer-Scherrer R and Schwarzinger I (2001) The new hematology analyzer Sysmex XE-2100; performance evaluation of a novel white blood cell differential technology. *Arch Pathol Lab Med*, **125**, 391–396.

53 Briggs C, Harrison P, Grant D, Staves J, and Machin SJ (2000) New quantitative parameters on a recently introduced automated blood cell counter—the XE 2100. *Clin Lab Haematol*, **22**, 345–350.

54 Grotto HZW and Noronha JFA (2004) Platelet larger cell ratio (P-LCR) in patients with dyslipidemia. *Clin Lab Haematol*, **26**, 347–349.

55 Kaito K, Otsubo H, Usui N, Yoshida M, Tanno J, Kurihara E *et al.* (2005) Platelet size deviation width, platelet large cell ratio, and mean platelet volume have sufficient sensitivity and specificity in the diagnosis of immune thrombocytopenia. *Br J Haematol*, **128**, 698–702.

56 Ansari-Lari MA, Kickler TS and Borowitz MJ (2003) Immature granulocyte measurement using the Sysmex XE-2100. *Am J Clin Pathol*, **120**, 795–799.

57 Otsubo H, Kaito K, Asai O, Usui N, Kobayashi M and Hoshi Y (2005) Persistent nucleated red blood cells in peripheral blood is a poor prognostic factor in patients undergoing stem cell transplantation. *Clin Lab Haematol*, **27**, 242–246.

58 Pollard Y, Watts MJ, Grant D, Chavda N, Linch DC and Machin SJ (1999) Use of the haemopoietic progenitor cell count of the Sysmex SE-9500 to refine apheresis timing of peripheral blood stem cells. *Br J Haematol*, **106**, 538–544.

59 Briggs C, Kunka S, Hart D, Oguni S and Machin SJ (2005) Assessment of an immature platelet fraction (IPF) in peripheral thrombocytopenia. *Br J Haematol*, **126**, 93–99.

60 Briggs C, Kunka A and Machin SJ (2004) The most accurate platelet count on the Sysmex XE-2100. Optical or impedance? *Clin Lab Haematol*, **26**, 157–158.

61 Banno S, Ito Y, Tanaka C, Hori T, Fujimoto K, Suzuki T *et al.* (2005) Quantification of red blood cell fragmentation by the automated hematology analyzer XE-2100 in patients with living donor liver transplantation. *Clin Lab Haematol*, **27**, 292–296.

62 Mohandas N, Kim YR, Tycko DH, Orlik J, Wyatt J and Groner W (1986) Accurate and independent measurement of volume and hemoglobin concentration of individual red cells by laser light scattering. *Blood*, **68**, 506–513.

63 von Feltan U, Furlan M, Frey R and Bucher U (1978) Test of a new method for hemoglobin determinations in automatic analysers. *Med Lab*, **31**, 223–231.

64 Breymann C, Rohling R, Krafft A, Huch A and Huch R (2000) 'Blood doping' with recombinant erythropoietin (rhEPO) and assessment of functional iron deficiency in healthy volunteers. *Br J Haematol*, **108**, 883–888.

65 Thomas C and Thomas L (2002) Biochemical markers and hematologic indices in the diagnosis of functional iron deficiency. *Clin Chem*, **8**, 1066–1076.

66 Tsakonas DP, Tsakona CP, Worman CP, Goldstone AH and Nicolaides KH (1994) Myeloperoxidase activity and nuclear segmentation of maternal neutrophils during normal pregnancy. *Clin Lab Haematol*, **16**, 337–342.

67 Chapman DH, Hardin J-A, Miers M, Moyle S and Kinney MC (2001) Reduction of the platelet review rate using two-dimensional platelet method. *Am J Clin Pathol*, **115**, 894–898.

68 Brummitt DR and Barker HF (2000) The determination of a reference range for new platelet parameters produced by the Bayer ADVIA™120 full blood count analyser. *Clin Lab Haematol*, **22**, 103–107.

69 Cornbleet PJ, Myrick D, Judkins S and Levy R (1992) Evaluation of the CELL-DYN 3000 differential. *Am J Clin Pathol*, **98**, 603–614.

70 Kim YR, Yee M, Metha S, Chupp V, Kendall R and Scott CS (1998) Simultaneous differentiation and quantification of erythroblasts and white blood cells on a high throughput clinical haematology analyser. *Clin Lab Haematol*, **20**, 21–29.

71 Grimaldi E and Scopacasa F (2000) Evaluation of the Abbott CELL-DYN 4000 hematology analyzer. *Am J Clin Pathol*, **113**, 497–505.

72 Hoedemakers RMJ, Pennings JMA and Hoffmann JJML (1999) Performance characteristics of blast flaging on the Cell-Dyn 4000 haematology analyser. *Clin Lab Haematol*, **21**, 347–351.

73 Hoffmann JJML and Hoedemakers RMJ (2004) Diagnostic performance of the variant lymphocyte flag of the Abbott Cell-Dyn 4000 haematology analyser. *Clin Lab Haematol*, **26**, 9–13.

74 Gill JE, Davis KA, Cowart WJ, Nepacena FU and Kim Y-T (2000) A rapid and accurate closed-tube immunoassay for platelets on an automated hematology analyzer. *Am J Clin Pathol*, **114**, 47–56.

75 Kunz D, Kunz WS, Scott CS and Gressner AM (2001) Automated CD61 immunoplatelet analysis of thrombocytopenic samples. *Br J Haematol*, **112**, 584–592.

76 Molera T, Roemer B, del Mar Perera Alvarez M, Lemes A, de la Iglesia Iñigo S, Palacios G and Scott CS (2005) Analysis and enumeration of T cells, B cells and NK cells using the monoclonal antibody fluorescence capability of a routine haematology analyser (Cell-Dyn CD4000). *Clin Lab Haematol*, **27**, 224–234.

77 Little BH, Robson R, Roemer B and Scott CS (2005) Immunocytometric quantitation of foeto-maternal haemorrhage with the Abbott Cell-Dyn CD4000 haematology analyser. *Clin Lab Haematol*, **27**, 21–31.

78 Scott CS, Zyl D, Ho E, Meyersfeld D, Ruivo L, Mendelow BV and Coetzer TL (2003) Automated detection of malaria-associated intraleucocytic haemozoin by Cell-Dyn CD4000 depolarization analysis. *Clin Lab Haematol*, **25**, 77–86.

79 Lacombe F, Lacoste L, Vial J-P, Briais A, Reiffers J, Boisseau MR and Bernard P (1999) Automated reticulocyte counting and immature reticulocyte fraction measurements. *Am J Clin Pathol*, **112**, 677–685.

80 Riley RS, Ben-Ezra JM and Tidwell A (2001) Reticulocyte enumeration: past & present. *Lab Med*, **10**, 599–608.

81 Watanabe K, Kawai Y, Takeuchi K, Shimizu N, Iri H, Ikeda Y and Houwen B (1994) Reticulocyte maturity as an indicator for estimating qualitative abnormality of erythropoiesis. *J Clin Pathol*, 47, 736–739.

82 Daliphard S, Bizet M, Callat MP, Beufe S, Latouche JB, Soufiani H and Monconduit M (1993) Evaluation of reticulocyte subtype distribution in myelodysplastic syndromes. *Am J Hematol*, **44**, 210–220.

83 Torres Gomez A, Casano J, Sanchez J, Madrigal E, Blanco F and Alvarez MA (2003) Utility of reticulocyte maturation parameters in the differential diagnosis of macrocytic anemias. *Clin Lab Haematol*, **25**, 283–288.

84 Kendall RG, Mellors I, Hardy J and McArdle B (2001) Patients with pulmonary and cardiac disease show an elevated proportion of immature reticulocytes. *Clin Lab Haematol*, **23**, 27–31.

85 Grotto HZW, Vigoritto AC, Noronha JFA and Lima GALM (1999) Immature reticulocyte fraction as a criterion for marrow engraftment. Evaluation of a semi-automated reticulocyte counting method. *Clin Lab Haematol*, **23**, 285–287.

86 Sica S, Sora F, Laurenti L, Piccirillo N, Salutari P, Chiusolo P, d'Onofrio G and Leone G (1999) Highly fluorescent reticulocyte count predicts haemopoietic recovery after immunosuppression for severe aplastic anaemia. *Clin Lab Haematol*, **21**, 387–389.

87 Briggs C, Grant D and Machin SJ (2001) Comparison of the automated reticulocyte counts and immature reticulocyte fraction measurements obtained with the ABX Pentra 120 Retic blood cell

analyzer and the Sysmex XE-2100 automated haematology analyzer. *Lab Haematol*, **7**, 1–6.

88 Franck S, Linssen J, Messinger M and Thomas L (2004) Potential utility of Ret-Y in the diagnosis of iron-restricted erythropoiesis. *Clin Chem*, **50**, 1240–1242.

89 Robinson M, Machin S, Mackie I and Harrison P (2000) *In vivo* biotinylation studies: specificity of labelling of reticulated platelets by thiazole orange and mepacrine. *Br J Haematol*, **108**, 859–864.

90 Robinson M, Mackie I, Machin S and Harrison P (2000) Technological methods: two colour analysis of reticulated platelets. *Clin Lab Haematol*, **22**, 211–213.

91 Romp KG, Peters WP and Hoffman M (1994) Reticulated platelet counts in patients undergoing autologous bone marrow transplantation: an aid in assessing marrow recovery. *Am J Hematol*, **46**, 319–324.

92 Kurata Y, Hayashi S, Kiyoi T, Kosugi S, Kashiwagi H, Honda S and Tomiyama Y (2001) Diagnostic value of tests for reticulated platelets, plasma glycocalicin, and thrombopoietin levels for discriminating between hyperdestructive and hypoplastic thrombocytopenia. *Am J Clin Pathol*, **115**, 656–664.

93 Koh K-R, Yamane T, Ohta K, Hino M, Takubo T and Tatsumi N (1999) Pathophysiological significance of simultaneous measurement of reticulated platelets, large platelets and serum thrombopoietin in non-neoplastic thrombocytopenic disorders. *Eur J Haematol*, **63**, 295–301.

94 Lewis SM, Scott GJ and Wynn KJ (1998) An inexpensive and reliable new haemoglobin colour scale for assessing anaemia. *J Clin Pathol*, **51**, 21–24.

95 Anonymous (2000) Hemoglobin, hematocrit, and WBCs in the microcirculation. *Lab Med*, **31**, 440–441.

96 Berrebi A and Fine I (1999) Non-invasive measurement of hemoglobin/hematocrit over a wide clinical range using a new optical signal processing method. *Blood*, **94**, Suppl. 1, Part 2, 10b.

97 Kinoshita Y, Yamane T, Takubo T, Kanashima H, Kamitani T, Tatsumi N and Hino M (2002) Measurement of hemoglobin concentrations using the Astrim™ non-invasive blood vessel monitoring apparatus. *Acta Haematol*, **108**, 109–110.

98 Saigo K, Imoto S, Hashimoto M, Mito H, Moriya J, Chinzei T *et al.* (2004) Noninvasive monitoring of hemoglobin: the effects of WBC counts on measurement. *Am J Clin Pathol*, **121**, 51–55.

99 Wood BL, Andrews J, Miller S and Sabath DE (1999) Refrigerated storage improves the stability of the complete blood count and automated differential. *Am J Clin Pathol*, **112**, 687–695.

Answers to test questions

Multiple choice questions

MCQ 2.1	FFFFT
MCQ 2.2	FFTTF
MCQ 2.3	TTTTF
MCQ 2.4	FFTTF
MCQ 2.5	TFTTT
MCQ 2.6	TTFFT

Extended matching questions

EMQ 2.1
1 B
2 D
3 A
4 C
5 F

EMQ 2.2
1 D
2 B
3 C
4 E
5 E

EMQ 2.3
1 G
2 B
3 A
4 B
5 G

3 Morphology of blood cells

Examining the blood film

Blood films should be examined in a systematic manner, as follows.

1 Patient identification should be checked and confirmed and the microscope slide matched with the corresponding full blood count (FBC) report. The sex and age of the patient should be noted since the blood film cannot be interpreted without this information. In a multiracial community it is also helpful to know the ethnic origin of the patient.

2 The film should be examined macroscopically to confirm adequate spreading and to look for any unusual spreading or staining characteristics. The commonest macroscopic abnormality is an increased blue coloration caused by hypergammaglobulinaemia (Fig. 3.1) due either to a paraprotein, e.g. in multiple myeloma and related conditions, or to a reactive increase in immunoglobulins, e.g. in cirrhosis or rheumatoid arthritis. Abnormal staining characteristics are also caused by the presence of foreign substances such as heparin, which conveys a pink tinge, or the vehicles of certain intravenous drugs. Occasionally, macroscopic abnormalities are caused by precipitation of cryoglobulin, gross red cell agglutination, platelet clumping or the presence of clumps of tumour cells (Figs 3.2–3.4).

3 The film should be examined microscopically, using a microscope correctly set up to give optimal illumination. Examination should take place first under a low power (e.g. with the × 10 or × 25 objective)

Fig. 3.2 Peripheral blood films from a patient with a potent cold agglutinin. The left hand film, which shows marked agglutination, was prepared from EDTA-anticoagulated blood that had been standing at room temperature. The right hand film, which shows no macroscopic agglutination, was prepared from blood warmed to 37°C.

Fig. 3.1 Peripheral blood film of a patient with multiple myeloma (left) compared with another blood film stained in the same batch (right). The deeper blue staining occurs because the high concentration of immunoglobulin leads to increased uptake of the basic component of the stain.

Fig. 3.3 Peripheral blood film from a patient with multiple myeloma showing cryoglobulin precipitates. Courtesy of Dr Sue Fairhead, London.

and then with a higher power (× 40 or × 50 objective) with an eyepiece magnification of × 10 or × 12. It is only necessary to use oil immersion and a × 100 objective when observation of fine detail is required or when searching for malaria parasites. Laboratories using unmounted films may find it useful to have a × 50 oil immersion objective in addition to a × 100. It should be noted that some immersion oils can cause contact dermatitis and care should therefore be exercised in their use [1]. The use of a relatively low power is important since it allows rapid scanning of a large part of the film and facilitates the detection

(a)

(b)

Fig. 3.4 Peripheral blood film showing visible aggregates of tumour cells. (a) Macroscopic photograph of slide. (b) Photomicrograph showing that the visible masses are clumps of tumour cells. Courtesy of Dr Sue Fairhead.

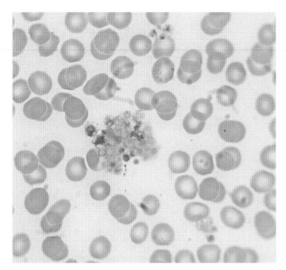

Fig. 3.5 Platelet aggregate in a peripheral blood film. The platelets have agglutinated and some have discharged their granule contents and thus appear grey.

Fig. 3.6 Fibrin strands in a peripheral blood film from a patient with a hypercoagulable state. The fibrin strands are very weakly basophilic and cause deformation of the red cells between which they pass. Fibrin strands can also form when there has been partial clotting of a blood specimen because of difficulty in venepuncture.

of abnormal cells when they are present at a low frequency. It is also useful in the appreciation of rouleaux and red cell and white cell agglutination. Examination of the blood film must also include examination of the edges and the tail since large abnormal cells and clumps of cells are often distributed preferentially in these areas. Platelet aggregates and fibrin strands, if present, are often found in the tail of the film.

On placing a film under the microscope the first decision to be made is whether or not it is suitable for further examination. Spreading, fixation and staining must be satisfactory and there should be no artefactual changes produced by excess ethylenediaminetetra-acetic acid (EDTA) or prolonged storage. It is unwise to give an opinion on an inadequate blood film. A well-spread film should have an appreciable area where cells are a monolayer, i.e. where they are touching but not overlapping. White cells should be distributed regularly without undue concentration along the edges or in the tail, such as occurs when the film is spread too thinly. Granulocytes are found preferentially along the edges and in the tail of a wedge-spread film and lymphocytes are preferentially in the centre but in a carefully spread film the difference is not great (see p. 28).

Blood films should be examined for platelet aggregates (Fig. 3.5), which may cause the platelet count to be falsely low, or fibrin strands (Fig. 3.6), which indicate partial clotting of the sample with the likelihood that the platelet count and possibly other variables are invalid. Platelets that have discharged their granules following aggregation may appear as pale blue masses not immediately identifiable as platelets.

Storage-induced artefacts

Blood films should be made without delay but laboratories that receive specimens by post or transported from a distance should be aware of the changes induced by storage. Prolonged storage of EDTA-anticoagulated blood causes loss of central pallor simulating spherocytosis [2], crenation or echinocytic changes in red cells (Fig. 3.7), degeneration of neutrophils (see Fig. 3.7) and lobulation of some lymphocyte nuclei (Fig. 3.8). Excess EDTA may itself cause crenation of red cells and also accelerates the development of storage changes. Degenerating neutrophils may have a similar

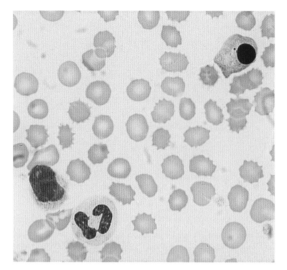

Fig. 3.7 Peripheral blood film showing storage artefact—crenation (echinocytosis), a disintegrated cell and a neutrophil with a rounded pyknotic nucleus.

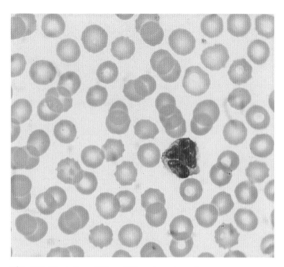

Fig. 3.8 Peripheral blood film showing storage artefact—mild crenation and lobulation of a lymphocyte nucleus.

appearance to necrobiotic neutrophils formed *in vivo* (see Fig. 3.89) or may be completely amorphous. If there has been prolonged delay in the blood specimen reaching the laboratory, e.g. 3 days or more, most of the neutrophils will have degenerated and the white blood cell count (WBC) will have fallen as a consequence. If an inexperienced laboratory worker does not recognize the storage artefact and attempts to perform a differential count, a factitious neutropenia and lymphocytosis will be recorded.

Inexperienced observers may also misclassify neutrophils with a single rounded nuclear mass as nucleated red blood cells (NRBC). Storage also leads to artefactual changes in other components of the automated blood count.

Another unusual artefactual change is produced by accidentally heating samples, e.g. by transporting a blood specimen in a hot car [3]. This causes dramatic fragmentation of red cells (Fig. 3.9), which can be confused with hereditary pyropoikilocytosis.

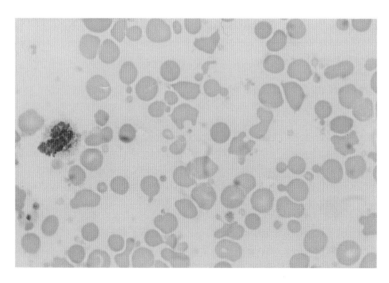

Fig. 3.9 Peripheral blood film from a blood specimen that has been transported in a hot motor vehicle, showing red cell budding and fragmentation.

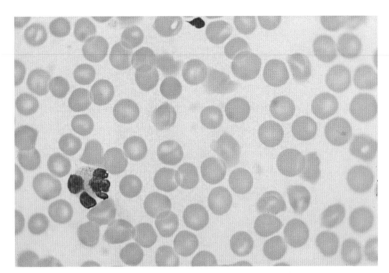

Fig. 3.10 Peripheral blood film from a patient with hyperlipidaemia showing misshapen red cells with fuzzy outlines and blurring of the outline of the lobes of a neutrophil consequent on the high concentration of lipids.

Fig. 3.11 Red cell agglutinates in the peripheral blood film of a patient with a high titre cold agglutinin.

If a blood film is regarded as suitable for further examination then all cell types and also the background staining should be evaluated systematically. The film appearances should be compared with the FBC and a judgement made as to whether the WBC, haemoglobin concentration (Hb), mean cell volume (MCV) and platelet count are consistent with the film, or whether there is some unusual feature that could invalidate them. If the FBC and the film are inconsistent with each other then the blood specimen should be inspected and the FBC—and if necessary the film—should be repeated. Such discrepancies may be due to: (i) a poorly mixed or partly clotted specimen; (ii) a specimen that is too small so that the instrument has aspirated an inadequate volume; or (iii) the blood film and FBC being derived from different blood specimens. If such technical errors are eliminated, discrepancy may be due to an abnormality in the specimen such as hyperlipidaemia or the presence of a cold agglutinin. Hyperlipidaemia may be suspected when there are blurred red cell outlines (Fig. 3.10) and red cell agglutinates are often present in the film when there is a cold agglutinin (Fig. 3.11). The validation of the blood count by comparison with the blood film and by other means is dealt with in Chapter 4.

Erythrocytes

The majority of normal red cells or erythrocytes are disciform in shape (Fig. 3.12) [4]; a minority are bowl-shaped. On a stained peripheral blood film they are approximately circular in outline and show only minor variations in shape and moderate variations in size (Fig. 3.13). The average diameter is about 7.5 μm. In the area of a film where cells form a monolayer, a paler central area occupies approximately the middle third of the cell.

The normal shape and flexibility of a red cell are dependent on the integrity of the cytoskeleton to which the lipid membrane is bound. An abnormal shape can be caused by a primary defect of the cytoskeleton or membrane or be secondary to red cell fragmentation or to polymerization, crystallization or precipitation of haemoglobin. The red cell membrane is a lipid bilayer crossed by several

Fig. 3.12 Scanning electron micrograph of a normal red cell (discocyte). Courtesy of Professor A. Polliack, Jerusalem, from Hoffbrand and Pettit [4].

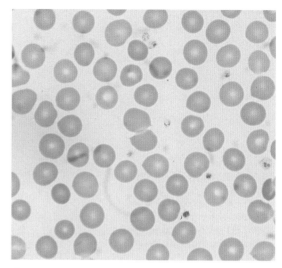

Fig. 3.13 Peripheral blood film of a healthy subject showing normal red cells and platelets. The red cells show little variation in size and shape. Some of the platelets show granules dispersed through the cytoplasm while others have a granulomere and a hyalomere.

transmembrane proteins, most importantly protein 3 and the glycophorins. The principal protein of the cytoskeleton is spectrin; heterodimers composed of α and β spectrin chains assemble into spectrin tetramers, which are bound to other spectrin tetramers to form a complex network. The cytoskeletal network is bound to the lipid bilayer by interactions of spectrin β chain with ankyrin and the transmembrane protein, band 3, and interactions of spectrin α and β chains with actin, protein 4.1 and the transmembrane protein, glycophorin C; the interaction of ankyrin with band 3 is modulated by protein 4.2 while the interaction of spectrin and actin is stabilized by interaction with protein 4.1 and adducin (see Fig. 8.30) [5].

Certain terms used to describe red cell morphology require definition. Two terms are used to describe cells of normal morphology: (i) normocytic, which means that the cells are of normal size; and (ii) normochromic, which means that the cells contain the normal amount of haemoglobin and therefore stain normally. Other descriptive terms imply that the morphology is abnormal and they should therefore not be used, when reporting blood films, to describe normal physiological variation. For example, the cells of a neonate should not be reported as 'macrocytic' since it is normal for the cells of a neonate to be larger than those of an adult. Similarly, the red cells of a healthy pregnant woman should not be reported as showing 'anisocytosis' or 'poikilocytosis' since no abnormality is present. Policy differs between laboratories as to whether every normal film is reported as being normocytic and normochromic or whether a comment on the red cell morphology is made only when it is abnormal or when it is particularly significant that it is normal. Either policy is acceptable as long as it is consistently applied and clinical staff are aware of it. If a patient is anaemic but the red cells are normocytic and normochromic it is useful to say so since this narrows the diagnostic possibilities.

Anisocytosis

Anisocytosis is an increase in the variability of erythrocyte size beyond that which is observed in a normal healthy subject. Anisocytosis is a common, non-specific abnormality in haematological disorders. In automated instrument counts an increase in the red cell distribution width (RDW) (see p. 36) is indicative of anisocytosis.

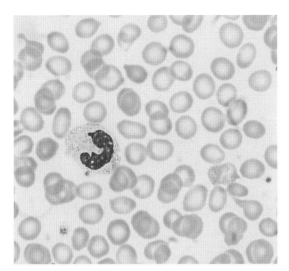

Fig. 3.14 Microcytosis in a patient with β thalassaemia trait; the MCV was 62 fl. The blood film also shows mild hypochromia, anisocytosis and poikilocytosis.

Microcytosis

Microcytosis is a decrease in the size of the erythrocytes. Microcytes are detected on a blood film by a reduction of red cell diameter to less than 7–7.2 μm (Fig. 3.14). The nucleus of a small lymphocyte, which has a diameter of approximately 8.5 μm, is a useful guide to the size of a red cell. Microcytosis may be general or there may be a population of small red cells. If all or most of the red cells are small there is a reduction in the MCV (see p. 26) but a small population of microcytes can be present without the MCV falling below the reference range. Some of the causes of microcytosis are listed in Table 3.1.

The red cells of healthy children are smaller than those of adults, whereas those of neonates are much larger, so that cell size must be interpreted in the light of the age of the subject. Microcytosis is uncommon in neonates but can occur in α thalassaemia disorders and when iron deficiency results from intrauterine blood loss; it is also likely that microcytosis is present at birth in congenital sideroblastic anaemia and atransferrinaemia. As a group, Black people have smaller red cells than white people; this is likely to be largely the result of a high prevalence of α thalassaemia trait, together with a lower prevalence of β thalassaemia trait, haemoglobin

Table 3.1 Some causes of microcytosis.

Inherited

β thalassaemia heterozygosity (β thalassaemia trait, β thalassaemia minor)

β thalassaemia homozygosity or compound heterozygosity (β thalassaemia major or intermedia)

δβ and γδβ thalassaemia heterozygosity or δβ thalassaemia homozygosity

Haemoglobin Lepore heterozygosity or homozygosity

Hereditary persistence of fetal haemoglobin homozygosity and some instances of heterozygosity

α^0 thalassaemia heterozygosity

α^+ thalassaemia homozygosity or, to a lesser extent, heterozygosity

Haemoglobin Constant Spring heterozygosity

Haemoglobin H disease

Sickle cell heterozygosity [6,7] (disputed, see p. 303)

Haemoglobin C heterozygosity [6,7] and homozygosity

Sickle cell/haemoglobin C disease [8]

Haemoglobin E heterozygosity [9] and homozygosity [10]

Haemoglobin D-Los Angeles (D-Punjab) heterozygosity

Heterozygosity for other rare abnormal haemoglobins producing thalassaemia-like conditions (e.g. haemoglobin Tak, haemoglobin Indianapolis)

Congenital sideroblastic anaemia

Atransferrinaemia

Ferrochelatase deficiency (erythropoietic protoporphyria) [11]

Hepatoerythropoietic porphyria [12]

Associated with iron overload but with absent bone marrow iron [13]

Associated with elliptocytosis [14]

Inherited iron malabsorption plus defect in incorporation of iron [15]

Acaeruloplasminaemia [16]

Copper deficiency [17]

Haem oxygenase deficiency [18]

Homozygosity for *DMT1* mutation [19]

Acquired

Iron deficiency (including bone marrow iron deficiency in pulmonary haemosiderosis)

Anaemia of chronic disease

Myelodysplastic syndromes, particularly but not only [20] associated with acquired haemoglobin H disease

Secondary acquired sideroblastic anaemia (e.g. caused by various drugs; some cases of lead poisoning and some cases of copper deficiency [21] or zinc excess with functional copper deficiency, e.g. ingestion of zinc-containing coins as a feature of mental illness [22–24]; ? hyperzincaemia with hypercalprotectinaemia (nature of anaemia not specified) [25]

Hyperthyroidism [26]

Ascorbic acid deficiency (rarely) [27]

Cadmium poisoning [28]

Aluminium poisoning

Antibody to erythroblast transferrin receptor [29]

Fig. 3.15 Macrocytosis associated with liver disease; the MCV was 105 fl. Several target cells are also present.

Fig. 3.16 Hypochromic red cells in a patient with iron deficiency anaemia. The film also shows anisochromasia.

C trait and other haemoglobinopathies which are associated with microcytosis, rather than to any intrinsic ethnic difference in red cell size.

Macrocytosis

Macrocytosis is an increase in the size of erythrocytes. The erythrocytes of neonates show a considerable degree of macrocytosis if they are assessed in relation to those of adults (see p. 131). Fetal red cells are also much larger than those of adults. A slight degree of macrocytosis is also seen as a physiological feature of pregnancy [30] and in older adults [31].

Macrocytosis is recognized on a blood film by an increase in cell diameter (Fig. 3.15). It may be a generalized change, in which case the MCV will be raised, or it may affect only a proportion of the red cells. Macrocytes may be round or oval in outline, the diagnostic significance being somewhat different. Some of the causes of macrocytosis are listed in Table 3.2.

Hypochromia

Hypochromia is a reduction of the staining of the red cell (Fig. 3.16); there is an increase in central pallor, which occupies more than the normal

approximate one-third of the red cell diameter. Hypochromia may be general or there may be a population of hypochromic cells. Severe hypochromia may be reflected in a reduction in the mean cell haemoglobin concentration (MCHC), but the sensitivity of this measurement to hypochromia depends on the method by which it is measured (see p. 40). Any of the conditions leading to microcytosis may also cause hypochromia, although in some subjects with α or β thalassaemia trait the blood film shows microcytosis without appreciable hypochromia and, in rare patients with copper deficiency, hypochromia is associated with macrocytosis [34]. Red cells of healthy children are often hypochromic if assessed in relation to the appearance of the red cells of adults. Since the intensity of staining of the red cell is determined by the thickness of the cell as well as by the concentration of haemoglobin, hypochromia can also be noted in cells that are thinner than normal, whether or not they have a normal volume and haemoglobin concentration; such cells are designated 'leptocytes'.

Hyperchromia

The term 'hyperchromia' is rarely used in describing blood films. It can be applied when cells are more intensely stained than normal but it is more

Table 3.2 Some causes of macrocytosis.

Associated with reticulocytosis
Haemolytic anaemia
Haemorrhage

Associated with megaloblastic erythropoiesis
Vitamin B_{12} deficiency and inactivation of vitamin B_{12} by chronic exposure to nitric oxide
Folic acid deficiency, antifolate drugs (including methotrexate, pentamidine, pyrimethamine and trimethoprim and
   including methotrexate administered intrathecally [32]), cough mixture abuse [33]
Scurvy
Drugs interfering with DNA synthesis—used as anticancer drugs, immunosuppressive agents and in the treatment of
   the acquired immunodeficiency syndrome (including doxorubicin, daunorubicin, azathioprine, mercaptopurine,
   cyclophosphamide, cytarabine, fluorouracil, hydroxycarbamide (previously known as hydroxyurea), procarbazine,
   thioguanine, zidovudine and stavudine)
Rare inherited defects of DNA synthesis (including hereditary orotic aciduria, thiamine-responsive anaemia, Wolfram's
   syndrome (also known as DIDMOAD—**D**iabetes **I**nsipidus, **D**iabetes **M**ellitus **O**ptic **A**trophy and
   Deafness—syndrome), and the Lesch–Nyhan syndrome)

Associated with megaloblastic or macronormoblastic erythropoiesis
Myelodysplastic syndromes including primary acquired sideroblastic anaemia
Some acute myeloid leukaemias
Multiple myeloma
Ethanol intake
Liver disease
Phenytoin therapy
Some cases of copper deficiency [34]
Arsenic poisoning [35]
? Familial macrocytosis [36]

Associated with macronormoblastic erythropoiesis
Some congenital dyserythropoietic anaemias, particularly type I
Pure red cell aplasia of infancy (Blackfan–Diamond syndrome) including a forme fruste with macrocytosis only [37]
Aplastic anaemia
Maternally inherited sideroblastic anaemia [38]
Pearson's syndrome
Anorexia nervosa [39]
Genetic haemochromatosis [40]

Uncertain mechanism
Cigarette smoking [31]
Chronic obstructive airways disease
Trisomy 18 [41]
Trisomy 21 (Down's syndrome) [41,42]
Triploidy [41,43]
Familial autoimmune/lymphoproliferative disorder [44]
Development of antibodies to thrombopoietin [45]
Imatinib therapy in chronic myeloid leukaemia [46]

Factitious
Cold agglutinins
Delay in measuring MCV in some types of hereditary stomatocytosis, particularly hereditary cryohydrocytosis [47]
Marked delay in measuring MCV with certain automated counters (see Chapter 4)

MCV, mean cell volume.

useful to indicate why a cell is hyperchromic. Spherocytes (see p. 72) and irregularly contracted cells (see p. 74) stain more intensely than normal; the MCHC may be increased, indicating that the hyperchromia is related not only to a change in the shape of the cell but also to a true increase in the haemoglobin concentration. Some macrocytes are thicker than normal and this causes them to be hyperchromic without any increase in haemoglobin concentration; central pallor may be totally lacking.

Anisochromasia

Anisochromasia describes an increased variability in the degree of staining or haemoglobinization of the red cell (see Fig. 3.16). In practice, it usually means that there is a spectrum of staining from hypochromic to normochromic. Anisochromasia commonly indicates a changing situation, such as iron deficiency developing or responding to treatment or anaemia of chronic disease developing or regressing. Anisochromasia is reflected in an elevated haemoglobin distribution width (HDW) measured by some automated instruments (see p. 44).

Dimorphism

Dimorphism indicates the presence of two distinct populations of red cells (Fig. 3.17). The term is most often applied when there is one population of hypo-

Fig. 3.17 A dimorphic peripheral blood film from a patient with sideroblastic anaemia as a consequence of a myelodysplastic syndrome. One population of cells is normocytic and normochromic while the other is microcytic and hypochromic. One of the poorly haemoglobinized red cells contains some Pappenheimer bodies.

chromic, microcytic cells and another population of normochromic cells, the latter being either normocytic or macrocytic. Since the term is a general one, it is necessary to describe the two populations. They may differ in their size, haemoglobin content or shape and this is relevant to the differential diagnosis. Automated counters may confirm the visual impression of dimorphism, although some instruments may be unable to distinguish between a difference in size and a difference in haemoglobin concentration (see p. 181). Causes of a dimorphic film included iron deficiency anaemia (following administration of iron or blood transfusion), sideroblastic anaemia, the heterozygous state for hereditary sideroblastic anaemia, macrocytic anaemia post-transfusion, double deficiency of iron and either vitamin B_{12} or folic acid, unmasking of iron deficiency following treatment of megaloblastic anaemia and delayed transfusion reactions. Rare causes include mosaicism for β thalassaemia trait associated with a constitutional chromosomal abnormality [48] and chimaerism post-stem cell transplantation when either the donor or the host has microcytosis with a genetic basis.

Polychromasia

Polychromasia or polychromatophilia describes red cells that are pinkish-blue as a consequence of uptake both of eosin (by haemoglobin) and of basic dyes (by residual ribosomal RNA). Since reticulocytes (see p. 30) are cells in which ribosomal RNA takes up a vital dye to form a visible reticulum it will be seen that there is likely to be a relationship between reticulocytes and polychromatic cells. Both are immature red cells newly released from the bone marrow. However, the number of polychromatic cells in a normal blood film is usually less than 0.1% [49], considerably less than the normal reticulocyte count of around 1–2%. This is because only the most immature (grade I) reticulocytes are polychromatic. In conditions of transient or persistent haemopoietic stress, when erythropoietin levels are high, immature reticulocytes are released from the bone marrow. They are considerably larger than mature erythrocytes and, as a consequence of a reduced haemoglobin concentration, are less dense. On average their diameter is about 28% greater than that of

Fig. 3.18 Scanning electron microscopy of a reticulocyte. Courtesy of Professor A. Polliack, from Hoffbrand and Pettit [4].

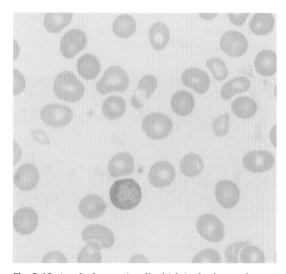

Fig. 3.19 A polychromatic cell which is also larger then a normal cell; it may be designated a polychromatic macrocyte. The film also shows anisocytosis and poikilocytosis.

a mature erythrocyte [49]. On scanning electron microscopy they have an irregular, multilobated surface (Fig. 3.18). They are readily recognized, in May-Grünwald–Giemsa (MGG)-stained films, by their greater diameter, their lack of central pallor and their polychromatic qualities (Fig. 3.19). They are often referred to as 'polychromatic macrocytes'. Late reticulocytes, which are the only forms present

in the blood of haematologically normal subjects, are cup-shaped and only slightly larger than mature erythrocytes. They are therefore difficult to recognize on an MGG-stained film.

The total number of reticulocytes, the proportion of early reticulocytes and the number of polychromatic macrocytes increase as a physiological response to increasing altitude or other hypoxic stimulus and as a normal response to anaemia when there are no factors limiting erythropoiesis. In severely anaemic patients, a lack of polychromasia is significant. It is absent in pure red cell aplasia and in aplastic anaemia and is inconspicuous in the anaemia of chronic disease and often in renal failure when the erythropoietin response is inadequate. The absence of polychromasia in a patient with sickle cell anaemia or other haemolytic anaemia is important since it may indicate complicating parvovirus-induced red cell aplasia.

Polychromatic erythrocytes are increased in myelofibrosis and in metastatic carcinoma of the bone marrow. In these conditions the number of polychromatic cells is greater than would be expected from the degree of anaemia and the polychromatic cells may be abnormal—more deeply basophilic than normal and not always increased in size [28].

When the reticulocyte count is increased, automated counters show an increased MCV and RDW. Bayer H.1 series instruments show, in addition, an increased HDW and reticulocytes are seen as hypochromic macrocytes on the red cell cytogram (see Fig. 8.56).

Poikilocytosis

A cell of abnormal shape is a poikilocyte. Poikilocytosis is therefore a state in which there is an increased proportion of cells of abnormal shape. High altitude produces some degree of poikilocytosis in haematologically normal subjects [50]. Poikilocytosis is also a common, often non-specific abnormality in many haematological disorders. It may result from the production of abnormal cells by the bone marrow or from damage to normal cells after release into the blood-stream. If poikilocytosis is very marked, diagnostic possibilities include myelofibrosis, congenital and acquired dyserythropoietic

Fig. 3.20 Peripheral blood film showing deformation of red cells by a precipitated cryoglobulin.

anaemias, hereditary pyropoikilocytosis and haemoglobin H disease. The presence of poikilocytes of certain specific shapes, e.g. spherocytes or elliptocytes, may have a particular significance (see below).

It is important not to confuse deformation of red cells due to a plasma abnormality with true poikilocytosis. The presence of cryoglobulin can lead to remarkable deformation of red cells (Fig. 3.20). Because the cryoglobulin may be only weakly basophilic it may not be readily apparent. The appearance of something extraneous indenting red cells provides a clue.

Spherocytosis

Spherocytes are cells that, rather than being disciform, are spherical or near-spherical in shape (Fig. 3.21) [51]. They are cells that have lost membrane without equivalent loss of cytosol, as a consequence of an inherited or acquired abnormality of the red cell cytoskeleton and membrane. In a stained blood film, spherocytes lack the normal central pallor. The diameter of a sphere is less than that of a disc-shaped object of the same volume, and thus a spherocyte may appear smaller than a discocyte. It is preferable, however, to restrict the term 'microspherocyte' to

Fig. 3.21 Scanning electron micrography of spherocytes and forms intermediate between discocytes and spherocytes. From Bessis [51].

Table 3.3 Some causes of spherocytosis.

Conditions that may be associated with numerous spherocytes
Hereditary spherocytosis
Warm autoimmune haemolytic anaemia
Delayed transfusion reactions
ABO haemolytic disease of the newborn
Administration of anti-D to Rh D-positive patients, e.g. in the treatment of autoimmune thrombocytopenic purpura
Clostridium perfringens (previously known as *Clostridium welchii*) sepsis
Drug-induced immune haemolytic anaemia (innocent bystander mechanism)
Zieve's syndrome*
Low erythrocyte ATP caused by phosphate deficiency [52,53]
Snake-bite induced haemolysis
Bartonellosis (Oroya fever)
Fresh-water drowning or intravenous infusion of water

Conditions that may be associated with smaller numbers of spherocytes
As an isolated feature
Immediate transfusion reaction
Acute cold autoimmune haemolytic anaemia
Chronic cold haemagglutinin disease
Rh haemolytic disease of the newborn
Penicillin-induced haemolytic anaemia
Acute attacks of paroxysmal cold haemoglobinuria
Infusion of large amounts of intravenous lipid [54]
Pyrimidine 5'-nucleotidase deficiency[†] [55]

In association with other poikilocytes
Normal neonate
Hyposplenism
Sickle cell anaemia
Microangiopathic haemolytic anaemia
Mechanical haemolytic anaemia
Heterozygosity for hereditary elliptocytosis with transient severe manifestations in infancy [56]
Hereditary pyropoikilocytosis (including homozygosity for mutations causing hereditary elliptocytosis)
Rh null phenotype

ATP, adenosine triphosphate.
* Irregularly contracted cells may be more characteristic.
† Spherocytes may be spiculated.

cells of reduced volume rather than merely reduced diameter. Macrospherocytes may be a feature of hereditary stomatocytosis (over-hydrated variant); they result from osmotic swelling. In examining a blood film for the presence of spherocytes it is important to examine that part of the film where the

cells are just touching, since normal cells may lack central pallor near the tail of the film. Overlapping cells can also give a false impression of spherocytosis. Spherocytes do not stack well into rouleaux.

The distinction between spherocytes and irregularly contracted cells (see below) is important since the diagnostic significance is different.

Some of the causes of spherocytosis are shown in Table 3.3. There are a variety of underlying mechanisms. In hereditary spherocytosis there is an abnormality of the cytoskeleton with a secondary destabilization and loss of membrane. In acquired conditions, spherocytosis can result from direct damage to the red cell membrane, e.g. by heat (Fig. 3.22), clostridial toxins (Fig. 3.23) or snake venoms. Loss of membrane can follow antibody coating of the cell by alloantibodies (Fig. 3.24), autoantibodies or drug-induced antibodies; the macrophages of the reticuloendothelial system recognize immunoglobulin or complement on the surface of the cell and remove pieces of membrane. When red cells fragment, those fragments with a relative lack of membrane form microspherocytes; this is the mechanism of formation of spherocytes in microangiopathic haemolytic anaemia, mechanical haemolytic anaemia and hereditary pyropoikilocytosis.

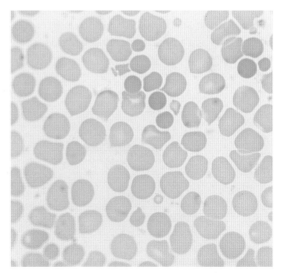

Fig. 3.22 Peripheral blood film of a patient with severe burns showing spherocytes, microspherocytes and red cells that appear to be budding off very small spherocytic fragments.

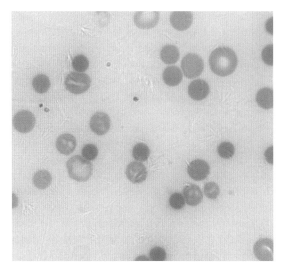

Fig. 3.23 Peripheral blood film of a patient with clostridial septicaemia showing many spherocytes. Courtesy of Professor H. Smith, Brisbane.

Erythrocytes stored for transfusion become sphero-echinocytes as the blood ages (see below). Rarely, marked spherocytosis has been described in hypophosphataemia, e.g. in liver disease [52], in acute diabetic ketoacidosis [53] and during over-vigorous correction of hyperphosphataemia [57]; the mechanism is likely to be adenosine triphosphate (ATP) depletion. In Heinz body haemolytic anaemias, although most abnormal cells are irregularly contracted cells (see below), there are usually also some spherocytes.

Irregularly contracted cells

Irregularly contracted cells lack central pallor and appear smaller and denser than normal erythrocytes without being as regular in shape as spherocytes (Fig. 3.25). Irregularly contracted cells are formed when there is oxidant damage to erythrocytes, or damage to red cell membranes by precipitation of unstable haemoglobin or free α or β chains. Blood films showing irregularly contracted cells often also show some spherocytes; these are formed when a red cell inclusion, such as a Heinz body, has been removed by the pitting action of splenic macrophages with associated loss of red cell membrane. Keratocytes (see below) may likewise be present as a result of the removal of a Heinz body. Blood films showing irregularly contracted cells may also show ghost cells and also hemighosts or blister cells. The latter are cells in which most of the haemoglobin has precipitated in half of the cell leaving the red cell membranes in apposition with each other in the other half of the cell; Heinz bodies may be present in the clear area as well as in the rest of the cell [58] (Figs 3.26 & 3.27). Some causes of irregularly contracted cells are shown in Table 3.4.

Elliptocytosis and ovalocytosis

Elliptocytosis indicates the presence of increased numbers of elliptocytes and ovalocytosis the presence of increased numbers of ovalocytes. These terms have not been used in any consistent manner

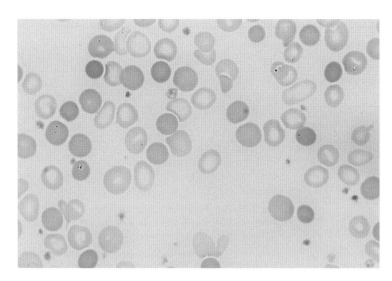

Fig. 3.24 Spherocytes in the peripheral blood film of an iron deficient patient who suffered a delayed transfusion reaction due to an anti-Rh D antibody; the film is dimorphic showing a mixture of the recipient's hypochromic microcytic cells and the donor cells which have become spherocytic.

Fig. 3.25 Peripheral blood film of a patient with haemoglobin C disease showing irregularly contracted cells and several target cells.

Fig. 3.27 Transmission electron micrograph showing a hemi-ghost cell containing Heinz bodies. Courtesy of Dr T.K. Chan and colleagues, Hong Kong, and the *British Journal of Haematology* [58].

Fig. 3.26 Scanning electron micrograph showing a hemi-ghost cell containing Heinz bodies. Courtesy of Dr T.K. Chan and colleagues, Hong Kong, and the *British Journal of Haematology* [58].

Table 3.4 Some conditions that are associated with irregularly contracted cells.

Conditions that may be associated with numerous irregularly contracted cells
Haemoglobin C disease
Haemoglobin C/β thalassaemia
Sickle cell/haemoglobin C disease
Unstable haemoglobins
Acute haemolysis in G6PD deficiency or other abnormalities of the pentose shunt
Severe oxidant stress (drugs or chemicals) in patients without abnormalities of the pentose shunt
Zieve's syndrome
Wilson's disease [59]

Conditions that may be associated with smaller numbers of irregularly contracted cells
Minor haemolytic episodes in G6PD deficiency
Moderate oxidant stress in patients without abnormalities of the pentose shunt
Defects in glutathione biosynthesis
Neonatal glutathione peroxidase deficiency (which is probably secondary to transient deficiency of selenium, an essential co-factor)
Haemoglobin C trait
Unstable haemoglobins
β thalassaemia trait
Haemoglobin H disease
Haemoglobin E disease or trait
Hereditary xerocytosis (dehydrated variant of hereditary stomatocytosis)
Congenital dyserythropoietic anaemia type II [60]

G6PD, glucose-6-phosphate dehydrogenase.

but it has been suggested that a cell with a long axis more than twice its short axis should be designated an elliptocyte while a cell with the long axis less than twice its short axis is designated an ovalocyte [61]. When elliptocytes or ovalocytes are numerous (Fig. 3.28) and are the dominant abnormality it is likely that the patient has an inherited abnormality affecting the red cell cytoskeleton, such as hereditary elliptocytosis (see p. 322). Smaller numbers of

Fig. 3.28 Peripheral blood film of a patient with hereditary elliptocytosis showing elliptocytes and ovalocytes.

elliptocytes or ovalocytes may be seen in iron deficiency, in some patients with β thalassaemia heterozygosity and homozygosity, megaloblastic anaemia, myelofibrosis and myelodysplastic syndromes and occasionally in inherited red cell enzyme abnormalities, e.g. pyruvate kinase deficiency; in these conditions it is likely that elliptocytes reflect dyserythropoiesis. Elliptocytosis in myelodysplastic syndromes has been linked to an acquired deficiency of protein 4.1 [62]. In Papua New Guinea, ovalocytosis has been associated with Gerbich negativity and a specific mutation in the gene encoding glycophorin

C [63]. Macrocytic ovalocytes or oval macrocytes are characteristic of megaloblastic anaemia and South-East Asian ovalocytosis (see p. 327) and are also seen in dyserythropoiesis, e.g. in idiopathic myelofibrosis. Elliptocytes are biconcave and thus are capable of forming rouleaux.

Teardrop cells (dacrocytes)

Teardrop or pear-shaped cells (dacrocytes) (Fig. 3.29) occur when there is bone marrow fibrosis or severe dyserythropoiesis and also in some haemolytic

Fig. 3.29 Peripheral blood film of a patient with idiopathic myelofibrosis showing teardrop poikilocytes (dacrocytes).

Fig. 3.30 Echinocytes in the peripheral blood film of a patient with chronic renal failure.

anaemias. They are particularly characteristic of megaloblastic anaemia, thalassaemia major and myelofibrosis—either idiopathic myelofibrosis or myelofibrosis secondary to metastatic carcinoma or other bone marrow infiltration. In both thalassaemia major and idiopathic myelofibrosis, the proportion of teardrop cells decreases following splenectomy suggesting either that they are the product of extra-medullary haemopoiesis or that they are formed when the spleen causes further damage to abnormal red cells. Teardrop cells that are present in occasional cases of autoimmune haemolytic anaemia [64], Heinz body haemolytic anaemia and β thalassaemia major are likely to be consequent on the action of splenic macrophages on abnormal erythrocytes, resulting from the removal of part of the red cell, Heinz bodies or α chain precipitates. Teardrop poikilocytes are common in patients with erythroleukaemia [65].

Spiculated cells

The terminology applied to spiculated cells is confused. In particular, the term 'burr cell' has been used by different authors to describe different cells and therefore is better abandoned. The terminology of Bessis [51] is recommended since it is based on careful study of abnormal cells by scanning electron microscopy and is clear and relatively easy to apply. Bessis divided spiculated cells into echinocytes, acanthocytes, keratocytes and schistocytes.

Echinocytes

Echinocytes are erythrocytes that have lost their disc shape and are covered with 10–30 short blunt spicules of fairly regular form (Figs 3.30 & 3.31). The main causes of echinocytosis are shown in Table 3.5. Echinocytes may be produced *in vitro* by exposure to fatty acids and certain drugs or simply by incubation. The end stage of a discocyte–echinocyte

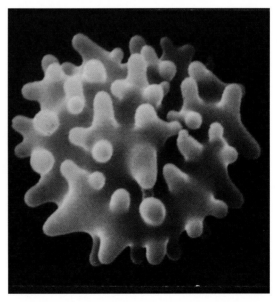

Fig. 3.31 Scanning electron micrograph of an echinocyte. Courtesy of Professor A. Polliak, from Hoffbrand and Pettit [4].

Table 3.5 Some causes of echinocytosis.

Storage artefact
Liver disease, particularly with coexisting renal failure
Nutritional or other phosphate deficiency [57]
Pyruvate kinase deficiency
Phosphoglycerate kinase deficiency
Aldolase deficiency [66]
Decompression phase of diving [67]
Haemolytic uraemic syndrome
Following burns
Following cardiopulmonary bypass
Post-transfusion (spheroechinocytes)

transformation is a spheroechinocyte. A sphero-echinocyte is also formed when a spherocyte undergoes an echinocytic change and, similarly, other abnormally shaped cells, e.g. acanthocytes, can undergo an echinocytic change.

When donor blood is stored for transfusion, cells become spheroechinocytes (Fig. 3.32) as lysolecithin is formed and as ATP concentration decreases; membrane lipid, both cholesterol and phospholipid, is then lost when microvesicles containing small amounts of haemoglobin are shed from the tips of the spicules. When blood is transfused and there is resynthesis of ATP many of the cells revert to cup-shaped stomatocytes rather than to discocytes; those that have lost a lot of membrane remain spherocytic.

In vivo, echinocyte formation may be related to increased plasma fatty acids (such as occurs during heparin therapy), ATP depletion and lysolecithin

formation. During echinocyte formation there is entry of calcium into cells with polymerization of spectrin. Echinocytosis is reversible *in vitro* and *in vivo*, e.g. by suspending cells in fresh plasma or by allowing ATP resynthesis.

In laboratories that make films from EDTA-anticoagulated blood rather than fresh blood by far the most common cause of echinocytosis is delay in making the blood film (see Fig. 3.7). This storage artefact, often referred to as 'crenation', is likely to be caused by a fall in ATP or by lysolecithin formation. Echinocytosis, other than as an artefactual change, is quite uncommon. The prevalence is greater in neonates [68]. It can occur in liver disease [68] but acanthocytosis (see below) is more common. It can occur in the early stages of the haemolytic uraemic syndrome but subsequently echinocytosis resolves leaving only the features of microangiopathic haemolytic anaemia. Echinocytosis, other than as a storage artefact, is probably most common in critically ill patients with multiorgan failure including both hepatic and renal failure.

Echinocytosis observed following the development of hypophosphataemia in patients on parenteral feeding is attributable to a fall in ATP concentration and this may also be the mechanism operating when echinocytes develop in hereditary pyruvate kinase deficiency and in phosphoglycerate kinase deficiency. Echinocytosis occurring in hypothermic, heparinized patients on cardiopulmonary bypass has been attributed to a rise of free fatty acid concentration.

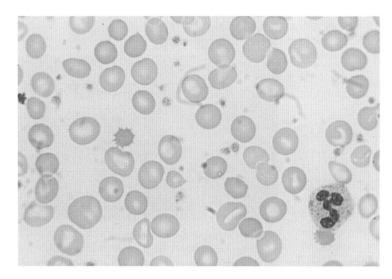

Fig. 3.32 Spheroechinocyte in a peripheral blood film made from blood taken shortly after a blood transfusion. The spheroechinocyte is a transfused cell.

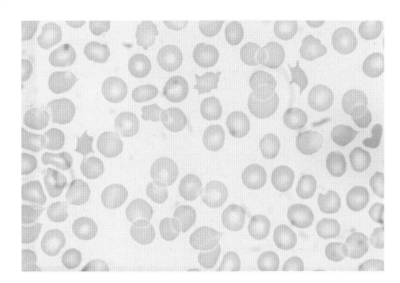

Fig. 3.33 Acanthocytes in a patient with anorexia nervosa.

The echinocytosis that has been noted as a delayed response in severely burned patients may be the result of lipid abnormalities.

Acanthocytes

Acanthocytes are cells of approximately spherical shape bearing between two and 20 spicules that are of unequal length and distributed irregularly over the red cell surface (Figs 3.33–3.38). Some of the spicules have club-shaped rather than pointed ends. Causes of acanthocytosis are shown in Table 3.6. Acanthocyte formation probably results from a preferential expansion of the outer leaflet of the lipid bilayer that comprises the red cell membrane [74]. Acanthocytes cannot form rouleaux.

Unlike echinocytosis, acanthocytosis is not reversible on suspending cells in fresh plasma. In acanthocytosis associated with abetalipoproteinaemia or liver disease the cholesterol : phospholipid ratio

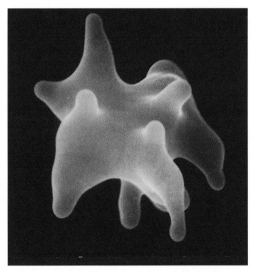

Fig. 3.34 Scanning electron micrograph of an acanthocyte. Courtesy of Professor A. Polliack, from Hoffbrand and Pettit [4].

Fig. 3.35 Scanning electron micrograph showing acanthocytes in a patient with the McLeod phenotype. Courtesy of Dr G. Lucas, Manchester.

Fig. 3.36 Unusually numerous acanthocytes in the peripheral blood film of a haematologically normal subject who has had a splenectomy. The film also shows a target cell.

in the red cells is increased. This is in contrast to the target cells associated with liver disease in which the cholesterol and phospholipid concentrations rise in parallel.

Acanthocytosis as an inherited phenomenon is associated with a number of different syndromes and its presence may help in their diagnosis. It was first described in association with retinitis pigmentosa, degenerative neurological disease, fat malabsorption and abetalipoproteinaemia [75]. Subsequently, it was recognized in association with several rare degenerative neurological diseases with normal β lipoproteins [76,77]. These conditions have been designated choreoacanthocytosis or neuroacanthocytosis. The acanthocytes may be more apparent on

Fig. 3.37 Numerous acanthocytes in a patient with abetalipoproteinaemia.

Fig. 3.38 Numerous acanthocytes in the blood film of a baby with infantile pyknocytosis.

Table 3.6 Some causes of acanthocytosis.

Conditions associated with large numbers of acanthocytes

Inherited

Hereditary abetalipoproteinaemia

Hereditary hypobetalipoproteinaemia (some cases)

Associated with degenerative neurological disease but
with normal lipoproteins—neuroacanthocytosis
(*CHAC* (*VPS13A*) or *JPH3* mutation)

McLeod red cell phenotype (mutation in the *KX* gene)

In(Lu) red cell phenotype (dominantly inherited Lu(a-b-
phenotype))

Associated with abnormal band 3 of red cell membrane
[69] resulting from a mutation in the *SLC4A1* (solute
carrier family 4, anion exchanger, member 1) gene [70]

Hereditary high red cell membrane phosphatidylcholine
haemolytic anaemia [71]

Acquired

Hypobetalipoproteinaemia caused by malnutrition or
lipid deprivation

'Spur cell' haemolytic anaemia associated with liver
disease (usually associated with alcoholic cirrhosis but
also occasionally with severe viral hepatitis, neonatal
hepatitis, cardiac cirrhosis, haemochromatosis or
advanced Wilson's disease)

Infantile pyknocytosis

Vitamin E deficiency in premature neonates

Myelodysplastic syndrome [72]

Conditions associated with small numbers of acanthocytes

Inherited

Heterozygotes for the McLeod phenotype

Pyruvate kinase deficiency

Woronet's trait

Dyserythropoiesis associated with a *GATA1* mutation [73]

Acquired

Post-splenectomy and hyposplenism

Anorexia nervosa and starvation

Myxoedema and panhypopituitarism

a wet preparation [78]. Most cases result from mutation in the *CHAC* or *VPS13A* gene [79]; inheritance
can be autosomal recessive or autosomal dominant.
A minority of cases represent Huntingdon-disease-
like 2 resulting from a mutation in the *JP3* (junc-
tophilin 3) gene [80]. Several inherited abnormalities
of red cell antigens are characterized by acanthocytosis. In the In(Lu) phenotype, in which there is
suppression of Lu and several other blood group
antigen systems, there are no associated abnormalities [81] whereas some cases of the McLeod pheno-

type, in which there is mutation in the *KX* gene and
Kell antigens are lacking, also have chronic granulomatous disease; female carriers of this mutation
have two populations of red cells, one acanthocytic
and one not. Acanthocytosis has also been associated
with a deficiency of band 3 protein [69].

Keratocytes

Keratocytes (or horned cells) (Fig. 3.39) are cells
with pairs of spicules—usually two but sometimes
four or six—which have been formed by the fusion
of opposing membranes to form a pseudovacuole
with subsequent rupture of the membrane at the cell
surface. They are formed when there is mechanical
damage to red cells, e.g. by fibrin strands or a
malfunctioning cardiac prosthesis. They have been
observed in microangiopathic haemolytic anaemia,
in disseminated intravascular coagulation and in
renal disease, e.g. glomerulonephritis, uraemia and
post-transplantation. They can also result from
removal of a Heinz body (Fig. 3.40) [82].

Schistocytes

Schistocytes are fragments of red cells formed either
by fragmentation of abnormal cells, e.g. in hereditary
pyropoikilocytosis, or following mechanical, toxin
or heat-induced damage of previously normal cells
(Fig. 3.41). When consequent on mechanical damage,
schistocytes often coexist with keratocytes. Many
schistocytes are spiculated. Others have been left
with too little membrane for their cytoplasmic volume and therefore have formed microspherocytes
(spheroschistocytes). In burnt patients, schistocytes
may be microdiscocytes as well as microspherocytes (see Fig. 3.78). An uncommon form of red
cell fragment, a linear or filamentous structure, is
observed in sickle cell anaemia [83] (Fig. 3.42).
The commonest causes of schistocyte formation
are microangiopathic and mechanical haemolytic
anaemias. Schistocytes may be a feature of the
myelodysplastic syndromes [84] and are common in
patients with erythroleukaemia [65].

Target cells

Target cells have an area of increased staining which
appears in the middle of the area of central pallor

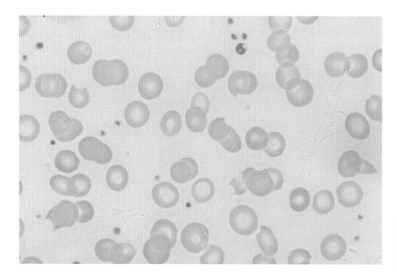

Fig. 3.39 Keratocytes in the peripheral blood film of a patient with microangiopathic haemolytic anaemia.

(Figs 3.43). Target cells are formed as a consequence of there being redundant membrane in relation to the volume of the cytoplasm. They may also be thinner than normal cells. *In vivo* they are bell-shaped and this can be demonstrated on scanning electron microscopy (Fig. 3.44). They flatten on spreading to form the characteristic cell seen on light microscopy. Target cells may be microcytic, normocytic or macrocytic, depending on the underlying abnormality and the mechanism of their formation. Some of the causes of target cell formation are shown in Table 3.7. Target cells may also be an artefact, as a result of using dirty slides [90].

Target cells may be formed because of an excess of red cell membrane, as when there is excess

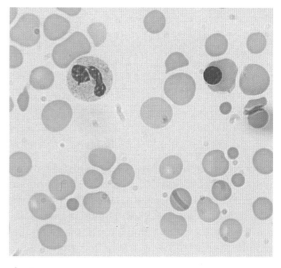

Fig. 3.40 Scanning electron micrograph of a keratocyte, formed by removal of a Heinz body. Courtesy of Dr M. Amare and colleagues and the *British Journal of Haematology* [82].

Fig. 3.41 Fragments including microspherocytes in the peripheral blood film of a patient with the haemolytic uraemic syndrome. The film also shows polychromasia and a nucleated red blood cell (NRBC).

Fig. 3.42 The blood film of a patient with sickle cell anaemia showing linear red cell fragments and increased numbers of irregularly contracted cells; the latter feature resulted from a severe pulmonary sickling crisis at the time the film was made.

Fig. 3.43 Peripheral blood film of a haematologically normal patient who has had a splenectomy, showing target cells and a Howell–Jolly body.

membrane lipid. This is the mechanism of formation in obstructive jaundice, severe parenchymal liver disease and hereditary deficiency of lecithin-cholesterol acyl transferase (LCAT). The ratio of membrane cholesterol to cholesterol ester is increased. Red cells lack enzymes for the synthesis of cholesterol and phospholipid and for the esterification of cholesterol so that changes in the membrane lipids are passive, reflecting changes in plasma lipids. When LCAT activity is reduced, the ratio of cholesterol to

Table 3.7 Some causes of target cell formation.

Conditions that are often associated with large numbers of target cells
Obstructive jaundice
Hereditary LCAT deficiency
Familial hypobetalipoproteinaemia [85]
Haemoglobin C disease
Sickle cell anaemia
Compound heterozygosity for haemoglobin S and
    haemoglobin C
Haemoglobin D disease
Haemoglobin O-Arab disease

Conditions that may be associated with moderate or small numbers of target cells
Parenchymal liver disease
Splenectomy and other hyposplenic states
Haemoglobin C trait
Haemoglobin S trait
Haemoglobin E trait and disease
Haemoglobin Lepore trait
β thalassaemia minor and major
Haemoglobin H disease
Iron deficiency
Sideroblastic anaemia
Hereditary xerocytosis (dehydrated variant of hereditary
    stomatocytosis) [86]
Analphalipoproteinaemia [87] and
    hypoalphalipoproteinaemia [88]
Hereditary phytosterolaemia [89]
Acquired phytosterolaemia as a result of parenteral
    nutrition [89]

LCAT, lecithin-cholesterol acyl transferase.

Fig. 3.44 Scanning electron micrographs of target cells. From Bessis [51].

cholesterol ester in the red cell membrane increases. There may also be an increase in total membrane cholesterol, with a proportionate increase in lecithin and with a decrease in ethanolamine. LCAT is synthesized in hepatocytes and so it may be reduced in liver disease. In obstructive jaundice very high levels of bile salts inhibit LCAT. This does not, however, appear to be the sole mechanism of target cell formation in obstructive jaundice since patients may have target cells without their plasma being able to inhibit the LCAT activity of normal plasma. When target cells are formed as a consequence of plasma lipid abnormalities they revert to a normal shape on being transfused into a subject with normal plasma lipids. If changes in membrane lipids that would normally cause target cell formation occur in patients with spherocytosis the cells become more disciform; this phenomenon may be observed when a patient with hereditary spherocytosis develops obstructive jaundice.

An alternative mechanism of target cell formation is a reduction of cytoplasmic content without a proportionate reduction in the quantity of membrane. This is the mechanism of target cell formation in a group of conditions such as iron deficiency, thalassaemias and haemoglobinopathies in which target cells are associated with hypochromia or microcytosis. Target cells are much less numerous in iron deficiency than in thalassaemias. The reason for this is not clear.

Stomatocytosis

Stomatocytes are cells that, on a stained blood film, have a central linear slit or stoma (Fig. 3.45). Occasionally such cells are seen in the blood films of healthy subjects. On scanning electron microscopy or in wet preparations with the cells suspended in plasma they are cup- or bowl-shaped (Fig. 3.46). Stomatocytes can be formed *in vitro*, e.g. in response to low pH or exposure to cationic lipid-soluble drugs such as chlorpromazine; the change in shape is reversible. The end stage of a discocyte–stomatocyte transformation is a spherostomatocyte. Stomatocytosis results from a variety of membrane abnormalities but probably essentially from expansion of the inner leaflet of the lipid bilayer that comprises the red cell membrane [74]. In liver disease, stomatocyte formation has been attributed to an increase of lysolecithin in the inner layer of the red cell membrane. In hereditary spherocytosis and autoimmune haemolytic anaemia, progressive loss of membrane leads to formation of stomatocytes, spherostomatocytes and spherocytes.

Stomatocytes have been associated with a great variety of clinical conditions [91,92] but an aetiological connection has not always been established. The commonest cause of stomatocytosis is alcohol excess and alcoholic liver disease; in these cases there is often associated macrocytosis and in those with very advanced liver disease there may also be

Fig. 3.45 Peripheral blood film showing stomatocytes.

Fig. 3.46 Scanning electron micrograph of stomatocytes. From Bessis [51].

triconcave cells [93]. The combination of stomatocytosis and macrocytosis is also seen in patients receiving hydroxycarbamide (previously known as hydroxyurea) and occasionally in the myelodysplastic syndromes. It is possible that chlorpromazine exposure can cause stomatocytosis *in vivo* as well as *in vitro* since an association has been observed [92]. Certain inherited erythrocyte membrane abnormalities are characterized by stomatocytes either alone in hereditary stomatocytosis and hereditary xerocytosis—or in association with other abnormalities in Rh_{null} or Rh_{MOD} syndromes [94] and South-East Asian ovalocytosis. Stomatocytosis in hereditary high red cell membrane phosphatidylcholine haemolytic anaemia is associated with

numerous target cells [71]; this condition is now thought to be identical to hereditary xerocytosis [95] (see p. 329). Stomatocytosis has been associated with some cases of hereditary haemolytic anaemia associated with adenosine deaminase overproduction [95]. Analphalipoproteinaemia (Tangier disease) [87] and hypoalphalipoproteinaemia [88] are associated with stomatocytosis. Increased stomatocytes have been reported in association with target cells in a single patient with familial hypobetalipoproteinaemia but in the published photograph the target cells are much more convincing than the stomatocytes [85]. LCAT deficiency shows both target cells and stomatocytes. An increased incidence of stomatocytosis has been reported in healthy Mediterranean (Greek and Italian) subjects in Australia [96]. This condition, designated Mediterranean stomatocytosis/macrothrombocytopenia, is now known to be a manifestation of hereditary phytosterolaemia (see p. 369) [97]. Similar morphological features, also associated with haemolytic anaemia and thrombocytopenia, occur in association with parenteral nutrition with soy-based lipid emulsions [89].

Sickle cells

A sickle cell is a very specific type of cell that is confined to sickle cell anaemia and other forms of sickle cell disease. Sickle cells are crescent- or sickle-shaped with pointed ends (Fig. 3.47). The characteristic shape is very apparent on scanning electron micrography (Fig. 3.48). The blood film in sickle cell anaemia may also show boat- or oat-shaped cells (see Fig. 3.46) that are not pathognomonic for the presence of haemoglobin S but are highly suggestive. Other highly characteristic poikilocytes formed in the presence of haemoglobin S are SC poikilocytes, formed when both haemoglobin S and haemoglobin C are present (Fig. 3.49) and 'Napoleon hat cells' that are characteristic of haemoglobin S-Oman (Fig. 3.50).

Pincer cells

Pincer or mushroom-shaped cells are a feature of hereditary spherocytes resulting from deficiency of band 3 (Fig. 3.51). They are also common in erythroleukaemia [65]. Similar cells can be seen in

Fig. 3.47 Peripheral blood film showing a sickle cell, boat-shaped cells and an NRBC.

oxidant-induced haemolysis, when they result from removal of two adjacent Heinz bodies.

Inclusions in erythrocytes

Howell–Jolly bodies

Howell–Jolly bodies (see Fig. 3.43) are medium sized, round, cytoplasmic red cell inclusions that have the same staining characteristics as a nucleus and can be demonstrated to be composed of DNA. A Howell–Jolly body is a fragment of nuclear mater-

ial. It can arise by karyorrhexis (the breaking up of a nucleus) or by incomplete nuclear expulsion, or can represent a chromosome that has separated from the mitotic spindle during abnormal mitosis. Some Howell–Jolly bodies are found in erythrocytes within the bone marrow in haematologically normal subjects but, since they are removed by the spleen, they are not seen in the peripheral blood. They appear in the blood following splenectomy and are also present in other hyposplenic states, including transient hyposplenic states resulting from reticuloendothelial overload. They can be a normal finding in neonates (in whom the spleen is functionally immature). The rate of formation of Howell–Jolly bodies is increased in megaloblastic

Fig. 3.49 Peripheral blood film from a patient with compound heterozygosity for haemoglobin S and haemoglobin C showing a characteristic SC poikilocyte.

Fig. 3.48 Scanning electron micrograph of a sickle cell. From Bessis [51].

Fig. 3.50 Peripheral blood film of a patient with compound heterozygosity for haemoglobin S and haemoglobin S-Oman showing the 'Napoleon hat' red cells that are characteristic of haemoglobin S-Oman. Courtesy of Dr R. A. Al Jahdamy and colleagues, Oman.

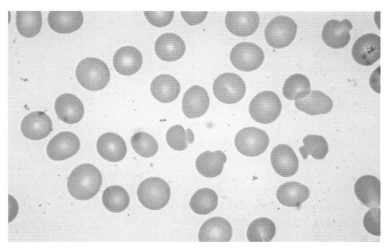

Fig. 3.51 Peripheral blood film of a patient with hereditary spherocytosis as a result of a band 3 mutation showing pincer or mushroom cells.

anaemias and, if the patient is also hyposplenic, large numbers of Howell–Jolly bodies will be seen in the peripheral blood.

Basophilic stippling

Basophilic stippling (Fig. 3.52) or punctate basophilia describes the presence in erythrocytes of considerable numbers of small basophilic inclusions that are dispersed through the erythrocyte cytoplasm and can be demonstrated to be RNA. They are composed of aggregates of ribosomes; degenerating mitochondria and siderosomes may be included in the aggregates but most such inclusions are negative with Perls' acid ferrocyanide stain for iron. Very occasional cells with basophilic stippling can be seen in normal subjects. Increased numbers are seen in the presence of thalassaemia minor (particularly β thalassaemia trait and α thalassaemia trait due to haemoglobin Constant Spring), thalassaemia major, megaloblastic anaemia, unstable haemoglobins, haemolytic anaemia, dyserythropoietic states in general (including congenital dyserythropoietic anaemia, sideroblastic anaemia, erythroleukaemia and idiopathic myelofibrosis), liver disease and poisoning by heavy metals such as lead, arsenic, bismuth, zinc, silver and mercury. Basophilic stippling is a prominent feature of hereditary deficiency of pyrimidine 5'-nucleotidase [98], an enzyme that is required for RNA degradation. Inhibition of this enzyme may also be responsible for the prominent basophilic stippling in some patients with lead

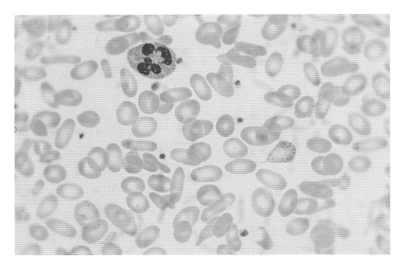

Fig. 3.52 Prominent basophilic stippling in the peripheral blood film of a patient who has inherited both β thalassaemia trait and hereditary elliptocytosis. The film also shows microcytosis and numerous elliptocytes and ovalocytes. One of the heavily stippled cells is a teardrop poikilocyte. Courtesy of Dr F. Toolis, Dumfries.

poisoning. Similar findings have been reported in a putative deficiency of CPD-choline phosphotransferase, resulting in accumulation of the pyrimidine phosphodiester, CPD-choline [99].

Pappenheimer bodies

Pappenheimer bodies (see Fig. 3.17) are basophilic inclusions that may be present in small numbers in erythrocytes; they often occur in small clusters towards the periphery of the cell and can be demonstrated to contain iron. They are composed of ferritin aggregates, or mitochondria or phagosomes containing aggregated ferritin. They stain on a Romanowsky stain because clumps of ribosomes are co-precipitated with the iron-containing organelles. A cell containing Pappenheimer bodies is a sidero-cyte. Reticulocytes often contain Pappenheimer bodies. Following splenectomy in a haematologically normal subject, small numbers of Pappenheimer bodies appear, these being ferritin aggregates. In pathological conditions, such as lead poisoning or sideroblastic anaemia, Pappenheimer bodies can also represent iron-laden mitochondria or phagosomes. If the patient has also had a splenectomy they will be present in much larger numbers.

Micro-organisms in erythrocytes

Both protozoan parasites (see pp. 142–155) and other micro-organisms (see p. 136) can be seen within red cells.

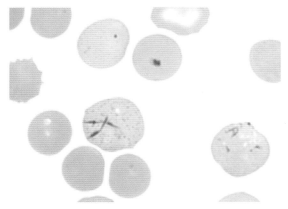

Fig. 3.53 Peripheral blood film of a patient with congenital erythropoietic porphyria showing radially arranged crystals in red cells. Courtesy of Dr Anna Merino and colleagues, Barcelona, and the *British Journal of Haematology* [100].

Crystals

Slender purple-violet crystals, often radially arranged, have been observed in red cells in congenital erythropoietic porphyria (Fig. 3.53) [100].

Circulating nucleated red blood cells

Except in the neonatal period and occasionally in pregnancy, the presence of NRBC (see Fig. 3.41) in the peripheral blood is abnormal, generally indicating hyperplastic erythropoiesis or bone marrow infiltration. In the neonatal period, an increased number of NRBC are seen in premature neonates and when there is growth retardation or the neonate has experienced hypoxia. An increased NRBC count at birth with a rise rather than a fall in the neonatal period has been found predictive of intraventricular haemorrhage in premature babies [101]. Increased numbers of NRBC can also be seen in babies with Down's syndrome.

If both NRBC and granulocyte precursors are present the film is described as leucoerythroblastic (see p. 233). NRBC in the peripheral blood may be morphologically abnormal; e.g. they may be mega-loblastic or show the features of iron deficient or sideroblastic erythropoiesis. An increased frequency of karyorrhexis in circulating NRBC may be seen in arsenic and lead poisoning [102] and in certain dyserythropoietic states such as erythroleukaemia and severe iron deficiency anaemia. Examination of a buffy coat film is helpful if assessment of morpho-logical abnormalities in NRBC is required.

Red cell agglutination, rouleaux formation and red cell rosetting

Red cell agglutinates (see Fig. 3.11) are irregular clumps of cells whereas rouleaux (Fig. 3.54) are stacks of erythrocytes resembling a pile of coins.

Reticulocytes may form agglutinates when their numbers are increased; this is a normal phe-nomenon. Mature red cells agglutinate when they are antibody-coated. Small agglutinates may be seen in warm autoimmune haemolytic anaemia whereas the presence of cold agglutinates may cause massive agglutination (see Fig. 3.2).

Rouleaux formation is increased when there is an increased plasma concentration of proteins of high molecular weight. The most common causes are pregnancy (in which fibrinogen concentration is increased), inflammatory conditions (in which polyclonal immunoglobulins, α_2 macroglobulin and fibrinogen are increased) and plasma cell dyscrasias such as multiple myeloma (in which increased immunoglobulin concentration is caused by the presence of a monoclonal paraprotein). Rouleaux formation may be artefactually increased if a drop of blood is left standing for too long on a microscope slide before the blood film is spread.

Abnormal clumping of red cells can also occur in patients receiving certain intravenous drugs that use polyethoxylated castor oils as a carrier (e.g. miconazole, phytomenadione and ciclosporin).

Rosetting of red cells around neutrophils (Fig. 3.55) is a rare phenomenon that is likely to be immunologically mediated.

Leucocytes

Normal peripheral blood leucocytes are classified either as polymorphonuclear leucocytes or as mononuclear cells, the latter term indicating lymphocytes and monocytes. Polymorphonuclear leucocytes are also referred to as polymorphonu-clear granulocytes, polymorphs or granulocytes. The term 'granulocyte' has also been used to refer more

Fig. 3.54 Peripheral blood film of a patient with multiple myeloma showing increased rouleaux formation consequent on the presence of a paraprotein; the film also shows increased background staining and a circulating myeloma cell.

Fig. 3.55 Red cell rosetting.

generally to both the mature polymorphonuclear leucocytes usually seen in the peripheral blood and their granulated precursors. Polymorphs have lobulated nuclei, which are very variable in shape, hence 'polymorphic', and prominent cytoplasmic granules, which differ in staining characteristics between the three classes—neutrophil, eosinophil and basophil. Mononuclear cells may also have granules; in the case of the monocyte they are inconspicuous, whereas in the lymphocyte they are sometimes prominent but are not numerous. In pathological conditions and in certain physiological conditions, such as pregnancy and during the neonatal period, precursors of polymorphs may appear in the peripheral blood. A variety of abnormal leucocytes may also be seen in certain disease states.

Granulocytes

The neutrophil

The mature neutrophil measures 12–15 µm in diameter. The cytoplasm is acidophilic with many fine granules. The nucleus has clumped chromatin and is divided into two to five distinct lobes by filaments, which are narrow strands of dense heterochromatin bordered by nuclear membrane (Fig. 3.56). The nucleus tends to follow an approximately

Fig. 3.56 Peripheral blood film of a healthy subject showing a normal polymorphonuclear neutrophil and normal small lymphocyte. The disposition of the nuclear lobes around the circumference of a circle is apparent.

Fig. 3.57 Peripheral blood film of a healthy female showing a normal neutrophil with a drumstick.

Fig. 3.58 A neutrophil band form. The nucleus is non-segmented and also has chromatin that is less condensed than that of the majority of segmented neutrophils.

circular form since in the living cell the nuclear lobes are arranged in a circle around the centrosome. In normal females a 'drumstick' may be seen protruding from the nucleus of a proportion of cells (Fig. 3.57). A normal neutrophil has granules spread evenly through the cytoplasm but there may be some agranular cytoplasm protruding at one margin of the cell. This may represent the advancing edge of a cell in active locomotion.

Characteristics of the nucleus

The neutrophil band form and left shift. A cell that otherwise resembles a mature neutrophil but that lacks nuclear lobes (Fig. 3.58) is referred to as a neutrophil band form or a 'stab' form (from the German *Stabzelle* referring to a shepherd's staff or crook). The Committee for the Clarification of Nomenclature of Cells and Diseases of the Blood Forming Organs has defined a band cell as 'any cell of the granulocyte series which has a nucleus which could be described as a curved or coiled band, no matter how marked the indentation, if it does not completely segment the nucleus into lobes separated by a filament'. A filament is a thread-like connection with 'no significant nuclear material' [103]. A band is differentiated from a metamyelocyte (see below) by having an appreciable amount of nucleus with parallel sides. Small numbers of band cells are seen in healthy subjects. An increase in the number of band cells in relation to normal neutrophils is known as a left shift. When a left shift occurs, neutrophil pre-

cursors more immature than band forms (metamyelocytes, myelocytes, promyelocytes and blast cells) may also be released into the blood. A left shift is a physiological occurrence in pregnancy. In the non-pregnant patient it often indicates response to infection or inflammation, or some other stimulus to the bone marrow. A left shift, including even a few blast cells, is produced by the administration of cytokines such as granulocyte colony-stimulating factor (G-CSF) and granulocyte macrophage colony-stimulating factor (GM-CSF).

The actual percentage or absolute number of band forms or the ratio of band forms to neutrophils that is regarded as normal is dependent on the precise definition of band form used and how the definition is applied in practice. Inconsistency between laboratories with regard to definition is common, as is variation between and within laboratories as to how definitions are applied.

Band cell counts have been employed in the detection of infection in neonates, but again various definitions have been applied [104,105]. For example, Akenzua *et al.* [104] defined a (segmented) neutrophil as a cell with lobes separated by a thin filament whose width is less than one-third the maximum diameter of the lobes whereas Christensen *et al.* [106] required the lobes to be separated by a definite nuclear filament.

The neutrophil lobe count and right shift. In normal blood, most neutrophils have one to five lobes. Six-lobed neutrophils are rare. A right shift is said to

Fig. 3.59 A hypersegmented neutrophil showing seven nuclear lobes. The film also shows anisocytosis with both microcytes and macrocytes.

be present if the average lobe count is increased or if there is an increased percentage of neutrophils with five or six lobes. The average lobe count of normal neutrophils varies between observers, with values of 2.5–3.3 obtained in different studies [107]. In practice, a formal lobe count is time-consuming and the presence of more than 3% of neutrophils with five lobes or more (Fig. 3.59) is a more practical indicator of right shift. This is also a more sensitive index of neutrophil hypersegmentation than the average lobe count and allows hypersegmentation to be detected in patients in whom a simultaneous increase in band forms means that the average lobe count is normal. A further index of right shift, which has been found to be more sensitive than either of the above, is the segmentation index:

$$\frac{\text{Number of neutrophils with 5 lobes or more} \times 100}{\text{Number of neutrophils with four lobes}}$$

Values of greater than 16.9 are abnormal [108]. A right shift or neutrophil hypersegmentation is seen in megaloblastic anaemia and in occasional patients with infection, uraemia or myelodysplastic syndrome. There is also a significant incidence in iron deficiency anaemia when other haematinic deficiencies are excluded [109]. Some hypersegmented neutrophils are seen following the administration of G-CSF [110]. Hypersegmented neutrophils are diploid cells; in patients with megaloblastic anaemia they are **not** derived from giant metamyelocytes [111]. Neutrophil hypersegmentation occurs as a rare hereditary characteristic with an autosomal dominant inheritance [112]. In the inherited condition known as myelokathexis there is neutropenia in association with a defect of neutrophil lobulation [113,114]. Neutrophils are hypersegmented with long chromatin filaments separating the lobes and with coarse, almost pyknotic chromatin; Döhle bodies, toxic granulation and neutrophil vacuolation have also been noted [114]. Rarely, a similar anomaly is seen in the myelodysplastic syndromes but at least some of these cases differ from the inherited condition in that the hypersegmented neutrophils are tetraploid (Fig. 3.60).

The presence of macropolycytes with more than five lobes (see p. 106) is not an indication of right shift since the increased number of lobes is consequent on an increased DNA content rather than on any abnormality of nuclear segmentation.

The neutrophil drumstick, sessile nodules and other nuclear projections. Some neutrophils in normal females have a drumstick-shaped nuclear appendage about 1.5 µm in diameter, which is linked to the rest of the nucleus by a filament [115] (see Fig. 3.57). These drumsticks represent the inactive X chromosome of the female. Similar projections with central pallor (racquet forms) are not drumsticks and do not have the same significance. In cells without drumsticks, the inactive X chromosome may be condensed

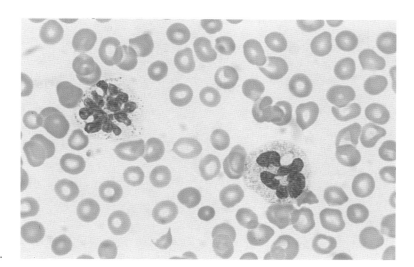

Fig. 3.60 Peripheral blood film of a patient with a myelodysplastic syndrome showing two neutrophils. Both are macropolycytes and one shows a defect of nuclear segmentation resembling myelokathexis. The size of the cells and the amount of nuclear material suggests that they are tetraploid cells.

Fig. 3.61 Peripheral blood film of a healthy female showing a band neutrophil with a sessile nodule.

beneath the nuclear membrane, where it can be detected in some neutrophil band forms [116], or it may protrude from the nucleus as a sessile nodule (Fig. 3.61). Like drumsticks, sessile nodules are usually only found in females. In one study the frequency of drumsticks was found to vary from one in 38 to one in 200 neutrophils, and to be characteristic of the individual but also proportional to the lobe count [115,117]. If a left shift occurs, the proportion of cells with drumsticks reduces, whereas in macropolycytes (see p. 106), and when there is right

shift due to megaloblastic anaemia or hereditary hypersegmentation of neutrophils, the frequency of drumsticks is increased.

The presence and frequency of drumsticks is related to the number of X chromosomes. They do not occur in normal males, in individuals with the testicular feminization syndrome who are phenotypically female but genetically (XY) male, or in Turner's syndrome (XO) females. In males with Klinefelter's syndrome (XXY) drumsticks are found but in lower numbers than in females. Paradoxically, XXX females rarely have cells with double drumsticks and on average their lobe count and frequency of drumsticks are lower than those of normal females; they have an increased incidence of sessile nodules and it has been suggested that the presence of an extra X chromosome inhibits nuclear segmentation [118]. However, triploidy, with the karyotype 69 XXY, is associated with the presence of drumsticks and in addition the nuclei are large and show increased sessile nodules and thorn-like and club-shaped projections [119]. Females with an isochromosome of the long arms of the X chromosome have larger and more frequent drumsticks, whereas females with deletions from the X chromosome have smaller drumsticks [112]. Natural human chimaeras whose cells are a mixture of cells of male and female origin have a drumstick frequency consistent with a male/female mixture of neutrophils [117] and, similarly, an alteration of the drumstick

Fig. 3.62 Peripheral blood film of a patient with chronic myelomonocytic leukaemia showing neutrophils with abnormal nuclear projections.

count may be seen after bone marrow transplantation when bone marrow from a female has been transplanted into a male or vice versa.

The proportion of neutrophils with drumsticks and sessile nodules is reduced in women with chronic granulocytic leukaemia (CGL) but returns to normal when the WBC falls on treatment [120].

The drumstick count (and the average lobe count) are reduced in Down's syndrome [121].

In addition to drumsticks and sessile nodules, neutrophil nuclei may have other projections that can have the shape of clubs, hooks or tags. These projections can also be seen in the neutrophils of males. Increased nuclear projections are a relatively uncommon feature of the myelodysplastic syndromes (Fig. 3.62). Several thread-like projections from the nuclei of most neutrophils is a characteristic features of congenital trisomy 13 syndrome [122,123].

Other abnormalities of neutrophil nuclei. Other abnormalities of neutrophil nuclei are shown in Table 3.8. Reduced neutrophil segmentation that is not consequent on temporary bone marrow stimulation with release of immature cells is seen as an inherited anomaly (the Pelger–Huët anomaly) or as an acquired anomaly (the pseudo-Pelger–Huët or acquired Pelger–Huët anomaly). The Pelger–Huët anomaly was first described by Pelger in 1928 and its familial nature was recognized by Huët in 1931 [140]. It is inherited as an autosomal dominant char-

acteristic with a prevalence between one in 100 and one in 10 000 in different communities [141]. It has been recognized in many ethnic groups including white and Black people, Chinese, Japanese and Indonesians. It results from a mutation in the *LBR* gene encoding the lamin B receptor [142]. The abnormality is distinctive. The majority of neutrophils have bilobed nuclei (Fig. 3.63a), the lobes being rounder than normal and the chromatin more condensed than would be expected for the degree of nuclear lobulation; a characteristic spectacle or *pince-nez* shape is common. Other nuclei are shaped like dumbells or peanuts (Fig. 3.63b). A small proportion of neutrophils, usually not more than 4%, have non-lobulated nuclei (Fig. 3.63c); they are distinguished from myelocytes by a lower nucleo-cytoplasmic ratio, the condensation of nuclear chromatin and the maturity of the cytoplasm. Subjects with the Pelger–Huët anomaly also show reduced lobulation of eosinophils and basophils [143]. In rare homozygotes with the Pelger–Huët anomaly all the neutrophils have round or oval nuclei. Neutrophils, eosinophils, basophils and monocytes are non-lobulated and there may also be mild neutropenia, giant platelets and mild thrombocytopenia [144]. Homozygotes may also show developmental delay, epilepsy and skeletal abnormalities [142]. The distinction between the Pelger–Huët anomaly and a left shift is important since heterozygosity for the inherited condition is of no clinical significance. If

Table 3.8 Some alterations and abnormalities that may be present in neutrophil nuclei.

Abnormality	Presence noted in
Left shift	Pregnancy, infection, hypoxia, shock
Hypersegmentation	Megaloblastic erythropoiesis Iron deficiency Uraemia Infection Hereditary neutrophil hypersegmentation Myelokathexis [113] Myelodysplastic syndrome [124]
Hyposegmentation	Pelger–Huët anomaly Bilobed neutrophils with reduced specific granules (lactoferrin deficiency) [125] Non-lobed neutrophils with other congenital anomalies (one case) [126] Acquired or pseudo-Pelger–Huët anomaly (myelodysplastic syndromes and acute myeloid leukaemia)
Increased nuclear projections	Trisomy 13 syndrome [122] Associated with large platelets (single family) [127] Associated with a large Y chromosome (drumstick-like) [128] Turner's syndrome [129] As an isolated defect [130] Myelodysplastic syndromes
Ring nuclei	Chronic granulocytic leukaemia [131] Acute myeloid leukaemia [132] Chronic neutrophilic leukaemia [133] Megaloblastic anaemia [134]
Botryoid nucleus	Heat stroke [135] Hyperthermia [136] Burns
Dense chromatin clumping	Myelodysplastic syndromes [137] Reversible effect of certain drugs (including mycophenolate mofetil) Myelokathexis [114]
Detached nuclear fragments	Dysplastic granulopoiesis due to HIV infection [138] or administration of drugs interfering with DNA synthesis [139], including chlorambucil, mycophenolate mofetil and tacrolimus

HIV, human immunodeficiency virus.

a left shift occurs in a patient with the Pelger–Huët anomaly the proportion of non-lobed neutrophils is further increased. If a subject with the Pelger–Huët anomaly develops megaloblastic erythropoiesis, a right shift occurs and neutrophils with three, four or even five lobes are seen [145]; megaloblastosis also causes loss of the characteristic dense clumping of the nuclear chromatin and drumsticks may become identifiable.

In another congenital anomaly, designated either 'lactoferrin deficiency' or 'specific granule deficiency', neutrophils with a marked reduction in the numbers of specific granules also have bilobed nuclei [125,146].

A single patient has been described in whom non-lobed neutrophils were associated with skeletal malformations, microthalmia and mental retardation [126].

The acquired Pelger–Huët anomaly (Fig. 3.64) is common in myelodysplastic syndromes and in acute myeloid leukaemias. It occurs occasionally in other haematological neoplasms, particularly idiopathic myelofibrosis and during the evolution of CGL. Features that help in making the distinction

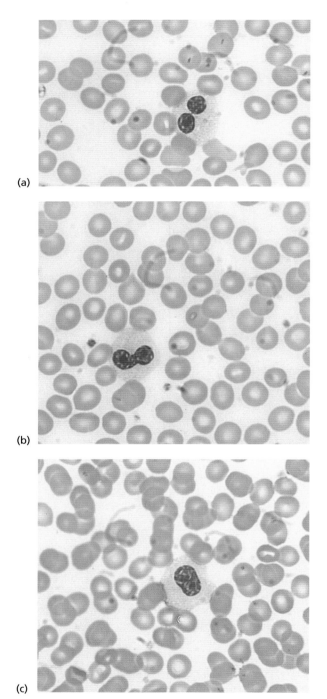

(a)

(b)

(c)

Fig. 3.63 Peripheral blood film of a patient with the inherited Pelger–Huët anomaly showing three neutrophils with: (a) bilobed nucleus; (b) peanut-shaped nucleus; and (c) non-lobed nucleus.

(a)

(b)

Fig. 3.64 Peripheral blood film of a patient with the acquired Pelger–Huët anomaly as part of a therapy-related myelodysplastic syndrome showing: (a) neutrophil with non-lobed nucleus; and (b) anisocytosis, poikilocytosis and neutrophil with bilobed nucleus.

from the inherited Pelger–Huët anomaly are that the percentage of affected neutrophils is usually less and there is commonly an association with neutropenia, hypogranularity of neutrophils, Döhle bodies (see p. 103) or dysplastic features in other lineages.

Reduced neutrophil lobulation is rarely seen in other circumstances but has been described in association with therapy with colchicine, ibuprofen [147], paclitaxel [148], docetaxel [148], mycophenolate

Fig. 3.65 Peripheral blood film from a patient with reversible myelodysplasia caused by mycophenolate mofetil. Both neutrophils have a non-segmented rounded nucleus with very coarse chromatin clumping; one also has a high nucleocytoplasmic ratio.

Fig. 3.66 Peripheral blood film of a patient with chronic granulocytic leukaemia (CGL) showing neutrophils and neutrophil precursors. There is one neutrophil with a ring-shaped nucleus.

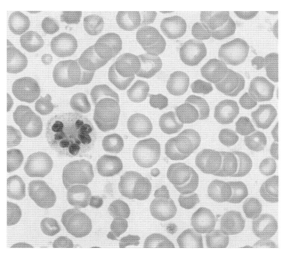

Fig. 3.67 Peripheral blood film from a patient with severe burns showing a neutrophil with a botryoid nucleus containing a small Döhle body.

mofetil [149] (Fig. 3.65) and other drugs, and in infectious mononucleosis, malaria, myxoedema, metastatic carcinoma involving the bone marrow, chronic lymphocytic leukaemia (CLL) and acute enteritis [112].

Neutrophils with ring or doughnut nuclei (Fig. 3.66) are seen occasionally in normal subjects. Their frequency is increased in CGL, in chronic neutrophilic leukaemia and probably in the myelodysplastic syndromes [131]; occasionally they are prominent in acute myeloid leukaemia (AML) [132].

Another acquired defect of the neutrophil nucleus is radial segmentation to form a 'botryoid' nucleus, i.e. a nucleus with a shape resembling a bunch of grapes. The change is consequent on contraction of microfilaments radiating from the centriole. Botryoid nuclei have been demonstrated in burns (Fig. 3.67), heat stroke [135] and in hyperthermia arising from brain stem haemorrhage [136].

Excessive clumping of the neutrophil nuclear chromatin is observed sometimes in the myelodysplastic syndromes and in AML and also in the reversible pseudo-Pelger–Huët anomaly associated with administration of various drugs.

Rarely, neutrophils have detached nuclear fragments (Fig. 3.68) equivalent to the Howell–Jolly bodies of erythrocytes; their nature can be confirmed by a Feulgen stain for DNA. Such inclusions are indicative of dysgranulopoiesis. They were first reported in a patient on azathioprine therapy [139]. They are also seen occasionally in patients on anticancer chemotherapeutic agents, in association with a reversible drug-induced pseudo-Pelger–Huët anomaly. They are not infrequently observed in

Fig. 3.68 Peripheral blood film of a patient on combination chemotherapy for lymphoma showing a neutrophil with a detached nuclear fragment (Howell–Jolly body-like inclusion).

HIV-positive individuals [138], the latter sometimes in the absence of any drug therapy.

The administration of G-CSF and GM-CSF can be associated with the appearance of a proportion of neutrophils with hypersegmented, hyposegmented and ring nuclei [150].

Neutrophils occasionally show features of apoptosis, i.e. the nucleus becomes homogeneous with peripheral chromatin condensation or, alternatively, the nucleus fragments into rounded homogeneous masses. This is a non-specific abnormality that may be seen in infective, inflammatory and autoimmune conditions or during cytotoxic chemotherapy [151]. Apoptosis should be distinguished from the morphologically similar degenerative changes that occur as an *in vitro* artefact on prolonged storage of blood (see pp. 63–64).

Abnormalities of neutrophil cytoplasm

Abnormalities of neutrophil cytoplasm are summarized in Table 3.9.

Reduced granulation. Reduced granulation of neutrophils occurs as a congenital anomaly, e.g. in lactoferrin (specific granule) deficiency, but this is rare. It is usually an acquired abnormality, most often as a feature of one of the myelodysplastic syndromes (Fig. 3.69). In HIV infection some neutrophils may show reduced granulation but this is

Fig. 3.69 Peripheral blood film of a patient with acute myeloid leukaemia (AML) showing three blasts and a hypogranular neutrophil.

not as marked as in the myelodysplastic syndromes. Reduced granulation may be apparent in severe infections, as a result of discharge of granules; residual granules may be prominent. Neutrophils produced in response to administration of G-CSF may be hypogranular [110].

Increased granulation. Increased granulation of neutrophils, with granules appearing both larger and more basophilic than normal, is designated toxic

Table 3.9 Some alterations and abnormalities of neutrophil cytoplasm.

Abnormality	Presence noted in	
Reduced granulation	Myelodysplastic syndromes and acute myeloid leukaemia Congenital lactoferrin (specific granule) deficiency [125] Grey platelet syndrome (some families) [152]	
Increased granulation	'Toxic' granulation—pregnancy, infection, inflammation, G-CSF and GM-CSF therapy [153,154] Aplastic anaemia Hypereosinophilic syndromes Alder–Reilly anomaly Chronic neutrophilic leukaemia [133] Myelodysplastic syndromes (uncommonly) [155] Myelokathexis [114]	
Abnormal granulation	Chédiak–Higashi syndrome and related anomalies [156,157] Alder–Reilly anomaly Acute myeloid leukaemia [158] and myelodysplastic syndromes [155]	
Vacuolation	Infection, G-CSF therapy, GM-CSF therapy Acute alcohol poisoning [159,160] Jordans' anomaly [161] Carnitine deficiency Kwashiorkor [162] Myelokathexis (some families) [114,163]	
Döhle bodies or similar inclusions	Infection, inflammation, burns, pregnancy, G-CSF therapy Myelodysplastic syndromes and acute myeloid leukaemia May–Hegglin anomaly Fechtner [164] and Sebastian syndromes Kwashiorkor [162] Myelokathexis [114]	
Actin inclusions	Congenital abnormality associated with anaemia and grey skin [165]	
Phagocytosed material	Bacteria and fungi	Bacterial and fungal infections
	Parasites	Leishmaniasis, malaria (rare)
	Cryoglobulin	Multiple myeloma and other cryoglobulinaemias
	Mucopolysaccharide	Various carcinomas [166] Wilms' tumour Hirschsprung's disease [167]
	Nucleoprotein	Systemic lupus erythematosus [168] ('LE cell')
	Melanin	Melanoma [169]
	Bilirubin crystals or amorphous deposits	Severe hyperbilirubinaemia [170,171]
	Cystine crystals	Cystinosis [172]
	Haemosiderin	Iron overload [173]
	Erythrocytes	Autoimmune haemolytic anaemia, paroxysmal cold haemoglobinuria [174], incompatible blood transfusion, potassium chlorate poisoning

G-CSF, granulocyte colony-stimulating factor; GM-CSF, granulocyte macrophage colony-stimulating factor.

Fig. 3.70 Three neutrophils in the peripheral blood film of a patient with bacterial infection showing toxic granulation and vacuolation.

Fig. 3.71 Peripheral blood film of a patient with the idiopathic hypereosinophilic syndrome showing a normal neutrophil, a neutrophil with abnormally heavy granulation and a hypogranular band eosinophil.

granulation (Fig. 3.70). When neutrophil maturation is normal, the azurophilic or primary granules become less strongly azurophilic as the cell matures so that, rather than staining reddish-purple, they stain violet or fail to stain at all. In a neutrophil showing toxic granulation the primary granules remain strongly azurophilic; this may be related to a higher concentration of acid mucosubstances than in normal neutrophils [175]. Degranulation may lead to neutrophils that show toxic granulation also having reduced numbers of granules. Although 'toxic' granulation is characteristic of infection it is non-specific being seen also in the presence of tissue damage of various types. It is also a feature of nor-

mal pregnancy and occurs with cytokine therapy (G-CSF and GM-CSF) even in the absence of infection. Other causes of heavy neutrophil granulation are shown in Figs 3.71 and 3.72 and in Table 3.9.

Abnormal granulation and Auer rods. Abnormal neutrophil granulation is seen in a number of inherited conditions including the Chédiak–Higashi syndrome and the heterogeneous group of conditions giving rise to the Alder–Reilly anomaly (Table 3.10). The Alder–Reilly anomaly occurs as an isolated abnormality, in association with an abnormal peroxidase [176] and as a feature of the mucopolysaccharidoses, Tay–Sachs disease or Batten–Spielmeyer–Vogt

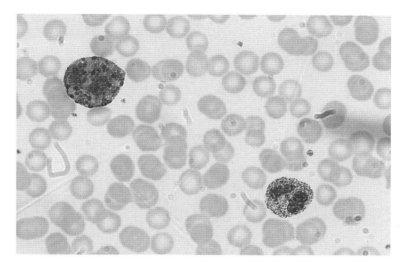

Fig. 3.72 Peripheral blood film of a patient with the Maroteaux–Lamy syndrome showing the Alder–Reilly anomaly of neutrophils. The neutrophil has granules that resemble 'toxic' granules. The other granulocyte is probably an eosinophil with granules having very abnormal staining characteristics. Courtesy of Mr A. Dean, Nottingham.

Table 3.10 Inherited conditions in which leucocytes have abnormal granules or cytoplasmic inclusions.

Abnormality	Associated features	Morphology of granules or inclusions	Nature of granules or inclusions	Nature of cells affected
Chédiak–Higashi anomaly*	Anaemia, neutropenia, thrombocytopenia, jaundice, neurological abnormalities, recurrent infections	Giant granules with colour ranging from grey to red	Giant secondary (specific) granules	Neutrophil, eosinophil, basophil, monocyte, lymphocyte, melanocyte, renal tubular cell, many other body cells
Alder–Reilly anomaly*†	Tay–Sachs disease, mucopolysaccharidoses (Hunter's syndrome†, Sanfilippo syndrome, Morquio's syndrome, Scheie's syndrome, Maroteaux–Lamy syndrome)	Dark red or purple inclusion which may resemble toxic granules, inclusions or vacuoles in lymphocytes	Mucopolysaccharide or other abnormal carbohydrate	Neutrophil, eosinophil, basophil, monocyte (rarely), lymphocyte
May–Hegglin anomaly‡	Thrombocytopenia, giant platelets	Resemble Döhle bodies	Amorphous areas of cytoplasm containing structures related to ribosomes	Neutrophil, eosinophil, basophil, monocyte

* Autosomal recessive.
† Hunter's syndrome is sex-linked recessive.
‡ Autosomal dominant.

disease. The abnormal neutrophils may have heavy granulation resembling toxic granulation or there may be large, clearly abnormal granules (see Fig. 3.72). In the Chédiak–Higashi syndrome (Fig. 3.73) the abnormal granules are quite variable in their staining characteristics and some may resemble Döhle bodies (see p. 103); at the ultrastructural level, however, they are abnormal granules rather than rough endoplasmic reticulum, being formed by the fusion of primary granules with each other and with secondary granules. There have been reports of abnormal neutrophil granulation resembling that of the Chédiak–Higashi syndrome but with atypical features [156]. In an apparently distinct syndrome, abnormal granulation of all mature myeloid cells was associated with bile duct atresia and livedo

Fig. 3.73 Peripheral blood film of a patient with the Chédiak–Higashi syndrome showing a neutrophil with giant and abnormally staining granules. Courtesy of Dr J. McCallum, Kirkaldy.

reticularis [171]. Giant bright blue inclusions composed of actin have been described in the neutrophils and other leucocytes of an infant with anaemia and grey skin discoloration [165] (Fig. 3.74) and in a second infant without associated abnormalities [177]. Occasional patients with myelodysplastic syndromes or with AML have giant granules in neutrophils, which are morphologically similar to those of the Chédiak–Higashi syndrome [158].

The Auer rod that is seen in haematological malignancies, specifically AML and refractory anaemia with excess of blasts in transformation (one of the myelodysplastic syndromes, as defined by the French–American–British (FAB) group), is formed by fusion of primary granules. Auer rods are usually confined to blast cells (Fig. 3.75) but occasionally they are seen in maturing cells, including neutrophils, which are part of the neoplastic clone.

Vacuolation. Neutrophil vacuolation may occur as the result of fusion of granules with a phagocytic vacuole with subsequent exocytosis of the contents of the secondary lysosome. This is usually a feature of infection (see Fig. 3.70) and partial degranulation of the neutrophil may also be apparent. Vacuolation of neutrophils can also occur as a toxic effect following ethanol ingestion [159] (Fig. 3.76) but this is much less often observed than ethanol-induced vacuolation of myeloid precursors; the vacuolation is attributed to both invagination of the membrane with inclusion of plasma and mitochondrial swelling and disruption [160]. A rare cause of neutrophil vacuolation (together with vacuolation of neutrophil precursors, monocytes and some eosinophils, basophils and lymphocytes) is a familial defect designated Jordans' anomaly [161,178]; cells contain neutral lipid which is stainable with oil red O and the vacuoles are due to dissolution of lipid [178]. Jordans' original patients may have had carnitine deficiency, which is known to cause lipid

Fig. 3.74 Bone marrow film of a patient with giant actin inclusions (Brandalise's syndrome) showing blue inclusions in a neutrophil and a promyelocyte. Similar inclusions were present in peripheral blood neutrophils and also in eosinophils, basophils, monocytes and lymphocytes. Courtesy of Dr. R.C. Ribeiro, Memphis.

Fig. 3.75 Peripheral blood film of a patient with AML showing blasts, one of which contains an Auer rod.

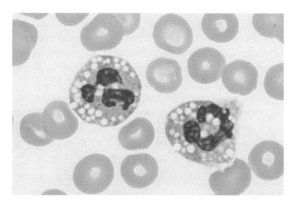

Fig. 3.76 Peripheral blood film of a patient with a heavy alcohol intake showing heavy vacuolation of neutrophils. Courtesy of Dr Wendy Erber, Cambridge.

storage myopathy with lipid vacuoles in neutrophils [179]. Similar lipid vacuoles in neutrophils occur in neutral lipid storage disease (also known as triglyceride storage disease with impaired long-chain fatty acid oxidation and as Dorfman–Chanarin syndrome [180,181]). Neutrophil vacuolation is also observed in some families with myelokathexis [163] and is a feature of the neutrophil dysplasia associated with the acquired chromosome anomaly, 17p–.

Döhle bodies and similar inclusions. Döhle bodies are small, pale-blue or blue-grey cytoplasmic inclusions,

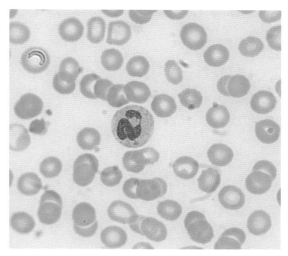

Fig. 3.77 Peripheral blood film of a patient with septicaemia showing a Döhle body in a neutrophil.

single or multiple, often found towards the periphery of the cell (Fig. 3.77). They usually measure only 1–2 μm in diameter but may be up to 5 μm. At the ultrastructural level, they are composed of stacks of endoplasmic reticulum together with glycogen granules. Their ribosomal component is indicated by pink staining with a methyl green–pyronin stain and by destruction by ribonuclease; they are seen better in films made from non-anticoagulated blood [182]. Döhle bodies are associated with pregnancy, infective and inflammatory states, burns (Fig. 3.78) and administration of cytokines such as G-CSF and GM-CSF. They may be seen in the myelodysplastic syndromes and in AML, and have been described in pernicious anaemia, polycythaemia rubra vera (PRV), CGL, haemolytic anaemia, Wegener's granulomatosis, and following use of anticancer chemotherapeutic agents [183].

Large inclusions resembling Döhle bodies, often numerous and sharply defined, are a feature of the May–Hegglin anomaly which is also characterized by thrombocytopenia and giant platelets (Fig. 3.79); they are often spindle- or crescent-shaped, randomly distributed in the cell rather than near the cell margin, and more intensely staining than Döhle bodies. At the ultrastructural level these inclusions differ from the Döhle bodies of reactive states; they appear as an amorphous area largely devoid of organelles, often incompletely surrounded by a single strand of

Fig. 3.78 Peripheral blood film from a patient with severe burns showing a prominent Döhle body. The red cells also show abnormalities attributable to burns.

Fig. 3.80 Peripheral blood film of a patient with *Plasmodium falciparum* malaria showing malarial pigment in a neutrophil and ring forms of the parasite within red cells.

Fig. 3.79 Peripheral blood film of a patient with the May–Hegglin anomaly showing a May–Hegglin inclusion, which resembles a Döhle body. Large platelets are also apparent. Courtesy of Dr N. Parker, London.

rough endoplasmic reticulum and containing a few dense rods and spherical particles which are probably ribosomes [184]. They are composed largely of a mutant form of the non-muscle myosin heavy chain IIa protein [185].

Inclusions resembling Döhle bodies but differing from them ultrastructurally have also been associated with the features of Alport's or Epstein's syndrome. The names Fechtner's syndrome [164] and Sebastian syndrome have been proposed for two of these genetically related conditions (see Table 8.13).

In normal subjects, Döhle bodies are rare. In one study they were seen in three of 20 healthy subjects with an average frequency of 0.1 per 100 cells [183]. In pregnancy, the number of Döhle bodies per 100 cells increases in parallel with the WBC [182]; the increased frequency persists into the post-partum period.

Exogenous neutrophil inclusions. Since neutrophils are phagocytes they may contain inclusions that represent phagocytosed material such as micro-organisms (see pp. 136–140) or cryoglobulin. Malarial pigment is occasionally observed in neutrophils (Fig. 3.80) but is more commonly present in mono-cytes. Less often malaria parasites are present (Fig. 3.81). Cryoglobulin (Fig. 3.82) may be seen as single or multiple round, weakly basophilic inclu-sions or as a single large inclusion that displaces the nucleus. Phagocytosis of cryoglobulin occurs *in vitro*, when the blood is left standing, rather than *in vivo* [186]. Abnormal mucopolysaccharide, which circulates in the blood of patients with malignant diseases, may be ingested by neutrophils; the blood

Fig. 3.81 Peripheral blood film of a patient with malaria showing microgametocytes of *Plasmodium vivax* that have been phagocytosed by neutrophils.

(a)   (b)

Fig. 3.82 Peripheral blood film of a patient with cryoglobulinaemia showing cryoglobulin that has been ingested by neutrophils and appears as: (a) small round inclusions; and (b) large masses filling the cytoplasm and displacing the nucleus. Some extracellular cryoglobulin is also present. Courtesy of Mr A. Dean.

film may also show amorphous or fibrillar deposits [166]. The formation of lupus erythematosus (LE) cells is usually an *in vitro* phenomenon but they may be seen in the peripheral blood (Fig. 3.83), e.g. in patients with severe lupus erythematosus [168]. Square or rectangular crystals of cystine can be seen in peripheral blood leucocytes in cystinosis but are more readily detected with phase-contrast microscopy [172]. Large cytoplasmic inclusions were observed in a case of colchicine poisoning

[187]. Refractile golden yellow haemosiderin inclusions were observed in a patient with thalassaemia major who had iron overload and sepsis [173].

Neutrophils may also ingest red cells, a phenomenon referred to as erythrophagocytosis. This has been observed in autoimmune haemolytic anaemia, paroxysmal cold haemoglobinuria, during acute exacerbations of chronic cold haemagglutinin disease, in other patients with a positive direct antiglobulin test and in haemolysis induced by

Fig. 3.83 Peripheral blood film showing a lupus erythematosus (LE) cell that has formed spontaneously.

Fig. 3.84 A neutrophil containing melanin in a patient with widely disseminated malignant melanoma. Courtesy of Dr J. Luckit, London, and Dr D. Swirsky, Leeds.

snake-bite, both with and without a positive direct antiglobulin test [188]. It is also seen in patients with defective red cells, as in sickle cell anaemia and sickle cell/haemoglobin C disease and in any severe haemolytic anaemia due to an intrinsic red cell defect. Erythrophagocytosis has been reported in a patient given G-CSF and GM-CSF; the latter agent appeared to be the principal cause [189]. Abnormal neutrophils showing marked erythrophagocytosis were reported in a patient with chronic myelomonocytic leukaemia (CMML) [190]. Ingestion of melanin has been seen in patients with metastatic melanoma (Fig. 3.84). Rarely, bilirubin crystals are seen within neutrophils of infants and children with a markedly elevated plasma bilirubin; they are refractile and faintly yellow (Fig. 3.85); they have been found to form *in vitro* when EDTA-anticoagulated blood is allowed to stand for at least 30 minutes [191].

Fig. 3.85 A neutrophil containing refractile bilirubin crystals. Courtesy of Dr Sudharma Vidyatilake, Colombo.

Other abnormalities of neutrophil morphology

Macropolycytes. A macropolycyte is about twice the size of a normal neutrophil (Fig. 3.86); its diameter is 15–25 μm rather than 12–15 μm and analysis of its DNA content shows that it is tetraploid rather than diploid, the number of lobes present being increased proportionately. Some macropolycytes are binucleated (Fig. 3.87). Occasional macropolycytes

are seen in the blood of healthy subjects. Increased numbers are seen in an inherited (autosomal dominant) condition in which 1–2% of neutrophils are giant with six- to 10-lobed nuclei, or with twin mirror-image nuclei [192]. Increased numbers, together with rather non-specific dysplastic features, have been described in DiGeorge's syndrome [193]. Macropolycytes, including binucleated cells, have been observed following the administration of

Fig. 3.86 Peripheral blood film of a patient with a myelodysplastic syndrome showing a macropolycyte, which is twice the size of the adjacent normal, neutrophil. The nucleus is also twice normal size and shows increased nuclear segmentation; it is likely that this is a tetraploid cell. In addition the film shows anisochromasia.

Fig. 3.87 Peripheral blood film of a patient with chronic lymphocytic leukaemia (CLL) and reversible chlorambucil-induced myelodysplasia showing a binucleated tetraploid neutrophil. Courtesy of the late Dr P.C. Srivastava, Burton-on-Trent.

G-CSF [153] and are present in increased numbers in megaloblastic anaemia. In megaloblastic anaemia they have a DNA content varying between diploid and tetraploid [111]; in contrast to hypersegmented

Fig. 3.88 Peripheral blood film of a patient with AIDS showing a hypogranular (probably tetraploid) giant metamyelocyte.

neutrophils, they are derived from giant metamyelocytes. They have also been reported in chronic infection, CGL and other myeloproliferative disorders, and following the administration of cytotoxic drugs and antimetabolites. Most macropolycytes have nuclear and cytoplasmic staining characteristics that are the same as those of other neutrophils but in megaloblastic anaemia macropolycytes may be seen which have a more open chromatin pattern and do not have an increased number of lobes [194]. Patients with HIV infection may have not only binucleate macropolycytes and macropolycytes with an open chromatin pattern but also circulating giant metamyelocytes (Fig. 3.88), cells that are characteristic of megaloblastic anaemia and are usually seen only in the bone marrow.

Necrobiotic (apoptotic) neutrophils and other myeloid cells. Necrobiotic neutrophils are cells that have died in the peripheral blood by a process known as apoptosis or 'programmed cell death'. Occasionally such cells are seen in the blood of healthy subjects and are recognized by their dense, homogeneous (pyknotic) nuclei, which eventually become completely round or fragment into multiple dense masses; the cytoplasm shows prominent acidophilia (Fig. 3.89). Infection is the most common cause of apoptotic

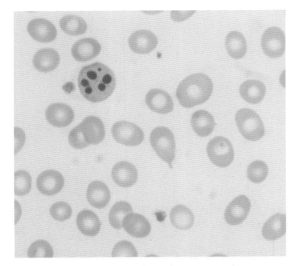

Fig. 3.89 Peripheral blood film of a patient with megaloblastic anaemia showing a necrobiotic (apoptotic) neutrophil. The chromatin has condensed and the nucleus has fragmented into rounded pyknotic masses. The film also shows anisocytosis, macrocytosis and a teardrop poikilocyte.

neutrophils [195]. Some patients with AML have numerous necrobiotic myeloid cells (Fig. 3.90). If blood is left at room temperature for a long time, a similar change can occur as an *in vitro* artefact (see p. 63). Leucocytes that have degenerated to the extent that nuclear material is no longer apparent have been designated necrotic; this is generally an artefact consequent on prolonged storage.

Fig. 3.90 Peripheral blood film of a patient with AML showing five apoptotic leukaemic cells.

Neutrophil aggregation. Aggregation of neutrophils with or without aggregation of platelets develops *in vitro* in some patients when EDTA-anticoagulated blood is allowed to stand. This is an antibody-mediated time-dependent phenomenon which is not of any clinical significance although it may lead to erroneous automated WBCs. Neutrophil aggregation has also been observed as a transient phenomenon in association with infectious mononucleosis [196] and in acute bacterial infection (Fig. 3.91). Occasionally, it is observed in a patient

Fig. 3.91 Peripheral blood film of a patient with overwhelming sepsis showing neutrophil aggregation, left shift, toxic granulation and neutrophil vacuolation.

Fig. 3.92 Peripheral blood film of a patient with rheumatoid arthritis showing neutrophil aggregation caused by a cold antibody. In this patient, *in vitro* neutrophil aggregation was observed for more than a decade and often led to inaccurate automated white blood cell counts (WBCs).

over many months or years and may then be associated with autoimmune disease (Fig. 3.92).

In some patients when the cause is a cold-acting antibody, red cell agglutinates coexist.

Neutrophil or other leucocyte fragments

Occasionally, circulating fragments of neutrophil cytoplasm are present in patients with sepsis [197] or in patients to whom G-CSF has been administered [110]. Fragmentation of neutrophils has been observed, in association with microangiopathic haemolytic anaemia, in a patient with clot formation at the tip of a dialysis catheter [198]. The mechanism is likely to have been mechanical damage to neutrophils. Neoplastic cells, such as leukaemic blast cells, are more prone to fragmentation than are normal cells and leucocyte fragmentation is not infrequently observed in AML (see Fig. 4.2).

The eosinophil

The eosinophil (Fig. 3.93) is slightly larger than the neutrophil with a diameter of 12–17 μm. The nucleus is usually bilobed but occasional nuclei are trilobed, the average lobe count being about 2.3. In females, eosinophils may have drumsticks (Fig. 3.94), but as the frequency of drumsticks is related to the degree of lobulation of the nucleus they are quite infrequent. Eosinophil granules are

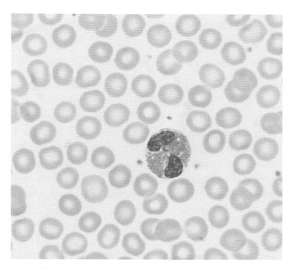

Fig. 3.93 An eosinophil in the peripheral blood film of a healthy subject.

spherical and considerably larger than those of neutrophils; they pack the cytoplasm and stain reddish-orange. The cytoplasm of eosinophils is weakly basophilic, ribosomes and rough endoplasmic reticulum being more abundant than in mature neutrophils; when degranulation occurs the pale blue cytoplasm is visible. Very occasional eosinophils in healthy subjects contain some granules with basophilic staining characteristics.

Fig. 3.94 Peripheral blood film of a female with idiopathic hypereosinophilic syndrome (HES) showing two eosinophils, one of which has a drumstick.

Fig. 3.95 Peripheral blood film of a patient with idiopathic HES showing eosinophil hypersegmentation. Both eosinophils have nuclei with four lobes.

Abnormalities of eosinophil nuclei

Eosinophils may show nuclear hypersegmentation (Fig. 3.95), hyposegmentation (Fig. 3.96) or ring-shaped nuclei (Fig. 3.97). Hypersegmentation can occur in megaloblastic anaemia. It can also be a hereditary phenomenon [199]; in one family hypersegmented eosinophils were also poorly granulated [200] without any apparent clinical defect. Increased lobulation has also been reported in Down's syndrome [201] and in myelokathexis [114]. Reduced eosinophil lobulation occurs in the Pelger–Huët anomaly (see Fig. 3.96) and has also been observed in lactoferrin (specific granule) deficiency [125].

Hypersegmentation, hyposegmentation and ring-shaped nuclei can all occur as acquired abnormalities. Hyposegmentation of eosinophil nuclei occurs as an acquired phenomenon in myeloproliferative disorders including idiopathic myelofibrosis and in the myelodysplastic syndromes (Fig. 3.98). In

Fig. 3.96 Peripheral blood film of a patient with the inherited Pelger–Huët anomaly showing a bilobed neutrophil and a nonlobed eosinophil.

Fig. 3.97 Peripheral blood film of a patient with cyclical oedema with eosinophilia showing an eosinophil with a ring-shaped nucleus.

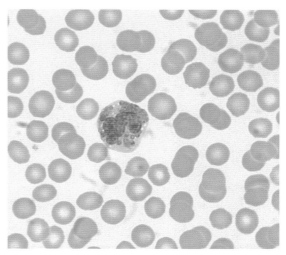

Fig. 3.99 Peripheral blood film of a patient with the Chédiak–Higashi syndrome showing an abnormally granulated eosinophil. Courtesy of Dr J. McCallum.

Fig. 3.98 Peripheral blood film of a patient with a myelodysplastic syndrome showing a non-lobulated and hypogranular eosinophil.

the latter group of disorders the chromatin may be clumped and the nuclei entirely or largely non-lobed [202]; this may be regarded as an acquired Pelger–Huët anomaly confined to eosinophils. Patients with eosinophilic leukaemia may have both hypersegmented and hyposegmented eosinophils. Hyposegmented eosinophils can be seen in reactive

eosinophilia [203]. Ring eosinophils are seen in a variety of conditions [204]; they appear to have no specific diagnostic significance.

Abnormalities of eosinophil granules and cytoplasm

Abnormal eosinophil granules may be seen, together with abnormal neutrophil granules in a variety of inherited conditions including the Chédiak–Higashi syndrome (Fig. 3.99) and the Alder–Reilly anomaly (see Fig. 3.72; Table 3.10). In the Alder–Reilly anomaly, eosinophil granules may be grey-green or purple on Romanowsky staining [140]. In the Chédiak–Higashi syndrome, some granules are blue-grey. A further abnormality, confined to eosinophils and basophils, has been noted in one family, the inheritance being autosomal dominant [199]; inclusions were grey or grey-blue. Cytoplasmic inclusions are present in eosinophils in the May–Hegglin anomaly and in the actin inclusion (Brandalise's) syndrome [165].

In acquired disorders of granulopoiesis it is not uncommon to see eosinophils in which some granules have basophilic staining characteristics. These are immature granules, sometimes designated 'pro-eosinophilic granules'. Such cells are increased

Fig. 3.100 Peripheral blood film of a patient with CGL showing a normal neutrophil and an eosinophil with some basophilic granules.

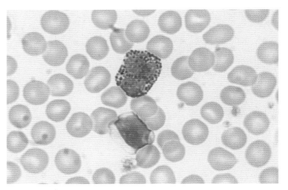

Fig. 3.101 A basophil and a small lymphocyte in the peripheral blood film of a healthy subject.

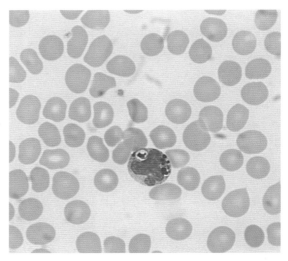

Fig. 3.102 Peripheral blood film of a patient with the Chédiak–Higashi syndrome showing an abnormal basophil. Courtesy of Dr J. McCallum.

in frequency in CGL (Fig. 3.100), eosinophilic leukaemia and certain categories of AML in which eosinophils are part of the leukaemic clone, particularly cases of acute myelomonocytic leukaemia with eosinophilia associated with inversion of chromosome 16. In all the above cases the abnormal granules are shown on ultrastructural examination to be eosinophil granules with unusual staining characteristics in some patients with CGL there are also hybrid cells with a mixture of granules of eosinophil type and basophil type [205].

In acquired disorders, eosinophils may be vacuolated or wholly or partly agranular. Hypogranularity could result from defective formation of eosinophil granules in dysmyelopoietic states but since it is usually accompanied by vacuolation it appears likely that in most instances it results from degranulation.

Vacuolation and hypogranularity are seen in some but not all cases of eosinophilic leukaemia. However, the changes are quite non-specific being also sometimes seen in reactive eosinophilia. For example, among seven patients with eosinophilia associated with B and T lymphoblastic leukaemia or lymphoma five had cytologically abnormal eosinophils [203].

The basophil

The basophil (Fig. 3.101) is of similar size to the neutrophil (10–14 μm in diameter). The nucleus is usually obscured by purple-black granules, which are intermediate in size between those of the neutrophil and those of the eosinophil. Basophils have abnormal granules in various inherited conditions (Fig. 3.102; also see Table 3.10).

Granules can be reduced in number in myeloproliferative disorders and in the myelodysplastic syndromes (Fig. 3.103), and degranulation can occur in acute allergic conditions (such as urticaria and

Fig. 3.103 Peripheral blood film of a patient with a myelodysplastic syndrome showing a hypogranular basophil.

anaphylactic shock), and during post-prandial hyperlipidaemia. A reduction in the number of granules can also be artefactual since basophil granules are highly water-soluble.

Lymphocytes and plasma cells

The lymphocyte

Peripheral blood lymphocytes vary in diameter from 10 to 16 μm. The smaller lymphocytes (10–12 μm), which predominate, usually have scanty cytoplasm and a round or slightly indented nucleus with condensed chromatin (Fig. 3.104). The larger lymphocytes (12–16 μm), which usually constitute about 10% of circulating lymphocytes, have more abundant cytoplasm and the nuclear chromatin is somewhat less condensed (Fig. 3.105). The smaller lymphocytes are usually circular in outline, whereas larger ones may be somewhat irregular. The cytoplasm, being weakly basophilic, stains pale blue. Lymphocytes may have small numbers of azurophilic granules, which contain lysosomal enzymes; occasional larger cells with more abundant cytoplasm have a dozen or so quite prominent granules. Such cells have been designated 'large granular lymphocytes' (Fig. 3.106). In healthy subjects they sometimes constitute as

Fig. 3.104 A small lymphocyte in the peripheral blood film of a healthy subject.

Fig. 3.105 A large lymphocyte in the peripheral blood film of a healthy subject.

Fig. 3.106 A large granular lymphocyte in the peripheral blood film of a healthy subject.

many as 10–15% of lymphocytes but usually they are less frequent.

Mature lymphocytes have a nucleolus but, because of the condensation of the chromatin, it is not usually visible in small lymphocytes. In large lymphocytes the nucleolus can sometimes be discerned. Because of the chromatin condensation, it is similarly difficult to detect sex chromatin in lymphocytes but sometimes it is visible condensed beneath the nuclear membrane in the larger lymphocytes with more dispersed chromatin [116]. The lymphocytes of infants and children are larger and more pleomorphic than those of adults. In general, the functional subsets of lymphocytes cannot be distinguished morphologically, but lymphokine-activated cytotoxic T cells and natural killer cells are found within the population of large granular lymphocytes.

Morphological abnormalities of lymphocytes in inherited conditions

Inclusions may be found in lymphocytes in the Chédiak–Higashi syndrome and Alder–Reilly anomaly (see Table 3.10). In the Chédiak–Higashi syndrome the lymphocyte inclusions can be very large (Fig. 3.107) but in the Alder–Reilly anomaly

Fig. 3.107 Peripheral blood film of a patient with the Chédiak–Higashi syndrome showing a lymphocyte with a large cytoplasmic inclusion. Courtesy of Dr J. McCallum.

(Fig. 3.108) they are only a little larger than the granules of normal large granular lymphocytes. Heterozygous carriers of the Chédiak–Higashi syndrome may also have lymphocyte inclusions but only in a small proportion of cells [206]. Occasionally, in the Alder–Reilly anomaly, inclusions are found in lymphocytes in the absence of neutrophil abnormalities. Lymphocyte inclusions are usually found when the Alder–Reilly anomaly is consequent on Tay–Sachs disease or on the mucopolysaccharidoses, although they are rare in Morquio's syndrome. Heterozygous carriers for Tay–Sachs disease may have lymphocyte inclusions [140], but in a much lower proportion of lymphocytes than in homozygotes. Alder–Reilly inclusions may be round or comma-shaped; they are sometimes surrounded by a halo, and tend to be clustered at one pole of the cell (see Fig. 3.108a). When the Alder–Reilly anomaly is due to one of the mucopolysaccharidoses the inclusions stain polychromatically with toluidine blue (see Fig. 3.108b) but when the underlying cause is Tay–Sachs disease they do not.

Lymphocyte vacuolation occurs in many inherited metabolic disorders including the following: I-cell disease (mucolipidosis type II) (Fig. 3.109), sialidosis (mucolipidosis type I), the mucopolysaccharidoses, Jordans' anomaly (see p. 102), Niemann–Pick disease type A, Wolman's disease, cholesteryl ester storage disease, GM1 gangliosidosis (small vacuoles in late infantile (type 2) disease and larger vacuoles in infantile (type 1) disease), mannosidosis, Pompe's disease, Tay–Sachs disease, juvenile Batten's disease (but not other types of Batten's disease), galactosidaemia (see Fig. 3.122), galactosialidosis (combined deficiency of β-galactosidase and α-neuraminidase), sialic acid storage disease and several other rare congenital disorders of metabolism [61,207–210]. In Tay–Sachs disease and Batten–Spielmeyer–Vogt disease, heterozygous carriers may also have lymphocyte vacuolation. The metabolic product responsible for vacuolation varies. In some conditions, e.g. Wolman's disease and cholesteryl ester storage disease, it is lipid and stains with oil red O, whereas in Pompe's disease it is glycogen and the periodic acid–Schiff (PAS) reaction is positive. In the mucopolysaccharidoses, vacuoles may result from dissolution of abnormal granules. The presence of a

(a)

(b)

Fig. 3.108 Peripheral blood film of a patient with the Sanfilippo syndrome showing: (a) abnormal lymphocyte inclusions, which are surrounded by a halo; and (b) blood film of the same patient stained with toluidine blue to show metachromatic staining of the lymphocyte inclusions. Courtesy of Mr A. Dean.

Fig. 3.109 Peripheral blood film of a child with I-cell disease. One of the two lymphocytes shows heavy cytoplasmic vacuolation.

Fig. 3.110 Peripheral blood film of a postoperative patient showing a plasma cell and a neutrophil with toxic granulation and a drumstick.

pink-staining ring around cytoplasmic vacuoles has been strongly associated with type II mucopolysaccharidosis (Hunter's disease) [211]. In I-cell disease, vacuoles were reported to be PAS and Sudan black B positive in one patient but were negative in another [212]. In the mucopolysaccharidoses there is variable staining with toluidine blue, depending on the specific metabolic defect present.

Reactive changes in lymphocytes

Lymphocytes can respond to viral infections and other immunological stimuli by an increase in number and cytological alterations. B lymphocytes can differentiate into plasma cells (Fig. 3.110). Intermediate stages are also seen and are designated

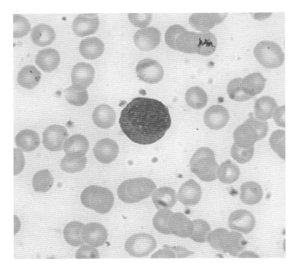

Fig. 3.111 The same peripheral blood film as shown in Fig. 3.110 showing a plasmacytoid lymphocyte.

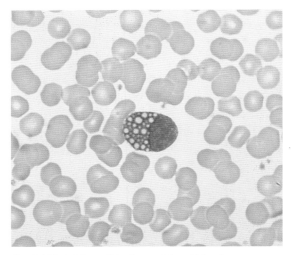

Fig. 3.112 A Mott cell in the peripheral blood.

plasmacytoid lymphocytes (Fig. 3.111) or Türk cells. Plasmacytoid lymphocytes may contain abundant globular inclusions (Fig. 3.112) composed of immunoglobulin. Such cells have been called 'Mott cells', 'morular cells' or 'grape cells'. Plasmacytoid lymphocytes may also contain crystals of immunoglobulin (Figs 3.113 & 3.114). Both T and B lymphocytes can also transform into immunoblasts —large cells with a central prominent nucleolus and abundant basophilic cytoplasm (Fig. 3.115). Cells

Fig. 3.113 A plasmacytoid lymphocyte containing crystals in the peripheral blood film of a patient with bacterial sepsis.

showing other less specific changes in lymphocyte morphology are subsumed under the designation 'atypical lymphocytes' or 'atypical mononuclear cells' (Fig. 3.116). Abnormalities include increased size of the cell, immaturity of the nucleus including lack of chromatin condensation and presence of a nucleolus, irregular nuclear outline or nuclear lobulation, cytoplasmic basophilia, cytoplasmic vacuolation and irregular cellular outline. Mitotic figures may be observed (Fig. 3.117). The commonest cause of large numbers of atypical lymphocytes is infectious mononucleosis, which is discussed, together with other causes of atypical lymphocytes, on p. 400. Multilobated lymphocyte nuclei, often with a clover leaf-shaped nucleus, are characteristic of adult T-cell leukaemia/lymphoma (ATLL) (see p. 453) but are also occasionally seen in carriers of the human T-cell lymphotropic virus (HTLV-I) and in infectious mononucleosis, HIV infection, cytomegalovirus (CMV) infection, rickettsial infection and toxoplasmosis [213,214]. Lymphocytes with convoluted nuclei, resembling Sézary cells, may occur in reactive conditions including HIV infection [215] and have been reported, together with skin infiltration, as an unusual reaction to hairy cell leukaemia [216]. Villous lymphocytes, resembling those of splenic lymphoma with villous lymphocytes, can

Fig. 3.114 A buffy coat film from the same patient whose peripheral blood film is shown in Fig. 3.113 showing one plasmacytoid lymphocyte containing globular inclusions and another containing a giant crystal.

Fig. 3.115 An immunoblast in the peripheral blood film of a patient with infectious mononucleosis.

occur in hyper-reactive malarial splenomegaly [217]. Binucleated lymphocytes have been reported after low-dose irradiation and binucleated lymphocytes and lymphocytes with bilobed nuclei are characteristic of chronic polyclonal B-cell lymphocytosis of cigarette smokers (Fig. 3.118). The number of large granular lymphocytes may also increase as a reactive phenomenon, e.g. in association with chronic viral infection, such as Epstein–Barr virus (EBV) infection [218] or hepatitis.

Occasionally, apparently normal lymphocytes appear in blood films in clumps [219].

Apoptotic lymphoid cells. Increased numbers of apoptotic lymphocytes may be present in reactive conditions, particularly infectious mononucleosis and other viral infections. They are recognized by peripheral condensation of the nucleus and a glassy appearance of the cytoplasm (Fig. 3.119).

Lymphocyte morphology in lymphoproliferative disorders

In most lymphoproliferative disorders the neoplastic cells are cytologically abnormal. Abnormalities show some overlap with those seen in reactive conditions but the majority of lymphoid neoplasms can be recognized as such on cytology alone. Typical features of different conditions are described in Chapter 9.

Lymphocyte aggregates. The presence of lymphocyte aggregates in the peripheral blood is an uncommon feature of lymphoproliferative disorders. It may represent an *in vitro* phenomenon [220] or, even more rarely, may indicate that the patient has an intravascular lymphoma [221]. As an *in vitro* artefact, this phenomenon has been associated particularly with splenic lymphoma with villous lymphocytes [220,222] and has also been observed in mantle cell lymphoma [223].

Fig. 3.116 Atypical lymphocytes in the peripheral blood film of a patient with cytomegalovirus infection.

Fig. 3.117 A peripheral blood lymphocyte in mitosis.

Fig. 3.118 A binucleated lymphocyte in the peripheral blood film of a female cigarette smoker with persistent polyclonal B-cell lymphocytosis.

The plasma cell

Plasma cells are usually tissue cells but, on occasion, they may be present in the peripheral blood, either as a feature of multiple myeloma or as a reactive phenomenon (see Figs 3.54 & 3.110). They are not seen in healthy subjects [224]. Reactive plasma cells are seen in the blood as a response to increased interleukin 6 secretion in infection, inflammation and cirrhosis and in various neoplasms (e.g. AML, carcinoma, lymphoma and cardiac myxoma) [225]. Occasionally, reactive plasma cells are present in large numbers, simulating plasma cell leukaemia. This has been reported following streptokinase therapy and in Castleman's disease, bacterial sepsis [226], rubella and dengue fever [227]. Plasma cells range in size from somewhat larger than a small lymphocyte (8–10 μm) up to a diameter of about 20 μm and are oval in shape with an eccentric nucleus, coarsely clumped chromatin, a moderate amount of strongly basophilic cytoplasm and a less

Fig. 3.119 An apoptotic lymphocyte in the peripheral blood of a patient with infectious mononucleosis. There are also red cell agglutinates.

Fig. 3.120 A normal monocyte in the peripheral blood film of a healthy subject.

basophilic Golgi zone adjacent to the nucleus. The clock-face chromatin pattern that is seen in tissue sections stained with haematoxylin and eosin is less apparent in circulating plasma cells stained with a Romanowsky stain. Plasma cells may contain secretory products, which appear as round or globular inclusions or, less often, crystals.

Circulating plasma cells are also sometimes seen in neoplastic disorders (multiple myeloma, plasma cell leukaemia and related conditions). The range of cytological abnormalities in these conditions is very broad.

Cells of monocyte lineage

The monocyte

The monocyte (Fig. 3.120) is the largest normal peripheral blood cell with a diameter of about 12–20 μm. It has an irregular, often lobulated nucleus and opaque greyish-blue cytoplasm with fine azurophilic granules. The cell outline is often irregular and the cytoplasm may be vacuolated. Sex chromatin may be seen condensed beneath the nuclear membrane [116].

Monocytes produced under conditions of bone marrow stimulation, e.g. infection or recovery from bone marrow suppression, show an increased

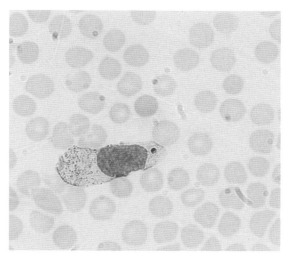

Fig. 3.121 Peripheral blood film of a patient with the Maroteaux–Lamy syndrome showing a monocyte with an abnormal cytoplasmic inclusion. Courtesy of Mr A. Dean.

nucleocytoplasmic ratio, a more delicate chromatin pattern, nucleoli and increased numbers of vacuoles [110]. Cytoplasmic basophilia and azurophilic granules may also be increased. The administration of G-CSF produces similar cytological changes [110].

Monocytes may contain abnormal inclusions in various inherited conditions (Fig. 3.121) (see also Table 3.10). In some metabolic disorders they may

Fig. 3.122 An abnormally vacuolated monocyte and a very heavily vacuolated lymphocyte in the peripheral blood of a patient with galactosidaemia. Courtesy of Dr G. Lucas, Manchester.

Fig. 3.124 Peripheral blood film of a patient with cryoglobulinaemia showing cryoglobulin within a monocyte. Courtesy of Mr A. Dean.

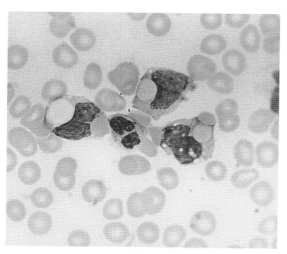

Fig. 3.123 Peripheral blood film of a patient with chronic renal failure taken during haemodialysis showing erythrocytes that have been phagocytosed by monocytes. The patient had a positive direct antiglobulin test but no overt haemolysis.

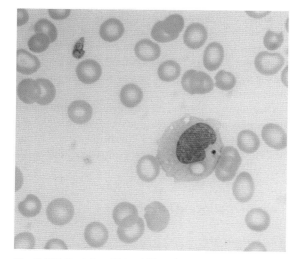

Fig. 3.125 Peripheral blood film of a patient with malaria showing malarial pigment within a monocyte. The film also shows a *Plasmodium falciparum* gametocyte.

be heavily vacuolated (Fig. 3.122). Since they are phagocytic they are occasionally found to have ingested red cells (Fig. 3.123), cryoglobulin (Fig. 3.124), micro-organisms (see pp. 136 and 140), malarial pigment (Fig. 3.125) and, rarely, melanin [169] or bilirubin [170]. Erythrophagocytosis by monocytes may be the result of abnormal red cells (as in sickle cell disease) or antibody or complement binding to red cells (as in paroxysmal cold haemoglobinuria or autoimmune haemolytic anaemia). Peripheral blood monocytes may contain parasitized red cells in malaria [228].

Monocyte precursors

Monocyte precursors, designated promonocytes and monoblasts, are not normally present in the peripheral blood. Monoblasts are very large cells with voluminous agranular cytoplasm and a large round nucleus. They are only seen in the peripheral blood in acute leukaemia with monocytic differentiation (see p. 417). Promonocytes, as defined by the FAB group and in the World Health Organization (WHO) classification of haematological neoplasms are very primitive cells (equivalent to a monoblast in significance) with a diffuse chromatin pattern but with lobulation or other irregularity of the nucleus. They need to be distinguished from the immature or abnormal monocytes that are present in reactive conditions (see above) and in chronic myeloid neoplasms.

The macrophage

Monocytes usually develop into macrophages (also called histiocytes) in tissues rather than in the blood. However, occasionally circulating cells with the characteristics of macrophages are seen (Fig. 3.126) [229]. They are associated with a variety of infective and inflammatory states (such as subacute bacterial endocarditis, tuberculosis and virus-associated haemophagocytic syndrome [230]), malignant disease and parasitic diseases. They may be a little larger than a monocyte or may be very large and multinucleated [170]. The cytoplasm may contain haemopoietic cells, recognizable cellular debris or amorphous debris. In certain inherited metabolic disorders foamy macrophages containing lipid are present in the peripheral blood [208]. Circulating phagocytic cells are also sometimes seen in malignant histiocytosis and acute monocytic leukaemia.

Granulocyte precursors

Granulocytes are generally produced in the bone marrow from myeloblasts, with the intervening stages being promyelocytes, myelocytes and metamyelocytes. On occasion, granulocyte precursors are seen in the blood. The appearance of appreciable numbers of such cells is designated a left shift. If NRBC are also present the blood film is described as leucoerythroblastic. The appearance in the peripheral blood of leucocytes of an earlier stage of development than the metamyelocyte is usually regarded as abnormal unless the blood is from a pregnant woman or a neonate. However, if buffy coat preparations are made, metamyelocytes and/or myelocytes are found in about 80% of healthy subjects with a frequency of about one in 1000 granulocytes [231].

The myeloblast

The myeloblast measures 12–20 μm and has a high nucleocytoplasmic ratio and a round or slightly oval

Fig. 3.126 A phagocytic macrophage in a peripheral blood film. Courtesy of Dr Z. Currimbhoy, Mumbai.

nucleus (see Fig. 3.69). The cell is usually somewhat oval and the outline may be slightly irregular. The nucleus has a diffuse chromatin pattern and one to five (most often two or three) not very prominent nucleoli. The cytoplasm is pale blue. A myeloblast is often defined as a cell that has no granules visible by light microscopy, although ultrastructural examination and cytochemistry show that granules are actually present. It is now becoming more common for cells with a relatively small number of granules but without the other characteristics of promyelocytes (see below) to also be included in the myeloblast category, in accordance with the recommendations made by the FAB group in relation to the diagnosis of AML [232], and subsequently supported by the WHO classification. Although a myeloblast does have characteristic cytological features it is not always possible to make the distinction between an agranular myeloblast and a lymphoblast on an MGG-stained film.

Circulating blast cells are very rare in healthy subjects; in one study they constituted, on average, 0.11% of mononuclear cells [224]. Circulating myeloblasts in haematological neoplasms may show abnormal cytological features such as the presence of Auer rods (see Fig. 3.75) or cytoplasmic vacuoles. The presence of even one blast cell with an Auer rod indicates the existence of a myeloid neoplasm.

The promyelocyte

The promyelocyte is larger than the myeloblast with a diameter of 15–25 μm (Fig. 3.127). The cell is round or slightly oval. In comparison with the myeloblast, the nucleocytoplasmic ratio is lower and the cytoplasm is more basophilic. The nuclear chromatin shows only slight condensation and nucleoli are apparent. (Clumped or condensed chromatin, known as heterochromatin, is genetically inactive, whereas diffuse euchromatin is genetically active; cellular maturation is associated with progressive condensation of chromatin.) The promyelocyte nucleus is oval with an indentation in one side. The Golgi zone is apparent as a much less basophilic area adjacent to the nuclear indentation. The promyelocyte contains primary or azurophilic granules, which surround the Golgi zone and are scattered through the remainder of the cytoplasm.

Fig. 3.127 A promyelocyte in the peripheral blood film of a patient with megaloblastic anaemia. The nucleolus and the Golgi zone are readily detectable. The film also shows anisocytosis and teardrop poikilocytes.

Morphologically abnormal promyelocytes may be seen in the peripheral blood in several subtypes of AML (see p. 415).

The myelocyte

The myelocyte is smaller than the promyelocyte, measuring 10–20 μm in diameter. It can be identified as belonging to the neutrophil, eosinophil or basophil lineage by the presence of specific or secondary granules with the staining characteristics of these cell lines (Figs 3.128–130). Eosinophil myelocytes may have some pro-eosinophilic granules with basophilic staining characteristics. The myelocyte nucleus is oval and sometimes has a slight indentation in one side. Chromatin shows a moderate degree of coarse clumping and nucleoli are not apparent. The cytoplasm is more acidophilic than that of the promyelocyte and the Golgi zone is much less apparent. Neutrophil and eosinophil myelocytes may appear in the blood in reactive conditions and in leukaemias. The presence of basophil myelocytes in the peripheral blood is essentially confined to the leukaemias. In acute leukaemias, circulating myelocytes may show morphological abnormalities such as hypogranularity or abnormally large granules.

Fig. 3.128 A neutrophil myelocyte in the peripheral blood film of a healthy pregnant woman.

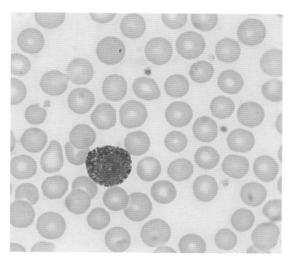

Fig. 3.130 A basophil myelocyte in the peripheral blood film of a patient with CGL.

Fig. 3.129 An eosinophil and an eosinophil myelocyte in the peripheral blood film of a patient with CGL.

Fig. 3.131 A metamyelocyte and two neutrophils in the peripheral blood film of a patient with CGL.

The metamyelocyte

The metamyelocyte measures 10–12 μm in diameter. Its chromatin is clumped and its nucleus is definitely indented or U-shaped (Fig. 3.131). Protein synthesis has stopped. A neutrophil metamyelocyte has acidophilic cytoplasm while that of an eosinophil myelocyte is weakly basophilic. Small numbers of neutrophil metamyelocytes are occa-

sionally seen in the blood in healthy subjects. They are commonly present in reactive conditions. Some eosinophil metamyelocytes may be seen in patients with eosinophilia.

The mast cell

Mast cells are essentially tissue cells. They are extremely rare in the peripheral blood of normal

Fig. 3.132 A mast cell in the peripheral blood film of a patient having a health check for non-specific symptoms.

subjects. They are large cells with a diameter of 20–30 μm. The cellular outline is somewhat irregular. The cytoplasm is packed with basophilic granules, which do not obscure the central nucleus (Fig. 3.132). The nucleus is relatively small and round or, more often, oval with a dispersed chromatin pattern. In systemic mastocytosis and in mast cell leukaemia (see p. 420) circulating mast cells are cytologically quite abnormal and may have lobulated nuclei, scanty granules or a denser chromatin pattern.

Disintegrated cells

The finding of more than a small percentage of disintegrated cells in a blood film is of significance.

It may indicate that several days have elapsed since the blood was taken from the patient and that the specimen is unfit for testing. When disintegration of cells is due to prolonged storage the granulocytes are smeared preferentially and, if an attempt is made to perform a differential count, there will appear to be neutropenia.

If disintegration of cells occurs in films made from fresh blood it indicates that cells are abnormally fragile. Disintegrated lymphocytes, usually called 'smear cells' or 'smudge cells', are common in CLL (Fig. 3.133). Their presence is of some use in diagnosis since they are not common in non-Hodgkin's lymphoma from which a distinction may have to be

made. The fact that these cells are intact *in vivo* and are smeared during preparation of the film is demonstrated by the fact that they are not present if a film of the same blood is made by centrifugation. Although smeared lymphocytes are characteristic of CLL they are not pathognomonic, being seen occasionally in non-Hodgkin's lymphoma and even sometimes in reactive conditions such as whooping cough. Other abnormal cells, e.g. blast cells in AML, may also disintegrate on spreading the blood film. The term 'basket cell' has been applied to a very large, spread out smear cell. Disintegrated cells, if at all frequent, should be included in the differential count (see p. 29). When the cell of origin is clear, e.g. as in CLL, they should be counted with intact cells of the same type.

Necrotic bone marrow cells

Necrotic bone marrow cells have been recognized in a venous blood sample from a patient with sickle cell crisis [233].

Platelets and circulating megakaryocytes

When platelets are examined in a blood film, an assessment should be made of their number (by relating them to the number of red cells), their size and their morphological features. The film should

Fig. 3.133 Intact lymphocytes and several disintegrated cells (smear cells or smudge cells) in the peripheral blood film of a patient with CLL.

be examined for platelet aggregates or platelet satellitism. Megakaryocytes are seen, although rarely, in the blood of healthy people. Their number is increased in certain disease states.

Platelets

The normal platelet measures 1.5–3 μm in diameter. Platelets contain fine azurophilic granules which may be dispersed throughout the cytoplasm or concentrated in the centre; in the latter case the central granule-containing cytoplasm is known as the granulomere and the peripheral, weakly basophilic agranular cytoplasm as the hyalomere (see Fig. 3.13). Platelets contain several different types of granules of which the α granules are the equivalent of the azurophilic granules seen on light microscopy.

In EDTA-anticoagulated blood, platelets generally remain separate from one another whereas in native blood they show a tendency to aggregate (see Figs 1.6–1.8). In Glanzmann's thrombasthenia, a severe inherited defect of platelet aggregation, the normal tendency of platelets to aggregate when films are made from native blood is completely absent.

Abnormalities of platelet size

Platelet size can be assessed by comparing the diameter of the platelets with the diameter of ery-

throcytes, or platelet diameter can be measured by means of an ocular micrometer.

Platelet size in healthy subjects varies inversely with the platelet count but this variation is not sufficiently great to be detected when a blood film is examined by light microscopy. A sufficient size increase to be detectable microscopically occurs in certain congenital abnormalities of thrombopoiesis and in certain disease states (Table 3.11). Large platelets (i.e. those with a diameter greater than 4 μm) are designated macrothrombocytes. Particularly large platelets with diameters similar to those of red cells or lymphocytes are often referred to as giant platelets (Fig. 3.134). When platelet turnover is increased, platelets are usually large. The absence of large platelets in patients with thrombocytopenia is therefore of diagnostic significance; it suggests that there is a defect of platelet production. Decreased platelet size is less common than increased size but it is a feature of the Wiskott–Aldrich syndrome (Fig. 3.135).

Other abnormalities of platelet morphology and distribution

Platelets that are lacking in α granules appear grey or pale blue. This occurs as a rare congenital defect known as the grey platelet syndrome resulting from an granule deficiency [238] or a deficiency of both α and δ granules [239]. There may be a mixture of normal and abnormal platelets. In some families

Table 3.11 Some causes of large platelets.

	Inheritance
Congenital	
Bernard–Soulier syndrome* [234]	AR
Heterozygous carriers of Bernard–Soulier syndrome/Mediterranean macrothrombocytopenia* [96,234]	AD
Mediterranean stomatocytosis/macrothrombocytopaenia (phytosterolaemia)	AR
Epstein's syndrome (associated with hereditary deafness and nephritis)* [185,235]	AD
Fechtner's syndrome* [236]	AD
Sebastian's syndrome* [236]	AD
Montreal platelet syndrome* [236]	
Chédiak–Higashi anomaly*	AR
May–Hegglin anomaly*	AD
Associated with increased nuclear projections in neutrophils [127]	AD
Marfan's syndrome and various other inherited connective tissue defects (in occasional families) [237]	
Platelet-type von Willebrand's syndrome [237]	
Grey platelet syndrome* [238]	AR
Hereditary thrombocytopenia with giant platelets but without other morphological abnormality or associated disease*	AR or AD
Acquired	
Immune thrombocytopenic purpura, primary and secondary*	
Thrombotic thrombocytopenic purpura*	
Disseminated intravascular coagulation*	
Myeloproliferative disorders—polycythaemia rubra vera, chronic granulocytic leukaemia (chronic phase or in transformation)*, idiopathic myelofibrosis*, essential thrombocy thaemia	
Myelodysplastic syndromes* and myelodysplastic/myeloproliferative disorders	
Megakaryoblastic leukaemia*	
Postsplenectomy and hyposplenic states (including sickle cell anaemia)	

AD, autosomal dominant; AR, autosomal recessive.
* May also have thrombocytopenia.

Fig. 3.134 A giant platelet, almost as large as the adjacent basophil, in the peripheral blood of a patient with idiopathic myelofibrosis. The film also shows a platelet of normal size. The red cells show poikilocytosis.

Fig. 3.135 The peripheral blood film of a patient with Wiskott–Aldrich syndrome showing thrombocytopenia and small platelets.

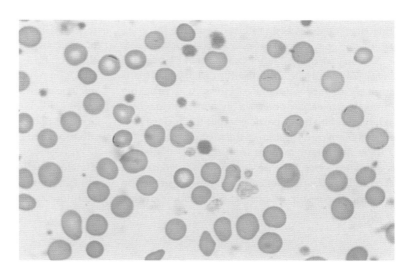

Fig. 3.136 The peripheral blood film of a patient with CGL showing a mixture of normally granulated and agranular platelets. There is also platelet anisocytosis.

with the grey platelet syndrome, neutrophils are also markedly hypogranular [152]. The grey platelet syndrome can occur as an isolated disorder but has also been reported in association with the Chédiak–Higashi syndrome, Hermansky–Pudlak syndrome, Wiskott–Aldrich syndrome and thrombocytopenia with absent radii [239]. Inherited causes of agranular platelets are all uncommon. More commonly, apparently agranular platelets result from discharge of platelet granules *in vivo* or *in vitro* or from formation of defective platelets by dysplastic megakaryocytes (Fig. 3.136). If venepuncture is difficult, stimulation of platelets may cause granule release.

This is sometimes associated with platelet aggregation so that masses of agranular platelets may be seen. Rarely, a similar phenomenon is caused by a plasma factor causing *in vitro* platelet degranulation and aggregation [240]; in one patient the factor originated from a leiomyosarcoma [241]. Degranulation may be confined to platelets in blood anticoagulated with EDTA, platelet morphology being normal when either heparin or citrate is used as an anticoagulant [242]. Cardiopulmonary bypass can cause release of α granules with the agranular platelets continuing to circulate. In hairy cell leukaemia, agranular platelets probably result from degranulation within abnormal vascular channels—pseudosinuses lined by hairy cells, which are present in the spleen and other organs. Some agranular platelets are commonly present in the myelodysplastic syndromes and are likely to indicate defective thrombopoiesis. Agranular platelets in the myeloproliferative disorders may result either from defective thrombopoiesis or from discharge of granules from hyperaggregable platelets. In both myelodysplastic and myeloproliferative conditions, platelets may be giant and of abnormal shape, features again indicative of abnormal thrombopoiesis. In the May–Hegglin anomaly, platelets may not only be larger than normal but also of unusual shape, e.g. cigar-shaped [243]. A population of platelets with one or more giant red granules on a Romanowsky-stained film has been reported in two members of a family with thrombocytopenia and an 11q23 deletion [244]; this syndrome has been referred to as the Jacobsen syndrome or as Paris–Trousseau thrombocytopenia.

Various particles, e.g. the parasites of *Plasmodium vivax* [245], may be found within platelets. This is unlikely to represent phagocytosis; it is probably equivalent to emperipolesis, a phenomenon in which white cells and other particles enter the surface connected membrane system of the megakaryocyte.

It is important to note the presence of platelet aggregates since they are often associated with a factitiously low platelet count. Platelet aggregation may be the result of platelet stimulation during skin-prick or venepuncture, or be immunoglobulin mediated. When there is incipient clotting of blood the platelets may be partly degranulated and the blood film may, in addition, show fibrin strands. Platelet aggregation occurring as an *in vitro* phenomenon, particularly in EDTA-anticoagulated blood, is mediated by a cold antibody with specificity against platelet glycoprotein IIb/IIIa [246]. This antibody is not known to be of any clinical significance. The phenomenon may be observed transiently in neonates, being attributable to the transplacental passage of the causative antibody [247]. EDTA-related platelet aggregation may be induced by therapy with antiglycoprotein IIb/IIIa monoclonal antibodies such as abciximab and can persist for several days after therapy [248].

Platelet satellitism (Fig. 3.137) is an *in vitro* phenomenon occurring particularly but not only in EDTA-anticoagulated blood. It is induced by a plasma factor, usually either immunoglobulin G (IgG) or IgM, which causes platelets to adhere to CD16 on neutrophils [249]. Platelets adhere to and encircle neutrophils and some may be phagocytosed [250]. Neutrophils can be joined together by a layer of platelets. Occasionally satellitism involves other normal cells, e.g. large granular lymphocytes [249], eosinophils [251], monocytes [251] or basophils. Platelet satellitism does not appear to be of any clinical significance, although it may lead to a factitiously low platelet count.

Fig. 3.137 Platelet satellitism.

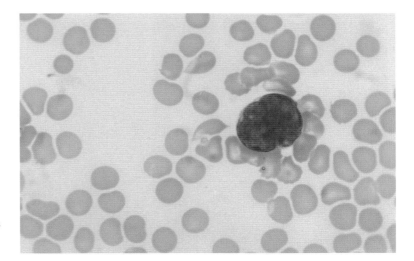

Fig. 3.138 A bare megakaryocyte nucleus in the peripheral blood film of a healthy subject; the size and lobulation of the nucleus indicates its origin from a polyploid megakaryocyte.

Platelet satellitism around lymphoma cells as a non-EDTA-dependent phenomenon has been reported in a single patient with mantle cell lymphoma [252].

Platelet satellitism can interfere with the immunophenotyping of cells that are encircled.

Megakaryocytes

Megakaryocytes are rarely seen in the blood of healthy adults. They are released by the bone marrow but most are trapped in the pulmonary capillaries. However, the fact that they are detectable, albeit in low numbers, in venous blood arising from parts of the body lacking haemopoietic marrow indicates that some can pass through the pulmonary capillaries. Since their concentration is, on average, only between five and seven per millilitre they are more likely to be seen in buffy coat preparations or when special concentration procedures are carried out. In healthy subjects, 99% of the megakaryocytes in peripheral venous blood are almost bereft of cytoplasm (Fig. 3.138) but rare cells with copious cytoplasm are seen. The number of megakaryocytes is increased in the blood of neonates and young infants and also postpartum, postoperatively and in patients with infection, inflammation, malignancy, disseminated intravascular coagulation and myeloproliferative disorders [253–256]. In neonates there is a correlation with prematurity and with respira-

tory distress syndrome [257]. The numbers of megakaryocytes in venous blood is increased during and after cardiopulmonary bypass [258]. The proportion of intact megakaryocytes with plentiful cytoplasm is increased in infants [254] and in patients with idiopathic myelofibrosis and CGL [256].

Abnormal megakaryocytes and megakaryoblasts

Abnormal megakaryocytes and megakaryoblasts may be seen in the blood in pathological conditions.

Micromegakaryocytes are seen in some patients with haematological neoplasms, e.g. idiopathic myelofibrosis (Fig. 3.139) and CGL, particularly CGL in transformation. They are small diploid mononuclear cells with a diameter of 7–10 μm, which are not always immediately identifiable as megakaryocytes. The nucleus is round or slightly irregular with dense chromatin. Cytoplasm varies from scanty to moderate in amount; when scanty, the nucleus may appear 'bare' but electron microscopy shows that such cells usually have a thin rim of cytoplasm. Cytoplasm is weakly basophilic. There may be cytoplasmic vacuolation or a few or numerous cytoplasmic granules. Sometimes there are small cytoplasmic protrusions or 'blebs' and sometimes platelets appear to be 'budding' from the surface. Somewhat larger micromegakaryocytes with well-developed granular cytoplasm may be

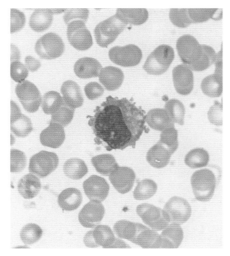

Fig. 3.139 A micromegakaryocyte in the peripheral blood film of a patient with idiopathic myelofibrosis.

Fig. 3.140 Micromegakaryocyte in a neonate with transient abnormal myelopoiesis of Down's syndrome.

seen in acute megakaryoblastic leukaemia including transient abnormal myelopoiesis of Down's syndrome (Fig. 3.140).

Megakaryoblasts (Fig. 3.141) vary from about 10 μm in diameter up to about 15–20 μm or larger. Smaller ones may resemble lymphoblasts and have no distinguishing features. Larger megakaryoblasts have a diffuse chromatin pattern and cytoplasmic basophilia varying from weak to moderately strong. Cytoplasm varies from scanty to moderate in

Fig. 3.141 Peripheral blood film of a patient with megakaryoblastic transformation of CGL showing three megakaryoblasts. One of these is large with no distinguishing features, another shows some maturation and has cytoplasm that resembles that of a platelet while the third resembles a lymphoblast. The lineage was confirmed by ultrastructural cytochemistry.

amount and may form blebs. Megakaryoblasts are often not identifiable as such by cytology alone.

Blood film in healthy subjects

Healthy adult

The blood film in a normal adult shows only slight variation in size and shape of red cells (see Figs 3.13 & 3.56). White cells that are normally present are neutrophils, neutrophil band forms, eosinophils, basophils, lymphocytes and monocytes. Metamyelocytes and myelocytes are rare. Megakaryocytes, usually in the form of almost bare nuclei, are very rare. Platelets are present in such numbers that the ratio of red cells to platelets is of the order of 10–40 : 1.

Pregnancy

During pregnancy, the red cells show more variation in size and shape than is seen in non-pregnant women. The MCV also increases, being greatest around 30–35 weeks' gestation. This change occurs independently of any deficiency of vitamin B_{12} or folic acid, although there is an increased need for folic acid during pregnancy. The Hb falls, the lowest concentration being at 30–34 weeks' gestation. Although both iron and folic acid deficiency have an increased prevalence during pregnancy this commonly observed fall in the Hb is not due to a deficiency state, and in fact occurs despite an increase in the total red cell mass. It is consequent on an even greater increase in the total plasma volume. The erythrocyte sedimentation rate (ESR) and rouleaux formation are also increased. Polychromatic cells are more numerous and the reticulocyte count is increased with peak levels of 6% at 25–30 weeks.

The WBC, neutrophil count and monocyte count rise with neutrophils commonly showing toxic granulation and Döhle bodies. A left shift occurs: band forms, metamyelocytes and myelocytes are common, and occasional promyelocytes and even myeloblasts may be seen. Small numbers of NRBC may be seen but it should be noted that small numbers of NRBC of fetal origin may also be present in the maternal circulation [259]. The WBC and neutrophil count continue to rise till term. The absolute lymphocyte and eosinophil counts fall. On Bayer H.1 series instruments, the lobularity index (LI) and mean peroxidase index (MPXI) are increased.

The platelet count and platelet size do not usually change during normal pregnancy, but the platelet count may fall and the mean platelet volume (MPV) may rise if pregnancy is complicated by pregnancy-associated hypertension ('toxaemia'). Pregnancy-associated thrombocytopenia of unknown mechanism occurs in a small proportion of women with an uncomplicated pregnancy. Normal ranges for haematological parameters during pregnancy are given in Table 5.13.

Infancy and childhood

In normal infants and children, red blood cells are hypochromic and microcytic, in comparison with those of adults, and the MCV and mean cell haemoglobin (MCH) are lower. Iron deficiency is common in infancy and childhood but the difference from adult norms is present even when there is

no iron deficiency. The male–female difference in Hb, red blood cell count (RBC) and packed cell volume/haematocrit (PCV/Hct) is not present before puberty.

The lymphocyte count of children is higher than that of adults and the lymphocyte percentage commonly exceeds the neutrophil percentage ('reversed differential'). A greater proportion of large lymphocytes is commonly observed and some of these may have visible nucleoli. Reactive changes in lymphocytes in response to infection and other immunological stimuli are far more common than in adults and even apparently completely healthy children may have a few 'atypical' lymphocytes.

Normal ranges for haematological parameters during infancy and childhood are given in Tables 5.10–5.12.

Neonate

The blood film of a healthy neonate may show hyposplenic features (see below), specifically Howell–Jolly bodies, acanthocytes and spherocytes. Spherocytes are, however, more numerous than in a hyposplenic adult. The WBC and the neutrophil, monocyte and lymphocyte counts are much higher in the neonate than in the older child or adult. NRBC are much more common and myelocytes are not uncommon. The number of circulating megakaryocytes is greater than in infants and children. The proportion of micromegakaryocytes is increased [260]. Hb, RBC and PCV are much higher than at any other time after birth and the resultant high viscosity of the blood leads to poor spreading so that the blood film appears 'packed'. This physiological polycythaemia also leads to a very low ESR. Red cell size is increased in comparison with that of infants, children and adults. The reticulocyte count is high during the first 3 days after birth [261].

Physiological changes in haematological variables occur in the first days and weeks of life. There is a rise, on average of about 60% of initial counts, in the WBC and the neutrophil count, with peak levels being reached at about 12 hours after birth [262]. By 72 hours the count has fallen back to below that observed at birth. The lymphocyte count falls to its lowest level at about 72 hours and then rises again

[262]. By the end of the first week, the number of neutrophils has usually fallen below the number of lymphocytes. If there has been late clamping of the umbilical cord there are also rises in Hb, PCV and RBC due to 'autotransfusion' from the placenta followed by reduction of plasma volume. NRBC usually disappear from the blood by about the fourth day in healthy term babies and by the end of the first week most of the myelocytes and metamyelocytes have also disappeared. Band forms are also more numerous during the first few days of life than thereafter, a plateau being reached by the fifth day.

Normal ranges for the neonatal period are given in Tables 5.8 and 5.9.

Premature neonate

Many haematological variables in premature babies differ from those of full-term babies (see above). Their blood films show greater numbers of NRBC, metamyelocytes, myelocytes, promyelocytes and myeloblasts. Hyposplenic features are much more marked than in term babies (Fig. 3.142) and may persist for the first few months of life. Premature

Fig. 3.142 Peripheral blood film from a premature but healthy infant, showing macrocytosis (relative to the film of an adult), a Howell–Jolly body in a polychromatic cell, target cells and a schistocyte.

babies often develop eosinophilia between the second and third weeks after birth [263].

Hyposplenism

Splenectomy in haematologically normal subjects produces characteristic abnormalities of the blood count and film. The same abnormalities are seen if the spleen is congenitally absent, suffers atrophy or extensive infarction, or becomes non-functional for any reason. Occasionally, if the spleen is heavily infiltrated by abnormal cells, features of hyposplenism are seen in the presence of splenomegaly.

Immediately after splenectomy there is thrombocytosis and a marked neutrophil leucocytosis. If infection occurs post-splenectomy, the neutrophilia and left shift are very marked. After recovery from surgery, the neutrophil count falls to nearly normal levels and the platelet count falls to high normal or somewhat elevated levels—platelet counts of around $500–600 \times 10^9/l$ may persist. A lymphocytosis and a monocytosis persist indefinitely—the lymphocytosis is usually moderate but levels up to $10 \times 10^9/l$ are occasionally seen [264]. Characteristically large granular lymphocytes are increased (see Fig. 9.10); immunophenotypically these are natural killer cells [265,266]; T and B cells may also be increased [267]. In normal subjects the Hb does not change postsplenectomy but the red cell morphology is altered (see Figs 3.36 & 3.45). Abnormal features include target cells, acanthocytes, Howell–Jolly bodies, small numbers of Pappenheimer bodies (the presence of siderotic granules being confirmed on a stain for iron), occasional NRBC and small numbers of spherocytes. Small vacuoles may be seen in Romanowsky-stained films; on interference phase-contrast microscopy these appear as 'pits' or 'craters' but in fact they are autophagic vacuoles [268]. The reticulocyte count is increased. Special stains show small numbers of Heinz bodies. Some large platelets may be noted and the MPV is higher, in relation to the platelet count, than in non-splenectomized subjects.

In patients with underlying haematological disorders a greater degree of abnormality is often seen post-splenectomy. When there is anaemia that persists post-splenectomy a marked degree of thrombocytosis is usual. If Heinz bodies are being formed

Table 3.12 Some causes of hyposplenism.

Physiological
Neonatal period (particularly in premature babies), old age

Pathological
Congenital
Congenital absence or hypoplasia (may be hereditary [269]; may be associated with situs inversus and cardiac anomalies; may be associated with anophthalmia and agenesis of the corpus callosum [270]; occurs in reticular agenesis and Fanconi's anaemia [271]; has been reported in Pearson's syndrome; may be caused by maternal coumarin intake)
Inherited (AD) early involution of the spleen
Congenital polysplenism [272]

Acquired
Splenectomy
Splenic infarction (sickle cell anaemia, sickle cell/haemoglobin C disease and other sickling disorders; essential thrombocythaemia; polycythaemia rubra vera; following splenic torsion; consequent on acute infection [273])
Splenic atrophy (associated with coeliac disease, dermatitis herpetiformis, ulcerative colitis [274], Crohn's disease [274] and tropical sprue [275]; autoimmune splenic atrophy including that associated with autoimmune thyroid disease, systemic lupus erythematosus [276] and autoimmune polyglandular disease [277]; graft-versus-host disease [278]; following splenic irradiation [279] or Thorotrast administration [280])
Splenic infiltration or replacement (amyloidosis, sarcoidosis, leukaemia and lymphoma (occasionally); carcinoma [281] and sarcoma [282] (rarely), granulomas caused by atypical mycobacterial infection in AIDS [283])
Functional asplenia, e.g. caused by reticuloendothelial overload (early in the course of sickle cell disease, severe haemolytic anaemia and immune-complex or autoimmune disease) [284]

AD, autosomal dominant; AIDS, acquired immunodeficiency syndrome.

(e.g. because of an unstable haemoglobin or because an oxidant drug is administered) large numbers are seen when the pitting action of the spleen is lacking. If there is erythroblast iron overload (e.g. in sideroblastic anaemia or in thalassaemia major) Pappenheimer bodies are very numerous. If the bone marrow is megaloblastic or dyserythropoietic, Howell–Jolly bodies are particularly large and numerous.

Some of the causes of hyposplenism are given in Table 3.12.

Blood film evidence of hyposplenism should be deliberately sought when children present with pneumococcal sepsis [285] or if coeliac disease is suspected.

Non-haemopoietic cells

Non-haemopoietic cells may appear in a blood sample or in a blood film made from a skin-prick sample either because they are present in the circulating blood or because the sample has become contaminated during the process of obtaining it.

Endothelial cells

Endothelial cells (Figs 3.143 & 3.144) are most likely to be detected if blood films are made from the first drop of blood in a needle; this was particularly noted when needles were re-used and were sometimes barbed [286]. Endothelial cells may appear singly or in clusters. They are large cells, often elongated, with diameters of 20–30 μm and a large amount of pale blue or blue-grey cytoplasm. The nucleus is round to oval with a diameter of 10–15 μm and one to three light blue nucleoli. Nuclei may appear grooved.

Increased numbers of endothelial cells are present in conditions with vascular injury (e.g. rickettsial infection, peripheral vascular disease, CMV infection, thrombotic thrombocytopenic purpura (TTP), sickle cell disease and following coronary angioplasty) but even in such circumstances they are very infrequent [287].

Virus-infected cells, interpreted as abnormal endothelial cells, have been detected in films of peripheral blood from patients with immunodeficiency and

Fig. 3.143 Endothelial cells obtained by scraping the vena cava during post-mortem examination. Courtesy of Dr Marjorie Walker, London.

active CMV infection [288]. They were 50–60 μm in diameter with abundant basophilic cytoplasm and a central granular eosinophilic zone that appeared to displace the nucleus.

Epithelial cells

When blood is obtained by skin puncture, epithelial cells from the skin may occasionally be present in the blood film. They are large cells with a small nucleus and large amounts of sky-blue featureless cytoplasm (Fig. 3.145a). Some are anucleate (Fig. 3.145b).

Fat cells

Occasionally, recognizable fat cells are present in a blood film (Fig. 3.146). It is likely that they are derived from subcutaneous fat that is penetrated by the phlebotomy needle.

Amniotic fluid cells

Amniotic fluid cells may be present if contamination occurs during fetal blood sampling.

Non-haemopoietic malignant cells

In various small cell tumours of childhood, tumour cells can circulate in the blood in appreciable numbers and be mistaken for the lymphoblasts of acute lymphoblastic leukaemia. Such circulating cells have been described in neuroblastoma, rhabdomyosarcoma and medulloblastoma [289–291]. In rhabdomyosarcoma, syncytial masses of tumour cells have been seen [292]. Rarely, circulating neuroblastoma cells are associated with neurofibrils [293]. Carcinoma cells can also circulate in the blood but usually in such small numbers that they are unlikely to be noted unless special concentration

Fig. 3.144 Endothelial cells in a peripheral blood film made from a venous blood sample.

(a)

(b)

Fig. 3.145 Epithelial cells in a peripheral blood film prepared from a drop of blood obtained by finger prick: (a) nucleated epithelial cell; and (b) anucleate epithelial cell.

Fig. 3.146 A clump of fat cells, likely to represent subcutaneous fat, in a blood film prepared from EDTA-anticoagulated venous blood (× 40 objective).

procedures are employed [294]. Rarely, they may be seen on routine blood films (Fig. 3.147). Even more rarely a 'leukaemia' of carcinoma cells occurs. 'Carcinocythaemia' has been most often observed in carcinoma of the lung and breast [295] (Fig. 3.148). Malignant cells in the blood may be in clusters, sometimes large enough clusters to be visible macroscopically (see Fig. 3.4). Rarely, melanoma cells are present in large numbers in the circulation [296]; when they are amelanotic there is a potential for confusion with acute leukaemia. Circulating

melanoma cells containing melanin are more readily identified [297] (Fig. 3.149).

In patients with advanced Hodgkin's disease small numbers of Reed–Sternberg cells and mononuclear Hodgkin's cells have rarely be noted in the blood [298]. Even more rarely, abnormal cells may be present in such numbers as to constitute a Reed–Sternberg cell leukaemia. In one such patient the total WBC was $140 \times 10^9/l$ with 92% malignant cells [299]. These included typical Reed–Sternberg cells (giant cells with a diameter of 12–40 μm with

Fig. 3.147 Malignant cells in the routine peripheral blood film of a patient subsequently found to have widespread metastatic adenocarcinoma.

Fig. 3.148 Malignant cells in the peripheral blood of a patient with a past history of carcinoma of the breast, subsequently found to have widespread metastatic disease.

mirror-image nuclei and giant nucleoli), and multi-nucleated and mononuclear Hodgkin's cells, also with giant nucleoli. However, it should be noted that there are no recent reports of circulating Reed–Sternberg or Hodgkin's cells, even in patients with HIV infection who often present with widespread disease; descriptions of such cells predate the availability of immunophenotyping techniques.

Micro-organisms in blood films

In patients with bacterial, fungal or parasitic infections micro-organisms may be observed free between cells or within red cells, neutrophils or monocytes.

They are visible on an MGG-stained film but special stains aid in their identification. The only micro-organisms that are observed fairly frequently are malarial parasites but the fortuitous observation of other micro-organisms in a blood film can also be diagnostically useful, leading to earlier diagnosis and treatment.

Bacteria

In louse- and tick-borne relapsing fevers the causative spirochetes, e.g. *Borrelia recurrentis*, *Borrelia duttoni*, *Borrelia turicata*, *Borrelia parkeri* or *Borrelia hermsii*, are observed free between cells (Fig. 3.150).

Fig. 3.149 Melanoma cell containing melanin in a buffy coat film from a patient with metastatic malignant melanoma and a leucoerythroblastic anaemia; the bone marrow was among the infiltrated tissues. Courtesy of Dr J. Luckit and Dr D. Swirsky.

Organisms can be detected in the peripheral blood film in 70% of cases of tick-borne relapsing fever [300]. When *Borrelia* species are being sought a thick film is useful.

It is quite uncommon for bacteria other than *Borrelia* to be noted in routine blood films. When present they are most often observed within neutrophils or, occasionally, free between cells. When they are being deliberately sought a buffy coat preparation makes detection more likely. Bacteria

Fig. 3.151 A neutrophil containing diplococci from a patient with fatal *Neisseria meningitidis* septicaemia.

are most often seen in hyposplenic or immunosuppressed subjects and in those with indwelling intravenous lines or overwhelming infections. Bacteria that have been observed within neutrophils in routine peripheral blood films include streptococci, staphylococci, *Streptococcus pneumoniae* (pneumococcus), *Neisseria meningitides* (meningococcus) (Fig. 3.151), *Clostridium perfringens* (previously known as *Clostridium welchii*), *Yersinia pestis*, *Bacteroides distasonis* [301], *Corynebacterium* species [301], *Capnocytophaga canimorsus* (previously known as the DF-2 organism) (Fig. 3.152) [302], *Escherichia coli* [303], *Klebsiella*

Fig. 3.150 *Borrelia* species in the peripheral blood of a child of a febrile North African child.

(a)

(b)

Fig. 3.152 Peripheral blood film from a patient who had been bitten by a dog showing *Capnocytophaga canimorsus*: (a) MGG stain; (b) Gram stain. Courtesy of Dr Ilsa Louw, Cape Town.

Fig. 3.153 Peripheral blood film showing multiple small rod-shaped bacilli associated with erythrocytes in a patient with bartonellosis. There is also a red cell containing a Howell–Jolly body. Courtesy of Dr D. Swirsky and the late Professor Sir John Dacie, London.

pneumoniae [303], *Klebsiella oxytoca* [304] and *Pseudomonas aeruginosa* [305].

In bartonellosis or Oroya fever (Fig. 3.153), a disease confined to South America, the causative organism, a flagellated bacillus, is present on the surface of red cells and infection leads to spherocytosis and haemolytic anaemia. The organisms, *Bartonella bacilliformis*, stain deep red or purple on an MGG stain [306]. *Bartonella quintana*, the causative organism of trench fever, has been detected in peripheral blood erythrocytes by immunofluores-

cence [307] so it is possible that the bacilli could be detected in an MGG-stained film. Haemotropic bacilli, *Tropheryma whipplei* (previously *Tropheryma whippelii*), have also been reported in Whipple's disease in hyposplenic subjects (Fig. 3.154) and have been recognized as PAS-positive inclusions in the monocytes of another patient [308]. Intraerythrocytic *Grahamella* species have been reported in three Eastern European patients [309]. Rod-shaped structures, apparently associated with red cells and suspected of being bacterial in nature, have been

Fig. 3.154 Peripheral blood film from a hyposplenic patient with Whipple's disease showing a red cell fragment, a red cell containing a Howell–Jolly body and several red cells with which are associated numerous delicate rod-shaped bacilli. Wright's stain. Courtesy of Dr B.J. Patterson, Toronto.

reported in some patients with thrombotic thrombocytopenic purpura [310].

Micro-organisms are occasionally seen in monocytes and even in lymphocytes and platelets. *Tropheryma whipplei* has been detected in monocytes by means of immunocytochemical staining of a buffy coat preparation [311]. In HIV infection, the observation of rod-shaped negative images within monocytes or neutrophils suggests *Mycobacterium avium intracellulare* infection [312]. Ehrlichia may be detected in neutrophils, monocytes and, occasionally, lymphocytes. They may appear as small single organisms or as morulae containing a number of elemental bodies (Fig. 3.155). In human granulocytic ehrlichiosis, caused by *Ehrlichia phagocytophila* (which forms a single species with *Ehrlichia equi* and is currently known as *Anaplasma phagocytophilum*), the organisms are in granulocytes [313]. *Ehrlichia ewingii*, an organism closely related to *Ehrlichia canis*, also infects man and is associated with morulae in granulocytes [313,314]. Human monocytic ehrlichiosis, caused by *Ehrlichia chaffeensis*, has organisms mainly in monocytes but occasionally in lymphocytes (which may be atypical) or neutrophils [315,316]. Ehrlichia inclusions in peripheral blood leucocytes are more often seen in human granulocytic ehrlichiosis than in human monocytic ehrlichiosis. Cases of ehrlichiosis have mainly been described in the USA but the disease also occurs Europe [317]. Ehrlichia have been described in the neutrophils of a neonate with transplacentally acquired human

Fig. 3.155 Peripheral blood of a patient with ehrlichiosis showing the morular form of the organism within a neutrophil. Courtesy of Dr Vandita Johari, Minneapolis.

granulocytic ehrlichiosis [318]. In Venezuela there is a species of Ehrlichia that appears predominantly in platelets, which has been detected in individuals who have had close contact with dogs [319]; one clinically affected patient has been described [320].

Bacteria in peripheral blood films may have characteristic features that give a clue to their identity. They can be identified as cocci or bacilli and, following a Gram stain, as Gram negative or Gram positive. Spore forming by Clostridia has been observed [321]. The plague bacillus, *Yersinia pestis*

Fig. 3.156 Peripheral blood film from a patient with plague showing the bipolar bacilli of *Yersinia pestis*. Courtesy of the American Society of Haematology Slide Bank.

(Fig. 3.156), is found extracellularly and may be bipolar in a Romanowsky stain [322]. Ehrlichia are distinctive (see above). Bacteria that have colonized indwelling venous lines despite antibiotic therapy may be morphologically abnormal, appearing filamentous as a consequence of failure of septation (Fig. 3.157) [322].

The finding of bacteria in a blood film is usually highly significant. The exception is with cord blood samples which are often collected in circumstances in which bacterial contamination is likely; if they are left at room temperature and delay occurs in delivery to the laboratory it is not uncommon to see bacteria in stained films.

Fungi

Fungi have also been observed in peripheral blood films, particularly in patients with indwelling central venous lines who are also neutropenic or have defective immunity. They may be observed free or within neutrophils or monocytes. Fungi which have been observed in neutrophils include *Candida albicans*, *Candida parapsilosis* [323] (Fig. 3.158), *Candida glabrata*, *Candida tropicalis* [324], *Candida krusei* [324], *Candida guilliermondii* [324], *Hansenula anomala* [325], *Histoplasma capsulatum* (Figs 3.159 and 3.160), *Cryp-tococcus neoformans* [326], *Penicillium marneffei* (Fig. 3.161) [327] and *Rhodotorula glutinis* [324] and in monocytes *Histoplasma capsulatum* and *Penicillium marneffei* [327]. *Malassezia furfur* has been observed extracellularly [328]. *Rhodotorula rubra* has also been observed in blood films [324]. In *Candida albicans* infection, both yeast forms and pseudo-hyphae have been observed [329]. In febrile neutropenic patients a search of the peripheral blood film can confirm a diagnosis of systemic fungal infection some days in advance of positive cultures in a significant proportion of patients [325].

Parasites

Some parasites, such as malaria parasites and babesiae, are predominantly blood parasites, while others, such as filariae, have part of their life cycle in the blood. Parasites that may be detected in the

Fig. 3.157 *Klebsiella oxytoca* in a film of blood obtained from an indwelling venous line, showing failure of septation: (a) MGG stain. *Continued*

(a)

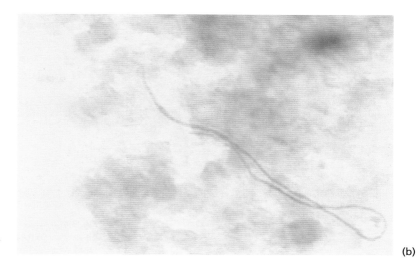

Fig. 3.157 *Continued* (b) Gram stain. Courtesy of Dr Carol Barton and Mr J. Kitaruth, Reading.

(b)

(a)

(b)

Fig. 3.158 *Candida parapsilosis* in a peripheral blood film: (a) within neutrophils; and (b) free between red cells. Several organisms are budding. Courtesy of Dr B. Vadher and Dr Marilyn Treacy, London.

blood film are listed with their geographical distribution in Tables 3.13 and 3.14.

Malaria and babesiosis

Although malaria parasites may be detected in MGG-stained blood films, their detection and identification is facilitated by Leishman or Giemsa staining at a higher pH. A thick film is preferable for detection of parasites and a thin film for iden-

tification of the species. A thick film should be examined for at least 5 minutes before being considered negative. If only a thin film is available it should not be considered negative until it has been examined for at least 15 minutes or until 200 high power fields or the whole blood film have been examined. Partially immune subjects are particularly likely to have a low parasite count so that a prolonged search may be required for parasite detection. In patients with a strong suspicion of

Fig. 3.159 A band neutrophil in a buffy coat film showing three *Histoplasma capsulatum*. Courtesy of Dr Sian Lewis, Oxford.

Fig. 3.160 Methenamine silver stain of *Histoplasma capsulatum* in the peripheral blood. Courtesy of Dr H. Musa, Minneapolis.

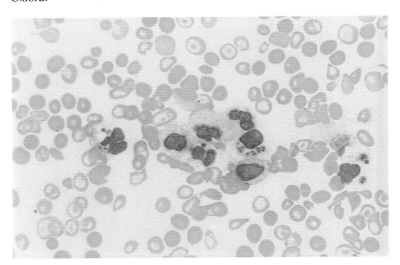

Fig. 3.161 *Penicillium marneffei* in the peripheral blood of a patient with AIDS. Courtesy of Dr K.F. Wong, Hong Kong.

malaria whose initial films are negative, repeated blood examinations may be needed. *Plasmodium falciparum* is associated with the highest parasite counts with sometimes 10–40% of red cells being parasitized; paradoxically, patients may be seriously ill with no parasites being detectable on initial blood examination. This is consequent on parasitized red cells being sequestered in tissues. When *P. falciparum* is detected, a count of the proportion of cells that are parasitized should be made to allow monitoring during therapy; a Miller graticule, as used for reticulocyte counts, facilitates this. Alternatively, parasites can be counted in a thick film, their numbers being related to the number of leucocytes, to produce an absolute count. A failure of the parasite count to fall indicates a drug-resistant parasite. Useful features in distinguishing between the four species are summarized in Fig. 3.162 and illustrated in Figs 3.163–3.166.

Table 3.13 Protozoan parasites that may be detected in blood films.

Parasite	Disease or common name	Usual distribution
Sporozoans		
Plasmodium falciparum	Malignant tertian malaria	Widespread in tropics and sub-tropics, particularly in Africa
Plasmodium vivax	Benign tertian malaria	Widespread in tropics and occurs also in some temperate zones; quite uncommon in West and Central Africa
Plasmodium malariae	Quartan malaria	Scattered in the tropics
Plasmodium ovale	Benign tertian malaria	Tropical West Africa; scattered foci elsewhere including tropical Asia, New Guinea and the Western Pacific
Plasmodium knowlesi		Malaysian Borneo [330]
Babesia microti	Babesiosis	North-Eastern coastal USA, West Coast and Mid-West
Babesia equi	Babesiosis	California
Babesia divergens	Babesiosis	Europe
Haemoflagellates		
Trypanosoma brucei rhodesiense	Sleeping sickness	East Africa
Trypanosoma brucei gambiense	Sleeping sickness	Tropical West and Central Africa
Trypanosoma cruzi	South American trypanosomiasis or Chagas' disease	Wide area of Central and South America
Trypanosoma rangeli	Non-pathogenic	Central and South America
Leishmania donovani	Visceral leishmaniasis or kala azar	India, China, Central Asia, Central and Northern Africa, Portugal, the Mediterranean littoral, Central and South America

Table 3.14 Nematode (family filariidae) parasites that may be detected in blood films.

Parasite	Disease or common name	Usual distribution
Wuchereria bancrofti	Filariasis—end stage may be elephantiasis	Widespread in tropics and sub-tropics, particularly Asia, Polynesia, New Guinea, Africa and Central and South America
Brugia malayi	Filariasis—end stage may be elephantiasis	India, South East Asia, China, Japan
Loa loa	Eye worm or Calabar swellings	African equatorial rainforest and its fringes
Mansonella perstans	Persistent filariasis, usually non-pathogenic	Tropical Africa, Central and South America
Mansonella ozzardi	Ozzard's filariasis, usually non-pathogenic	Central and South America, West Indies
Onchocerca volvulus	Onchocerciasis (river blindness)	Central and West Africa and Sudan, Central America

	General features and changes in red cells	Early trophozoite (ring form)	Mature trophozoite
Plasmodium vivax	Red cells much enlarged, irregular and pale with fine red stippling (Schüffner's dots); usually low or moderate parasitaemia; all stages of life cycle often present; sometimes multiple parasites per cell	Thick rings, 1/3–1/2 the diameter of the red cell A few Schüffner's dots Accolé (shoulder) forms and double dots less common than with *P. falciparum*	Ameboid rings, 1/2–2/3 the diameter of the red cell Pale blue or lilac parasite with prominent central valuole Indistinct outline Scattered fine yellowish-brown pigment granules or rods
Plasmodium ovale	Red cells enlarged but not as much as with *P. vivax*; cells pale and some are oval or pear-shaped; some are ragged (fimbriated) at one or both ends; fine to coarse red stippling (Schüffner's dots); low parasitaemia; often fewer stages present than with *P. vivax*	Thick, compact rings, 1/3–1/2 the diameter of the red cell Numerous Schüffner's dots but paler than with *P. vivax*	Thick rings, less irregular than those of *P. vivax*, 1/3–1/2 the diameter of the red cell Less prominent vacuole, distinct outline Yellowish-brown pigment which is coarser and darker than that of *P. vivax* Schüffner's dots prominent
Plasmodium falciparum	Cells not enlarged; staining characteristics usually unaltered but sometimes there are some pale cells; sometimes multiple parasites per cell and heavy parasitaemia (10–40% of cells); often only ring forms are present	Delicate rings, 1/6–1/4 the diameter of the red cell Double dots and accolé forms common	Fairly delicate rings, 1/3–1/2 the diameter of the red cell Red-mauve stippling (Maurer's dots or clefts) may be present Mature trophozoites are less often present in peripheral blood than ring forms
Plasmodium malariae	Cells not enlarged, sometimes contracted; staining characteristics not altered; lowest degree of parasitaemia; multiple parasites per cell rare; no stippling unless overstained; all stages usually present	Small, thick, compact rings Small chromatin dot which may be inside the ring Double dots and accolé forms rare	Ameboid form more compact than *P. vivax* Sometimes angular or band forms Heavy, dark yellow-brown pigment No stippling unless overstained

(a)

Fig. 3.162 Features that are useful in distinguishing between the different species of malaria parasites.

Early schizont	Late schizont	Gametocyte	
		Macrogametocyte	**Microgametocyte**
Rounded or irregular Ameboid Loose central mass of fine yellowish-brown pigment Schizont almost fills cell Schüffner's dots	12–24 (usually 16–24) medium-sized merozoites 1–2 clumps of peripheral pigment Schizont almost fills cell Schüffner's dots	Round or ovoid, almost fills enlarged cell Blue cytoplasm Eccentric compact red nucleus Scattered pigment	Round or ovoid, as large as a normal red cell but does not fill the enlarged red cell Faintly staining Larger, lighter red central or eccentric nucleus Fine, scattered pigment
Round, compact Darkish brown pigment, heavier and coarser than that of *P. vivax* Schüffner's dots	6–12 (usually 8) large merozoites arranged irregularly like a bunch of grapes Central pigment Schüffner's dots	Similar to *P. vivax* but somewhat smaller Pigment coarser and blacker, scattered but mainly near the periphery	Similar to *P. vivax* but smaller
Not usually seen in blood Very small, ameboid Scattered light brown to black pigment	Not usually seen in blood 8–32 (usually few) very small merozoites; grouped irregularly Peripheral clump of coarse dark brown pigment	Sickle or crescent shaped Deforms cell which often appears empty of haemoglobin Blue cytoplasm Compact central nucleus with pigment aggregated around it	Oval or crescentic with blunted ends Pale blue or pink Large pale nucleus with pigment more scattered than in macrogametocyte
Compact, round, fills red cell Coarse dark yellow-brown pigment	6–12 (usually 8–10) large merozoites, arranged symmetrically, often in a rosette or daisy head formation Central coarse dark yellowish-brown pigment	Similar to *P. vivax* but smaller, round or oval, almost fills cell, blue with a dark nucleus Prominent pigment concentrated at centre and periphery	Similar to *P. vivax* but smaller, pink or paler blue than macrogametocyte with a larger, paler nucleus Prominent pigment

(b)

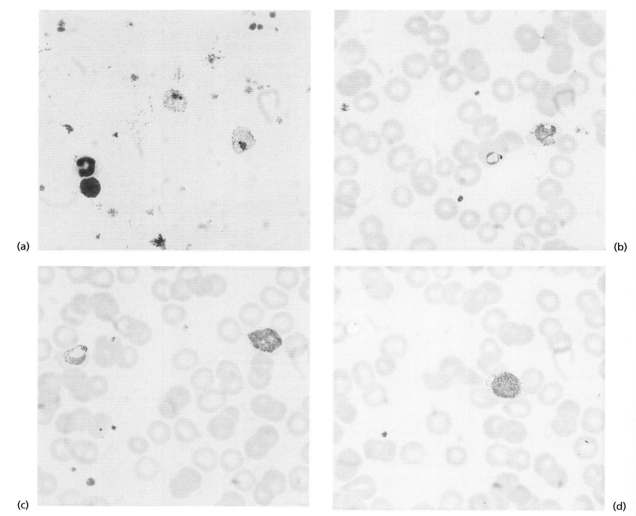

(a)

(b)

(c)

(d)

Fig. 3.163 Stages in the life cycle of *Plasmodium vivax* shown in Giemsa-stained peripheral blood thick (a) and thin (b–h) films: (a) two ring forms within red cell ghosts; (b) a ring form and an ameboid trophozoite; both the parasitized cells are enlarged and decolorized and contain faint Schüffner's dots; (c) a ring form and an early schizont containing two chromatin masses; both parasitized cells are decolorized and contain faint Schüffner's dots; (d) a microgametocyte—the pigment is fine and scattered and the parasite does not completely fill the cell. (e) a macrogametocyte—the pigment is fine and scattered and the parasite completely fills the cell and is larger than the non-parasitized red cells; (f) exflagellation of microgametes from a gametocyte—this stage of the parasite life cycle usually occurs in the stomach of the mosquito; (g) microgametes—this stage of the parasite life cycle usually occurs in the stomach of the mosquito; (h) microgametes clustered around three macrogametes—it appears that one microgamete has fertilized a macrogamete since its nucleus appears to have penetrated the macrogamete—this stage of the parasite life cycle usually occurs in the stomach of the mosquito; (i) ookinete—this stage of the malaria parasite life cycle usually occurs in the stomach of the mosquito and is very rarely seen in the peripheral blood of man. Courtesy of Dr Wendi Bailey, Liverpool.

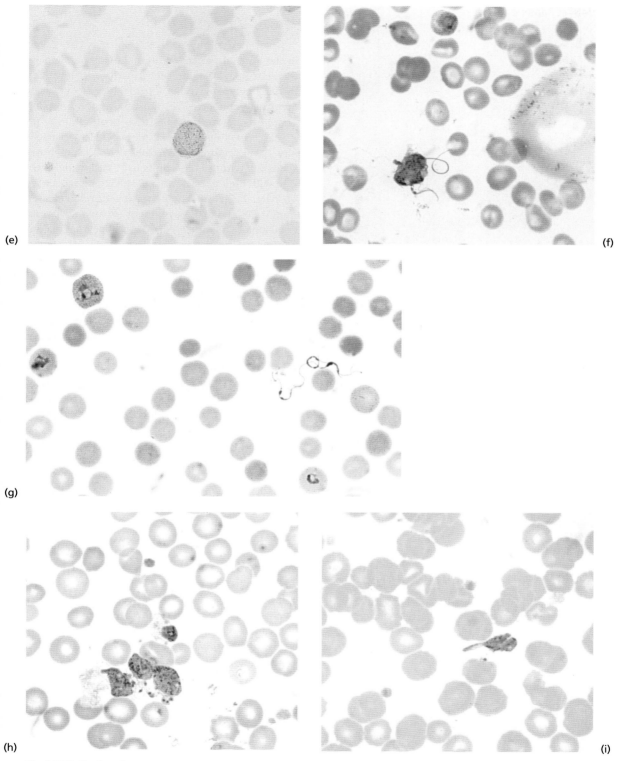

(e)

(f)

(g)

(h)

(i)

Fig. 3.163 *Continued*

(a)

(b)

Fig. 3.164 Stages in the life cycle of *Plasmodium ovale* in Giemsa-stained thin films: (a) a late trophozoite in an enlarged, decolorized and oval red cell which has a fimbriated end; pigment is coarser and darker than in *Plasmodium vivax*, the parasite is more compact and Schüffner's dots are more prominent; (b) a schizont containing eight merozoites; coarse pigment is clustered centrally.

In addition to these four species, a focus of human infection with the simian parasite, *Plasmodium knowlesi*, has been described in Malaysian Borneo [330]; morphologically this parasite is difficult to distinguish from *Plasmodium malariae*.

Associated abnormalities that may be noted in the films of patients with malaria are anaemia—the reticulocyte count being inappropriately low, thrombocytopenia, lymphopenia, lymphocytosis or atypical lymphocytes, eosinopenia (and suppression of pre-existing eosinophilia), early neutrophilia (with *P. falciparum*), neutropenia, monocytosis, occasionally phagocytosed merozoites and sometimes schizonts within neutrophils in *P. falciparum* infection with high parasitaemia [331,332], phagocytosis of parasitized and non-parasitized red cells by monocytes and malaria pigment—in monocytes and occasionally in neutrophils. Thrombocytopenia can be a diagnostically useful feature, alerting the laboratory or the clinician to the likelihood of malaria. In one study of children presenting to an Accident and Emergency Department in London one-quarter of patients with a platelet count of less than $150 \times 10^9/l$ were found to have malaria [333]; thrombocytopenia was seen in association with both falciparum and vivax malaria. Malaria pigment in leucocytes is mainly associated with *P. falciparum* malaria. The pigment is haemozoin, a degradation product of haemoglobin. It can be visualized readily in stained or unstained films and is birefringent when polarized light is used [334]. The pigment is released into the plasma during schizogony [331] and is then phagocytosed. The percentage of leucocytes containing pigment therefore reflects the sequestered parasite burden and has been found to be of prognostic significance [331]. Monocytes containing malarial pigment can often be found in the blood for many days after parasitized red cells have disappeared; this can be useful in making a retrospective diagnosis of malaria [335]. Leucocytosis, neutrophilia, lymphocytosis and monocytosis correlate with severity of malaria [332]. In multivariate analysis leucocytosis, lymphocytosis and monocytopenia correlate with a higher rate of death [332].

The histograms or scatter plots of automated full blood counters may be abnormal in the presence of malarial parasites.

Babesiosis is an uncommon tick-borne parasitic disease [336], which can easily be confused with malaria. *Babesia microti* is endemic in southern New England, southern New York state, Wisconsin and Minnesota. *Babesia divergens* infection occurs sporadically in the USA, Europe (including Ireland) and

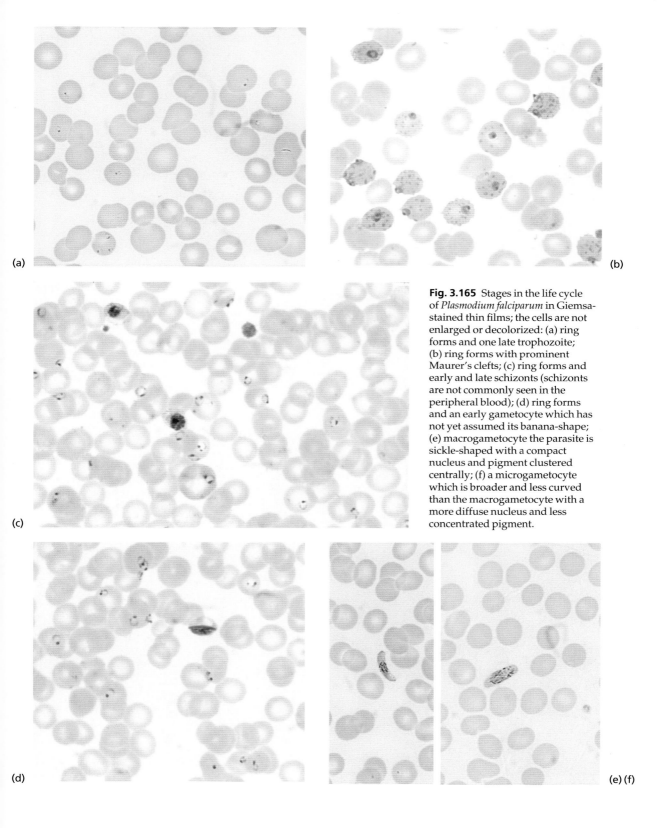

Fig. 3.165 Stages in the life cycle of *Plasmodium falciparum* in Giemsa-stained thin films; the cells are not enlarged or decolorized: (a) ring forms and one late trophozoite; (b) ring forms with prominent Maurer's clefts; (c) ring forms and early and late schizonts (schizonts are not commonly seen in the peripheral blood); (d) ring forms and an early gametocyte which has not yet assumed its banana-shape; (e) macrogametocyte the parasite is sickle-shaped with a compact nucleus and pigment clustered centrally; (f) a microgametocyte which is broader and less curved than the macrogametocyte with a more diffuse nucleus and less concentrated pigment.

(a)

(b)

(c)

(d)

(e) (f)

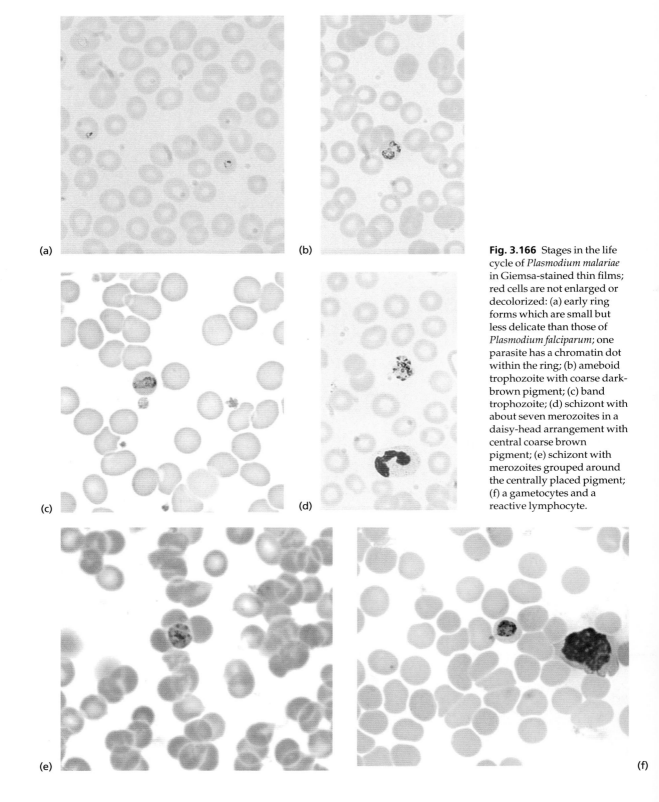

Fig. 3.166 Stages in the life cycle of *Plasmodium malariae* in Giemsa-stained thin films; red cells are not enlarged or decolorized: (a) early ring forms which are small but less delicate than those of *Plasmodium falciparum*; one parasite has a chromatin dot within the ring; (b) ameboid trophozoite with coarse dark-brown pigment; (c) band trophozoite; (d) schizont with about seven merozoites in a daisy-head arrangement with central coarse brown pigment; (e) schizont with merozoites grouped around the centrally placed pigment; (f) a gametocytes and a reactive lymphocyte.

Asia. About 30 human cases have been described in Europe, more than three-quarters of them in hyposplenic patients [337]. *Babesia bovis* infection also occurs in Europe [338]. The trophozoites of *Babesia* species are small rings, similar to those of *P. falciparum*, 1–5 μm in diameter with one, two or three chromatin dots and scanty cytoplasm. Sometimes they are pyriform (pear-shaped) and either paired (Fig. 3.167a) or have the pointed ends of four parasites being in contact to give a Maltese cross formation (Fig. 3.167b). Extracellular parasites are sometimes seen [339] and may form clusters [338]. *Babesia microti* is associated with Maltese cross and ring forms, the latter with small to large cytoplasmic vacuoles [340]. The ring forms of *Babesia* species may be even smaller than those of *P. falciparum* (Fig. 3.168); this and the vacuolation of the parasite, the pleomorphism of the ring forms, the presence of extracellular trophozoites and the absence of haemozoin ('malarial pigment'), can help in making

(a)   (b)

Fig. 3.167 Blood film from a splenectomized monkey parasitized by *Babesia microti*: (a) a single ring form and a pair of pyriform parasites; (b) a single ring form and four pyriform parasites in a tetrad or Maltese cross formation. Courtesy of Mr J. Williams, London.

Fig. 3.168 Blood film from a hyposplenic patient with babesiosis caused by *Babesia divergens* showing numerous parasites including a Maltese cross formation and paired pyriform parasites. Courtesy of Mr C. Murphy, Cork.

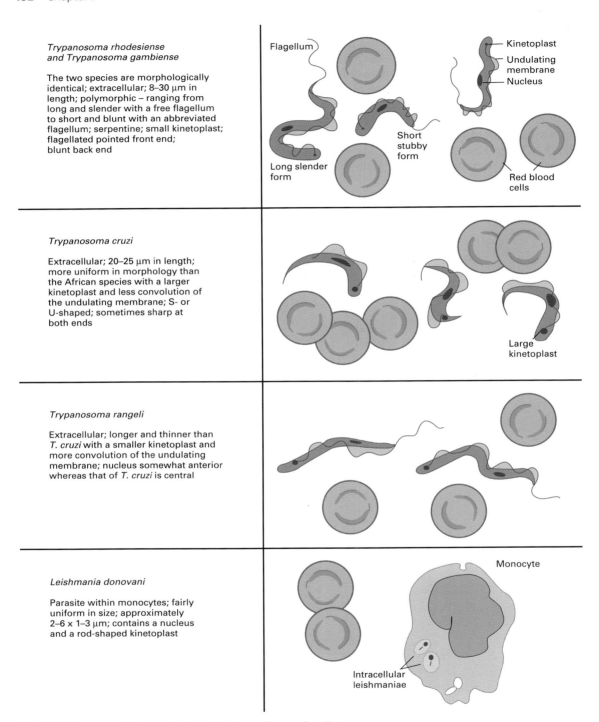

*Trypanosoma rhodesiense
and Trypanosoma gambiense*

The two species are morphologically
identical; extracellular; 8–30 μm in
length; polymorphic – ranging from
long and slender with a free flagellum
to short and blunt with an abbreviated
flagellum; serpentine; small kinetoplast;
flagellated pointed front end;
blunt back end

Trypanosoma cruzi

Extracellular; 20–25 μm in length;
more uniform in morphology than
the African species with a larger
kinetoplast and less convolution of
the undulating membrane; S- or
U-shaped; sometimes sharp at
both ends

Trypanosoma rangeli

Extracellular; longer and thinner than
T. cruzi with a smaller kinetoplast and
more convolution of the undulating
membrane; nucleus somewhat anterior
whereas that of *T. cruzi* is central

Leishmania donovani

Parasite within monocytes; fairly
uniform in size; approximately
2–6 x 1–3 μm; contains a nucleus
and a rod-shaped kinetoplast

Fig. 3.169 Summary of the morphological features of haemoflagellates.

the distinction. *Babesia divergens* usually has pyriform pairs of parasites at the periphery of the erythrocyte [340]. Babesiosis occurs particularly but not exclusively in hyposplenic subjects in whom 25% or more of cells may be parasitized. In those with a functioning spleen the level of parasitaemia is usually low but in HIV-positive and immunosuppressed patients more severe infection occurs [339]. The method of detection is by thick and thin film examination, as for malaria. There is often associated thrombocytopenia.

Other tests

Malaria can be diagnosed immunologically using commercially available strips for immunochromatographic detection of either a *P. falciparum* antigen, histidine-rich protein 2, or parasitic lactate dehydrogenase (pLDH) [340]. The strips for detection of pLDH distinguish between *P. falciparum* and other malaria parasites but do not distinguish other malaria parasites from each other. They are sensitive and specific for the detection of *P. falciparum* and are sensitive for the detection of *P. vivax*; however, only around half of cases of *P. ovale* or *P. malariae* infection are detected [341]. Tests for histidine-rich protein 2 remain positive for some time after an acute infection whereas positivity for pLDH correlates with the presence of viable organisms and may give a clue to a drug-resistant infection. False positive tests may be observed in patients with rheumatoid arthritis with both types of kit [342].

Babesiosis can be diagnosed serologically (although cross-reactivity with malaria can occur) and by polymerase chain reaction (PCR) [339].

Toxoplasmosis

Rarely *Toxoplasma gondii* has been identified in the peripheral blood in patients with toxoplasmosis and underlying immune deficiency [343,344]. Organisms may be extracellular or within neutrophils [344].

Infection by haemoflagellates

The morphological features of haemoflagellates that may be found in the peripheral blood are summarized in Fig. 3.169. Trypanosomes may be detected in the peripheral blood as motile, extracellular parasites [345]. They have a slender body and move by means of a flagellum extending from the kinetoplast at the rear end of the parasite to the front end where the flagellum is free (Figs 3.170 & 3.171); the flagellum is joined to the body by an undulating membrane. The parasite may be seen moving in a wet preparation when a drop of anticoagulated blood is placed on a slide, beneath a coverslip, for microscopic examination. They may also be detected in fixed preparations such as thick or thin films or buffy coat films. Scanty parasites are more readily detected by examining the sediment of 10–20 ml of haemolysed blood. *Trypanosoma brucei rhodesiense* and *Trypanosoma brucei gambiense* (see Fig. 3.170) are morphologically identical but their geographical distributions differ (see Table 3.13). Examination of the peripheral blood is more likely to be useful in the case of *T. brucei rhodesiense*. Concentration techniques may be needed with *T. brucei gambiense*, or parasites may be undetectable in the blood, lymph node puncture being required for diagnosis. Patients with trypanosomiasis often have a normocytic normochromic anaemia and thrombocytopenia [346].

Trypanosoma cruzi (see Fig. 3.171), the causative agent of Chagas' disease, differs morphologically from the African parasites. It is rarely detected by direct examination of the blood, concentration procedures usually being required. Examining a wet preparation of buffy coat for motile parasites can be useful. It can be distinguished on morphological grounds from the non-pathogenic *Trypanosoma rangeli*, which has a similar geographical distribution (see Fig. 3.169). Lymphocytosis and mild anaemia may be observed in the acute phase of Chagas' disease.

Leishmania donovani, the causative organism of kala azar, may be detected in monocytes or neutrophils in the peripheral blood, in thick or thin films or in buffy coat preparations (Fig. 3.172). Examination of a peripheral blood film may avoid the need for a bone marrow or splenic aspiration but these procedures are much more sensitive than peripheral blood examination. Both peripheral blood and bone marrow culture are more sensitive than microscopy. Associated features that may be noted in patients with kala azar are anaemia, leucopenia, neutropenia, thrombocytopenia and

Fig. 3.170 *Trypanosoma brucei gambiense*; the parasites are serpentine with a small kinetoplast (× 40 objective).

(a)

Fig. 3.171 *Trypanosoma cruzi*; the parasite is curved but not usually serpentine and has a large kinetoplast (× 40 objective).

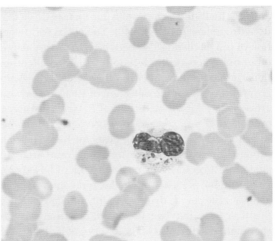

(b)

Fig. 3.172 *Leishmania donovani* in: (a) a monocyte; and (b) a neutrophil in the peripheral blood of a patient with AIDS.

increased rouleaux formation. A cryoglobulin may be present and paraproteins can occur.

Other tests

Rapid immunological methods are available for the detection of *T. brucei gambiense* and *T. brucei rhode-*

siense antigens [340]. Immunological techniques are also applicable to chronic *T. cruzi* infection. A variety of sensitive immunological tests are also available for the diagnosis of leishmaniasis.

Filariasis

In filariasis, adult worms reside in tissues and release microfilariae into the blood-stream.

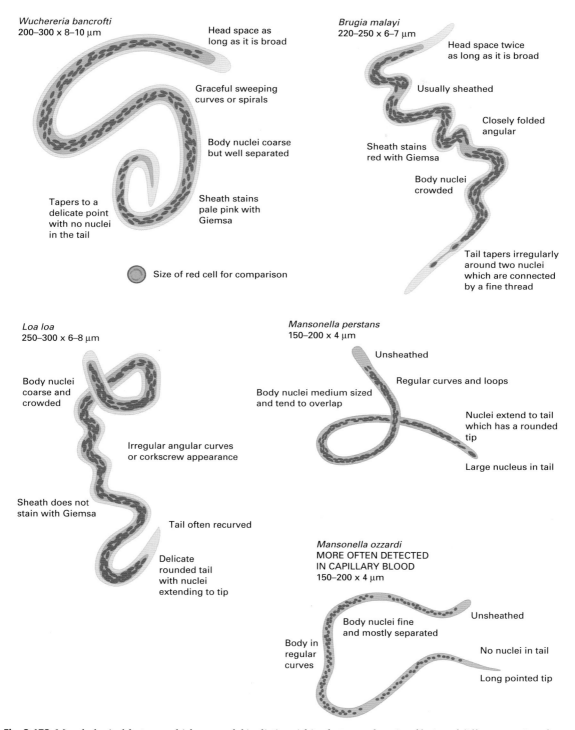

Wuchereria bancrofti
200–300 x 8–10 μm

Head space as long as it is broad

Graceful sweeping curves or spirals

Body nuclei coarse but well separated

Tapers to a delicate point with no nuclei in the tail

Sheath stains pale pink with Giemsa

Size of red cell for comparison

Brugia malayi
220–250 x 6–7 μm

Head space twice as long as it is broad

Usually sheathed

Closely folded angular

Sheath stains red with Giemsa

Body nuclei crowded

Tail tapers irregularly around two nuclei which are connected by a fine thread

Loa loa
250–300 x 6–8 μm

Body nuclei coarse and crowded

Irregular angular curves or corkscrew appearance

Sheath does not stain with Giemsa

Tail often recurved

Delicate rounded tail with nuclei extending to tip

Mansonella perstans
150–200 x 4 μm

Unsheathed

Regular curves and loops

Body nuclei medium sized and tend to overlap

Nuclei extend to tail which has a rounded tip

Large nucleus in tail

Mansonella ozzardi
MORE OFTEN DETECTED IN CAPILLARY BLOOD
150–200 x 4 μm

Body nuclei fine and mostly separated

Unsheathed

Body in regular curves

No nuclei in tail

Long pointed tip

Fig. 3.173 Morphological features which are useful in distinguishing between the microfilariae of different species of filaria.

(a)

(b)

Fig. 3.174 Microfilariae of *Wuchereria bancrofti* in thick films: (a) microfilaria showing the negative impression of the sheath (× 40 objective); (b) tail of a microfilaria showing that the nuclei do not extend into the tail.

Microfilariae are detectable during the acute phase of the disease, but are not detectable in patients with chronic tissue damage but without active disease. As the microfilariae are motile, examination of a wet preparation is often useful; they can also be detected in thick and thin films. Repeated blood examinations may be needed and blood specimens must be obtained at an appropriate time for the species being sought: *Wuchereria bancrofti* and *Brugia malayi* release their microfilariae at night, whereas those of *Loa loa* are released during the day. *Mansonella ozzardi* is non-periodic. It lives in skin capillaries so may be more readily identified in capillary blood [347]. *Mansonella perstans* is usually non-periodic but release may be nocturnal or, less often, diurnal.

Morphological features that are useful in distinguishing the various microfilariae are summarized in Fig. 3.173 and illustrated in Figs 3.174–3.177. In general, pathogenic filariae are sheathed and non-pathogenic are non-sheathed. However, *B. malayi* is sometimes seen unsheathed [347]. *Brugia timori*, which is confined to Lesser Sunda Island of Indonesia, is similar to *B. malayi* but it is longer with fewer body kinks, a longer space at the head end, less dense nuclei and less intense staining [347]. *Onchocerca volvulus* is occasionally seen in the blood, especially in heavy infections and after therapy [347].

Fig. 3.175 Microfilariae of *Brugia malayi* in thick film showing the widely separated tail nuclei. Courtesy of Dr S. Abdalla, London.

(a)

Fig. 3.176 Microfilariae of *Loa loa*: (a) a thick film showing the head and tail of microfilariae; nuclei extend to the tail (× 40 objective); (b) the tail of a microfilaria in a thin film showing the negative impression of the sheath; the nuclei extend to the tail.

(b)

Fig. 3.177 Microfilaria of *Mansonella perstans* in a thin film. Courtesy of Dr S. Abdalla.

Microfilariae moving through tissues are responsible for the syndrome known as tropical eosinophilia in which respiratory symptoms are associated with eosinophilia, increased rouleaux formation and an elevated ESR. However, microfilariae are not usually detectable in the blood of patients with tropical eosinophilia.

Other tests

Rapid simple immunological tests for the detection of *Wuchereria bancrofti* antigens are available [340]. Tests for *Loa loa* are under development.

Further learning resources for blood film morphology

Lewis SM, Bain BJ and Swirsky DM. *Bench Aids in the Morphological Diagnosis of Anaemia*. World Health Organization, Geneva, 2001. ISBN 92-4-154532-1

Bain BJ (2005) Diagnosis from the blood smear. *N Engl J Med*, **353**, 498–507.

Bain BJ, *Interactive Haematology Imagebank* (CD-ROM). Blackwell Science, Oxford, 1999.

For images of malaria and other parasites see www.med.cmu.ac.th/dept/parasite/default.htm (Chiang Mai University, Thailand) and then click on 'Image' or 'parasite web link' (both useful) or www.biosci.ohio-state.edu/~parasite/malaria_images.html (Ohio State University) or www.dpd.cdc.gov/dpdx/HTML/Image_Library.htm (Centers of Disease Control and Prevention, USA) or www.rph.wa.gov.au (Royal Perth Hospital, West Australia, click on malaria information for learn and test yourself site).

Tropical Health Technology, Doddington, Cambridgeshire www.tht.ndirect.co.uk (low cost books and bench aids for developing countries):
Learning Bench Aid No 1. Malaria
Learning Bench Aid No 2. African and S. American Trypanosomiasis—Leishmaniasis
Learning Bench Aid No 3. Microscopical Diagnosis of Lymphatic Filariasis, Loiasis, Onchocerciasis
Learning Bench Aid No 7. Blood: Normal cells—Anaemias—Infections—Leukaemias

Test your knowledge

Multiple choice questions (MCQs)

(1–5 answers may be correct)

MCQ 3.1 Elliptocytosis is normal in
(a) Camels
(b) Elephants
(c) Lizards
(d) Llamas
(e) Penguins

MCQ 3.2 Acanthocytes can result from
(a) Prolonged storage of EDTA-anticoagulated blood
(b) Abetalipoproteinaemia
(c) The McLeod phenotype
(d) Rh null disease
(e) Liver failure

MCQ 3.3 Neutrophil hypersegmentation can result from
(a) Iron deficiency
(b) Vitamin B$_{12}$ deficiency
(c) Folic acid deficiency
(d) Renal failure
(e) Liver failure

MCQ 3.4 Persistent or transient hyposplenism can result from
(a) Coeliac disease
(b) Severe autoimmune haemolytic anaemia
(c) Autoimmune thrombocytopenic purpura
(d) Splenic infarction
(e) Congenital absence of the spleen

MCQ 3.5 Features of hyposplenism include
(a) Thrombocytopenia
(b) Acanthocytes
(c) Howell–Jolly bodies in red cells
(d) Döhle bodies in neutrophils
(e) Target cells

Extended matching questions (EMQs)

Select the single most appropriate response from the options listed for each of the stems. Each option may be used once, more than once or not at all.

EMQ 3.1
Theme: leucocyte morphology
Options
A HIV infection
B Bacterial infection
C Pelger–Huët anomaly
D Anticancer chemotherapy
E Burns
F Acute myeloid leukaemia
G Chédiak–Higashi syndrome
H Viral infection
I Hyperthermia

Select the option that best explains the leucocyte abnormality

Abnormality	Matching option
1 Toxic granulation	
2 Neutrophil vacuolation	
3 Detached nuclear fragments in neutrophils	
4 Auer rods	
5 Radial segmentation of neutrophil nuclei	

EMQ 3.2
Theme: red cell morphology
Options
A Haemoglobin H disease
B β thalassaemia major
C Hydroxycarbamide therapy
D Sideroblastic anaemia
E Hereditary poikilocytosis
F β thalassaemia trait
G Anaemia of chronic disease
H High affinity haemoglobin
I Lead poisoning
J Low affinity haemoglobin

Select the diagnosis providing a probable explanation of the red cell abnormality

Abnormality	Matching option
1 Basophilic stippling	
2 Pappenheimer bodies	
3 Dimorphic red cells	
4 Macrocytosis	
5 Polycythaemia	

EMQ 3.3
Theme: red cell morphology
Options
A Alcoholic liver disease
B Autoimmune haemolytic anaemia
C Microangiopathic haemolytic anaemia
D Oxidant-induced haemolysis
E Low affinity haemoglobin
F Anaemia of chronic disease
G Renal failure
H Obstructive jaundice

Select the option providing the best explanation of the morphological abnormality

Morphological abnormality	Matching option
1 Spherocytes	
2 Stomatocytes	
3 Irregularly contracted cells	
4 Target cells	
5 Schistocytes	

EMQ 3.4

Theme: inherited anomalies

Options

A Large platelets
B Thrombocytopenia
C Macropolycytes
D Giant abnormally staining neutrophil granules
E Neutrophil hyposegmentation
F Hypogranular platelets
G Very long filaments separating nuclear lobes of neutrophils
H Abnormally small platelets

From the options, select the abnormality likely to be seen in the following conditions

Anomaly	Matching option
1 May–Hegglin anomaly	
2 Chédiak–Higashi anomaly	
3 Bernard–Soulier syndrome	
4 Pelger–Huët anomaly	
5 Myelokathexis	

EMQ 3.5

Theme: red and white cell morphology

Options

A Oxidant-induced haemolytic anaemia
B β thalassaemia trait
C Pyruvate kinase deficiency
D Pyrimidine 5′-nucleotidase deficiency
E Congenital sideroblastic anaemia
F Viral infection
G Bacterial infection
H Hyposplenism
I Acquired sideroblastic anaemia

Select the option providing the most likely explanation of the morphological abnormality

Morphological abnormality	Matching option
1 Basophilic stippling	
2 Pappenheimer bodies plus macrocytosis	
3 Heinz bodies	
4 Howell–Jolly bodies	
5 Döhle bodies	

EMQ 3.6

Theme: white cell abnormalities

Options

A Neutrophilia
B Neutropenia
C Leucoerythroblastic anaemia
D Non-lobulated neutrophils
E Right shift
F Blast cells
G Atypical lymphocytes
H Plasmacytoid lymphocytes

For each clinical situation select the most likely haematological abnormality

Clinical situation	Matching option
1 Pregnancy	
2 Bacterial infection	
3 Infectious mononucleosis	
4 Folic acid deficiency	
5 Administration of corticosteroids	

References

1 Le Coz C and Goosens A (1998) Contact dermatitis from an immersion oil for microscopy. *N Engl J Med*, **339**, 406–407.

2 Nguyen D and Diamond L. *Diagnostic Hematology: a Pattern Approach*. Butterworth-Heinemann, Oxford, 2000.

3 Bain BJ and Liesner R (1996) Pseudopyropoikilocytosis: a striking artefact. *J Clin Pathol*, **49**, 772–773.

4 Hoffbrand AV and Pettit JE. *Sandoz Atlas of Clinical Haematology*. Gower, London, 1988.

5 Mohandas N and Gascard P (2000) What do mouse gene knockouts tell us about the structure and function of the red cell membrane? *Clin Haematol*, **12**, 605–620.

6 Sheehan RG and Frenkel EP (1983) Influence of hemoglobin phenotype on the mean erythrocyte volume. *Acta Haematol*, **69**, 260–265.

7 Maggio A, Gagliano F and Siciliano S (1984) Hemoglobin phenotype and mean erythrocyte volume in Sicilian people. *Acta Haematol*, **71**, 214.

8 Kaplan E, Zuelzer WW and Neel JV (1953) Further studies on haemoglobin C alone and in combination with sickle cell anemia. *Blood*, **8**, 735–746.

9 Fairbanks VF, Gilchrist GS, Brimhall B, Jereb JA and Goldston EC (1979) Hemoglobin E trait reexamined: a cause of microcytosis and erythrocytosis. *Blood*, **53**, 109–115.

10 Bird AR, Wood K, Leisegang F, Mathew CG, Ellis P, Hartley PS and Karabus CD (1984) Hemoglobin E variants: a clinical, haematological and biosynthetic study of four South African families. *Acta Haematol*, **72**, 135–137.

11 Stavem P, Romslo I, Hovig T, Rootwelt K and Emblem R (1985) Ferrochelatase deficiency of the bone marrow in a syndrome of congenital microcytic anaemia with iron overload of the liver and hyperferraemia. *Scand J Haematol*, **34**, 204–206.

12 Horina JH and Wolf P (2000) Epoetin for severe anemia in hepatoerythropoietic porphyria. *N Engl J Med*, **342**, 1294–1295.

13 Shahidi NT, Nathan DE and Diamond LK (1945) Iron deficiency anemia associated with an error of iron metabolism. *J Clin Invest*, **43**, 510–521.

14 Cooley TB (1945) A severe form of hereditary anemia with elliptocytosis: interesting sequence of splenectomy. *Am J Med Sci*, **209**, 561–568.

15 Hartman KR and Barker JA (1996) Microcytic anemia with iron malabsorption: an inherited disorder of iron metabolism. *Am J Hematol*, **51**, 269–275.

16 Andrews NC (1998) Disorders of iron metabolism. *N Engl J Med*, **341**, 1986–1995.

17 Miyoshi I, Saito T and Iwahara Y (2004) Copper deficiency anaemia. *Br J Haematol*, **125**, 106.

18 Yachie A, Niida Y, Toma T, Shimura S, Ohta K, Fujimoto K *et al.* (2000) What did we learn from the first case of human heme oxygenase deficiency? *Acta Haematol*, **103**, Suppl. 1, 82.

19 Priwitzerova M, Pospisilova D, Prchal JT, Hlobilkova A, Mihal V, Indrak K *et al.* (2003) The first human mutation of DMT1 (Nramp2) causes severe defect of erythropoiesis that can be rescued in vitro by Fe-SIH. *Blood*, **102**, 156a.

20 Tulliez M, Testa U, Rochant H, Henri A, Vainchenker W, Toubol J *et al.* (1982) Reticulocytosis, hypochromia, and microcytosis: an unusual presentation of the preleukemic syndrome. *Blood*, **59**, 293–299.

21 Ruocco L, Baldi A, Cecconi N, Marini A, Azzarà A, Ambrogi F and Grassi B (1986) Severe pancytopenia due to copper deficiency. *Acta Haematol*, **76**, 224–226.

22 Simon SR, Branda RF, Tindle BF and Burns SL (1988) Copper deficiency and sideroblastic anemia associated with zinc ingestion. *Am J Hematol*, **28**, 181–183.

23 Ramadurai J, Shapiro C, Kozloff M and Telfer M (1993) Zinc abuse and sideroblastic anemia. *Am J Hematol*, **42**, 227–228.

24 Kumar A and Jazieh AR (2001) Case report of sideroblastic anemia caused by ingestion of coins. *Am J Hematol*, **66**, 126–129.

25 Sampson B, Fagerhol MK, Sunderkötter C, Golden BE, Richmond P, Klein N *et al.* (2003) Hyperzincaemia with hypercalprotectinaemia: a new disorder of zinc metabolism. *Lancet*, **360**, 1742–1745.

26 How J, Davidson RJL and Bewsher PD (1979) Red cell changes in hyperthyroidism. *Scand J Haematol*, **23**, 323–328.

27 Ural AU (1997) Anemia related to ascorbic acid deficiency. *Am J Hematol*, **56**, 69.

28 Hillman RS and Finch CA. *Red Cell Manual*, 5th Edn. FA Davis, Philadelphia, 1985.

29 Larrick JW and Hyman ES (1984) Acquired iron deficiency anemia caused by an antibody against the transferrin receptor. *N Engl J Med*, **311**, 214–218.

30 Cauchi MN and Smith MB (1981) Quantitative aspects of red cell size variation during pregnancy. *Clin Lab Haematol*, **4**, 149–154.

31 Helman N and Rubenstein LS (1975) The effects of age, sex, and smoking on erythrocytes and leukocytes. *Am J Clin Pathol*, **63**, 35–44.

32 Sallah S, Hanrahan LR and Phillips DL (1999) Intrathecal methotrexate-induced megaloblastic anemia in patients with acute leukemia. *Arch Pathol Lab Med*, **123**, 774–777.

33 Au WY, Tsang J, Cheng TS, Chow WS, Woo YC, Ma SK and Tam S (2003) Cough mixture abuse as

a novel cause of megaloblastic anaemia and peripheral neuropathy. *Br J Haematol*, **123**, 956–957.

34 Porter KG, McMaster D, Elmes ME and Love AHG (1977) Anaemia and low serum copper during zinc therapy. *Lancet*, **ii**, 774.

35 Heaven R, Duncan M and Vukelja SJ (1994) Arsenic intoxication presenting with macrocytosis and peripheral neuropathy, without anemia. *Acta Haematol*, **92**, 142–143.

36 Sechi LA, De Carli S, Catena C, Zingaro L and Bartoli E (1996) Benign familial macrocytosis. *Clin Lab Haematol*, **18**, 41–43.

37 Willig T-N, Draptchinskaia N, Dianzani I, Ball S, Niemeyer C, Ramenghi U *et al.* (1999) Mutations in ribosomal protein S19 gene and Diamond–Blackfan anemia: wide variations in phenotypic expression. *Blood*, **94**, 4294–4306.

38 Tuckfield A, Ratnaike S, Hussein S and Metz J (1997) A novel form of hereditary sideroblastic anaemia with macrocytosis. *Br J Haematol*, **97**, 279–285.

39 Mehler PS and Howe SE (1995) Serous fat atrophy with leukopenia in severe anorexia nervosa. *Am J Hematol*, **49**, 171–172.

40 Barton JC, Bertoli LF and Rothenberg BE (2000) Peripheral blood erythrocyte parameters in hemochromatosis: evidence for increased erythrocyte hemoglobin content. *J Lab Clin Med*, **135**, 96–104.

41 Sipes SL, Weiner CP, Wenstrom KD, Williamson RA and Grant SS (1991) The association between fetal karyotype and mean corpuscular volume. *Am J Obstet Gynecol*, **165**, 1371–1376.

42 Eastham RD and Jancar J (1970) Macrocytosis in Down's syndrome and during long term anticonvulsant therapy. *J Clin Pathol*, **23**, 296–298.

43 Pai GS, Grush OC and Shuman C (1982) Hematological abnormalities in triploidy. *Am J Dis Child*, **136**, 367–369.

44 Bader-Meunier B, Rieux-Laucat F, Croisille L, Yvart J, Mielot F, Dommergues JP *et al.* (2000) Dyserythropoiesis associated with a fas-deficient condition in childhood. *Br J Haematol*, **108**, 300–304.

45 Li J, Yang C, Xia Y, Bertino A, Glaspy J, Roberts M and Kuter DJ (2001) Thrombocytopenia caused by the development of antibodies to thrombopoietin. *Blood*, **98**, 3241–3248.

46 Voglová J, Poznarová A, Chrovák L, Vogel J, Faber E and Cikhart M (2003) Mean cell volume changes in CML treated with Glivec. *Leuk Lymphoma*, **44**, Suppl. S75–S76.

47 Stewart GW and Turner EJH (2000) The hereditary stomatocytoses and allied disorders of erythrocyte membrane permeability to Na and K. *Baillière's Clin Haematol*, **12**, 707–727.

48 Rees MI, Worwood M, Thompson PW, Gilbertson C and May A (1994) Red cell dimorphism in a young man with a constitutional chromosomal translocation t(11;22) (p15.5;q11.21). *Br J Haematol*, **87**, 386–395.

49 Perrotta AL and Finch CA (1972) The polychromatophilic erythrocyte. *Am J Clin Pathol*, **57**, 471–477.

50 Rowles PM and Williams ES (1983) Abnormal red cell morphology in venous blood of men climbing at high altitude. *BMJ*, **286**, 1396.

51 Bessis M. *Living Blood Cells and their Ultrastructure*, trans. Weed RI. Springer-Verlag, Berlin, 1973.

52 Wolf PL and Koett J (1980) Hemolytic anemia in hepatic disease with decreased erythrocyte adenosine triphosphate. *Am J Clin Pathol*, **73**, 785–788.

53 Shilo S, Werner D and Hershko C (1985) Acute hemolytic anemia caused by severe hypophosphatemia in diabetic ketoacidosis. *Acta Haematol*, **73**, 55–57.

54 McGrath KM, Zalcberg JR, Slonin J and Wiley JS (1982) Intralipid induced haemolysis. *Br J Haematol*, **50**, 376–378.

55 Bianchi P, Fermo E, Alfinito F, Vercellati C, Baserga M, Ferraro F *et al.* (2003) Molecular characterization of six unrelated Italian patients affected by pyrimidine 5'-nucleotidase deficiency. *Br J Haematol*, **122**, 847–851.

56 Austin RF and Desforges JF (1969) Hereditary elliptocytosis: an unusual presentation of hemolysis in the newborn associated with transient morphologic abnormalities. *Pediatrics*, **44**, 196–200.

57 Melvin JD and Watts RG (2002) Severe hypophosphatemia: a rare cause of intravascular hemolysis. *Am J Hematol*, **69**, 223–224.

58 Chan TK, Chan WC and Weed RI (1982) Erythrocyte hemighosts: a hallmark of severe oxidative injury *in vivo*. *Br J Haematol*, **50**, 573–582.

59 Bain BJ (1999) Images in Haematology: Heinz body haemolytic anaemia in Wilson's disease. *Br J Haematol*, **104**, 647.

60 Wickramasinghe SN (1998) Congenital dyserythropoietic anaemias: clinical features, haemato-

logical morphology and new biochemical data. *Blood Rev*, **12**, 178–200.

61 Nurse GT, Coetzer TL and Palek J (1992) The elliptocytoses, ovalocytoses and related disorders. *Baillière's Clin Haematol*, **5**, 187–207.

62 Hur M, Lee KM, Cho HC, Park YI, Kim SH, Chang YM *et al.* (2004) Protein 4.1 deficiency and deletion of chromosome 20q are associated with acquired elliptocytosis in myelodysplastic syndrome. *Clin Lab Haematol*, **26**, 69–72.

63 Patel SS, Mehlotra RK, Kastens W, Mgone CS, Kazura JW and Zimmerman PA (2001) The association of the glycophorin C exon 3 deletion with ovalocytosis and malaria susceptibility in the Wosera, Papua New Guinea. *Blood*, **98**, 3489–3491.

64 Farolino DL, Rustagi PK, Currie MS, Doeblin TD and Logue GL (1986) Teardrop-shaped cells in autoimmune hemolytic anemia. *Am J Hematol*, **21**, 415–418.

65 Domingo-Claros A, Larriba I, Rozman M, Irriguible D, Vallespi T, Aventin A *et al.* (2002) Acute erythroid neoplastic proliferations. A biological study based on 62 patients. *Haematologica*, **87**, 148–153.

66 Miwa S, Fujii H, Tani K, Takahashi K, Takegawa S, Fujinami N *et al.* (1981) Two cases of red cell aldolase deficiency associated with hereditary hemolytic anemia in a Japanese family. *Am J Hematol*, **11**, 425–437.

67 Carlyle RF, Nichols G and Rowles PM (1979) Abnormal red cells in blood of men subjected to simulated dives. *Lancet*, **i**, 1114–1116.

68 Feo CT, Tchernia G, Subtil E and Leblond PF (1978) Observations of echinocytosis in eight patients: a phase contrast and SEM study. *Br J Haematol*, **40**, 519–526.

69 Kay MM, Bosman GJ and Lawrence C (1988) Functional topography of band 3: specific structural alteration linked to functional aberrations in human erythrocytes. *Proc Natl Acad Sci USA*, **85**, 492–496.

70 Bruce LJ, Kay MM, Lawrence C and Tanner MJ (2000) Band 3HT, a human red-cell variant associated with acanthocytosis and increased anion transport carries the mutation Pro-868→Leu in the membrane domain of band 3. *Biochem J*, **292**, 317–320.

71 Yawata Y, Kanzaki A, Yawata A, Kaku M, Takezono M, Sugihara T *et al.* (1997) Hereditary

xerocytosis is a phenotypically different entity from hereditary high red cell membrane phosphatidyl choline hemolytic anemia. *Blood*, **90**, Suppl. 1, 5a.

72 Doll DC, Lest AF, Dayhoff DA, Loy TS, Ringenberg QS and Yarbro JW (1989) Acanthocytosis associated with myelodysplasia. *J Clin Oncol*, **7**, 1569–1572.

73 Freson K, Devriendt K, Matthijs G, Van Hoof A, De Vos R, Thys C *et al.* (2001) Platelet characteristics in patients with X-linked macrothrombocytopenia because of a novel *GATA1* mutation. *Blood*, **98**, 85–92.

74 Palek J and Jarolim P (1993) Clinical expression and laboratory detection of red blood cell membrane protein mutations. *Semin Hematol*, **30**, 249–283.

75 Bassen FA and Kornzweig AL (1950) Malformation of the erythrocytes in a case of atypical retinitis pigmentosa. *Blood*, **5**, 381–387.

76 Estes JW, Morley TJ, Levine IM and Emerson CF (1967) A new hereditary acanthocytosis syndrome. *Am J Med*, **42**, 868–881.

77 Sakai T, Mawatari S, Iwashita H, Goto I and Kuroiwa Y (1981) Choreoacanthocytosis. *Arch Neurol*, **38**, 335.

78 Chowdhury F, Saward R and Erber W (2005) Neuroacanthocytosis. *Br J Haematol*, **131**, 285.

79 Rampoldi L, Dobson-Stone C, Rubio JP, Danek A, Chalmers RM, Wood NW *et al.* (2001) A conserved sorting-associated protein is mutant in choreaacanthocytosis. *Nat Genet*, **28**, 119–120.

80 Walker RH, Rasmussen A, Rudnicki D, Holmes SE, Alonso E, Matsuura T *et al.* (2003) Huntington's disease-like 2 can present as choreaacanthocytosis. *Neurology*, **61**, 1002–1004.

81 Udden MM, Umeda M, Hirano Y and Marcus DM (1987) New abnormalities in the morphology, cell surface receptors and electrolyte balance in In(lu) erythrocytes. *Blood*, **69**, 52–57.

82 Amare M, Lawson B and Larsen WE (1972) Active extrusion of Heinz bodies in drug-induced haemolytic anaemia. *Br J Haematol*, **23**, 215–219.

83 Ward PC, Smith CM and White JG (1979) Erythrocytic ecdysis. An unusual morphologic finding in a case of sickle cell anemia with intercurrent cold-agglutinin syndrome. *Am J Clin Pathol*, **72**, 479–485.

84 Samson RE, Abdalla DH and Bain BJ (1998) Teaching cases from the Royal Marsden and St Mary's Hospitals. Case 18. Severe anaemia and

thrombocytopenia with red cell fragmentation. *Leuk Lymphoma*, 31, 433–435.

85 Crook M, Williams A and Schey S (1998) Target cells and stomatocytes in heterozygous familial hypobetalipoproteinaemia. *Eur J Haematol*, **60**, 68–69.

86 McGrath KM, Collecutt MF, Gordon A, Sawers RJ and Faragher BS (1984) Dehydrated hereditary stomatocytosis—a report of two families and a review of the literature. *Pathology*, **16**, 146–150.

87 Reinhardt WH, Gössi U, Bütikofer P, Ott P, Sigrist H, Schatzmann H-J *et al.* (1989) Haemolytic anaemia in analpha-lipoproteinaemia (Tangier disease): morphological, biochemical, and biophysical properties of the red blood cell. *Br J Haematol*, **72**, 272–277.

88 Godin DV, Garnett ME, Hoag G, Wadsworth LD and Frohlich J (1988) Erythrocyte abnormalities in hypoalphalipoproteinemia syndrome resembling fish eye disease. *Eur J Haematol*, **41**, 176–181.

89 Clayton PT, Bowron A, Mills KA, Massoud A, Casteels M and Milla PJ (1993) Phytosterolaemia in children with parenteral nutrition-associated cholestatic liver disease. *Gastroenterology*, **105**, 1806–1813.

90 Exner M and Schwarzinger I (2001) Targeting the dust. *Br J Haematol*, **114**, 739.

91 Miller DR, Rickles FR, Lichtman MA, La Celle PL, Bates J and Weed R (1971) A new variant of hereditary hemolytic anemia with stomatocytosis and erythrocyte cation abnormality. *Blood*, **38**, 184–204.

92 Davidson RJ, How J and Lessels S (1977) Acquired stomatocytosis: its prevalence and significance in routine haematology. *Scand J Haematol*, **19**, 47–53.

93 Wislöff F and Boman D (1979) Acquired stomatocytosis in alcoholic liver disease. *Scand J Haematol*, **23**, 43–50.

94 Mallory DM, Rosenfield RE, Wong KY, Heller C, Rubinstein P, Allen FH *et al.* (1976) Rh$_{mod}$, a second kindred (Craig). *Vox Sang*, **30**, 430–440.

95 Gallagher PG and Lux SE, Disorders of the erythrocyte membrane. In: Nathan DG, Orkin SH, Ginsburg D and Look AT, *Nathan and Oski's Hematology of Infancy and Childhood*, 6th Edn. Saunders, Philadelphia, 2003.

96 von Behrens WE (1975) Splenomegaly, macrothrombocytopenia and stomatocytosis in healthy Mediterranean subjects. *Scand J Haematol*, **14**, 258–267.

97 Rees DC, Iolascon A, Carella M, O'Marcaigh AS, Kendra JR, Jowitt SN *et al.* (2005) Stomatocytic haemolysis and macrothrombocytopenia (Mediterranean stomatocytosis/macrothrombocytopenia) is the haematological presentation of phytosterolaemia. *Br J Haematol*, **130**, 297–309.

98 Valentine WN (1979) Hemolytic anemia and inborn errors of metabolism. *Blood*, **54**, 549–559.

99 Paglia DE, Valentine WN, Nakatani M and Rauth BJ (1983) Selective accumulation of cytosol CDP-choline as an isolated erythrocyte defect in chronic hemolysis. *Proc Natl Acad Sci U S A*, **80**, 3081–3085.

100 Merino A, To-Figueras J and Herrero C (2006) Atypical red cell inclusions in congenital erythropoietic porphyria. *Br J Haematol*, **132**, 124.

101 Green DW, Hendon B and Mimouni FR (1995) Nucleated erythrocytes and intraventricular hemorrhage in preterm neonates. *Pediatrics*, **96**, 475–478.

102 Eichner ER (1984) Erythroid karyorrhexis in the peripheral blood smear in severe arsenic poisoning: a comparison with lead poisoning. *Am J Clin Pathol*, **81**, 533–537.

103 Mathy KA and Koepke JA (1974) The clinical usefulness of segmented vs. stab neutrophil criteria for differential leukocyte counts. *Am J Clin Pathol*, **61**, 947–958.

104 Akenzua GI, Hui YT, Milner R and Zipursky A (1974) Neutrophil and band counts in the diagnosis of neonatal infections. *Pediatrics*, **54**, 38–42.

105 Christensen RD and Rothstein G (1978) Pitfalls in the interpretation of leukocyte counts of newborn infants. *Am J Clin Pathol*, **72**, 608–611.

106 Christensen RD, Rothstein G, Anstall HB and Bybee B (1981) Granulocyte transfusions in neonates with bacterial infection, neutropenia, and depletion of mature bone marrow neutrophils. *Pediatrics*, **70**, 1–6.

107 Chanarin I. *Megaloblastic Anaemias*, 2nd Edn. CV Mosby, St Louis, 1979.

108 Edwin E (1967) The segmentation of polymorphonuclear neutrophils. *Acta Med Scand*, **182**, 401–410.

109 Westerman DA, Evans D and Metz J (1999) Neutrophil hypersegmentation in iron deficiency anaemia: a case–control study. *Br J Haematol*, **107**, 512–515.

110 Kerrigan DP, Castillo A, Foucar K, Townsend K and Neidhart J (1989) Peripheral blood morphologic changes after high-dose antineoplastic chemotherapy and recombinant human granulocyte

colony-stimulating factor administration. *Am J Clin Pathol*, **92**, 280–285.

111 Wickramasinghe SN (1999) The wide spectrum and unresolved issues of megaloblastic anemia. *Semin Hematol*, **36**, 3–18.

112 Davidson WM (1968) Inherited variations in leukocytes. *Semin Haematol*, **5**, 255–274.

113 Hess U, Ganser A, Schnürch H-G, Seipelt G, Ottman OG, Falk S *et al.* (1992) Myelokathexis treated with recombinant human granulocyte-macrophage colony-stimulating factor (rhGM-CSF). *Br J Haematol*, **80**, 254–256.

114 Gorlin RJ, Gelb B, Diaz GA, Lofsness KG, Pittelkow MR and Fenyk JR (2000) WHIM syndrome, an autosomal dominant disorder: clinical, hematological, and molecular studies. *Am J Med Genet*, **91**, 368–376.

115 Davidson WM and Smith DR (1954) A morphological sex difference in the polymorphonuclear neutrophil leucocytcs. *BMJ*, **ii**, 6–7.

116 Murthy MSN and von Emmerich H (1958) The occurrence of the sex chromatin in white blood cells of young adults. *Am J Clin Pathol*, **30**, 216–227.

117 Davidson WM, Fowler JF and Smith DR (1958) Sexing the neutrophil leucocytes in natural and artificial chimaeras. *Br J Haematol*, **4**, 231–238.

118 Mittwoch U (1963) The incidence of drumsticks in patients with three X chromosomes. *Cytogenetics*, **2**, 24–33.

119 Pai GS, Grush OC and Shuman C (1982) Hematological abnormalities in triploidy. *Am J Dis Child*, **136**, 367–369.

120 Tomonaga M, Matsuura G, Watanabe B, Kamochi Y and Ozono N (1961) Leukocyte drumsticks in chronic granulocytic leukaemia and related disorders. *Blood*, **18**, 581–590.

121 Archer RK, Engisch HJC, Gaha T and Ruxton J (1971) The eosinophil leucocyte in the blood and bone marrow of patients with Down's anomaly. *Br J Haematol*, **21**, 271–276.

122 Huehns ER, Lutzner M and Hecht F (1964) Nuclear abnormalities of the neutrophils in D$_1$(13–15)-trisomy syndrome. *Lancet*, **i**, 589–590.

123 Salama ME, Shah V, Lebel RR and VanDyke DL (2004) Aberrant nuclear projections of neutrophils in Trisomy 13. *Arch Pathol Lab Med*, **128**, 243–244.

124 Davey FR, Erber WN, Gatter KC and Mason DY (1988) Abnormal neutrophil morphology in acute myeloid leukaemia and myelodysplastic syndrome. *Hum Pathol*, **19**, 454–459.

125 Strauss RG, Bove KE, Jones JF, Mauer AM and Fulginiti VA (1974) An anomaly of neutrophil morphology with impaired function. *N Engl J Med*, **290**, 478–484.

126 Plum CM, Warburg M and Danielsen J (1978) Defective maturation of granulocytes, retinal cysts and multiple skeletal malformations in a mentally retarded girl. *Acta Haematol*, **59**, 53–63.

127 Girolami A, Fabris F, Caronato A and Randi ML (1980) Increased numbers of pseudodrumsticks in neutrophils and large platelets. A 'new' congenital leukocyte and platelet morphological abnormality. *Acta Haematol*, **64**, 324–330.

128 Moore CM and Weinger RS (1980) Pseudo-drumsticks in granulocytes of a male with a Yqh+ polymorphism. *Am J Hematol*, **8**, 411–414.

129 Gibson BES. Inherited disorders. In: Hann IM, Gibson BES and Letsky EA, eds. *Fetal and Neonatal Haematology*. Baillière Tindall, London, 1991.

130 Seman G (1959) Sur une anomalie constitutionnelle héréditaire du noyau des polynucléaires neutrophiles. *Rev Hématol*, **14**, 409–412.

131 Langenhuijsen MMAC (1984) Neutrophils with ring shaped nuclei in myeloproliferative disorders. *Br J Haematol*, **58**, 227–230.

132 Stavem P, Hjort PF, Vogt E and Van der Hagen CB (1969) Ring-shaped nuclei of granulocytes in a patient with acute erythroleukaemia. *Scand J Haematol*, **6**, 31–32.

133 Kabob T, Saigo K and Yamagishi M (1986) Neutrophils with ring-shaped nuclei in chronic neutrophilic leukaemia. *Am J Clin Pathol*, **86**, 748–751.

134 Craig A (1988) Ring neutrophils in megaloblastic anaemia. *Br J Haematol*, **67**, 247–248.

135 Hernandez JA, Aldred SW, Bruce JR, Vanatta PR, Mattingly TL and Sheehan WW (1980) 'Botryoid' nuclei in neutrophils of patients with heat stroke. *Lancet*; **ii**, 642–643.

136 Neftel KA and Müller OM (1981) Heat-induced radial segmentation of leucocyte nuclei: a non-specific phenomenon accompanying inflammatory and necrotizing diseases. *Br J Haematol*, **48**, 377–382.

137 Gustke SS, Becker GA, Garancis JC, Geimer NF and Pisciotta AV (1970) Chromatin clumping in mature leukocytes: a hitherto unrecognized abnormality. *Blood*, **35**, 637–658.

138 Ozanne C, Bain B and Catovsky D (1996) Teaching cases from the Royal Marsden and St Mary's Hospitals Case 11: Dysplastic neutrophils in an African woman. *Leuk Lymphoma*, **18**, 351–352.

139 Bain BJ. *Blood Cells: A Practical Guide*, 1st Edn. Gower Medical Publishing, London, 1989.

140 Brunning RD (1970) Morphologic alterations in nucleated blood and marrow cells in genetic disorders. *Hum Pathol*, **1**, 99–124.

141 Skendzel LP and Hoffman GC (1962) The Pelger anomaly of leukocytes: forty cases in seven families. *Am J Clin Pathol*, **37**, 294–301.

142 Hoffmann K, Dreger CK, Olins AL, Olins DE, Shultz LD, Lucke B et al. (2002) Mutations in the gene encoding the lamin B receptor produce an altered nuclear morphology in granulocytes (Pelger–Huët anomaly). *Nat Genet*, **31**, 410–414.

143 Klein A, Hussar AE and Bornstein S (1955) Pelger–Huët anomaly of leukocytes. *N Engl J Med*, **253**, 1057–1062.

144 Erice JG, Pérez JM and Pericás FS (1999) Homozygous form of the Pelger–Huët anomaly. *Haematologica*, **84**, 748.

145 Ardeman S, Chanarin I and Frankland AW (1963) The Pelger–Huët anomaly and megaloblastic anemia. *Blood*, **22**, 472–476.

146 Parmley RT, Tzeng DY, Baehner R and Boxer LA (1983) Abnormal distribution of complex carbohydrates in neutrophils of a patient with lactoferrin deficiency. *Blood*, **62**, 538–548.

147 Deutsch PH and Mandell GL (1985) Reversible Pelger–Huët anomaly associated with ibuprofen therapy. *Arch Intern Med*, **145**, 166.

148 Juneja SK, Matthews JP, Luzinat R, Fan Y, Michael M, Rischin D et al. (1996) Association of acquired Pelger–Huët anomaly with taxoid therapy. *Br J Haematol*, **93**, 139–141.

149 Banerjee R, Halil O, Bain BJ, Cummins D and Banner N (2001) Neutrophil dysplasia caused by mycophenolate mofetil, *Transplantation*, **77**, 1608–1610.

150 Schmitz LL, McClure JS, Letz CE, Dayton V, Weisdorf DJ, Parkin IL and Brunning RD (1994) Morphologic and quantitative changes in blood and marrow cells following growth factor therapy. *Am J Clin Pathol*, **101**, 67–75.

151 Lach-Szyrma V and Brito-Babapulle F (1997) The significance of apoptotic cells in peripheral blood smears. *Br J Haematol*, **97**, Suppl. 1, 70.

152 Drouin A, Favier R, Massé J-M, Debili N, Schmitt A, Elbin C et al. (2001) Newly recognized cellular abnormalities in the gray platelet syndrome. *Blood*, **98**, 1382–1391.

153 Campbell LJ, Maher DW, Tay DLM, Boyd AW, Rockmart S, McGrath K et al. (1992) Marrow proliferation and the appearance of giant neutrophils in response to recombinant human granulocyte colony stimulating factor (rhG-CSF). *Br J Haematol*, **80**, 298–304.

154 Ryder JW, Lazarus HM and Farhi DC (1992) Bone marrow and blood findings after marrow transplantation and rhGM-CSF therapy. *Am J Clin Pathol*, **97**, 631–637.

155 Ghandi MK, Howard MR and Hamilton PJ (1996) The Alder–Reilly anomaly in association with the myelodysplastic syndrome. *Clin Lab Haematol*, **18**, 39–40.

156 Gale PF, Parkin JL, Quie PG, Pettitt RE, Nelson RP and Brunning RD (1986) Leukocyte granulation abnormality associated with normal neutrophil function and neurological abnormality. *Am J Clin Pathol*, **86**, 33–49.

157 Newburger PE, Robinson JM, Pryzwansky KB, Rosoff PM, Greenberger JS and Tauber AI (1983) Human neutrophil dysfunction with giant granules and defective activation of the respiratory burst. *Blood*, **61**, 1247–1257.

158 Van Slyck El and Rebuck JW (1974) Pseudo-Chediak–Higashi anomaly in acute leukemia. *Am J Clin Pathol*, **62**, 673–678.

159 Davidson RJ and McPhie JL (1980) Cytoplasmic vacuolation of peripheral blood cells in acute alcoholism. *J Clin Pathol*, **33**, 1193–1196.

160 Chetty-Raju N, Cook R and Erber W (2005) Vacuolated neutrophils in ethanol toxicity. *Br J Haematol*, **127**, 478.

161 Jordans GHW (1953) The familial occurrence of fat containing vacuoles in the leucocytes diagnosed in two brothers suffering from dystrophic musculorum progressiva. *Acta Med Scand*, **145**, 419–423.

162 Schopfer K and Douglas SD (1976) Fine structural studies of peripheral blood leucocytes from children with kwashiorkor: morphological and functional studies. *Br J Haematol*, **32**, 573–577.

163 Aprikyan AAG, Liles WC, Park JR, Jonas M, Chi EY and Dale DC (2000) Myelokathexis, a congenital disorder of severe neutropenia characterized by accelerated apoptosis and defective expression of *bcl-x* in neutrophil precursors. *Blood*, **95**, 320–327.

164 Peterson LC, Rao KV, Crosson JT and White JG (1985) Fechtner syndrome—a variant of Alport's

syndrome with leukocyte inclusions and macro-thrombocytopenia. *Blood*, **65**, 397–406.

165 Ribeiro RC, Howard TH, Brandalise S, Behm FG, Parham DM, Wang WC *et al.* (1994) Giant actin inclusions in hematopoietic cells associated with transfusion-dependent anemia and grey skin coloration. *Blood*, **83**, 3717–3726.

166 Nosanchuk J, Terzian J and Posso M (1987) Circulating mucopolysaccharide (mucin) in two adults with metastatic adenocarcinoma. *Arch Pathol Lab Med*, **111**, 545–548.

167 Yu PH and Wong KF (1996) Circulating leukocytes with ingested mucin in a child with Hirschsprung's disease. *Am J Hematol*, **52**, 240.

168 Chomet B, Kirshen MM, Schaefer G and Mudrik P (1953) The finding of the LE (lupus erythematosus) cells in smears of untreated, freshly drawn peripheral blood. *Blood*, **8**, 1107–1109.

169 Weil SC, Holt S, Hrisinko MA, Little L and De Backer N (1985) Melanin inclusions in peripheral blood leukocytes of a patient with malignant melanoma. *Am J Clin Pathol*, **84**, 679–681.

170 Sen Gupta PC, Ghosal SP, Mukherjee AK and Maity TR (1983) Bilirubin crystals in neutrophils of jaundiced neonates and infants. *Acta Haematol*, **70**, 69–70.

171 Smith H (1967) Unidentified inclusions in haemopoietic cells, congenital atresia of the bile ducts and livedo reticularis in an infant. A new syndrome? *Br J Haematol*, **13**, 695–705.

172 Miale JB. *Laboratory Medicine: Hematology*, 6th Edn. CV Mosby, St Louis, 1982.

173 Roberts GT, Perry JL, Al-Jefri A and Scott CS (2005) Intra-leukocytic hemosiderin inclusions detected as pseudoeosinophils by automated depolarization analysis in a patient with beta-thalassaemia major and immune hemolysis. *Blood Cells Mol Dis*, **34**, 162–165.

174 Hernandez JA and Steane SM (1984) Erythrophagocytosis by segmented neutrophils in paroxysmal cold hemoglobinuria. *Am J Clin Pathol*, **81**, 787–789.

175 Schofield KP, Stone PCW, Beddall AC and Stuart J (1983) Quantitative cytochemistry of the toxic granulation blood neutrophil. *Br J Haematol*, **53**, 15–22.

176 Presentey B (1986) Alder anomaly accompanied by a mutation of the myeloperoxidase structural gene. *Acta Haematol*, **75**, 157–159.

177 Doocey R, Thula R and Jackson S (2002) Giant actin inclusions in hematopoietic cells: a variant of Brandalise syndrome. *J Pediatr Hematol Oncol*, **24**, 781–782.

178 Rosenszajn L, Klajman A, Yaffe D and Efrati P (1966) Jordans anomaly in white blood cells. *Blood*, **28**, 258–265.

179 Markesbery WR, McQuillen MP, Procopis PG, Harrison AR and Engel AG (1974) Muscle carnitine deficiency: association with lipid myopathy, vacuolar neuropathy, and vacuolated leukocytes. *Arch Neurol*, **31**, 320–324.

180 Dorfman ML, Hershko C, Eisenberg S and Sagher F (1974) Ichthyosiform dermatosis with systemic lipidosis. *Arch Dermatol*, **110**, 261–266.

181 Chanarin I, Patel A, Slavin G, Wills EJ, Andrews TM and Stewart G (1975) Neutral-lipid storage disease: A new disorder of lipid metabolism. *BMJ*, **i**, 553–555.

182 Abernathy MR (1966) Döhle bodies associated with uncomplicated pregnancy. *Blood*, **27**, 380–385.

183 Itoga T and Laszlo J (1962) Döhle bodies and other granulocytic alterations during chemotherapy with cyclophosphamide. *Blood*, **20**, 668–674.

184 Jenis EH, Takeuchi A, Dillon DE, Ruymann FB and Rivkin S (1971) The May–Hegglin anomaly: ultrastructure of the granulocyte inclusion. *Am J Clin Pathol*, **55**, 187–196.

185 Drachman JG (2004) Inherited thrombocytopenia: when a low platelet count does not mean ITP. *Blood*, **103**, 390–398.

186 Volpé R and Ogryzlo MA (1955) The cryoglobulin inclusion cell. *Blood*, **10**, 493–496.

187 Powell HC and Wolf PL (1976) Neutrophilic leukocyte inclusions in colchicine intoxication. *Arch Pathol Lab Med*, **100**, 136–138.

188 Williams ST, Khare VK, Johnston GA and Blackall DP (1995) Severe intravascular hemolysis associated with brown recluse spider envenomation. *Am J Clin Pathol*, **104**, 463–467.

189 Au WY and Kwong YL (1999) Haemophagocytosis in the peripheral blood. *Br J Haematol*, **105**, 321.

190 Etzell J, Lu CM, Browne LW and Wang E (2005) Erythrophagocytosis by dysplastic neutrophils in chronic myelomonocytic leukemia and subsequent transformation to acute myeloid leukemia. *Am J Hematol*, **79**, 340–342.

191 Sen Gupta PC, Ghosal SP, Mukherjee AK and Maity TR (1983) Bilirubin crystals in neutrophils of

jaundiced neonates and infants. *Acta Haematol*, **70**, 69–70.

192 Kapff CT and Jandl JH. *Blood: Atlas and Sourcebook of Hematology*, Little Brown, Boston, 1981.

193 Özbek N, Derbent M, Olcay L, Yilmaz Z and Tokel K (2004) Dysplastic changes in the peripheral blood in children with microdeletion 22q11.2. *Am J Hematol*, **77**, 126–131.

194 Cooke WE (1927) The macropolycyte. *BMJ*, **i**, 12–13.

195 Shidham VB and Swami VK (2000) Evaluation of apoptotic leukocytes in peripheral blood smears. *Arch Pathol Lab Med*, **124**, 1291–1294.

196 Guibaud S, Plumet-Leger A and Frobert Y (1971) Transient neutrophil aggregation in a patient with infectious mononucleosis. *Am J Clin Pathol*, **80**, 883–884.

197 Foucar K, *Bone Marrow Pathology*, 2nd Edn. ASCP Press, Chicago, 2001.

198 Nand S, Bansal VK, Kozeny G, Vertuno L, Remlinger KA and Jordan JV (1985) Red cell fragmentation syndrome with the use of subclavian hemodialysis catheters. *Arch Intern Med*, **145**, 1421–1423.

199 Tracey R and Smith H (1978) An inherited anomaly of human eosinophils and basophils. *Blood Cells*, **4**, 291–300.

200 Presentey BZ (1968) A new anomaly of eosinophilic granulocytes. *Am J Clin Pathol*, **49**, 887–890.

201 Archer RK, Engisch HJC. Gaha T and Ruxton J (1971) The eosinophil leucocytes in the blood and bone marrow of patients with Down's anomaly. *Br J Haematol*, **21**, 271–276.

202 Kay NE, Nelson DA and Gottlieb AJ (1973) Eosinophilic Pelger–Huët anomaly with myeloproliferative disorder. *Am J Clin Pathol*, **60**, 663–668.

203 Catovsky D, Bernasconi C, Verdonck PJ, Postma A, Hows J, ven der Does-van den Berg A *et al.* (1980) The association of eosinophilia with lymphoblastic leukaemia or lymphoma: a study of seven patients. *Br J Haematol*, **45**, 523–534.

204 Bain BJ (1989) The significance of ring eosinophils in humans. *Br J Haematol*, **73**, 580–581.

205 Weil SC and Hrisinko MA (1987) A hybrid eosinophilic–basophilic granulocyte in chronic granulocytic leukaemia. *Am J Clin Pathol*, **87**, 66–70.

206 Douglas SD, Blume RS and Wolff SM (1969) Fine structural studies of leukocytes from patients and heterozygotes with the Chediak–Higashi syndrome. *Blood*, **33**, 527–540.

207 Groover RV, Burke EC, Gordon H and Berdon WE (1972) The genetic mucopolysaccharidoses. *Semin Haematol*, **9**, 371–402.

208 Kolodny EH (1972) Clinical and biochemical genetics of the lipidoses. *Semin Haematol*, **9**, 251–271.

209 Forestier F, Hohlfeld P, Vial Y, Olin V, Andreux J-P and Tissot J-D (1996) Blood smears and prenatal diagnosis. *Br J Haematol*, **95**, 278–280.

210 Patel MS, Callahan JW, Zhang S, Chan AKJ, Unger S, Levin AV *et al.* (1999) Early-infantile galactosialidosis: prenatal presentation and postnatal follow-up. *Am J Med Genet*, **85**, 38–47.

211 Maier-Redelsperger M, Stern M-H and Maroteaux P (1988) Pink rings lymphocyte: a new cytologic abnormality characteristic of mucopolysaccharidosis type II Hunter disease. *Pediatrics*, **82**, 286–287.

212 van der Meer W, Jakobs BS, Bocca G, Smeitink JAM, Schuurmans Steckhoven JH and de Keijzer MH (2001) Peripheral blood lymphocyte appearance in a case of I cell disease. *J Clin Pathol*, **54**, 724–726.

213 Iwasaki H, Ueda T, Uchida M, Nakamura T, Takada N and Mahara F (1991) Atypical lymphocytes with a multilobated nucleus from a patient with tsutsugamushi disease (scrub typhus) in Japan. *Am J Hematol*, **36**, 150–151.

214 Huhn KM, Dalal BI, Naiman SC and Buskard NA (1995) Case of chronic B-lymphocytic leukemia with clover leaf nuclei. *Am J Hematol*, **49**, 360–361.

215 Bachelez H, Hadida F and Gorochov G (1996) Massive infiltration of the skin by HIV-specific cytotoxic CD8-positive T cells. *N Engl J Med*, **335**, 61–62.

216 Wulf GG, Schulz H, Hallermann C, Kunze E and Wörmann B (2001) Reactive polyclonal T-cell lymphocytosis mimicking Sezary syndrome in a patient with hairy cell leukemia. *Haematologica*, **86**, E27.

217 Bates I, Bedu-Addo G, Bevan D and Rutherford T (1996) Circulating villous lymphocytes—the link between reactive malarial splenomegaly and splenic lymphoma. *Br J Haematol*, **93**, Suppl. 1, 69.

218 Kanegane H, Wado T, Nunogami K, Seki H, Taniguchi N and Tosato G (1996) Chronic persistent Epstein–Barr virus infection of natural killer cells and B cells associated with granular lymphocyte expansion. *Br J Haematol*, **95**, 116–122.

219 Lesesve J-F and Troussard X (2001) EDTA-dependent lymphoagglutination. *Br J Haematol*, **115**, 237.

220 Shelton JB and Frank IN (2000) Splenic B cell lymphoma with lymphocyte clusters in peripheral blood smears. *J Clin Pathol*, **53**, 228–230.

221 Cobcroft R (1999) Diagnosis of angiotropic large B-cell lymphoma from a peripheral blood film. *Br J Haematol*, **104**, 429.

222 Imbing F, Kumar D, Kumar S, Yuoh G and Gardner F (1995) Splenic lymphoma with circulating villous lymphocytes. *J Clin Pathol*, **48**, 584–587.

223 Wenburg JJ and Go RS (2003) EDTA-dependent lymphocyte clumping. *Haematologica*, **88**, EIM09.

224 Oertel J, Oertel B, Schleicher J and Huhn D (1998) Detection of small numbers of immature cells in the blood of healthy subjects. *J Clin Pathol*, **51**, 886–890.

225 Pellat-Deceunynck C, Jego G, Robilard N, Accard F, Amiot M and Bataille R (2000) Reactive plasmacytoses, a model for studying the biology of human plasma cell progenitors and precursors. *Hematol J*, **1**, 362–366.

226 Shtalrid M, Shvidel L and Vorst E (2003) Polyclonal reactive peripheral blood lymphocytosis mimicking plasma cell leukemia in a patient with staphylococcal sepsis. *Leuk Lymphoma*, **44**, 379–380.

227 Gawoski JM and Ooi WW (2003) Dengue fever mimicking plasma cell leukemia. *Arch Pathol Lab Med*, **127**, 1026–1027.

228 La Raja M (2002) Erythrophagocytosis by peripheral monocytes in *Plasmodium falciparum* malaria. *Haematologica*, **87**, EIM14.

229 Currimbhoy Z (1991) An outbreak of an infection associated with circulating activated monocytes and haemophagocytes in children in Bombay, India. *Am J Pediatr Hematol Oncol*, **13**, 274–279.

230 Tsuda H (1997) The use of cyclosporin-A in the treatment of virus–associated haemophagocytic syndrome in adults. *Leuk Lymphoma*, **28**, 73–82.

231 Efrati P and Rozenszajn L (1960) The morphology of buffy coats in normal human adults. *Blood*, **15**, 1012–1019.

232 Bennett IM, Catovsky D, Daniel MT, Flandrin G, Galton DAG, Gralnick HR and Sultan C (1982) Proposals for the classification of the myclodysplastic syndromes. *Br J Haematol*, **51**, 189–199.

233 van Hoeven KH, Wanner JL and Ballas SK (1997) Cytologic diagnosis of fat emboli in peripheral blood during sickle cell infarctive crisis. *Diagn Cytopathol*, **17**, 54–56.

234 Hicsönmez G and Ozkaynak F (1984) Diagnosis of heterozygous state for Bernard–Soulier disease. *Acta Haematol*, **71**, 285–286.

235 Epstein CJ, Sahud MA, Piel CF, Goodman JR, Bernfield MR, Kushner JH and Ablin AR (1972) Hereditary macrothrombocytopathia, nephritis and deafness. *Am J Med*, **52**, 299–310.

236 Bellucci S (1997) Megakaryocytes and inherited thrombocytopenias. *Baillière's Clin Haematol*, **10**, 149–162.

237 Estes JW (1968) Platelet size and function in the hereditable disorders of connective tissues. *Ann Intern Med*, **68**, 1237–1249.

238 Raccuglia G (1971) Gray platelet syndrome. A variety of qualitative platelet disorder. *Am J Med*, **51**, 818–827.

239 Biddle DA, Neto TG and Nguyen AND (2001) Platelet storage pool deficiency of α and δ granules. *Arch Pathol Lab Med*, **125**, 1125–1126.

240 Mant MJ, Doery JCG, Gauldie J and Sims H (1975) Pseudothrombocytopenia due to platelet aggregation and degranulation in blood collected in EDTA. *Scand J Haematol*, **15**, 161–170.

241 Stavem P and Kjaerheim A (1977) *In vitro* platelet stain preventing (degranulating) effect of various substances. *Scand J Haematol*, **18**, 170–176.

242 Cockbill SR, Burmester HB and Heptinstall S (1988) Pseudo grey platelet syndrome—grey platelets due to degranulation of platelets in blood collected into EDTA. *Eur J Haematol*, **41**, 326–333.

243 Hamilton RW, Shaikh BS, Ottic JN, Storch AE, Saleem A and White JG (1980) Platelet function, ultrastructure and survival in the May–Hegglin anomaly. *Am J Clin Pathol*, **74**, 663–668.

244 Breton-Gorius J, Favier R, Guichard J, Cherif D, Berger R, Debili N, Vainchenker W and Douay L (1995) A new congenital dysmegakaryopoietic thrombocytopenia (Paris–Trousseau) associated with giant platelet α-granules and chromosome 11 deletion at 11q23. *Blood*, **85**, 1805–1814.

245 Fajardo LF and Tallent C (1974) Malaria parasites within human platelets. *JAMA*, **229**, 1205–1207.

246 Casonato A, Bertomoro A, Pontara E, Dannhauser D, Lazzaro AR and Girolami A (1994) EDTA dependent pseudothrombocytopenia caused by antibodies against the cytoadhesive receptor of platelet gpIIB/IIIA. *J Clin Pathol*, **47**, 625–630.

247 Chiurazzi F, Villa MR and Rotoli B (1999) Transplacental transmission of EDTA-dependent pseudothrombocytopenia. *Haematologica*, **84**, 664.

248 Stiegler HM, Fischer Y and Steiner S (1999) Thrombocytopenia and glycoprotein IIb-IIIa receptor antagonists. *Lancet*, **353**, 1185.

249 Español I, Muñiz-Diaz E and Domingo-Clarós A (2000) The irreplaceable image: Platelet satellitism to granulated lymphocytes. *Haematologica*, **85**, 1322.

250 Yoo D, Weems H and Lessin LS (1982) Platelet to leukocyte adherence phenomenon. *Acta Haematol*, **68**, 142–148.

251 Lazo-Langner A, Piedras J, Romero-Lagarza P, Lome-Maldonado C, Sánchez-Guerrero J and López-Karpovitch X (2002) Platelet satellitism, spurious neutropenia, and cutaneous vasculitis: casual or causal association? *Am J Hematol*, **70**, 246–249.

252 Cesca C, Ben-Ezra J and Riley RS (2001) Platelet satellitism as presenting finding in mantle cell lymphoma. *Am J Clin Pathol*, **115**, 567–570.

253 Hansen M and Pedersen NT (1979) Circulating megakaryocytes in patients with pulmonary inflammation and in patients subjected to cholecystectomy. *Scand J Haematol*, **23**, 211–216.

254 Pederson NT and Petersen S (1980) Megakaryocytes in the foetal circulation and in cubital venous blood in the mother before and after delivery. *Scand J Haematol*, **25**, 5–11.

255 Pederson NT and Cohn J (1981) Intact megakaryocytes in the venous blood as a marker for thrombopoiesis. *Scand J Haematol*, **27**, 57–63.

256 Pederson NT and Laursen B (1983) Megakaryocytes in cubital venous blood in patients with chronic myeloproliferative disorders. *Scand J Haematol*, **30**, 50–58.

257 Swami VK, Solomon-Pestcoe F and Chen X (1996) Significance of circulating megakaryocytes in neonates: a prospective study of 68 cases. *Am J Clin Pathol*, **105**, 513–514.

258 Wilde NT, Burgess R, Keenan DJM and Lucas GS (1997) The effect of cardiopulmonary bypass on circulating megakaryocytes. *Br J Haematol*, **98**, 322–327.

259 Bianchi DW (1999) Fetal cells in the maternal circulation: feasibility in prenatal diagnosis. *Br J Haematol*, **105**, 574–583.

260 Levine RF, Olson TA, Shoff PK, Miller MK and Weisman LE (1996) Mature micromegakaryocytes: an unusual developmental pattern in term infants. *Br J Haematol*, **94**, 391–399.

261 Lowenstein ML (1959) The mammalian reticulocyte. *Int Rev Cytol*, **9**, 135–174.

262 Xanthou M (1970) Leucocyte blood picture in full-term and premature babies during neonatal period. *Arch Dis Child*, **45**, 242–249.

263 Gibson EL, Vaucher Y and Corrigan JJ (1984) Eosinophilia in premature infants: relationship to weight gain. *J Pediatr*, **95**, 99–101.

264 Wilkinson LS, Tang A and Gjedsted A (1983) Marked lymphocytosis suggesting chronic lymphocytic leukemia in three patients with hyposplenism. *Am J Med*, **75**, 1053–1056.

265 Kelemen E, Gergely P, Lehoczky D, Triska E, Demeter J and Vargha P (1986) Permanent large granular lymphocytosis in the blood of splenectomized individuals without concomitant increase of *in vitro* natural killer cell cytotoxicity. *Clin Exp Immunol*, **163**, 696–702.

266 Demeter J (1995) Persistent lymphocytosis of natural killer cells after splenectomy. *Br J Haematol*, **91**, 253–254.

267 Millard RE and Banerjee DK (1979) Changes in T and B blood lymphocytes after splenectomy. *J Clin Pathol*, **32**, 1045–1049.

268 Holyroyde CP and Gardner FH (1970) Acquisition of autophagic vacuoles by human erythrocytes: physiological role of the spleen. *Blood*, **36**, 566–575.

269 Kevy SV, Tefft M, Vawter GF and Rosen FS (1968) Hereditary splenic hypoplasia. *Pediatrics*, **42**, 752–757.

270 Devriendt K, Naulaers G, Matthijs G, Van Houdt K, Devlieger H, Gewillig M and Fryns JP (1997) Agenesis of corpus callosum and anophthalmia in the asplenia syndrome. A recognisable association? *Ann Genet*, **40**, 14–17.

271 Garriga S and Crosby WH (1959) The incidence of leukemia in families of patients with hypoplasia of the marrow. *Blood*, **14**, 1008–1114.

272 Rodin AE, Sloan JA and Nghiem QX (1972) Polysplenia with severe congenital heart disease and Howell–Jolly bodies. *Am J Clin Pathol*, **58**, 127–134.

273 Eshel Y, Sarova-Pinhas I, Lampl Y and Jedwab M (1991) Autosplenectomy complicating pneumococcal meningitis in an adult. *Arch Intern Med*, **151**, 998–999.

274 Ryan FP, Smart RC, Holdsworth CD and Preston FE (1978) Hyposplenism in inflammatory bowel disease. *Gut*, **19**, 50–55.

275 Corazza GR and Gasbarrini G (1983) Defective spleen function and its relation to bowel disease. *Clin Gastroenterol*, **12**, 651–669.

276 Dillon AM, Stein HB and English RA (1982) Splenic atrophy in systemic lupus erythematosus. *Ann Intern Med*, **96**, 40–43.

277 Friedman TC, Thomas PM, Fleisher TA, Feuillan P, Parker RI, Cassorla F and Chrousos GP (1991) Frequent occurrence of asplenia and cholelithiasis in patients with autoimmune polyglandular disease type 1. *Am J Med*, **91**, 625–630.

278 Kahls P, Panzer S, Kletter K, Minar E, Stain-Kos M, Walter R *et al.* (1988) Functional asplenia after bone marrow transplantation: a late complication related to extensive chronic graft-versus-host disease. *Ann Intern Med*, **109**, 461–464.

279 Dailey MO, Coleman CN and Fajardo LF (1981) Splenic injury caused by therapeutic irradiation. *Am J Surg Pathol*, **5**, 325–331.

280 Bensinger TA, Keller AR, Merrell LF and O'Leary DS (1971) Thorotrast-induced reticuloendothelial blockade in man. *Am J Med*, **51**, 663–668.

281 Kurth D, Deiss A and Cartwright GE (1969) Circulating siderocytes in human subjects. *Blood*, **34**, 754–764.

282 Steinberg MH, Gatling RR and Tavassoli M (1983) Evidence of hyposplenism, in the presence of splenomegaly. *Scand J Haematol*, **31**, 437–439.

283 Khan AM, Harrington RD, Nadel M and Greenberg BR (1998) Hyposplenism from *Mycobacterium avium* complex infection in a patient with AIDS and immune thrombocytopenia. *Acta Haematol*, **99**, 44–48.

284 Sunder-Plassmann G, Geissler K and Penner E (1992) Functional asplenia and vasculitis associated with antineutrophil cytoplasmic antibodies. *N Engl J Med*, **327**, 437–438.

285 Fadel M, Luyt D, Pandya H, Nichani S and Jenkins D (2004) Pneumococcal sepsis: should we look for asplenia? *J R Soc Med*, **97**, 582–583.

286 Shanberge IN (1954) Accidental occurrence of endothelial cells in peripheral blood smears. *Am J Clin Pathol*, **25**, 460–464.

287 George F, Brouqui P, Bofta M-C, Mutin M, Drancourt M, Brisson C *et al.* (1993) Demonstration of *Rickettsia conorii*-induced endothelial injury *in vivo* by measuring circulating endothelial cells, thrombomodulin, and von Willebrand factor in patients with Mediterranean spotted fever. *Blood*, **82**, 2109–2116.

288 Pooley R, Peterson L, Finn W and Kroft S (1998) Cytomegalovirus-infected cells in routinely prepared peripheral blood films of immunosuppressed patients. *Am J Clin Pathol*, **112**, 108–112.

289 Christensen WN, Ultmann JE and Mohos SC (1956) Disseminated neuroblastoma in an adult presenting with the picture of thrombocytopenic purpura. *Blood*, **11**, 273–278.

290 Nunez C, Abboud SL, Leman NC and Kemp JA (1983) Ovarian rhabdomyosarcoma presenting as leukemia. *Cancer*, **52**, 297–300.

291 Pollak ER, Miller HJ and Vye MV (1981) Medulloblastoma presenting as leukemia. *Am J Clin Pathol*, **76**, 98–103.

292 Krause JR (1979) Carcinocythemia. *Arch Pathol Lab Med*, **103**, 98.

293 Moodley V and Pool R (2003) Circulating neuroblastoma cells in peripheral blood. *Br J Haematol*, **123**, 2.

294 Melamed MR, Cliffton EE and Seal SH (1962) Cancer cells in the peripheral venous blood. A quantitative study of cells of problematic origin. *Am J Clin Pathol*, **37**, 381–388.

295 Brace W, Bain B, Walker M and Catovsky D (1995) Teaching cases from the Royal Marsden Hospital Case 9: an elderly patient with unusual circulating cells, *Leuk Lymphoma*, **18**, 529–530.

296 Trefzer U, Schlegel C, Sterry W, Späth-Schwalbe E, Possinger K and Denkert C (1999) Fulminant intravascular malignant melanoma mimicking acute leukemia. *Blood*, **94**, 1483–1484.

297 Swirsky D and Luckit J (1999) Images in haematology: the peripheral blood in metastatic melanoma. *Br J Haematol*, **107**, 219.

298 Bouroncle BA (1966) Sternberg–Reed cells in the peripheral blood of patients with Hodgkin's disease. *Blood*, **27**, 544–56.

299 Sinks LF and Clein GP (1966) The cytogenetics and cell metabolism of circulating Reed–Sternberg cells. *Br J Haematol*, **12**, 447–53.

300 Le CT (1980) Tick-borne relapsing fever in children. *Pediatrics*, **66**, 963–966.

301 Lawrence C, Brown ST and Freundlich LF (1988) Peripheral blood smear bacillemia. *Am J Med*, **85**, 111–113.

302 Yu RK, Shepherd LE and Rapson DA (2000) *Capnocytophaga canimorsus*, a potential emerging microorganism in splenectomized patients. *Br J Haematol*, **109**, 679.

303 Gloster ES, Strauss RA, Jimenez JF, Neuberg RW, Berry DH and Turner EJ (1985) Spurious elevated

platelet counts associated with bacteremia. *Am J Hematol*, **18**, 329–332.

304 Fife A, Hill D, Barton C and Burden P (1993) Gram negative septicaemia diagnosed on peripheral blood smear appearances. *J Clin Pathol*, **47**, 82–84.

305 Torlakovic E, Hibbs JR, Miller JS and Litz CE (1996) Intracellular bacteria in blood smears in patients with central venous catheters. *Arch Intern Med*, **155**, 1547–1550.

306 Dooley JR (1980) Haemotropic bacteria in man. *Lancet*, **ii**, 1237–1239.

307 Rolain J-M, Foucault C, Guieu R, La Scola B, Brouqui P and Raoult D (2002) *Bartonella quintana* in human erythrocytes. *Lancet*, **360**, 226–228.

308 Invernizzi R, Travaglino E and Perfetti V (2003) PAS positive monocytes in Whipple's disease. *Haematologica*, **88**, EIM16.

309 Puntariæ V, Borčič D, Bejuk D, Vrhovec B, Madić J, Busch K and Richter B (1994) Haemotropic bacteria in man, *Lancet*, **343**, 359–360.

310 Tarantolo SR, Landmark JD, Iwen PC, Kessinger A, Chan WC and Hinrichs SH (1997) *Bartonella*-like erythrocyte inclusions in thrombotic thrombocytopenic purpura. *Lancet*, **350**, 1602.

311 Raoult D, Lepidi H and Harle JR (2001) *Tropheryma whipplei* circulating in blood monocytes. *N Engl J Med*, **345**, 548.

312 Godwin JH, Stopeck A, Chang VT and Godwin TA (1991) Mycobacteremia in acquired immune deficiency syndrome. Rapid diagnosis based on inclusions in the peripheral blood smear. *Am J Clin Pathol*, **95**, 369–375.

313 Buller RS, Areno M, Hmiel SP, Paddock CD, Sumner JW, Rikihisa Y *et al.* (1999) *Ehrlichia ewingii*, a newly recognized agent of human ehrlichiosis. *N Engl J Med*, **341**, 148–155.

314 Chen S-M, Dumler JS, Bakken JS and Walker DH (1994) Identification of a granulocytotropic Ehrlichia species as the etiologic-agent of human disease. *J Clin Microbiol*, **32**, 589–595.

315 Rynkiewicz DL and Liu LX (1994) Human ehrlichiosis in New England. *N Engl J Med*, **330**, 292–293.

316 McDade JE (1990) Ehrlichiosis—a disease of animals and humans. *J Infect Dis*, **161**, 609–617.

317 Morais JD, Dawson JE, Greene C, Filipe AP, Galhardas LC and Bacellar F (1991) First European case of ehrlichiosis. *Lancet*, **338**, 633–634.

318 Horowitz HW, Kilchevsky E, Haber S, Aguero-Rosenfeld M, Kranwinkel R, James EK *et al.* (1998) Perinatal transmission of the agent of human granulocytic ehrlichiosis. *N Engl J Med*, **339**, 375–378.

319 Tamí I, Martinez JI, Tamí M, Redondo MC, Finol H and Simonovis N (1966) Identification of *Ehrlichia* species in blood smear. *Inf Dis Clin Practice*, **5**, 555–557.

320 Arraga-Alvarado C, Montero-Ojeda M, Bernardoni A, Anderson BE and Parra O (1996) [Human ehrlichiosis: report of the 1st case in Venezuela] (Article in Spanish). *Invest Clin*, **37**, 35–49.

321 Kuberski TT (1977) Intraleukocytic spore formation and leukocytic vacuolization during *Clostridium perfringens* septicemia. *Am J Clin Pathol*, **68**, 794–796.

322 Mann JM, Hull HF, Schmid GP and Droke WE (1984) Plague and the peripheral smear. *JAMA*, **251**, 953.

323 Monihan JM, Jewell TW and Weir GT (1986) Candida parapsilosis diagnosed by peripheral blood smear. *Arch Pathol Lab Med*, **110**, 1180–1181.

324 Yera H, Poulain D, Lefebvre A, Camus D and Sendid B (2004) Polymicrobial candidaemia revealed by the peripheral blood smear and chromogenic medium. *J Clin Pathol*, **57**, 196–198.

325 Girmenia C and Jaalouk G (1994) Detection of Candida in blood smears of patients with hematologic malignancies. *Eur J Haematol*, **52**, 124–125.

326 Yao YDC, Arkin CF, Doweiko JP and Hammer SM (1990) Disseminated cryptococcosis diagnosed on peripheral blood smear in a patient with acquired immunodeficiency syndrome. *Am J Med*, **89**, 100–102.

327 Wong KF, Tsang DNC and Chan JKC (1994) Bone marrow diagnosis of penicilliosis. *N Engl J Med*, **330**, 717–718.

328 Nayar R, Marley EF, Laban NLC and Campos JM (1995) Clinical pathology rounds: early diagnosis of fungemia in children. *Lab Med*, **26**, 381–383.

329 Berrouane Y, Bisiau H, Le Baron F, Cattoen C, Duthilleul P and Dei Cas E (1998) *Candida albicans* blastoconidia in peripheral blood smears from non-neutropenic surgical patients. *J Clin Pathol*, **51**, 537–538.

330 Singh B, Kim Sung L, Matusop A, Radhakrishnan A, Shamsul SS, Cox-Singh J, Thomas A and Conway DJ (2004) A large focus of naturally acquired *Plasmodium knowlesi* infections in human beings. *Lancet*, **363**, 1017–1024.

331 Wickramasinghe SN and Abdalla SH (2000) Blood and bone marrow changes in malaria. *Baillière's Clin Haematol*, **13**, 277–299.

332 Ladhani S, Lowe B, Cole AO, Kowuondo K and Newton CRJC (2003) Changes in white blood cells and platelets in children with falciparum malaria: relationship to disease outcome. *Br J Haematol*, **119**, 839–847.

333 Ladhani S, Khatri P, El-Bashir H and Shingadia D (2005) Imported malaria is a major cause of thrombocytopenia in children presenting to the emergency department in east London. *Br J Haematol*, **129**, 707–709.

334 Lawrence C (1999) Laveran remembered: malaria haemozoin in leucocytes. *Lancet*, **353**, 1852.

335 Day NPJ, Diep PT, Ly PT, Sinh DX, Chuong LV, Chau TTH *et al.* (1996) Clearance kinetics of parasites and pigment-containing leukocytes in severe malaria. *Blood*, **88**, 4694–4700.

336 Spach DH, Liles WC, Campbell GL, Quick RE, Anderson DE and Fritsche TR (1993) Tick-borne diseases in the United States. *N Engl J Med*, **329**, 936–947.

337 Rajpal DR, Murray DR, Morrell DR and O'Dwyer DR (2005) Human babesiosis: an unusual cause of haemolytic anaemia. *Br J Haematol*, **129**, Suppl. 1, 51.

338 Setty S, Khalil Z, Schori P, Azar M and Ferrieri P (2003) Babesiosis: two atypical cases from Minnesota and a review. *Am J Clin Pathol*, **120**, 554–559.

339 Pantanowitz L, Ballesteros E and de Girolami P (2001) Laboratory diagnosis of babesiosis. *Lab Med*, **32**, 184–188.

340 Moody AH and Chiodini PL (2000) Methods for the detection of blood parasites. *Clin Lab Haematol*, **22**, 189–202.

341 Moody A, Hunt-Cooke A, Gabbett E and Chiodini P (2000) Performance of the OptiMAL malaria antigen capture dipstick for malaria diagnosis and treatment monitoring at the Hospital for Tropical Diseases, London. *Br J Haematol*, **109**, 891–894.

342 Grobusch MP, Alpermann U, Schwenke S, Jelinek T and Warhurst DC (1999) False-positive rapid tests for malaria in patients with rheumatoid factor. *Lancet*, **353**, 297.

343 Albrecht H, Sobottka I, Stellbrink H-J, van Lunzen J and Greten H (1996) Diagnosis of disseminated toxoplasmosis using a peripheral blood smear. *AIDS*, **10**, 799–800.

344 Arnold SJ, Kinney MC, McCormick MS, Dunmer S and Scott MA (1997) Disseminated toxoplasmosis: unusual presentations in the immunocompromised host. *Arch Pathol Lab Med*, **121**, 869–873.

345 http://www.dpd.cdc.gov/dpdx/html/try-panosomiasisafrican.htm

346 Moore AC, Ryan ET and Waldron MA (2002) A 37-year-old man with fever, hepatosplenomegaly and a cutaneous foot lesion after a trip to Africa. *N Engl J Med*, **346**, 2069–2077.

347 Learning Bench Aid No 3. *Microscopical Diagnosis of Lymphatic Filariasis, Loiasis, Onchocerciasis.* Tropical Health Technology, Doddington, Cambridgeshire.

Answers to test questions

Multiple choice questions

MCQ 3.1	TFTTT
MCQ 3.2	FTTFT
MCQ 3.3	TTTTF
MCQ 3.4	TTFTT
MCQ 3.5	FTTFT

Extended matching questions

EMQ 3.1
1 B
2 B
3 A
4 F
5 E

EMQ 3.2
1 I
2 D
3 D
4 C
5 H

EMQ 3.3
1 B
2 A
3 D
4 H
5 C

EMQ 3.4

1 A
2 D
3 A
4 E
5 G

EMQ 3.5

1 D
2 I
3 A
4 H
5 G

EMQ 3.6

1 A
2 A
3 G
4 E
5 A

4 Detecting erroneous blood counts

The sources of errors in blood counts

Errors in blood counts may be pre-analytical, analytical or post-analytical. Pre-analytical errors are those that precede the analysis of the sample and include errors in producing a request form, errors during venesection and errors in transport and storage of the specimen (Table 4.1). Analytical errors are those that occur during the analysis of the sample (Table 4.2). Post-analytical errors are those that occur after analysis is completed and involve mishandling of data (Table 4.3). Sometimes an error at one stage of the process gives rise to

an error at another. Thus, incomplete or erroneous patient identification details or clinical information may lead to a result being issued with a wrong reference range or to interpretative comments being misleading.

The detection of errors in automated blood counts

Since automated blood counts may be inaccurate, it is the responsibility of the laboratory staff performing a count or authorizing a report to detect inaccuracies whenever possible.

Table 4.1 Some pre-analytical sources of errors in blood counts.

Type of error	Examples
Clerical errors	Patient's name, age or gender missing from request form Ethnic origin not supplied when it is essential for interpretation of a test result Information about pregnancy not given Location of patient or relevant clinician details missing
Unannounced blood transfusion	Previous blood transfusion, unknown to laboratory staff
Fault during patient identification or phlebotomy	Blood from wrong patient; blood specimen and request form relate to different patients Maternal and neonatal samples confused Specimen diluted (e.g. taken from above intravenous infusion or excess liquid EDTA relative to volume of blood) Specimen taken into wrong anticoagulant Specimen taken into too high a concentration of EDTA Specimen haemoconcentrated due to prolonged application of tourniquet Specimen partly clotted Specimen haemolysed Specimen too small leading to 'short sample'
Fault during fetal blood sampling	Contamination with amniotic fluid [1]
Fault during specimen transport or storage	Specimen inadvertently heated [2] or frozen Aged blood Specimen contaminated with subcutaneous fat [3]

EDTA, ethylenediaminetetra-acetic acid.

Table 4.2 Some analytical sources of errors in blood counts.

Type of error	Examples
Faulty sampling	Failure to prime instrument Inadequate mixing Aspiration probe blocked, e.g. by clot from previous sample 'Short sample' or clotted sample not detected Carryover from preceding very abnormal specimen (minor with modern instruments)
Faulty calibration Faulty maintenance, other instrument malfunction, reagent failure	Use of control material as calibrant or error in assigning values to calibrant
Inaccuracy inherent in specific methodologies	Underestimation of MCV by impedance counters in the presence of hypochromia Failure of identification of cells caused by peroxidase deficiency
Inaccuracy due to unusual characteristics of specimen	Error in Hb or red cell indices caused by presence of cold agglutinins, cryoglobulinaemia, hyperlipidaemia or (rarely) rosetting of red cells around neutrophils Error in platelet count caused by platelet aggregation or satellitism Factitious 'neutropenia' or other cytopenia caused by peroxidase deficiency

Hb, haemoglobin concentration; MCV, mean cell volume.

Table 4.3 Some post-analytical sources of errors in blood counts.

Type of error

Transcription error in laboratory
Transcription error in ward or outpatient department when results are telephoned
Results not issued in a timely manner
Results never reach intended destination
Results filed in wrong patient's notes and so applied to wrong patient
Results issued with incorrect reference range or no reference range
Results issued with inappropriate interpretation

The validation of an automated count requires: (i) knowledge that an instrument is capable of measuring all variables accurately, that it has been correctly calibrated and that quality control procedures indicate normal functioning; and (ii) assessment of each individual count as to whether it is likely to be correct or that, alternatively, it requires further review. If the first set of conditions has been met then it may be possible to validate counts by means of a computer program, either built into the automated counter or developed to fit the specifications of an individual laboratory. Counts can be computer-validated if: (i) all measurements fall within predetermined limits (which may be somewhat wider than the reference limits for that measurement) and there are no 'flags'; or (ii) measurements fall outside predetermined limits but nevertheless have not changed significantly in comparison with previous measurements on that individual. When results do not meet either set of criteria they should be individually assessed in relation to the clinical details and, if necessary, further steps should be taken to validate the results. These further steps may include: (i) examination of the histograms produced by an automated instrument to establish the likely reason for anomalous results or 'flags'; (ii) examination of the blood specimen, e.g. to check the date and time when venesection was performed, to confirm that the specimen was of adequate volume and to detect clots, fibrin strands, hyperlipidaemia or haemolysis; (iii) examination of a blood film; or (iv) various combinations of these procedures. Which procedures are necessary depends on the nature of the abnormality shown on the automated count and the safeguards that are already built into the instrumentation, e.g. to confirm the identity of the patient and detect specimens of inadequate volume or containing clots. Opinions differ as to whether blood films should always be examined in conjunction with the initial blood count from a patient or whether an automated count with no 'flags' can be accepted as valid evidence that there is no significant haematological abnormality. The latter policy will miss some abnormalities of clinical significance but not many. Regrettably, the time when it was possible to examine a blood film in conjunction with all blood counts appears to have passed, under the pressure of economic factors. Validation of a count before it is released also includes ensuring that results have been produced for all tests required, i.e. that no result has been 'voted out' because of poor replicate counts or because it is beyond the linearity limits of the instrument.

Blood count results should be assessed as to probability in the light of the clinical details. For example, cytopenia could be accepted without further review in a patient known to have had recent chemotherapy. Similarly, an increased white blood cell count (WBC) with a 'left shift' flag could be accepted in a postpartum or postoperative patient. Counts that have 'flags' indicating the presence of blast cells, atypical lymphocytes or nucleated red blood cells (NRBC) require microscopic review. Whether flags for 'left shift' or 'immature granulocytes' always require review is a matter of individual laboratory policy. Blood count results that are unexpected or that fall a long way outside reference limits generally require further attention. An abnormal mean cell haemoglobin concentration (MCHC) is a useful indicator of factitious results since it is derived from all measured red cell variables, i.e. haemoglobin concentration (Hb), red blood cell count (RBC) and mean cell volume (MCV) or haematocrit (Hct). It is thus sensitive to erroneous measurements in any of these variables caused, for example, by hyperlipidaemia, intravascular haemolysis, non-lysis of red cells in the Hb channel and red cell agglutination. A markedly elevated MCV is also often factitious. Some types of factitious result occur with all instruments while others are specific to a methodology. Laboratory workers should be familiar with the factitious results that are likely with the particular instrument they are operating. The rest of this chapter will deal with factitious results other than those consequent on technical errors or instrument and reagent malfunction.

When contamination with amniotic fluid leads to an inaccurate fetal blood count two mechanisms are operating. One is simple dilution, which affects all variables. The other is activation of coagulation in the sample, which has a disproportionate effect on the platelet count. A related blood film may show platelet aggregates and amniotic fluid cells [1].

It should be noted that factitious results are more likely to have been reported for instruments that have been in use for a long time or have been studied in detail. The lack of reported factitious results for other instruments does not indicate that they do not occur.

Errors in automated WBC

Errors that may occur in automated WBCs are summarized in Tables 4.4 and 4.5 and instrument printouts from a sample producing an erroneous count because of contamination with subcutaneous fat are shown in Fig. 4.1 [3]. The only common causes of erroneous counts are factitiously high counts caused by NRBC, platelet aggregates or non-lysis of red cells. Factitiously low counts are uncommon, unless the blood has taken many days to reach the laboratory. When a low WBC is the result of neutrophil aggregation it may be ethylenediaminetetra-acetic acid (EDTA)-dependent, temperature-dependent or dependent on both [8]. The former may be reversed by addition of kanamycin in a final concentration of 30 mg/ml [8].

Erroneous WBCs are usually detected because of instrument 'flags' and improbable results for the WBC or other measurements, or by abnormalities detectable on instrument scatter plots or histograms. For example, an erroneous WBC consequent on a cold agglutinin would usually be accompanied by an improbably high MCV and MCHC. Neutrophil aggregation may be indicated by an abnormal cloud at the top of the neutrophil area of the Coulter STKS or Bayer H.1 series instruments.

For many instruments, if significant numbers of NRBC are present and an accurate WBC is needed, it is necessary to correct the total nucleated cell count for the number of NRBC by counting their percentage on a blood film. However, it is also possible to accept the total nucleated cell count as a definitive measurement and calculate the absolute count of NRBC and each leucocyte type from the manual differential count. Non-lysis of red cells is mainly a problem when the WBC is measured by light-scattering technology. Impedance counters usually

Table 4.4 Some causes of a falsely high WBC.

Cause	Instruments on which fault can occur
Presence of NRBC	All instruments
Numerous giant platelets	All instruments
Non-lysis of red cells	
Uraemia	Bayer H.1 series*
Fetal and neonatal specimens	Bayer H.1 series*, Cell-Dyn instruments (optical channels), some Sysmex instruments, Coulter STKS
Abnormal haemoglobins (e.g. AS, SS, AC, AE, AD, AO-Arab)	Bayer H.1 series*, some Sysmex Instruments
Liver disease	Coulter and some Sysmex instruments
Cold agglutinins	Coulter instruments
Myelodysplastic syndromes	Coulter STKS
Megaloblastic anaemia	Coulter
Post-splenectomy	Coulter
Platelet aggregates	Coulter, Bayer and ABX instruments
Platelet phagocytosis by neutrophils	Abbott Cell-Dyn 3500 (impedance count accurate, optical count inaccurate) [4]
Cryoglobulinaemia and cryofibrinogenaemia	Coulter, Sysmex instruments and Bayer instruments [5]
Paraproteinaemia	Coulter and Sysmex instruments
Fibrin strands	Coulter instruments
Hyperlipidaemia	Coulter instruments
Contamination of specimen with subcutaneous fat	Bayer H.1 series [3]
Malarial parasites	Coulter and Sysmex instruments
Unstable haemoglobin	Coulter instruments

NRBC, nucleated red blood cell; WBC, white blood cell count.
* Basophil channel gives accurate WBC but differential counts are erroneous.

Table 4.5 Some causes of a falsely low WBC.

Cause	Instruments on which abnormality can occur
Cell lysis caused when blood is more than 3 days old	Coulter instruments, Cobas Argos 5 Diff and probably other instruments
Storage at room temperature for 24 hours or more	Cell-Dyn 3500—fall in optical WBC, impedance WBC stable [6]
Storage at 4°C for more than 24 hours	ABX instruments
Leucocyte or leucocyte and platelet aggregation due to an antibody or to alteration of the cell membrane or to the presence of neoplastic cells with abnormal characteristics (e.g. antibody-mediated aggregation of neutrophils, mucin-induced aggregation in adenocarcinoma, aggregation of lymphoma cells or neoplastic plasma cells); leucocyte rosetting around other cells [7]	Coulter instruments, Sysmex instruments, Bayer H.1 series instruments
Potent cold agglutinin	Coulter instruments

WBC, white blood cell count.

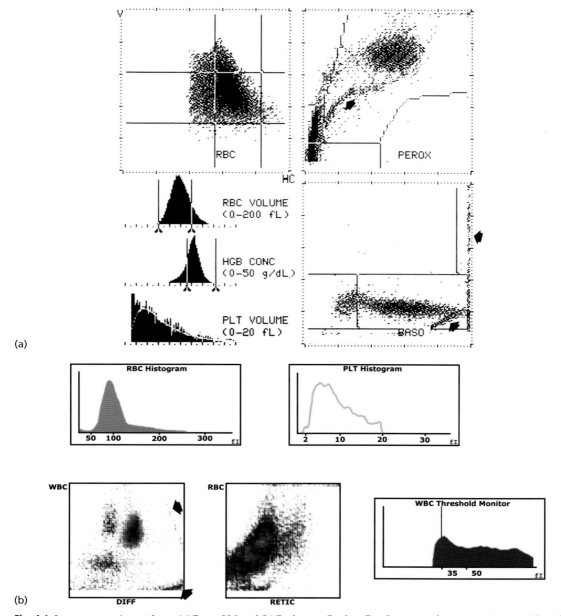

Fig. 4.1 Instrument printout from: (a) Bayer H.2 and (b) Beckman–Coulter Gen S counters from a specimen accidentally contaminated with subcutaneous fat [3]. The signals generated by the fat are arrowed. The H.2 count was inaccurate whereas the Gen S count was accurate.

produce an accurate result. The observation of factitious elevation of the WBC caused by non-lysis of red cells can be clinically useful since it may be indicative of a previously undiagnosed haemoglobinopathy. This has been noted with H.1 series instruments and on the differential count channel of Sysmex instruments.

Factitious counts caused by aggregation of platelets can usually be prevented by taking the blood specimen into citrate rather than into EDTA. Erroneous counts caused by cryoproteins and cold agglutinins can be rectified by keeping the specimen warm. Aggregation of leucocytes is often time-dependent [9] and is sometimes caused by a cold antibody, so that keeping the specimen warm and performing the blood count rapidly after phlebotomy can produce an accurate count. When erroneous counts are due to causes other than white cell clumping, haemocytometer counts will be accurate.

Errors in haemoglobin concentration and red cell indices

Haemoglobin concentration

Errors that can occur in automated measurements of the Hb and red cell indices are shown in Tables 4.6–4.8. Such erroneous results are usually suspected from a markedly elevated MCV, a markedly abnormal MCHC or a discrepancy between MCHC and cellular haemoglobin concentration mean (CHCM).

Erroneous estimations of Hb (see Table 4.6) most often result from turbidity caused by a high WBC or lipid in the plasma, either endogenous lipid [15] or that consequent on parenteral nutrition [16]. The degree of elevation of the WBC that causes an erroneous Hb varies greatly between instruments since it is dependent on the strength of the lytic agent that is employed in the WBC/Hb channel. The problem

can be circumvented if separate channels are used for the WBC and the Hb, as in recent Sysmex instruments, since a more powerful lytic agent can then be used. The instrument operator should be aware of the degree of leucocytosis that is likely to make the Hb erroneous on a specific instrument and results should then be checked by manual techniques. The haemolysate is centrifuged before absorbance is read so that turbidity caused by the presence of cellular debris does not affect the reading. Erroneous results from hyperlipidaemia may be suspected when red cell indices are improbable or red cells on stained blood films have fuzzy outlines. This error can be confirmed by examining the plasma, after either centrifugation or red cell sedimentation, and noting the milky appearance. The problem can be dealt with by performing a microhaematocrit and a 'blank' measurement using the patient's plasma. A correction is then as follows:

$$\text{True Hb} = \text{measured Hb} - ['Hb' \text{ of lipaemic plasma} \times (1 - \text{Hct})]$$

Alternatively, the plasma can be carefully removed and replaced by an equal volume of isotonic fluid before repeating the automated count. Similarly, the use of a plasma blank permits the correction of errors caused by the presence of a paraprotein or polyclonal hypergammaglobulinaemia (Table 4.9). With the Bayer H.1 series and Advia 120 instruments,

Table 4.6 Some causes of a falsely high Hb estimate.

Cause	Instruments on which fault can occur	Detection
High WBC	All, but to a variable extent	Check whenever WBC is very high
Hyperlipidaemia, endogenous or due to parenteral nutrition	Coulter and Bayer instruments, Cell-Dyn instruments but error eliminated by modified reagent [10]	Improbable results for MCH and MCHC or flagging of MCHC/CHCM discrepancy; fuzzy red cell outlines on blood films
Paraprotein or hypergammaglobulinaemia	Coulter instruments, Sysmex NE-8000	MCH and MCHC slightly elevated [11]
Cryoglobulinaemia	Coulter instruments	MCH and MCHC slightly elevated
High concentration of carboxyhaemoglobin [7] Turbidity resulting from non-lysis of red cells [7]		

CHCM, cellular haemoglobin concentration mean; MCH, mean cell haemoglobin; MCHC, mean cell haemoglobin concentration; WBC, white blood cell count.

Table 4.7 Some causes of inaccurate estimates of RBC, MCV and Hct estimations.

Fault	Cause	Instruments on which fault can occur
Falsely high RBC	WBC very high	Coulter and Bayer instruments
	Numerous large platelets	Coulter instruments
	Hyperlipidaemia (not consistently)	Coulter instruments, Bayer instruments
	Cryoglobulinaemia	(if concentration very high) [10]
	Cryofibrinogenaemia	Coulter instruments
Falsely low RBC	Cold agglutinins	Coulter and Bayer instruments
	EDTA-dependent panagglutination	Coulter instruments
	In vitro red cell lysis due to mishandling of specimen or very abnormal red cells	All instruments
	Extreme microcytosis or fragmentation causing red cells to fall below the lower threshold	Coulter (and probably other) instruments
Falsely high MCV	Storage of blood at room temperature	Most instruments, to a varying extent but particularly Bayer instruments (see text)
	Cold agglutinins and EDTA-dependent red cell agglutination	Coulter and Bayer instruments
	WBC very high	Coulter instruments
	Hyperosmolar states	Coulter instruments
	Excess K_2EDTA	Bayer H.1 series
Falsely low MCV	Hypochromic red cells	Some impedance instruments (Coulter STKR and earlier Coulter instruments, K-1000 to a lesser extent but not Sysmex NE-8000) [12]
	Increase in ambient temperature	Coulter instruments
	Hypo-osmolar states	Coulter instruments
	Repeated mixing of sample leading to increased oxygenation	Sysmex instruments [13] and probably also other impedance counters
Falsely high Hct	Factitious elevation of MCV (except when due to a cold agglutinin)	See above
	Factitious reduction of RBC	See above
Falsely low Hct	Factitious reduction of MCV	See above
	Factitious reduction of RBC by extreme microcytosis or *in vitro* red cell lysis	See above
	Cold agglutinin	Coulter instruments
	Repeated mixing of sample leading to increased oxygenation	Sysmex instruments [13] and probably also other impedance counters

EDTA, ethylenediametetra-acetic acid; Hct, haematocrit; MCV, mean cell volume; RBC, red blood cell count; WBC, white blood cell count.

a correct Hb can be calculated from the CHCM and a microhaematocrit when there is lipid or other interfering substances in the plasma. The errors introduced into the Hb estimation by marked hyperbilirubinaemia and the presence of high levels of carboxyhaemoglobin are not of such magnitude as to be of practical importance and can therefore be ignored.

A falsely low Hb is a much less frequent observation that a falsely high estimate, but has been reported with a Bayer H.2 instrument in three patients with a very high WBC (243, 348 and 850 × 10^9/l) [17]. There

was an associated factitious reduction of the MCHC leading to a discrepancy between the MCHC (calculated from the Hb) and the CHCM (measured directly). An unstable colour reaction was postulated as the cause of this observation.

RBC, MCV and Hct

Errors in the RBC, MCV and Hct are summarized in Table 4.7. Impedance and earlier light-scattering instruments have an intrinsic error that leads to the

Table 4.8 Some causes of inaccurate MCH and MCHC estimations.

Fault	Cause	Instruments on which fault can occur
MCH falsely high	Factitious elevation of Hb	See Table 4.6
	Factitious reduction of RBC	See Table 4.7
	Intravascular haemolysis with free haemoglobin in plasma (e.g. in *Clostridium perfringens* sepsis)	All instruments
	Administration of haemoglobin-based oxygen carriers [14]	All instruments
MCHC falsely high or true fall of MCHC masked	Factitious elevation of Hb	See Table 4.6
	Intravascular haemolysis with free haemoglobin in plasma or *in vitro* lysis of red cells	All instruments
	Factitious reduction in Hct or the product of the MCV and RBC	See Table 4.7
	Hypo-osmolar states	Coulter instruments
	Administration of haemoglobin-based oxygen carriers [14]	All instruments
MCHC falsely low	Factitious elevation of MCV (except when caused by cold agglutinins)	See Table 4.7
	Factitious elevation of RBC by numerous giant platelets	All instruments
	Hyperosmolar states	Coulter instruments
	Falsely low Hb caused by extreme leucocytosis	Bayer H.2 [5]

Hb, haemoglobin concentration; Hct, haematocrit; MCH, mean cell haemoglobin; MCHC, mean cell haemoglobin concentration; MCV, mean cell volume; RBC, red blood cell count.

MCV of hypochromic cells being underestimated and their MCHC being overestimated. This can also lead to two apparent populations on a red cell size histogram with blood samples that, on Bayer H.1 series and Advia 120 instruments, show a single population of cells on a histogram of red cell size but two populations on a histogram of red cell haemoglobinization.

Storage of blood at room temperature may cause errors in the MCV and Hct. Coulter instruments usually give stable measurements unless blood has been stored for several days but a 6 fl rise by 24 hours has been observed with another impedance counter, the Sysmex NE-8000 [18]. With the Abbott Cell-Dyn 2500 a rise of 2–3 fl by 24 hours was observed [6].

The MCV on the Cobas Argos Diff 5 rises by about 2 fl by 24 hours [19]. Marked changes are seen with Bayer H.1 series instruments (and it is likely that they also occur with the Advia 120); a rise in the MCV starts after about 8 hours and by 24 hours the average rise varies between 4–5 and 7–8 fl, depending on the ambient temperature. A low MCHC, without any corresponding hypochromia being detectable on a blood film, can indicate that an elevation in the MCV is caused by red cell swelling as a consequence of storage. A factitious rise in the Hct occurs in parallel with the rise in the MCV.

When blood samples are processed without delay, errors in the RBC, MCV and Hct (excluding those which are intrinsic to the methodology) are most

	FBC on whole blood	'FBC' of EDTA-plasma	FBC on washed and resuspended red cells
RBC ($\times 10^{-12}$/l)	2.68	0.02	2.62
Hb (g/dl)	10.1	1.7	8.2
MCV (fl)	94.3	88.2	95.5
MCH (pg)	37.6	++++	31.4
MCHC (g/dl)	39.9	++++	32.9

Table 4.9 Erroneous estimates of haemoglobin on Coulter Gen S counter caused by a paraprotein.

EDTA, ethylenediaminetetra-acetic acid; FBC, full blood count; Hb, haemoglobin concentration; MCH, mean cell haemoglobin; MCHC, mean cell haemoglobin concentration; MCV, mean cell volume; RBC, red blood cell count.

often caused by cold agglutinins. Impedance counters are prone to more major errors for this reason than are current Bayer light-scattering instruments. The factitious elevation of MCV is consequent on the doublets and triplets that pass through the aperture being counted and sized as if they were single cells. The RBC is factitiously low both for this reason and because, with some counters, larger agglutinates are above the upper threshold for red cells and are excluded from the count. The size of doublets and triplets is also underestimated. For these reasons although MCV (Hct × 1000/RBC) is overestimated, Hct is underestimated. The underestimation of Hct means that there is a factitious elevation of mean cell haemoglobin (MCH) and MCHC. Erroneous counts can generally be eliminated by warming the sample before processing. When the cold agglutinin is very potent it may be necessary to both warm the blood specimen and predilute the sample for analysis in warmed diluent.

Other causes of factitious errors in the RBC, MCV and Hct are uncommon. Various changes in plasma osmolality lead to artefacts in MCV measurement by impedance counters. If a cell is in a hyperosmolar environment *in vivo* due, e.g. to severe hypernatraemia or severe hyperglycaemia, then the cytoplasm of the cell will also be hyperosmolar. When the blood is diluted within the automated counter in a medium of much lower osmolality then the more rapid movement of water than of electrolytes, glucose or urea across the cell membrane will lead to acute swelling of the cell which is reflected in the measured MCV. Since the Hct is calculated from the MCV it will also be increased whereas the MCHC is correspondingly reduced. This phenomenon may occur in hypernatraemic dehydration [20], severe uraemia [20] and in hyperglycaemia, e.g. due to uncontrolled diabetes mellitus [21]. Not only may factitious macrocytosis be produced but true microcytosis may be masked. The converse error of a falsely low MCV and Hct with elevation of the MCHC may be seen in patients with hyponatraemia [20] such as may be seen in chronic alcoholics and patients with inappropriate secretion of antidiuretic hormone. The factitious reduction of MCV in hypo-osmolar states can lead to masking of a true macrocytosis as well as factitious microcytosis. This error can be eliminated in instruments with a predilute mode by diluting the sample and allowing time for equilibration of solutes across the red cell membrane. A control sample should be prediluted and tested in parallel since, although the osmolality of the recommended diluent differs between instruments, it is often somewhat hypertonic so that the MCV of cells from normal subjects may also alter on predilution.

With the Bayer H.1 series of instruments, factitious macrocytosis can result from cell swelling that is induced by taking a small volume of blood into excess K_2EDTA. A hypochromia 'flag' also occurs [22].

If microcytosis is severe, some red cells may fall below the lower threshold of the instrument and, as these cells are excluded from the measurements, the MCV is overestimated. In the case of impedance counters this is usually more than counteracted by the fact that the cells are likely to be hypochromic and the inherent error of the methodology leads to the size of those cells that fall above the threshold being underestimated (see p. 35). If there are normochromic red cell fragments falling below the lower threshold the MCV will be overestimated without any counterbalancing effect being expected. Neither of these artefacts is of practical importance.

Inaccuracies in the Hct are those expected from inaccuracies in the RBC and MCV.

MCH, MCHC and RDW

Errors that may occur in the MCH and MCHC are summarized in Table 4.8. Errors in these variables are consequent on errors in the primary measurements from which they are derived. Mechanisms have been explained above. The inherent error of impedance counting leads to the MCHC being a very stable variable which fails to reflect true changes occurring in red cells. This is paradoxically useful since abnormalities of the MCHC are commonly factitious and therefore serve to alert the laboratory worker to the possibility of an erroneous result. In the case of current Bayer instruments, true abnormality of the MCHC is more common but so is a factitious reduction consequent on swelling of cells as blood ages. A discrepancy between MCHC and CHCM serves as a flag since the latter variable is measured directly and thus is not affected by errors in Hb estimation.

With the Coulter instruments, and probably with others, the RDW rises with room temperature storage. In the case of the Coulter Gen S the rise starts from day 2 [23].

Errors in platelet counts

The causes of erroneous platelet counts are summarized in Table 4.10. Many instruments are inaccurate in the measurement of low platelet counts. A small inaccuracy can be clinically significant when a platelet count of $10 \times 10^9/l$ is used as a trigger for

platelet transfusion, e.g. in patients with acute leukaemia. In one study, one immunological method (Cell-Dyn) and one optical method (XE-2100) were accurate whereas another impedance method (LH750) and four optical methods (H.3, Advia, Cell-Dyn and XE-2100) overestimated by $2–5 \times 10^9/l$ [31]. The Pentra 120 impedance method underestimated by about $4 \times 10^9/l$. In addition to these errors, intrinsic to the technology, major errors in the platelet count can result from characteristics of the blood sample. Factitiously low platelet counts are quite common as a result either of partial clotting of the specimen

Table 4.10 Some causes of inaccurate automated platelet counts.

Cause	Instrument on which observed
Falsely low platelet counts	
Partial clotting of specimen	All instruments
Activation of platelets during venepuncture with consequent aggregation	All instruments
EDTA-induced platelet aggregation	All instruments
Platelet satellitism	All instruments
Storage of blood at 4°C for more than 24 hours	ABX instruments
EDTA-induced platelet phagocytosis by neutrophils and monocytes	Observed with Cell-Dyn 3500 but would be expected to occur with all instruments [4]
Giant platelets falling above upper threshold for platelet count	All instruments
Falsely high platelet counts	
Microcytic red cells or red cell fragments falling below upper threshold for the platelet count	All instruments
White cell fragments counted as platelets (fragments of leukaemic blast cells, hairy cells or lymphoma cells)	All instruments
Haemoglobin H disease	Coulter instruments
Cryoglobulin*	Coulter instruments, Bayer H.1 series, Cell-Dyn 4000 (impedance count inaccurate; optical count accurate) [24]
Hypertriglyceridaemia or hyperlipidaemia	Sysmex NE-8000, Bayer H.1 series [10,25], impedance counters
Bacteria in blood sample, either in patients with bacteraemia [26,27] or due to delay in processing in a hot climate [28]	Ortho ELT8 [26], Cell-Dyn 4000 [27]
Fungi in blood sample, often from fungal growth on indwelling intravenous line	Bayer H.1 series [29]
Inadvertent heating of blood sample	Bayer H.1 series [2]
Parasitized red cells in malaria	Cell-Dyn 4000, optical and impedance channels [30]

EDTA, ethylenediaminetetra-acetic acid.
* Platelet count and histograms of platelet size become normal on warming the blood.

or of platelet aggregation or satellitism (see p. 128). Platelet aggregation may be due to activation of platelets during a difficult venepuncture or may be mediated by an antibody, which is either an immunoglobulin G (IgG) or IgM EDTA-dependent antibody or an EDTA-independent antibody. IgG-dependent platelet antibodies are directed at a crypto-antigen on platelet glycoprotein IIb [32]. EDTA-dependent platelet aggregation can be a transient phenomenon, e.g. occurring during infectious mononucleosis [33]. Platelet aggregation often leads to instrument 'flags', abnormal histograms of platelet distribution and abnormal white cell scatter plots. Platelet satellitism is also an antibody-mediated EDTA-dependent phenomenon. Neither *in vitro* aggregation nor platelet satellitism is of any significance *in vivo* but the detection of all factitiously low platelet counts is very important in order to avoid unnecessary investigation and treatment of the patient. There have been instances in which a factitiously low platelet count has led to a mistaken diagnosis of 'idiopathic' (i.e. autoimmune) thrombocytopenic purpura (ITP) and consequent corticosteroid treatment and even splenectomy. Accurate platelet counts in subjects with EDTA-dependent platelet aggregation can be achieved by adding 20 mg of kanamycin either to the EDTA into which blood is taken or to the EDTA-anticoagulated blood sample [34] or by adding excess EDTA to cause disaggregation. Alternatively, blood can be taken into sodium citrate or a finger-prick sample can be collected using an alternative anticoagulant, e.g. Unopette (Becton Dickinson) containing ammonium oxalate.

The accuracy of any unexpectedly low platelet counts must always be confirmed. The specimen should be examined with an orange stick to detect any small clots or fibrin strands and the instrument histograms and scatter plots should be assessed. Some instruments are able to detect fibrin strands or small clots and flag their presence. The presence of platelet aggregates may also be flagged and an abnormal cluster or band of particles may be apparent in scattergrams. The presence of an abnormal cluster along the top of the neutrophil box with the Bayer H.1 series instruments may indicate the occurrence of platelet satellitism. However, not all falsely

low platelet counts are flagged or associated with abnormal scattergrams. For example, platelet aggregates may be so large that they are the same size as white cells and are thus not identified. It is therefore important to examine a blood film for the presence of fibrin strands, platelet aggregates, platelet satellitism and giant platelets whenever a platelet count is unexpectedly low. Falsely low counts should be deleted from reports since clinical staff often do not realize that a comment such as 'platelet aggregates' is likely to mean that the platelet count is wrong. When platelet aggregation is antibody-mediated, accurate counts can usually be obtained on specimens taken into citrate or heparin rather than EDTA (but the effect of dilution must be allowed for). Some such antibodies are cold antibodies, so performing a count rapidly on a specimen that has been kept warm can also produce a valid count. Alternatively, if the platelet count is clearly normal, the comment 'platelet count normal on film' may be acceptable and obviate the need to obtain a further blood specimen. Laboratories should be alert to platelet aggregation induced by therapy with monoclonal antibodies, such as abciximab, directed at platelet antigens since these agents may also cause true thrombocytopenia [35,36].

It may be impossible to obtain an accurate automated platelet count in the presence of numerous giant platelets, in which case a haemocytometer count is required.

If a low platelet count is supported by the blood film, but is nevertheless unexpected, a repeat specimen should be obtained with careful attention to venepuncture technique before the count is regarded as a valid result on which management decisions should be based.

Falsely elevated platelet counts are much less common than falsely reduced counts. They are usually due to the presence of marked microcytosis (e.g. in haemoglobin H disease) or to the presence of red cell fragments (e.g. in microangiopathic haemolytic anaemia or severe burns) so that a significant number of red cells fall below the upper threshold for platelets. Factitious elevation of the platelet count can also be produced by red cell fragmentation produced *in vitro* by inadvertent heating of a blood sample [2]. Even with variable thresholds and fitted curves it may not be possible to separate very small red cells or fragments from platelets. An accurate platelet count despite the presence of red cell fragments or microcytes can be produced by a Sysmex R-1000 Reticulocyte Analyzer. The RNA of both platelets and reticulocytes is stained with the fluorescent dye, auramine, and the two populations are then separated by gating [37]. Microcytic red cells do not take up the dye since they do not contain RNA.

Occasionally, falsely elevated platelet counts are caused by other particles of a similar size to platelets. The counting of fragments of white cell cytoplasm as platelets has been described in acute myeloid leukaemias [38,39] (Fig. 4.2), acute lymphoblastic leukaemia [39], hairy cell leukaemia [40] and lymphoma [41]. In patients with acute leukaemia this phenomenon is actually quite common [39]. The counting of red and white cell fragments [42] or extraneous particles such as fungi [29] (Fig. 4.3) as platelets may have serious implications in acute leukaemia as a severe thrombocytopenia may be masked and left untreated.

When platelets are distributed evenly in a blood film, the platelet count can be validated by counting the ratio of platelets to red cells and calculating the platelet count indirectly from the RBC.

Fig. 4.2 Peripheral blood film of a patient with acute monoblastic leukaemia (M5 acute myeloid leukaemia). Despite only a slight reduction of the 'platelet' count the patient had major bleeding. Inspection of the film showed that there were many fragments of cytoplasm derived from leukaemic cells that were of similar size to platelets and accounted for an erroneous Beckman–Coulter Gen S platelet count.

Fig. 4.3 Peripheral blood film of a patient with persistent pancytopenia after intensive chemotherapy for acute myeloid leukaemia. After many weeks of platelet dependency the 'platelet' count suddenly rose. Inspection of the film showed that platelets continued to be very sparse; the particles that were counted as platelets were fungi, subsequently identified as *Candida glabrata*, originating from the patients indwelling central intravenous line [29].

With Coulter instruments, and probably with others, the MPV rises with room temperature storage of the blood sample. In the case of the Coulter Gen S, the rise starts from day 2 of storage [23].

Errors in automated differential counts

Automated differential counts should be regarded as a means of screening blood samples for an abnormality and producing a differential count when there are only numerical abnormalities. Instruments may show systematic inaccuracies or may be inaccurate only with abnormal specimens of various types.

When mean automated counts for different leucocyte categories are compared with mean manual counts it is not uncommon for automated instruments to show inaccuracies that are statistically significant but too small to be of practical importance. Even when a discrepancy is larger it is not necessarily a practical problem as long as differential counts on patient samples are compared with a carefully derived reference range for the same instrument.

It is often not possible to obtain an accurate automated count on blood specimens with abnormal characteristics, e.g. if there are cells present for which the instrument does not have recognition criteria. The philosophy differs between instrument manufacturers as to whether counts on such samples are usually rejected (STKS and Sysmex NE-8000) or whether a count is usually produced but is 'flagged' (Bayer H.1 series and Cell-Dyn 3000) [43]. A possible disadvantage of the latter policy is that there are some laboratory workers with an inclination to believe any figure produced by a laboratory instrument, even if it is flagged. However, of more concern is the occurrence of inaccurate counts that are not flagged. All instruments fail to flag some samples containing NRBC, immature granulocytes, atypical lymphocytes and even, occasionally, blast cells.

Storage of blood at room temperature, e.g. during transport from outlying clinics or satellite hospitals, leads to inaccurate measurements but the time taken for such inaccuracy to occur differs according to the instruments and the cell type. Storage effects are generally greater with impedance counters than with cytochemical light-scattering instruments. The effect of storage is a great deal less if the specimen

can be stored at 4°C when any delay in analysis is anticipated.

Two-part and three-part differential counts on impedance-based automated full blood counters

Inevitably, two-part and three-part differential counts do not identify an increase of eosinophils or basophils and two-part differential counts do not identify monocytosis. The loss of clinically useful information is not great since most differential counts are performed to detect abnormalities of neutrophil or lymphocyte counts. The 'monocyte' or 'mononuclear cell' count is also not very accurate since some eosinophils, basophils and neutrophils are counted in this category [44]. Automated three-part differential counts on Coulter counters and other impedance instruments may be inaccurate within 30 minutes of venesection and become inaccurate again when the blood has been stored at room temperature for more than 6 hours. There is then a fall in the neutrophil count and a rise in the 'mononuclear cell' count, which is progressive with time.

The majority of (but not all) specimens containing NRBC, blast cells, immature granulocytes and atypical lymphocytes are flagged by impedance-based three-part automated differential counters.

Five- to seven-part differential counts

Differential count of Bayer H.1 series and Advia 120 instruments

Since the Bayer H.1 series and Advia instruments base the differential WBC on peroxidase cytochemistry in addition to light scattering they can produce erroneous counts as a result of inherited or acquired deficiency of peroxidase in neutrophils, eosinophils or monocytes. Some of the factitious results that have been observed with these instruments are shown in Table 4.11 and illustrated in Figs 4.4–4.9. A systematic underestimation of the monocyte count, in comparison with that obtained by flow cytometry with anti-CD14/CD45 monoclonal antibodies was observed in one study [49]. Storage effects are relatively minor with Bayer H.1 series and Advia automated differential counts. On average

Table 4.11 Some causes of inaccurate differential white cell counts on Bayer H.1 series and Advia 120 instruments.

Mechanism	Nature of factitious result
Non-lysis of red cells	Elevation of 'lymphocyte' count and reduction of neutrophil count (Fig. 4.4)
Neutrophil peroxidase deficiency	Reduction of neutrophil count; increase of monocyte and LUC (large unstained cell) counts (Fig. 4.5)
Eosinophil peroxidase deficiency	Reduction of eosinophil count; increase of neutrophil, monocyte or LUC count (Fig. 4.6)
Monocyte peroxidase deficiency	Reduction of monocyte count and increase of LUC count (Fig. 4.7)
Dysplastic monocytes misidentified as neutrophils	Reduction of monocyte count and increase of neutrophil count [45]
Neutrophil cluster misidentified as eosinophils	Reduction of neutrophil count and elevation of eosinophil count (Fig. 4.8)
Leukaemic blasts with strong peroxidase activity misidentified as eosinophils	Increase in eosinophil count [46]
Hypergranular promyelocytes misclassified as eosinophils	Increase in eosinophil count
Eosinophil cluster not recognized, sometimes but not always caused by reduced numbers of granules in eosinophils	Reduction of eosinophil count and elevation of neutrophil count [47]
Large cell residues in basophil channel due to presence of NRBC, blast cells, lymphoma cells, myeloma cells [45] or other abnormal cells or caused by coincidence, presence of heparin or storage of the sample at 4°C [48]	Elevation of 'basophil' count (Fig. 4.9)
Contamination of specimen with subcutaneous fat	Elevation of lymphocyte, monocyte and neutrophil counts [3]
Ageing of sample (more than 24 h)	'Left shift' flag

LUC, large unstained cells; NRBC, nucleated red blood cell.

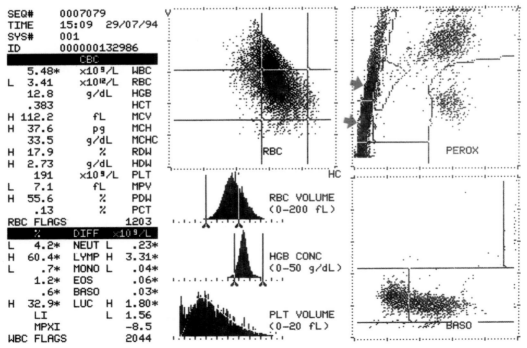

Fig. 4.4 Bayer H.2 histograms and scatter plots showing an erroneous differential count caused by failure of lysis of neonatal red cells. The peroxidase channel WBC of 75.8×10^9/l has been rejected in favour of the basophil channel WBC of 5.48×10^9/l but the differential count has been derived from the peroxidase channel where many of the non-lysed red cells have been counted as lymphocytes or large unstained cells (LUC). This has led to a factitious neutropenia. The erroneous differential count was flagged. The plots also illustrate the increased size of fetal red cells.

Fig. 4.5 Bayer H.2 white cell scatter plots from a patient with severe neutrophil peroxidase deficiency leading to an erroneous neutrophil count. Virtually all the neutrophils have been classified as large unstained (i.e. peroxidase-negative) cells and the neutrophil count was zero. The basophil lobularity channel, however, shows a normal number of granulocytes.

SEQ#	0000410		
TIME	12:00	20/07/88	
SYS#	901		
ID			

		CBC	
	4.52	×10⁹/L	WBC
L	3.86	×10¹²/L	RBC
	12.8	g/dL	HGB
	.385		HCT
H	99.9	fL	MCV
H	33.1	pg	MCH
	33.2	g/dL	MCHC
	14.2	%	RDW
	2.53	g/dL	HDW
L	114	×10⁹/L	PLT
	8.1	fL	MPV
	56.1	%	PDW
L	.09	%	PCT
RBC FLAGS			0200

%	DIFF	10⁹/L
67.7	NEUT	3.06
L 17.1	LYMP L	.77
4.6	MONO	.21
6.8	EOS	.31
.8	BASO	.04
3.0	LUC	.14
LI	L	1.21*
MPXI		-3.5
WBC FLAGS		4000

MORPHOLOGY FLAGS

PARAMETER	SUSP	VERIFY
ANISO		
MICRO		
MACRO	++	
VAR		
HYPO		
HYPER		
L SHIFT	+	
ATYP		
BLASTS		
OTHER		
OTHER	IG	

RBC VOLUME (0–200 fL)

HGB CONC (0–50 g/dL)

PLT VOLUME (0–20 fL)

Fig. 4.6 Bayer H.2 white cell scatter plots from a patient with partial eosinophil peroxidase deficiency showing an eosinophil cluster that has not been recognized. About two-thirds of the eosinophils have been classified as neutrophils.

Fig. 4.7 Bayer H.2 white cell scatter plots from a healthy subject with monocyte peroxidase deficiency causing an erroneous monocyte count. Almost all the monocytes have been counted as large unstained cells (LUC). The automated monocyte count was 0.09×10^9/l while the manual count was 0.5×10^9/l.

Fig. 4.8 Bayer H.1 white cell scatter plots showing neutrophils which have caused less forward light scatter than normal and have been misclassified as eosinophils.

Fig. 4.9 Bayer H.2 white cell scatter plots from a patient with follicular lymphoma showing pseudobasophilia as a consequence of lymphoma cells being misclassified as basophils.

there is no more than 1–2% change in any category of leucocyte by 72 hours.

Five-part differential counts on Coulter, Sysmex and other instruments

Some systematic inaccuracies in counts have been reported. One study of the Coulter STKS five-part differential [43] found an overestimation of lymphocyte numbers and an underestimation of monocyte numbers. In another study, the STKS gave less accurate granulocyte and lymphocyte counts in patients infected with the human immunodeficiency virus (HIV) than in other subjects [50]; some granulocyte counts were falsely low and lymphocyte counts were more scattered than with a Coulter S Plus IV. Three-part differential Cobas instruments have been observed to overestimate monocyte counts [51] whereas the Beckman–Coulter LH750 showed good agreement with the count obtained by flow cytometry with anti-CD14/CD45 monoclonal antibodies study [49].

Storage effects differ between instruments. The accuracy of the Coulter STKS differential count shows some deterioration after 6–8 hours of room temperature storage with a significant fall in the monocyte and eosinophil counts and a rise in the lymphocyte count [52] whereas, as noted above, counts on Bayer instruments are relatively stable. With the Coulter Gen S, there is a rise in the neutrophil, lymphocyte and eosinophil counts and a fall in the monocyte count, the inaccuracies appearing from day 1 to 2 of room temperature storage [23]. Some Sysmex instruments, e.g. the NE-8000, have shown a marked rise in the monocyte count after 8 hours room temperature storage and a rise in the neutrophil count after 24 hours [53]. The Cobas Argos 5 Diff shows a significant rise in the lymphocyte count and a fall in the counts of other types of leucocyte between 6 and 24 hours [54]. The effects of storage may differ for certain types of specimen. A study with the Sysmex NE-8000 counter found that in HIV-positive patients the lymphocyte count fell after 24 hours of room temperature storage [55].

Blood specimens with abnormal characteristics can give rise to inaccurate counts, as shown in Table 4.12.

Table 4.12 Some causes of inaccurate automated differential white cell counts on impedance and impedance/light-scattering instruments*.

Fault	Effect	Instrument on which observed
Some or many neutrophils counted as monocytes, particularly after 24 h storage of blood	Falsely high monocyte count and falsely low neutrophil count	Sysmex NE-1500 and NE-8000 [56,57]
Storage effects at room temperature	Falsely low neutrophil and monocyte counts, falsely high lymphocyte counts after 24 h at room temperature	Abbott Cell-Dyn 3500 [6]
	Falsely low neutrophil count and falsely high lymphocyte count after more than 18 h storage	Coulter STKS [58]
	Falsely low neutrophil count and falsely high monocyte count	Sysmex NE-1500 and NE-8000 (see above)
	Lymphocyte count rises significantly with less than 24 hours storage and eosinophil count falls	Cobas Argos 5 Diff [54]
Neutrophil aggregation	Falsely low WBC and neutrophil percentage, falsely high lymphocyte percentage	All instruments
Lymphocyte aggregation	Falsely high neutrophil percentage	Coulter STKS [59]
Non-lysis of red cells	Falsely high WBC and lymphocyte count	
Neonatal red cells		Coulter STKS [60]
Hyperlipidaemia		Coulter STKS
Abnormal haemoglobins (e.g. C, S, D, G)		Sysmex NE-8000
Obstructive jaundice		Sysmex NE-8000
Myelodysplastic syndrome		Coulter STKS
Malaria parasites	Falsely high lymphocyte and monocyte counts	Sysmex NE-8000
Malaria (neutrophils containing malaria pigment counted as eosinophils; rarely pigment-containing parasites in non-lysed red cells similarly counted)	Falsely high eosinophil count and falsely low neutrophil counts as malarial pigment polarizes light	Cell-Dyn 3500 [61,62]
Plasma interference	Falsely high eosinophil count	Coulter STKS [52]
Neutrophils containing haemosiderin counted as eosinophils	Falsely high eosinophil count and falsely low neutrophil count	Cell-Dyn CD3700 [63]
Hypogranular eosinophils counted as neutrophils	Falsely low eosinophil count; falsely high neutrophil count	Sysmex NE-8000 [47] Coulter STKS [64]
Hypogranular or hypolobated neutrophils counted as lymphocytes	Falsely low neutrophil count	ABX instruments
Other cells counted as basophils	Falsely high basophil count (pseudobasophilia)	
Abnormal lymphocytes in HIV-infected subjects		Coulter STKS [65]
Type of cell not specified		Coulter STKS [52]
Myeloblasts		Sysmex NE-8000 [66]
Promyelocytes in acute		Sysmex NE-8000 [67]

Continued p. 192

Table 4.12 *Continued*

Fault	Effect	Instrument on which observed
promyelocytic leukaemia		
Various abnormal cells		Cell-Dyn 3000 [68]
Lymphoblasts and myeloblasts		Coulter STKS [69]
Dysplastic neutrophils		Coulter STKS [45]
Atypical lymphocytes, lymphoma cells, myeloblasts, leukaemic promyelocytes		ABX instruments
Basophils counted as lymphocytes in some cases of CGL	Falsely low basophil count	Coulter STKS [52]
Various abnormal cells counted as monocytes—lymphocytes in chronic lymphocytic leukaemia, lymphoma cells, myeloblasts, lymphoblasts and hypergranular promyelocytes	Falsely high monocyte count	ABX instruments
Lymphocytes of infectious mononucleosis		Coulter STKS and Sysmex NE-8000 [70]
Myeloma cells		Sysmex SE-9000 [45]
Poor separation of leucocyte clusters	Some eosinophils sometimes counted as neutrophils, some neutrophils sometimes counted as monocytes, pseudobasophilia	Coulter STKS [54,71]
Giant platelets counted as lymphocytes	Falsely high lymphocyte count	Coulter STKS [71]
Nucleated red blood cells counted as lymphocytes	Falsely high lymphocyte count	ABX instruments
Some neutrophils counted as monocytes in patients with left shift	Falsely high monocyte count; falsely low neutrophil count	ABX instruments

CGL, chronic granulocytic leukaemia; CLL, chronic myeloid leukaemia; HIV, human immunodeficiency virus; WBC, white blood cell count.
* This list of errors should not be regarded as exhaustive.

Errors in automated reticulocyte counts and other reticulocyte measurements

Automated reticulocyte counts may be falsely elevated when there is autofluorescence or when fluorescence is produced by binding of the fluorochrome to something other than the RNA of reticulocytes, usually DNA or RNA in other cells. Less information is available on erroneous counts with non-fluorescent nucleic acid stains. However, a tendency to underestimate the reticulocyte count with technology based on 'new methylene blue' staining has been noted in haemoglobin H disease [72] and a factitious elevation was found in the presence of a high NRBC count,

using an oxazine 750 method [73]. With the new methylene blue method, factitiously elevated counts were also observed in some samples but only when a longer than recommended period of incubation was used [72]. Some known causes of falsely elevated reticulocyte counts are shown in Table 4.13. Inaccuracy of reticulocyte counts in the presence of nucleated red cells is method dependent, in one study being more likely with the XE-2100 than with the Pentra 120 Retic [81]. Malarial parasites within red cells may lead to a bimodal reticulocyte histogram, suggesting this diagnosis [82,83]. In the presence of malaria parasites there is also a factitious elevation of the immature reticulocyte fraction [83].

Table 4.13 Some causes of falsely elevated automated reticulocyte counts.

Increased autofluorescence
Neonatal samples and post-splenectomy [74]
Heinz bodies [75]

Binding of fluorescent dye to something other than RNA of reticulocytes
High WBC or NRBC count and/or abnormal leucocytes, e.g. in chronic lymphocytic leukaemia [76]
Howell–Jolly bodies [77]
Irreversibly sickled cells [76]
Cold agglutinins [74]
Large platelets [74]
Malaria parasites [78]
Heinz bodies [79]

Binding of non-fluorescent dye to something other than RNA of reticulocytes
NRBC [73]
Microcytic red cells [80]

NRBC, nucleated red blood cell; WBC, white blood cell count.

Erroneously low reticulocyte counts have been observed if blood is obtained from a patient after fluorescent retinal angiography has been performed [84].

Quantification of high fluorescence reticulocytes is affected by the presence of white cells and is likely to be erroneous when the white cell count is elevated [85].

Reticulocyte indices may be inaccurate when large platelets are present [86].

Test your knowledge

Multiple choice questions (MCQs)

(1–5 answers may be correct)

MCQ 4.1 An erroneous automated differential count with some instruments can result from
(a) Neutrophil peroxidase deficiency
(b) Degranulation of eosinophils
(c) Non-lysis of red cells
(d) The presence of nucleated red blood cells
(e) The presence of malaria parasites or malaria pigment

MCQ 4.2 A falsely high estimate of haemoglobin concentration with some instruments can result from

(a) The presence of giant platelets
(b) Reticulocytosis
(c) Hyperlipidaemia
(d) Paraproteinaemia
(e) Marked elevation of the white cell count

MCQ 4.3 A falsely high white cell count with some instruments can result from
(a) Leucocyte aggregation
(b) The presence of nucleated red blood cells
(c) The presence of giant platelets
(d) Ageing of the blood sample
(e) Non-lysis of red blood cells

MCQ 4.4 A falsely low platelet count with some instruments can result from
(a) Platelet aggregation
(b) Platelet satellitism
(c) The presence of giant platelets
(d) Microcytosis
(e) Hyperlipidaemia

MCQ 4.5 A falsely high MCV with some instruments can result from
(a) The presence of a cold agglutinin
(b) The presence of a warm autoantibody
(c) Hyperosmolar states
(d) Marked elevation of the white cell count
(e) Red cell hypochromia

Extended matching question (EMQs)

Select the most likely option for each of the stems. Each option may be used once, more than once or not at all.

EMQ 4.1
Theme: erroneous automated blood counts
Options
A Red cell fragmentation
B Malaria
C Hyperlidaemia
D Myeloperoxidase deficiency
E May–Hegglin anomaly
F Platelet satellitism
G Very high white cell count with 90% blast cells
H Platelet aggregation
I High titre cold agglutinin

J   Chédiak–Higashi syndrome
K   Bernard–Soulier syndrome
L   Megaloblastic anaemia

For each factitious result, select the most likely explanation from the options listed.

Variable	Matching option
1 Falsely low platelet count and blood film showing blue-grey inclusions in neutrophils	
2 Falsely elevated reticulocyte count and falsely elevated eosinophil count	
3 Falsely high RBC, Hb and MCV in a patient with bruising and blurred vision	
4 Falsely high Hb and fuzzy red cell outlines on blood film	
5 Falsely high MCV and MCH and falsely low RBC	

References

1 Hohlfeld P, Forestier F, Kaplan C, Tissot JD and Daffos F (1994) Fetal thrombocytopenia: a retrospective survey of 5,194 fetal blood samplings. *Blood*, **84**, 1851–1856.

2 Bain BJ and Liesner R (1996) Pseudopyropoikilocytosis: a striking artefact. *J Clin Pathol*, **49**, 772–773.

3 Whiteway A and Bain BJ (1999) Artefactual elevation of an automated white cell count following femoral vein puncture. *Clin Lab Haematol*, **21**, 65–68.

4 Criswell KA, Breider MA and Bleavins MR (2001) EDTA-dependent platelet phagocytosis: a cytochemical, ultrastructural, and functional characterization. *Am J Clin Pathol*, **115**, 376–384.

5 Fohlen-Walter A, Jacob C, Lecompte T and Lesesve J-F (2002) Laboratory identificaton of cryoglobulinemia from automated blood cell counts, fresh blood samples, and blood films. *Am J Clin Pathol*, **117**, 606–614.

6 Wood BL, Andrews J, Miller S and Sabath DE (1999) Refrigerated storage improves the stability of the complete blood count and automated differential. *Am J Clin Pathol*, **112**, 687–695.

7 Brigden ML and Dalal BI (1999) Cell counter-related abnormalities. *Lab Med*, **30**, 325–334.

8 Hoffmann EDTA-induced pseudo-neutropenia resolved with kanamycin. *Clin Lab Haematol*, **23**, 193–196.

9 Bizzaro N (1993) Granulocyte aggregation is edetic acid and temperature dependent. *Arch Pathol Lab Med*, **117**, 528–530.

10 Grimaldi E and Scopacasa F (2000) Evaluation of the Abbott CELL-DYN 4000 hematology analyzer. *Am J Clin Pathol*, **113**, 497–505.

11 McMullin MF, Wilkin HJ and Elder E (1999) Inaccurate haemoglobin estimation in Waldenström's macroglobulinaemia. *J Clin Pathol*, **48**, 787.

12 Paterakis GS, Laoutaris NP, Alexia SV, Siourounis PV, Stamulakatou AK, Premitis EE *et al.* (1993) The effect of red cell shape on the measurement of red cell volume. A proposed method for the comparative assessment of this effect among various haematology analysers. *Clin Lab Haematol*, **16**, 235–245.

13 Bryner MA, Houwen B, Westengard J and Klein O (1997) The spun micro-haematocrit and mean red cell volume are affected by changes in the oxygenation state of red blood cells. *Clin Lab Haematol*, **19**, 99–103.

14 Ali CYA (2000) Blood substitutes—clinical applications and impact of the laboratory. Paper presented at 24th World Congress of Medical Technology, Vancouver, Canada.

15 Nosanchuk JS, Roark MF and Wanser C (1974) Anemia masked by triglyceridemia. *Am J Clin Pathol*, **62**, 838–839.

16 Nicholls PD (1977) The erroneous haemoglobin–hyperlipidaemia relationship. *J Clin Pathol*, **30**, 638–640.

17 Fohlen-Walter A, Goupil JJ, Lecompte T and Lesesve J-F (2002) Underestimation of haemoglobin concentration in blood samples with high hyperleukocytosis: case report and alternative method for determination on blood cells automated analysers. *Haematologica*, **87**, ELT40.

18 Brigden ML, Page NE and Graydon C (1993) Evaluation of the Sysmex NE-8000 automated hematology analyzer in a high-volume outpatient laboratory. *Am J Clin Pathol*, **100**, 618–625.

19 Lewis SM, Bainbridge I, McTaggart P, Garvey BJ, England JM and Perry TE (1992) MDD Evaluation Report: Cobas Argos 5 Diff Automated Hematology Analyser. London: Medical Devices Directorate.

20 Beautyman W and Bills T (1974) Osmotic error in measurements of red cell volume. *Lancet*, **ii**, 905–906.

21 Strauchen JA, Alston W, Anderson J, Gustafson Z and Fajardo LF (1981) Inaccuracy in automated measurement of hematocrit and corpuscular indices in the presence of severe hyperglycemia. *Blood*, **57**, 1065–1067.

22 Hinchliffe RF, Bellamy GJ and Lilleyman JS (1992) Use of the Technicon H1 hypochromia flag in detecting spurious macrocytosis induced by excessive K$_2$EDTA concentration. *Clin Lab Haematol*, **14**, 268–269.

23 Gulati GL, Hyland LJ, Kocher W and Schwarting R (2002) Changes in automated complete blood cell count and differential leukocyte count results induced by storage of blood at room temperature. *Arch Pathol Lab Med*, **126**, 336–342.

24 Delgado J, Jiminez C, Larrocha C and Viloria A (2002) Cryoglobulinemia detected as a PIC/POC discrepancy of the automated complete blood count. *Eur J Haematol*, **69**, 65–66.

25 Kabutomori O, Iwatani Y and Kabutomori M (1999) Effects of hypertriglyceridemia on platelet counts in automated hematologic analysis. *Ann Intern Med*, **130**, 1152.

26 Gloster ES, Strauss RA, Jimenez JF, Neuberg RW, Berry DH and Turner EJ (1985) Spurious elevated platelet counts associated with bacteremia. *Am J Hematol*, **18**, 329–332.

27 Latif S, Veillon DM, Brown D, Kaltenbach J, Curry S, Linscott AJ et al. (2003) Spurious automated platelet count: enumeration of yeast forms as platelets by the Cell-DYN 4000. *Am J Clin Pathol*, **120**, 882–885.

28 Kakkar N (2004) Spurious rise in the automated platelet count because of bacteraemia. *J Clin Pathol*, **57**, 1096–1097.

29 Arnold JA, Jowzi Z and Bain BJ (1999) Images in haematology: *Candida glabrata* in a blood film. *Br J Haematol*, **104**, 1.

30 Crabbe G, van Poucke M and Cantineaux B (2002) Artefactually-normal automated platelet counts due to malaria-infected RBC. *Clin Lab Haematol*, **24**, 179–182.

31 Segal HC, Briggs C, Kunka S, Casbard A, Harrison P, Machin SJ and Murphy MF (2005) Accuracy of platelet counting haematology analysers in severe thrombocytopenia and potential impact on platelet transfusion. *Br J Haematol*, **128**, 520–525.

32 Fiorin F, Steffan A, Pradella P, Bizzaro N, Potenza R and de Angelis V (1998) IgG platelet antibodies in EDTA-dependent pseudothrombocytopenia bind to membrane glycoprotein IIb. *Am J Clin Pathol*, **110**, 178–183.

33 Hsieh AT, Chao TY and Chen YC (2003) Pseudothrombocytopenia associated with infectious mononucleosis. *Arch Pathol Lab Med*, **127**, e17–e18.

34 Sakurai S, Shiojima I, Tanigawa T and Nakahara K (1997) Aminoglycosides prevent and dissociate the aggregation of platelets in patients with EDTA-dependent pseudothrombocytopenia. *Br J Haematol*, **99**, 817–823.

35 Stiegler HM, Fischer Y and Steiner S (1999) Thrombocytopenia and glycoprotein IIb-IIIa receptor antagonists. *Lancet*, **353**, 1185.

36 Jubelirer SJ, Koenig BA and Bates MC (1999) Acute profound thrombocytopenia following C7E3 Fab (Abciximab) therapy: case reports, review of the literature and implications for therapy. *Am J Hematol*, **61**, 205–208.

37 Paterakis G, Konstantopoulos K and Loukopoulos D (1994) Spuriously increased platelet count due to microcyte interference: value of the R-1000 (Sysmex) Reticulocyte Analyzer. *Am J Hematol*, **45**, 57–58.

38 Shulman G and Yapit MK (1980) Whole blood platelet counts with impedance type particle counter. *Am J Clin Pathol*, **73**, 104–106.

39 van der Meer W, MacKenzie MA, Dinnissen JWB and de Keijzer MH (2003) Pseudoplatelets: a retrospective study of their incidence and interference with platelet counting. *J Clin Pathol*, **56**, 772–774.

40 Stass SA, Holloway ML, Slease RB and Schumacher HR (1977) Spurious platelet counts in hairy cell leukemia. *Am J Clin Pathol*, **68**, 530–531.

41 Stass SA, Holloway ML, Peterson V, Creegan WJ, Gallivan M and Schumacher HR (1979) Cytoplasmic fragments causing spurious platelet counts in the leukemic phase of poorly differentiated lymphocytic lymphoma. *Am J Clin Pathol*, **71**, 125–128.

42 Hammerstrom J (1992) Spurious platelet counts in acute leukaemia with DIC due to cell fragmentation. *Clin Lab Haematol*, **14**, 239–243.

43 Bentley SA, Johnson A and Bishop CA (1993) A parallel evaluation of four automated hematology analyzers. *Am J Clin Pathol*, **100**, 626–632.

44 Bain BJ (1986) An assessment of the three-population differential count on the Coulter Counter Model S Plus IV. *Clin Lab Haematol*, **8**, 347–359.

45 Hur M, Lee YK, Lee KM, Kim HJ and Cho HI (2004) Pseudobasophilia as an erroneous white blood cell differential count with a discrepancy between

automated cell counters: report of two cases. *Clin Lab Haematol*, **26**, 287–290.

46 Merino A and Esteve J (2005) Acute myeloid leukaemia with peculiar blast cell inclusions and pseudoeosinophilia. *Br J Haematol*, **131**, 286.

47 Kabutomori O and Iwatani Y (1997) Unusual eosinophilia not detected by an automated analyser in a patient with liver cirrhosis. *J Clin Pathol*, **50**, 967–968.

48 Bizzaro N (1996) Pseudobasophilia in the Technicon automated cell counters. *Clin Lab Haematol*, **18**, 298–299.

49 Grimaldi E, Carandente P, Scopacasa F, Romano MF, Pellegrino M, Bisogni R and de Caterina M (2005) Evaluation of the monocyte counting by two automated haematology analysers compared with flow cytometry. *Clin Lab Haematol*, **27**, 91–97.

50 Cohen AI, Peerschkc EIB and Steigbigel RT (1993) A comparison of the Coulter STKS, Coulter S+IV, and manual analysis of white cell differential counts in a human immunodeficiency virus-infected population. *Am J Clin Pathol*, **100**, 611–617.

51 Bentley SA, Johnson TS, Sohier CH and Bishop CA (1994) Flow cytometric differential leucocyte analysis with quantification of neutrophil left shift: an evaluation of the Cobas-Helios Analyzer. *Am J Clin Pathol*, **102**, 223–230.

52 Robertson EP, Lai HW and Wei DCC (1992) An evaluation of leucocyte analysis on the Coulter STKS. *Clin Lab Haematol*, **14**, 53–68.

53 Hu C-Y, Wang C-H, Chuang H-M and Shen M-C (1993) Evaluation of performance for automated differential leucocyte counting on Sysmcx NE-8000 by NCCLS recommended protocol H20-T. *Clin Lab Haematol*, **15**, 287–299.

54 Sheridan BL, Lollo M, Howe S and Bergeron N (1994) Evaluation of the Roche Cobas Argos 5 Diff automated haematology analyser with comparison with Coulter STKS. *Clin Lab Haematol*, **16**, 117–130.

55 Koepke JA and Smith-Jones M (1992) Lymphocyte counting in HIV-positive individuals. *Sysmex J Int*, **2**, 71–74.

56 Theodorsen L (1995) Evaluation of monocyte counting with two automated instruments by the use of CD14-specific immunomagnetic Dynabeads. *Clin Lab Haematol*, **17**, 225–229.

57 Bartels PCM and Schoorl M (1998) Time dependent increase of differential monocyte count on the Sysmex NE-2000. *Clin Lab Haematol*, **20**, 165–168.

58 Warner BA and Reardon DM (1991) Field evaluation of the Coulter STKS. *Am J Clin Pathol*, **95**, 207–217.

59 Shelton JB and Frank IN (2000) Splenic B lymphoma with lymphocyte clusters in peripheral blood smears. *J Clin Pathol*, **53**, 228–230.

60 Fournier M, Adenis C, Fontaine H, Camaille B and Goudemand J (1994) Evaluation and use of the white blood cell differential provided by the Coulter STKS in a children's hospital. *Clin Lab Haematol*, **16**, 33–42.

61 Mendelow BV, Lyons C, Nhlangothi P, Tana M, Munster M, Wypkema E *et al.* (1997) Automated malaria ascertainment by depolarization of laser light. *Proceedings of the 37th Annual Congress of the Federation of South African Societies of Pathology*, 145.

62 Hanscheid T, Pinto BG, Cristino JM and Grobusch MP (2000) Malaria diagnosis with the haematology analyser Cell-Dyn 3500; what does the instrument detect? *Clin Lab Haematol*, **22**, 259–261.

63 Roberts GT, Perry JL, Al-Jefri A and Scott CS (2005) Intra-leukocytic hemosiderin inclusions detected as pseudoeosinophils by automated depolarization analysis in a patient with beta-thalassaemia major and immune hemolysis. *Blood Cells Mol Dis*, **34**, 162–165.

64 Kim HJ, Lee YJ, Lee DS and Cho HI (1999) A case of idiopathic hypereosinophilic syndrome with hypersegmented and hypogranular eosinophils. *Clin Lab Haematol*, **21**, 428–430.

65 Germain PR and Lammers DB (1994) False basophil counts on the Coulter STKS. *Lab Med*, **25**, 376–379.

66 Sivakumaran M, Allen B and Wood JK (1994) Automated differential leucocyte counting on the Sysmex NE8000 analyser. *Clin Lab Haematol*, **16**, 206–207.

67 Meyepa LC, Tsoi G and Gan TE (1995) A new approach to the study of the blast suspect flag of the Sysmex NE8000. *Aust NZ J Med*, **25**, 74.

68 Cornbleet PJ, Myrick D, Judkins S and Levy R (1992) Evaluation of the CELL-DYN 3000 differential. *Am J Clin Pathol*, **98**, 603–614.

69 Pettit AR, Grace P and Chu P (1995) An assessment of the Coulter VCS automated differential counter scatterplots in the recognition of specific acute leukaemia variants. *Clin Lab Haematol*, **17**, 125–129.

70 Brigden ML, Au S, Thompson S, Brigden S, Doyle P and Tsaparas Y (1999) Infectious mononucleosis in an outpatient population: diagnostic utility of 2 automated hematology analyzers and the sensitivity and specificity of Hoagland's criteria in heterophile-positive patients. *Arch Pathol Lab Med*, **123**, 875–881.

71 Cornbleet PJ, Myrick D and Levy R (1993) Evaluation of the Coulter STKS five-part differential. *Am J Clin Pathol*, **99**, 72–81.

72 Lai SK, Yow CMN and Benzil IFF (1999) Interference of Hb-H disease in automated reticulocyte counting. *Clin Lab Haematol*, **21**, 261–264.

73 Brugnara C, Hipps MJ, Irving PJ, Lathrop H, Lee PA, Minchello EM and Winkelman J (1994) Automated reticulocyte counting and measurement of reticulocyte cellular indices: evaluation of the Miles H3 blood analyzer. *Am J Clin Pathol*, **102**, 623–632.

74 Chin-Yee I, Keeney M and Lohmann RC (1991) Flow cytometric reticulocyte analysis using thiazole orange; clinical experience and technical limitations. *Clin Lab Haematol*, **13**, 177–188.

75 Hinchliffe RF (1993) Error in automated reticulocyte counts due to Heinz bodies. *J Clin Pathol*, **46**, 878–879.

76 Ferguson DJ, Lee S-F and Gordon PA (1990) Evaluation of reticulocyte counts by flow cytometry in a routine laboratory. *Am J Hematol*, **33**, 13–17.

77 Lofsness KG, Kohnke ML and Geier NA (1994) Evaluation of automated reticulocyte counts and their reliability in the presence of Howell–Jolly bodies. *Am J Clin Pathol*, **101**, 85–90.

78 Hoffman JJML and Pennings JMA (1999) Pseudo-reticulocytosis as a result of malaria parasites. *Clin Lab Haematol*, **21**, 257–260.

79 Español I, Pedro C and Remache AF (1999) Heinz bodies interfere with automated reticulocyte counts. *Haematologica*, **84**, 373–374.

80 Buttarello M, Bulian P, Farina G, Temporin V, Toffolo L, Trabuio E and Rizzotti P (2000) Flow cytometric reticulocyte counting: parallel evaluation of five fully automated analyzers: an NCCLS-ICSH approach. *Am J Clin Pathol*, **115**, 100–111.

81 Briggs C, Grant D and Machin SJ (2001) Comparison of the automated reticulocyte counts and immature reticulocyte fraction measurements obtained with the ABX Pentra 120 Retic blood cell analyzer and the Sysmex XE-2100 automated haematology analyzer. *Lab Haematol*, **7**, 1–6.

82 Mellors I, Hardy J, Lambert J, Kendall R and McArdle B (2001) Detection of intra-erythrocyte

malarial parasites by an automated haematology analyser—a case study. *Br J Haematol*, **113**, Suppl. 1, 50.

83 Scott CS, van Zyl D, Ho E, Ruivo L, Kunz D and Coetzer TL (2002) Patterns of pseudo-reticulocytosis in malaria: fluorescent analysis with the Cell-Dyn® CD4000. *Clin Lab Haematol*, **24**, 15–20.

84 Hirata R, Morita Y, Hirai N, Seki M, Imanishi A, Toriumi J *et al.* (1992) The effects of fluorescent substances on the measurement of reticulocytes—using automated reticulocyte analyzers R-1000 and R-3000. *Sysmex J Int*, **2**, 10–15.

85 Villamor N, Kirsch A, Huhn D, Vives-Corrons JL and Serke S (1996) Interference of blood leucocytes in the measurements of immature red cells (reticulocytes) by two different (semi-) automated flow-cytometry technologies. *Clin Lab Haematol*, **18**, 89–94.

86 Bowen D, Williams K, Phillips I and Cavill I (1996) Cytometric analysis and maturation characteristics of reticulocytes from myelodysplastic patients. *Clin Lab Haematol*, **18**, 155–160.

Answers to test questions

Multiple choice questions

MCQ 4.1	TTTTT
MCQ 4.2	FFTTT
MCQ 4.3	FTTFT
MCQ 4.4	TTTFF
MCQ 4.5	TFTTF

Extended matching questions

EMQ 4.1

1 E
2 B
3 G
4 C
5 I

5 Normal ranges

The interpretation of any laboratory test result requires assessment as to whether or not the result is normal. 'Normal' means that the results are those expected in that individual when in a state of optimal health (assuming that the person does not have any inherited disorder affecting the blood). Since one rarely has the information to make this assessment, it is necessary instead to consider whether the result is what would be expected in a healthy subject as biologically similar to the particular individual as possible. Test results are conventionally compared with normal ranges, such ranges often being derived from textbooks and sometimes being of obscure origin. More recently, test results have been compared with reference ranges. The concepts underlying the derivation of a reference range are as follows.

A reference individual is one selected using defined criteria and coming from a population that includes all individuals who meet those criteria. A reference sample is a number of reference individuals chosen to represent the reference population. Reference values are test results derived from the reference individuals and can be analysed and statistically described: they will fall within certain limits; and they will have a certain distribution with a mean, a median and a mode. The usual method of describing a collection of reference values is in terms of the reference limits that exclude 2.5% of the values at either end of the observed range, i.e. the reference interval represents the central 95% of the observed values. Such a reference interval derived from the sample individuals will be representative of the reference interval of the population from which it is derived; the closeness of fit of the two intervals can be represented by the confidence limits of the mean and each of the reference limits. Closeness of fit is determined by the size of the sample and by whether the reference individuals have been chosen from the reference population in a way that is free of bias. Reference individuals can be derived from the reference population by random sampling or carefully selected to reflect the mix of age, gender, social class and other variables in the reference population. Reference intervals are commonly referred to as 'reference ranges', a readily understandable term although it is not officially recommended.

A reference individual is not necessarily healthy, but if a good state of health is included as a criterion for selection then it is clear that the reference interval may be very similar to a traditional 'normal range', although more carefully defined.

If reference ranges are to be useful in assessing haematology results they should take account of whether test results are influenced by age, gender or ethnic origin and separate ranges should be derived when necessary. Pregnant women would normally be excluded unless deriving a range for application during pregnancy. Reference ranges are often derived from test results obtained in carefully controlled conditions with fasting and rested subjects who have abstained from alcohol, cigarettes and drugs and whose blood specimens are taken at a defined time of day. Such conditions are not often met by patient populations and it may be more useful to use ambulant, non-fasting individuals whose habits reflect those of the population from which they and the patients are drawn. The site of blood sampling and other variations in the technique of obtaining a blood sample affect results of haematological tests (Table 5.1). For this reason blood specimens should be taken in the same manner and using the same anticoagulant (dry or liquid) as in the patient population.

Establishing reference ranges on a population sample is a difficult and expensive procedure, which is often beyond the resources of an individual laboratory. Nevertheless, laboratories should, whenever

Table 5.1 Some effects of the method of obtaining a blood specimen on haematological variables*.

Site of obtaining blood specimen
During the first week of life, the Hb, PCV/Hct and RBC are approximately 15% higher in heel-prick than in venous specimens[†]; the difference may be greater in babies with sepsis with poor peripheral circulation [3]; the MCV, MCH and RDW do not differ but the MCHC is higher [3]; in older infants, children and adults no consistent differences have been observed between finger-prick and venous specimens but ear-lobe capillary specimens have Hb, PCV/Hct and RBC values 6–17% higher than finger-prick or venous specimens
In neonates, heel-prick specimens have WBC, neutrophil and lymphocyte counts about 20% higher than arterial or venous samples; counts are most likely to approximate to those of venous blood if there is a free flow of blood and if early drops, excluding the first, are used for the count; in adults, the WBC and the neutrophil count are significantly higher in finger-prick samples than in venous samples with a progressive fall occurring with successive drops [4]
In neonates the platelet count and MCV are higher in venous samples than in capillary samples [3]

Position of the arm
Hb, PCV/Hct and RBC are 2–3% higher if the arm is hanging down than if it is at the level of the atrium of the heart

Use of tourniquet
Hb, PCV and RBC are increased by 2–3% by prolonged application of a tourniquet

Nature of anticoagulant
The dilution caused by using a liquid anticoagulant causes a slight reduction of cell counts, Hb and PCV/Hct

Oxygenation of the blood
Oxygenation of the blood lowers the PCV/Hct and MCV and raises the MCHC [5]

Prior rest
The Hb, PCV/Hct and RBC fall by 5–8% after as little as half an hour's bed rest; rest lowers the lymphocyte count [6]

Hb, haemoglobin concentration; Hct, haematocrit; MCH, mean cell haemoglobin; MCHC, mean cell haemoglobin concentration; MCV mean cell volume; MPV, mean platelet volume; PCV, packed cell volume; RBC, red blood cell count; RDW, red cell distribution width; WBC, white blood cell count.
* For other relevant references the reader is referred to the first edition of this book [1].
[†] It has been reported that, at birth, capillary Hb is higher than cord blood Hb [2] but it appears likely that this observation was the result of the 20–60 minutes delay that occurred before the capillary sample was obtained.

possible, establish their own ranges using their own techniques and instrumentation. Normal ranges can be derived from healthy volunteers, from subjects attending health screening clinics or having annual medical examinations or from staff having pre-employment testing. Hospital staff may not be ideal because their average age is likely to be considerably lower than that of the patient population. First-time blood donors are satisfactory but those who have donated regularly in the past may have depleted iron stores, which will affect haematological test results. It is also possible to derive normal ranges from data on patients, based on the assumption that the test results for any measurement will represent a normal and an abnormal population with some overlap. Large numbers are necessary and the statistics are fairly complex [7]. Particular problems exist in deriving ranges for elderly people because of the high prevalence of known and occult

disease. It is desirable, if possible, to separate the effects of the increasing incidence of disease from the effects of the ageing process itself. Similarly, it may be difficult in a developing country to select an adequate population sample that is not adversely affected by malnutrition and subclinical disease. In such circumstances it may be necessary to derive normal ranges from 'elite' individuals such as the army, police force, medical students, doctors, nurses and laboratory workers; such individuals will not be typical of the communities from which they are drawn, but their test results will more closely approximate to those that would be expected in an optimal state of health. Problems also occur in populations with a high prevalence of genetic disease. In deriving ranges for red cell variables it is necessary to exclude subjects with haemoglobinopathies and α and β thalassaemia trait. Exclusion of β thalassaemia trait and haemoglobinopathies is not difficult since diagnosis is usually easy but exclusion of α thalassaemia trait requires DNA analysis. However, unless this is done it is not possible to distinguish genuine ethnic differences from differences caused by a high prevalence of a genetic abnormality. Thus, subtle differences in haemoglobin concentration (Hb) and red cell indices between Afro-Americans and white Americans are attributable in part to the 25–30% prevalence of thalassaemia trait among Afro-Americans; however, when the effects of α thalassaemia and iron deficiency are excluded, haemoglobin concentration is about 0.34 g/dl lower in Afro-American men and about 0.32 g/dl lower in Afro-American women that in Caucasians [8]; this residual difference is not explained by sickle cell trait of by socio-economic differences or differences in renal function. These differences are sufficient to lead to 6% of Afro-American women and 8% of Afro-American men being classified as anaemic if Caucasian reference ranges are used [8]. In deriving reference ranges for children it is desirable to exclude subclinical iron deficiency. Even in adults, subtle differences in iron status may affect population means. For example, heterozygosity for mutations associated with genetic haemochromatosis is common among Northern European populations (around 12%) and has been found to be associated with a slightly but significantly higher Hb, the difference between carriers and non-carriers being of the order of 0.4–0.6 g/dl [9]. Hb, haematocrit (Hct), mean cell volume (MCV), mean cell haemoglobin (MCH) and mean cell haemoglobin concentration (MCHC) have all been found to be higher in patients with untreated haemochromatosis, probably as a result of enhanced delivery of iron to erythroblasts [10].

Once test results are available they must be dealt with by statistical techniques that are appropriate for the distribution of the data. If data have a normal (Gaussian) distribution then a mean and standard deviation (SD) can be estimated and the mean ± 1.96 SD will represent the central 95% of the data. The commonly used mean ± 2 SD represents 95.4% of the data. The Hb and the other red cell variables can be treated as if they have a Gaussian distribution, although they are not strictly Gaussian [11]. Various other haematological variables have a skewed distribution with a tail of higher values; this is true for the white blood cell count (WBC) and the absolute counts of various types of leucocytes. If data with this type of distribution are treated inappropriately, as if they were Gaussian, the estimates for both the upper and lower limits will be too low and the lower limit will often be negative. A logarithmic transformation may be appropriate or a more complex transformation may be necessary [12]. If a Gaussian distribution cannot be produced by transformation of the data, a non-parametric analysis must be carried out, i.e. one which makes no assumptions about the distribution. The advantages of using transformation to a Gaussian distribution is that a smaller sample size is adequate, of the order of 36 samples in contrast with the 120 samples which is the smallest adequate sample for non-parametric analysis [13].

Use of the central 95% range is arbitrary but gives a reasonable balance between missing a clinically significant abnormality and misclassifying a normal subject as abnormal. However, comparison of an observed value in a patient with a laboratory's normal range should be done with the constant awareness that for each test 5% of values of healthy subjects will fall outside the 'normal' range. Conversely, an individual may, as a result of a pathological process, have an alteration in a test result away from his or her own normal value while still remaining within the 'normal' range. When previous results are available on patients some attention should be paid to them as well as to whether a result falls outside the laboratory's normal range.

If a laboratory does not derive its own normal ranges but adopts those of others it is incumbent on it to be certain not only that the type of population is similar and the appropriate statistical techniques have been applied but also that the blood sampling techniques and laboratory methods, including the methods of calibrating instruments, are identical.

Haematological variables are affected not only by age, gender, ethnic origin and altitude but also by a number of other biological factors and extraneous influences (Tables 5.2 & 5.3).

Normal ranges for adults

Some reference ranges for red cell variables for Caucasian adults are shown in Table 5.4 and some data for Black adults in Table 5.5. Ranges for Caucasian

Table 5.2 Some demographic factors affecting haematological variables*.

Gender
RBC, Hb and PCV/Hct are higher in men than in women
Women in the reproductive age range have a higher WBC and neutrophil count than men, whereas in post-menopausal women the WBC is lower than in men
The platelet count is higher in women than in men

Age
Normal values of neonates, infants and children differ widely from those of adults (see Tables 5.8–5.12)
Hb rises in women and falls in men between the ages of 40–50 and 70–80 years
Between the ages of 70 and 88 years the Hb falls further in men but not in women so that after the age of 85 years there is no difference [14]
The lymphocyte counts fall in old age

Ethnic origin
The WBC and neutrophil counts are lower in Black people than in Caucasians, are lower in Africans than in Afro-Caribbeans or Afro-Americans (see Table 5.7) and are also lower in Yemenite Jews than in other Caucasians. The lower WBC in Black people is not apparent at birth but has appeared by the age of 1 year. The absolute lymphocyte count of Afro-Americans is slightly but significantly higher than that of American White people [8]. WBC and differential counts of Indians, Chinese and South-East Asian populations are the same as those of Northern European Caucasians. Eosinophil counts do not differ between healthy subjects of different ethnic groups
Black people have lower platelet counts than Caucasians
Afro-Americans have a lower Hb than White Americans by about 0.32 g/dl in women and 0.34 g/dl in men, when iron deficiency and α thalassaemia trait have been eliminated [8]

Geographical location
RBC, Hb and PCV/Hct are increased at higher altitude; in one study the response to moderate altitude was a rise in RBC alone with the MCV being lower whereas at a greater altitude Hb and PCV also rose [15]. In another study of the acute effects of changing altitude the rise in RBC and Hb at 14 days was proportionately greater than the rise in PCV [16]; during this time the mean MCV had risen from 85 to 93 fl. The platelet count is significantly higher at altitude [16,17]. Babies born at a high altitude have a higher WBC and neutrophil count [18]

Season
Overall, Hb and PCV are somewhat lower in summer [19]. In non-smokers, Hb and PCV are lower in summer, due to an increase in plasma volume [20]; in smokers the MCHC is lower and the PCV and RBC are higher in summer; the plasma volume is unchanged [20]

Hb, haemoglobin concentration; Hct, haematocrit; MCHC, mean cell haemoglobin concentration; MCV mean cell volume; PCV, packed cell volume; RBC, red blood cell count; WBC, white blood cell count.
* For further relevant references the reader is referred to the first edition of this book [1].

adults can also be applied to Indians, Chinese and South-East Asian populations. Indigenous Greenlanders have been found to have a lower Hb than Danish subjects, the difference not being explicable on the basis of diet, cigarette smoking or the prevalence of iron deficiency [25]. The gender difference in the Hb and related variables lessens after the menopause but, at any given ferritin concentration or transferrin saturation, values continue to differ by about 1 g/dl [29]. The Hb in men falls by about 1 g/dl between youth and old age, particularly after the age of 60 years, whereas the Hb in women is fairly stable [29].

White cell variables for Caucasian adults are shown in Table 5.6. For leucocyte counts, particularly neutrophil counts, it is necessary to have specific reference ranges applicable to Africans and Afro-Caribbeans (Table 5.7). The lower WBC and neutrophil counts observed in these ethnic groups may be partly explicable on the basis of diet and other extraneous influences but a true biological difference appears to exist [22,23,30]. However, the higher eosinophil counts previously reported in Africans and Indians do not represent a biological difference from Caucasians; eosinophilia observed was explicable on the basis of subclinical disease, particularly

Table 5.3 Some biological factors and common extraneous influences affecting haematological variables*.

Diurnal variation
The Hb and PCV are higher in the morning than the evening
The WBC and neutrophil counts are higher in the afternoon than in the morning. The eosinophil count is lowest at 10 a.m. to mid-day, and up to twice as high between midnight and 4 a.m. The lymphocyte count is lowest in the morning and highest in the evening [21]
The platelet count is higher in the afternoon and evening

Pregnancy (see Table 5.13)
RBC, Hb and PCV/Hct fall; MCV rises, on average about 6 fl
The WBC, neutrophil count and monocyte count rise during pregnancy; a left shift occurs; lymphocyte, eosinophil and basophil counts fall
The neutrophil alkaline phosphatase score rises
The platelet count has been observed to fall during pregnancy but if subjects with pregnancy-related hypertension are excluded there is usually no fall
The ESR rises

Labour
During labour there is a further marked rise in the WBC and the neutrophil count together with a steep fall in the eosinophil count and a slight further fall of the lymphocyte count

Postpartum
RBC, Hb and PCV/Hct fall to the lowest level at 3–4 days postpartum
WBC and neutrophil count remain markedly elevated for some days postpartum then fall gradually over 4–6 weeks

Menstruation
WBC, neutrophil count and monocyte count fall steeply during menstruation; a reciprocal change is seen in the eosinophil count; the basophil count falls mid-cycle.

Menopause
The Hb rises post-menopausally
The WBC and the neutrophil count fall

Exercise
The WBC and absolute counts of all leucocyte types rise as a response to vigorous exercise; the absolute rise in the WBC and neutrophil count is less in Black people than in Caucasians [22]
The RBC, Hb and PCV rise as a response to vigorous exercise
Intensive training leads to a fall in the lymphocyte count [23]

Cigarette smoking [24]
The RBC, Hb, PCV/Hct, MCV and MCH are higher in smokers
The WBC, neutrophil count and monocyte count are higher
The platelet count is higher
The ESR is higher

Alcohol intake
Alcohol consumption may be associated with an increased Hb [25] but heavy alcohol intake can cause anaemia, leucopenia and thrombocytopenia
The MCV and MCH are higher and RBC is lower

Obesity
WBC correlates with body fat [26] and is increased in morbid obesity [27]

ESR, erythrocyte sedimentation rate; Hb, haemoglobin concentration; Hct, haematocrit; MCH, mean cell haemoglobin; MCV mean cell volume; PCV, packed cell volume; RBC, red blood cell count; WBC, white blood cell count.
* For further relevant references the reader is referred to the first edition of this book [1].

Table 5.4 Ninety-five per cent ranges for red cell variables in Caucasian adults in three large series of subjects.

	Male				Female			
RBC × 10⁻¹²/l	4.32–5.66*				3.88–4.99*			
Hb (g/dl)	13.3–16.7*	13.3–17.6†	13.2–18.0‡	13.2–16.9§	11.8–14.8*	12–15.8†	12.2–16.5‡	11.5–15.4§
PCV (Hct) (l/l)	0.39–0.50*		0.39–0.51‡		0.36–0.44*		0.36–0.48‡	
MCV (fl)	82–98¶			82–99§	82–98¶			81–99§
MCH (pg)	27.3–32.6				27.3–32.6			
MCHC (g/dl)	31.6–34.9				31.6–34.9			
RDW	9.9–15.5¶				9.9–15.5¶			
	11.6–13.9††				11.6–13.9††			
HDW	1.82–2.64††				1.82–2.64††			

Hb, haemoglobin concentration; Hct, haematocrit; HDW haemoglobin distribution width; MCH, mean cell haemoglobin; MCHC, mean cell haemoglobin concentration; MCV mean cell volume; PCV, packed cell volume; RBC, red blood cell count; RDW, red cell distribution width; WBC, white blood cell count.

* Based on 700 healthy subjects, aged between 18 and 60 years, studied by the author: 350 were male and 350 female; half were studied on Coulter instruments (S and S Plus IV) and half on Bayer-Technicon instruments (Hemalog 8 and H.2); except where indicated, the ranges are derived from all 750 subjects.
† Based on 1379 iron-replete Danish males and 1003 iron-replete Danish females [25].
‡ Based on 1382 males and 1837 females for Hb and 1368 males and, 1818 females for Hct [28].
§ Based on 6240 males and 5780 females having health screening, iron deficiency was excluded [8]. MCV is very dependent on the technology used and the method of instrument calibration so that derivation of normal ranges for individual laboratories is important.
¶ Coulter S Plus IV, n = 200.
†† Bayer-Technicon H.2. n = 200.

Table 5.5 Haemoglobin concentration and MCV in Afro-Americans in whom iron deficiency and α thalassaemia trait were excluded [8]; 95% range and mean are shown*.

	Male (n = 172)	Females (n = 42)
Hb (g/dl)	12.7–16.7	11.3–14.9
MCV (fl)	80–99	81.5–99

Hb, haemoglobin concentration; MCV mean cell volume.
* Hb was significantly lower than that of Caucasians whereas MCV was not; sickle cell trait did not have any influence on the Hb or MCV.

parasitic infection. Because of superior precision, reference ranges for automated differential leucocyte counts are narrower than those for manual differential counts (see Table 5.6). They are also dependent on methodology and thus need to be derived specifically for individual models of instrument. Not even all instruments operating on the same principles give identical results. Locally derived reference ranges are needed for red cell variables for populations living at high altitude. Above 2000 m the Hb is elevated by 1–1.5 g/dl and RBC and PCV/Hct are also elevated [15].

Normal ranges for neonates and fetuses

Some normal ranges for haematological variables in neonates are shown in Tables 5.8 and 5.9. Ranges applicable to the fetus from 8 weeks' gestation onwards have also been published [46–49] (Fig. 5.1). The platelet count in the fetus has a mean value of around 250 × 10⁹/l and does not change between 17 weeks' gestation and term [50]; in this study of 5194 fetuses, the 95% range was 138–344 × 10⁹/l but fetuses with significant abnormalities causing thrombocytopenia were not excluded from the analysis. An unexpectedly high eosinophil count is sometimes observed in healthy fetuses [51]. Published ranges for red cell variables in Indian babies [52] and in Jamaican babies in whom haemoglobinopathies and β thalassaemia trait had been excluded [37] are similar to those for European neonates whereas Nigerian babies have been observed to have lower RBCs, Hbs and PCVs [38]. Since haemoglobinopathies and thalassaemia trait were not excluded in the latter group, it may be more appropriate to apply ranges for red cell variables derived for Caucasian babies to all ethnic groups, including

Table 5.6 Ninety-five per cent ranges for automated and manual leucocyte counts in Caucasian adults, derived by the author, using data from 700 healthy subjects aged between 18 and 60 years.

	Male		Female	Method and number of subjects (n)
WBC $\times 10^{-9}$/l	3.7–9.5		3.9–11.1	Various methods, n = 750
Neutrophils $\times 10^{-9}$/l	1.7–6.1		1.7–7.5	Automated counts, Bayer-Technicon H.2, n = 200
Lymphocytes $\times 10^{-9}$/l		1.0–3.2		
Monocytes $\times 10^{-9}$/l		0.2–0.6		
Eosinophils $\times 10^{-9}$/l		0.03–0.46		
Basophils $\times 10^{-9}$/l		0.02–0.09		
LUC* $\times 10^{-9}$/l		0.09–0.29		
Granulocytes $\times 10^{-9}$/l	1.8–7.5		2.1–8.9	Automated counts, Coulter S Plus IV, n = 200
Lymphocytes $\times 10^{-9}$/l		1.15–3.25		"
Mononuclear cells $\times 10^{-9}$/l		0.18–0.86		"
Neutrophils $\times 10^{-9}$/l	1.5–6.5		1.8–7.4	WBC on Coulter S or S IV; 500-cell manual differential count, n = 400
Lymphocytes $\times 10^{-9}$/l		1.1–3.5		"
Monocytes $\times 10^{-9}$/l		0.21–0.92		"
Eosinophils $\times 10^{-9}$/l		0.02–0.67		"
Basophils $\times 10^{-9}$/l		0.00–0.13		"

* LUC, large unstained (peroxidase-negative) cells; WBC, white blood cell count.

Table 5.7 Ninety-five per cent ranges for automated leucocyte counts in adult Africans and Afro-Caribbeans derived by the author.

	Male			Female		
	WBC $\times 10^{-9}$/l	Neutrophil count $\times 10^{-9}$/l	Number	WBC $\times 10^{-9}$/l	Neutrophil count $\times 10^{-9}$/l	Number
African	2.8–7.2	0.9–4.2	57	3.0–7.4	1.3–3.7	29
Afro-Caribbean	3.1–9.4	1.2–5.6	38	3.2–10.6	1.3–7.1	39

WBC, white blood cell count.

Table 5.8 Ninety-five per cent ranges for red cell variables in healthy full term babies during the first month of life.

	RBC $\times 10^{-12}$/l	Hb (g/dl)	PCV (l/l)	MCV (fl)
Caucasian				
Cord blood (early cord clamping) [31]	3.5–6.7	13.7–20.1	0.47–0.59	90–118
Cord blood (time of cord clamping not specified)* [32]	3.13–4.85	11.3–17.6		99–115
Birth-96 h (early cord clamping) [33,34]	3.8–6.5	14.2–24	0.46–0.75	101–137
(late cord clamping) [34]		16.1–24		
'Newborn' [35]	4.1–6.7	15–24	0.44–0.70	102–115
1–2 weeks (early cord clamping) [33]	3.2–6.4	12.8–21.8	0.38–0.70	75–149
3–4 weeks (early cord clamping) [33,36]	2.8–5.3	10.1–18.3	0.32–0.55	90–120
Jamaican				
1 day [37]	4.6–7.6	15.7–27.5		90–118
1 week [37]	4.0–6.9	13.4–22.4		88–116
4 weeks [37]	3.1–5.9	9.5–18.1		83–107
Nigerian				
1 day [38]	2.7–5.3	11.6–19.6	0.32–0.58	113 (mean)
2 weeks [38]	2.35–4.55	9.4–16.8	0.31–0.47	113 (mean)
4 weeks [38]	2.1–3.95	7.5–13.6	0.24–0.41	108 (mean)

Hb, haemoglobin concentration; MCV mean cell volume; PCV, packed cell volume; RBC, red blood cell count.
* Brazilian, from Porto Alegre, so likely to be essentially Caucasian.

Table 5.9 Ninety or 95% ranges for white cell and NRBC counts for full term Caucasian babies during the first month of life*.

Age	WBC × 10^{-9}/l	Neutrophils × 10^{-9}/l	Lymphocytes × 10^{-9}/l	Monocytes × 10^{-9}/l	Eosinophils × 10^{-9}/l	NRBC × 10^{-9}/l
Cord blood [31,32,39,42]	5–23	1.7–19	1–11	0.1–3.7	0.05–2.0	0.03–5.4
Half hour [41,43]		1.9–5.8				
12 hours [39,41]		6.6–23.5				
24 hours [39,41]		4.8–17.1				
'Newborn' [35]	9.1–34	6–23.5	2.5–10	< 3.5	< 2.0	< 0.4
48 hours [39,41]		3.8–13.4				
0–60 hours [40]			2–7.3	0–1.9	0–0.8	
72 hours [39,41]		2.0–9.4				
4 days [39,41,43]		1.3–8.0	2.2–7.1	0.2–1.8	0.2–1.9	
60 hours–5 days [40,41]		2.0–6.0	1.9–6.6	0–1.7	0–0.8	
7–8 days [39,41,44]	9–18.4	1.8–8	3–9	0.03–0.98	0.16–0.94	0.03–0.11
2 weeks [39,41]		1.7–6				
5 days–4 weeks [40,41]		1.8–5.4	2.8–9.1	0.09–1.7	0–0.8	
3–4 weeks [39,41]		1.6–5.8				
4 weeks [45]	5–19.5	1–9	4–13.5			

NRBC, nucleated red blood cells; WBC, white blood cell count.

* Data from different series have been amalgamated to include the lowest and highest limits found in different studies. The ranges of Gregory and Hey [39] and Weinberg et al. [40] are 90% rather than 95% ranges while the scatter plots of Manroe et al. [41] show the full range of counts.

Fig. 5.1 Haemoglobin concentrations in 265 healthy fetuses and reference range derived from the data, modified from Mari et al. 2000 [49].

Africans. The lower neutrophil count that is noted in Africans and Afro-Caribbeans later in life is not apparent in the neonatal period so that the same reference ranges for leucocyte counts can be applied to neonates of all ethnic groups [41,42,53]. The lymphocyte count in the neonatal period is of considerable importance in suggesting the possibility of congenital immunodeficiency. In severe combined immunodeficiency the count is almost invariably less than 2.8×10^9/l and it has been suggested that investigation is mandatory if the lymphocyte count is less than 1.0×10^9/l.

The Hb, PCV/Hct and RBC in the neonate are considerably influenced by the time of umbilical cord clamping (see Table 5.8), since inflow from the placenta increases the blood volume of the neonate by up to 50–60% during the first few minutes after birth. The rate of transfer of placental blood to the neonate is increased if oxytocin is administered to the mother to stimulate uterine contraction and is decreased if the baby is held above the level of the mother immediately after delivery. During the first few hours of life, plasma volume decreases so that the Hb, PCV/Hct and RBC rise appreciably, particularly when late clamping has been practised. Nucleated red blood cells (NRBC) may be present in appreciable numbers at birth but the count falls rapidly in the first 24 hours. By 4 days they are infrequent. NRBC are more numerous in the cord blood of premature infants and the infants of diabetic mothers [54]. They are also increased when there has been fetal blood loss, haemolysis or intrauterine hypoxia. The reticulocyte count at birth is higher than at any other time of life but it drops markedly after birth. There is a steady decline in the RBC, Hb and PCV/Hct but, as shown in Table 5.8, an Hb of less than 14 g/dl in the first week of life is indicative of anaemia. The WBC at birth is influenced by the mode of delivery, being lower after an elective caesarean section than after vaginal delivery or when a caesarean section has been performed after labour has commenced [55]. The WBC and neutrophil counts rise after birth to a peak level at about 12 hours and thereafter fall sharply [41]. The lymphocyte count falls in the first few days of life [43]. The neutrophil count is initially higher than the lymphocyte count. This is reversed between the fourth and seventh days of life.

Maternal smoking causes a small increase in the neonatal Hb, PCV/Hct and MCV and a more substantial decrease in the neutrophil count which persists for at least the first few days after birth [56]. Babies that are small for their gestational age also have lower neutrophil counts [57]. Other maternal and fetal factors influencing the neutrophil count in the neonate are shown in Tables 6.5 and 6.23 and causes of polycythaemia and anaemia in the neonatal period in Tables 6.2 and 6.20. Increased circulating NRBC on the first day of life have been found predictive of intraventricular haemorrhage in premature neonates [58].

Premature babies have a lower WBC and lower neutrophil and lymphocyte counts than term babies; NRBC and immature myeloid cells are more numerous and the reticulocyte count is higher [43,59]. At birth, the Hb and PCV/Hct are similar to those of term babies but the RBC is lower and the MCV higher [60]. Neutrophil and lymphocyte counts reach the levels of term babies by about 1 week [43,59]. In premature babies the eosinophil count often becomes elevated 2–3 weeks after birth.

Normal ranges in infants and children

Normal ranges applicable to infants and children are shown in Tables 5.10 and 5.11. The steady decline in RBC, Hb and PCV/Hct that follows the early peak continues to a nadir around 2 months of age. There is a simultaneous rapid fall in MCV and MCH. In premature babies the postnatal decline in Hb is more rapid and continues for longer, 8–12 weeks rather than 4–8 weeks; the nadir is lower (Table 5.12).

The exclusion of children with iron deficiency is important in deriving paediatric normal ranges since one of the purposes of such ranges is to facilitate the diagnosis of iron deficiency. The iron stores of the neonate are adequate to sustain erythropoiesis for 3–5 months, depending on whether the infant was full term or premature and on whether the cord was clamped early or late. Thereafter, iron deficiency is common. Iron deficiency can be excluded by requiring a normal serum ferritin or transferrin saturation, or a normal red cell protoporphyrin concentration, or by administering iron supplements before testing. Population studies often show a lower limit of normal that is lower than figures appearing in textbooks. For example, Emond *et al.* carried out a study on 1075 infants in Bristol (of whom only 1.2% had a serum ferritin concentration less than 12 µg/l) and found the fifth percentile for Hb to be as low as 9.7 g/dl [66]. In another UK study in which iron deficiency was not excluded, 83 infants aged 9 months had a mean Hb of 9.8 g/dl (95% range approximately 7.2–12.3 g/dl) [68].

Girls have a higher neutrophil count than boys from puberty onwards [70]. The lower WBC and neutrophil counts noted in Black adults have been observed in children between the age of 1 and 5

Table 5.10 Ninety-five per cent (or 90%) ranges for red cell variables for Caucasian infants and children*.

	RBC × 10⁻¹²/l	Hb (g/dl)	PCV/Hct (l/l)	MCV (fl)	MCH (pg)
2 months [36,41]	2.6–4.3	8.9–13.2	0.26–0.40	75–125[†] [41] 84–106[‡] [36]	
3 months [41,65]	3.1–4.3	9.3–13.8	0.27–0.39	73–103	
4 months [36]	3.5–5.1	10.3–14.1	0.32–0.44	76–97	
6 months [36,65]	3.9–5.5	9.9*–14.1	0.31–0.41	68–85	
8 months [66]		9.7–13.6[§]			
1 year [36,65]	4.1–5.3	9.8*–14.1	0.33–0.41	71–84	
1 year [67]		10–13.4[§]			
18 months [65]		9.7*–15.1			
18 months [67]		10.2–13[§]			
18 months [68]		9.1–14.7 (cow's milk); 9.8–14.7 (unfortified formula), 9.1–14.7 (iron-fortified formula)			
1–23 months [35]	3.8–5.4	10.5–14.0	0.32–0.42	72–88	
1–2 years [63]		10.7–13.3			
1–4 years[¶] [69]	3.5–5.3	10.7–15.1	0.31–0.45	72–100	23.8–34.2
3–5 years [63]		10.9–13.7			
2–5/6 years [36,45,61]	4.23–5.03	9.6*–14.8	0.34–0.40	73–86	
2–9 years [35]	4–5.3	11.5–14.5	0.30–0.43	76–90	
5–8 years[¶] [69]	3.45–5.49	10.3–15.1	0.31–0.44	71–99	24.6–33.4
5/6–9 years [45,62,70]	3.93–5.11	10.7–14.6	0.33–0.42	75–89.5	
6–11 [63]		11.5–14.5			
8–12 years [71]	4.34–5.74	12.1–14.5	0.366–0.452	76.5–92.1	
9–12 years [45,62,70]	4.08–5.11	11.5–15.4	0.34–0.42	76–91	
9–12 years[¶] [69]	4.11–5.49	11.3–15.3	0.34–0.44	72–99.6	24–34
12–14/15 years					
Males	4.19–5.54	11.5–15.8	0.36–0.46	76–92	
Females [45,61–63,70]	4.00–5.09	11.5–15.3	0.35–0.44	77–92.5	
13/14–18 years					
Male	4.34–5.88	12.7–17	0.37–0.49	77–95.6	
Female [45,62,70,71]	3.90–5.42	11.3–15.4	0.35–0.46	75–93.8	

Hb, haemoglobin concentration; MCV mean cell volume; PCV, packed cell volume; RBC, red blood cell count.
* Data have been amalgamated to include the highest and lowest limits in different series. Iron deficiency was largely excluded in most series [36,45,61,63]. Others have reported that the Hb is rarely less than 11 g/dl in children who are not iron deficient [64] and the data of Castriota-Scanderberg *et al.* [61] and early data of Dallman and Siimes [45] support this. In more recent investigations the Hb was sometimes below 11 g/dl in children of less than 5 years of age [63].
[†] MCV calculated from microhaematocrit and RBC [41].
[‡] MCV measured by impedance counter [36].
[§] Ninety per cent rather than 95% range, low prevalence of iron deficiency, Hb measured by Haemocue on heel-prick sample; at 18 months of age girls had a significantly higher Hb than boys but the magnitude of the difference was trivial (0.141 g/dl).
[¶] Central America, altitude 0–750 metres, Hb by haemoglobinometry, microhaematocrit and RBC on Coulter Counter Model B [69].

years [77] and in infants by 9–12 months of age [78]. Published reference ranges for Melanesian children show lower Hbs and MCVs than for Caucasians, even though α and β thalassaemia trait were excluded and iron deficiency was uncommon [79]; this probably reflects a high prevalence of malnutrition and malaria in the population studied.

Normal ranges in pregnancy

The changes in haematological variables that occur during pregnancy are discussed on p. 131. Normal ranges are given in Table 5.13. The Hb usually remains above 10 g/dl unless there is iron deficiency or some other complication.

Table 5.11 Ninety-four or 95% ranges for total and differential white cell counts for Caucasian infants, children and adolescents.

Age	9 days–1 year*	2 months†	5 months†	1 year*	1 year‡	13 months†
WBC × 10^{-9}/l	7.3–16.6	5.1–15.4	5.9–16.6	5.6–17	6.0–17.5	5.9–16.1
Neutrophils × 10^{-9}/l	1.5–6.9	0.7–4.7	1.1–5.6	1.5–6.9	1.5–8.5	1.0–7.6
Lymphocytes × 10^{-9}/l	3.4–9.4	3.0–9.9	3.2–10.6	2.5–8.6	4.0–10.5	3.1–9.6
		(3.3–10.5)	(3.4–11.3)			(3.5–10.4)
Monocytes × 10^{-9}/l	0.21–1.64	0.36–1.2	0.25–1.2	0.15–1.28		0.25–0.91
Eosinophils × 10^{-9}/l	0.06–0.62	0.09–0.84	0.1–1.0	0.06–0.62		0.05–0.88
Basophils × 10^{-9}/l	0.02–0.17	0.02–0.13	0.02–0.18	0.02–0.12		0.02–0.13
Large unstained cells × 10^{-9}/l	0.09–0.61	0.17–0.91	0.17–1.00	0.13–0.72		0.20–1.1

Age	2 years*	2 years‡	3 years*	4 years*	4 years‡	5 years*
WBC × 10^{-9}/l	5.6–17.0	6.0–17.0	4.9–12.9	4.9–12.9	5.5–15.5	4.9–12.9
Neutrophils × 10^{-9}/l	1.5–6.9	1.5–8.5	1.5–6.9	1.8–7.7	1.5–8.5	1.8–7.7
Lymphocytes × 10^{-9}/l	2.2–7.7	3.0–9.5	1.7–5.5	1.7–5.5	2.0–8.0	1.6–4.3
Monocytes × 10^{-9}/l	0.15–1.28		0.15–1.28	0.15–1.28		0.15–1.28
Eosinophils × 10^{-9}/l	0.04–1.19		0.04–1.19	0.9–1.40		0.9–1.40
Basophils × 10^{-9}/l	0.02–0.12		0.02–0.12	0.03–0.12		0.03–0.12
Large unstained cells × 10^{-9}/l	0.11–0.68		0.09–0.48	0.09–0.38		0.08–0.32

Age	6 years*	6 years‡	4–6 years§	4–7 years¶	7 years*	7–8 years§
WBC × 10^{-9}/l	4.4–10.6	5.0–14.5	4.8–12.1	6.3–16.2	4.4–10.6	4.5–11.7
Neutrophils × 10^{-9}/l	1.5–5.9	1.5–8.9	1.7–7.6	1.6–9.0	1.5–5.9	1.7–7.4
Lymphocytes × 10^{-9}/l	1.6–4.3	1.5–7.0	1.6–4.2	2.2–9.8	1.6–4.3	1.7–4.3
Monocytes × 10^{-9}/l	0.15–1.28		0.33–1.16	0.06–1.00	0.15–1.28	0.32–1.21
Eosinophils × 10^{-9}/l	0.08–1.10		0.06–0.95	0–1.4	0.08–1.01	0.08–1.00
Basophils × 10^{-9}/l	0.02–0.12		0.00–0.73	0.00–0.026	0.02–0.12	0.02–0.51
Large unstained cells × 10^{-9}/l	0.07–0.26				0.07–0.26	

Age	8 years*	8 years‡	9–10 years*	9–10 years§	10 years‡	
WBC × 10^{-9}/l	3.9–9.9	4.5–13.5	3.9–9.9	4.4–10.6	4.5–13.5	
Neutrophils × 10^{-9}/l	1.5–5.9	1.5–8.0	1.5–5.9	1.7–6.4	1.8–8.0	
Lymphocytes × 10^{-9}/l	1.4–3.8	1.5–6.8	1.4–3.8	1.7–3.9	1.5–6.5	
Monocytes × 10^{-9}/l	0.15–1.28		0.15–1.28	0.33–0.99		
Eosinophils × 10^{-9}/l	0.08–1.01		0.08–1.01	0.06–1.03		
Basophils × 10^{-9}/l	0.02–0.12		0.02–0.12	0.01–0.54		
Large unstained cells × 10^{-9}/l	0.07–0.26		0.07–0.26			

Age	11 years*	11–12 years§	12–13 years*	13–14 years§	14 years*	15–16 years*
WBC × 10^{-9}/l	3.9–9.9	4.0–10.4	3.9–9.9	4.2–10.7	3.9–9.9	3.9–9.9
Neutrophils × 10^{-9}/l	1.5–5.9	1.6–6.2	1.5–5.9	1.7–7.2	1.4–5.6	1.7–5.7
Lymphocytes × 10^{-9}/l	1.4–3.8	1.5–3.7	1.4–3.8	1.4–3.6	1.4–3.8	1.4–3.8
Monocytes × 10^{-9}/l	0.15–1.28	0.31–1.00	0.15–1.28	0.26–1.0	0.15–1.28	0.15–1.28
Eosinophils × 10^{-9}/l	0.04–0.76	0.06–1.12	0.04–0.76	0.05–0.61	0.04–0.76	0.04–0.76
Basophils × 10^{-9}/l	0.02–0.12	0.01–0.38	0.02–0.1	0.01–0.43	0.07–0.1	0.02–0.10
Large unstained cells × 10^{-9}/l	0.07–0.26		0.02–0.1		0.07–0.26	0.07–0.26

WBC, white blood cell count.

* Differential count performed on a Hemalog D automated differential counter [44]; 'large unstained cells' are large peroxidase-negative cells which, in healthy infants and children, represent mainly large lymphocytes.

† Differential count performed on a Bayer H.1 analyser [72]; 'large unstained cells' are large peroxidase-negative cells which, in healthy infants and children, represent mainly large lymphocytes; for the lymphocyte count the figures in parentheses represent lymphocytes plus large unstained cells.

‡ 100-cell manual differential count [73].

§ Differential count performed on Coulter STKS; figures for males and females have been amalgamated [70].

¶ 200-cell manual differential count, recalculated to make allowance for skewed distribution [74,75].

Table 5.12 Ninety-five per cent ranges for haemoglobin concentration (Hb) (g/dl) in pre-term but iron-replete babies in the first 6 months of life [76].

	Birthweight 1000–1500 g	Birthweight 1501–2000 g
2 weeks	11.7–18.4	11.8–19.6
4 weeks	8.7–15.2	8.2–15
2 months	7.1–11.5	8.0–11.4
3 months	8.9–11.2	9.3–11.8
4 months	9.1–13.1	9.1–13.1
6 months	9.4–13.8	10.7–12.6

Normal ranges for platelet counts

The manual platelet count is imprecise and both manual and automated platelet counts are prone to inaccuracy. As a consequence there are considerable discrepancies in published ranges (Table 5.14). It is therefore important for laboratories to establish their own reference ranges for their own methodologies. Platelet counts in Africans have been observed to be lower than those of Caucasians [93,94] but this is less true of Afro-Caribbeans and of Africans living in Britain [87]. This suggests that the low platelet counts observed in Africa are in part genetic but in part caused by dietary factors or sub-clinical disease.

The platelet count correlates with body weight, being higher in obese subjects [95].

In early studies, infants and children were reported to have similar platelet counts to adults [47,96]. Similarly, neonates, both premature and full term, were reported to have similar platelet counts to older children and adults [47,57,96] although babies that were small for gestational age [57] and many sick babies had lower counts. However, in more recent studies children have been observed to have higher counts than adults (Table 5.15). By adolescence, counts are similar to those of adults.

Normal ranges for reticulocyte counts

When reticulocyte counts are expressed as a percentage, reported normal ranges have been between 0.4 and 2% in one study [98] and 0.8–2.5% and 0.8–4.1% for males and females respectively in another [99]. Later studies with automated reticulocyte counts have not generally found any gender difference in the percentage of reticulocytes. Reticulocyte counts are more meaningfully expressed as

Table 5.13 Ninety-five per cent ranges for haematological variables during pregnancy.

Period of gestation	7–14 weeks	15–22 weeks	23–30 weeks	31–38 weeks
Hb (g/dl)	12.8–13.6*	11.4–13.8*	10.9–13.8*	11.1–13.6*

Period of gestation	First trimester	Second trimester	Third trimester
RBC $\times 10^{-12}$/l	3.52–4.52	3.2–4.41	3.1–4.44
Hb (g/dl)	11–14.3	10–13.7	9.8–13.7
PCV/Hct (l/l)	0.31–0.41	0.30–0.38	0.28–0.39
MCV (fl)	81–96	82–97	81–99
WBC $\times 10^{-9}$/l	5.7–13.6	6.2–14.8	5.9–16.9, 5.9–13.7[†]
Neutrophil count $\times 10^{-9}$/l	3.6–10.1	3.8–12.3	3.9–13.1, 3.7–10.8[†]
Lymphocyte count $\times 10^{-9}$/l	1.1–3.5	0.9–3.9	1–3.6, 1–3.1[†]
Monocyte count $\times 10^{-9}$/l	0–1	0.1–1.1	0.1–1.1, 0.3–1.1[†]
Eosinophil count $\times 10^{-9}$/l	0–0.6	0–0.6	0–0.6, 0.02–0.33[†]
Basophil count $\times 10^{-9}$/l	0–0.1	0–0.1	0–0.1, 0–0.09[†]
Platelet count $\times 10^{-9}$/l	174–391	171–409	155–429

Hb, haemoglobin concentration; Hct, haematocrit; MCV mean cell volume; PCV, packed cell volume; WBC, white blood cell count.
All data derived from Balloch *et al.* [7] except for data derived from Cruikshank [80]* and from England and Bain [81][†].

Table 5.14 Ninety-five per cent ranges for platelet counts ($\times 10^{-9}$/l) in healthy adults of differing ethnic origins.

Method	Male		Female	Reference
Caucasians				
Microscopy	140–440			[82]
Microscopy	127–351		165–359	[83]
		140–340		[83]
Microscopy		145–375		[84]
Impedance counting in platelet-rich plasma	143–179		156–417	[85]
Impedance counting in whole blood		170–430		[86]
"	168–411		188–445	[87]
"	184–370		196–451	[88]
"	157–365		164–384	[89]
Light-scattering in whole blood				
Hemalog 8		162–346		*
H.1	143–332		169–358	*
Advia 120	144–328		137–347	[90]
"		159–376 (aged 18–45 y)		[91]
"	156–300 (aged 45–65 y)		156–351 (aged 45–65 y)	[91]
		139–363 (aged > 65 y)		[91]
Japanese				
Light-scattering in whole blood		130–350		[92]
Africans and Afro-Caribbeans				
Microscopy (Nigerians)	95–278			[93]
"	114–322			[93]
Impedance counting (Zambians)	36–258			[94]
Impedance counting				
(Africans in London)	128–365		166–377	[87]
(Afro-Caribbeans in London)	210–351		160–411	[87]
Light-scattering				
(Africans in London)	118–297*		149–332	*
(Afro-Caribbeans in London)	134–332*		165–368	*

* Unpublished observations of the author.

absolute numbers. In one study, a mean of 88×10^9/l and a range of $18–158 \times 10^9$/l were found [100]. Reference ranges reported for automated reticulocyte counts have varied considerably, from $19–59 \times 10^9$/l [101] to $40–140 \times 10^9$/l [102]. The higher values reported by Chin-Yee *et at.* [102] appear more acceptable since, in this study, automated and manual counts were similar. These and other reported reference ranges for reticulocyte counts are summarized in Table 5.16. A higher range, approximately $94–222 \times 10^9$/l, has been reported in the neonatal period [32]; these were automated counts using an Abbott Cell-Dyn 4000 instrument.

Test your knowledge

Multiple choice questions (MCQs)

(1–5 answers may be correct)

MCQ 5.1 The absolute eosinophil count
(a) Is higher in healthy Indians than in northern European Caucasians
(b) Falls during pregnancy
(c) Shows diurnal variation
(d) Falls during labour
(e) Rises as a response to vigorous exercise

Table 5.15 Ninety-four per cent ranges for platelet counts ($\times 10^{-9}$/l) in healthy Caucasian children and adolescents.

Age	Male	Female
Cord blood* [32]	180–428	
2 months[†] [97]	214–648	
5 months[†] [97]	210–560	
13 months[†] [97]	202–550	
4–6 years[‡]	213–429	220–443
7–8 years[‡]	211–422	218–396
9–10 years[‡]	166–429	197–406
1–10 years[†] [91]	220–422	
11–12 years[‡]	175–375	174–374
13–14 years[‡]	166–360	192–439
15–19 years[‡]	171–370	171–356
8–14 years[‡]	193–445	183–410
15–18 years[‡]	145–330	163–361
10–18 years[†] [91]	165–396	

* Brazilian, from Porto Alegre, so likely to be essentially Caucasian; Abbott Cell-Dyn 4000.
[†] Bayer H.1 [97] or Advia 120 [91].
[‡] Coulter STKS [70,71].

MCQ 5.2 The haemoglobin in the neonate is affected by
(a) Maternal cigarette smoking
(b) Administration of oxytocin to the mother during labour
(c) The time of cord blood clamping
(d) Ethnic origin
(e) The prevalence of inherited disorders of globin chain synthesis

MCQ 5.3 Living at a high altitude leads to an increase in
(a) The white cell count
(b) The red cell count
(c) The haemoglobin concentration
(d) The haematocrit
(e) The platelet count

MCQ 5.4 Old age leads to
(a) A fall in the lymphocyte count
(b) In men, a fall in the haemoglobin concentration
(c) A rise in the platelet count
(d) A fall in the MCV
(e) A fall in the MCHC

Table 5.16 Reported reference ranges for manual and automated reticulocyte counts.

Method	95% range (median) of percentage reticulocytes	95% range (median) or [mean] of absolute reticulocyte count ($\times 10^{-9}$/L)	Reference
Manual		18–158 (88)	[100]
Manual	0.8–2.5 (males)		[99]
	0.8–4.1 (females)		[98]
Manual	0.4–2.0	19–111 (46)	[103]
Manual	0.4–2.3 (1.0)	19–59	[101]
		40–140	[102]
Bayer Advia 120	0.6–2.5 (1.2)	27–125 (58)	[103]
		16–72 [44]	[104]
Abbott Cell Dyn 4000	0.4–2.2 (1.3)	25–108 (57)	[103]
		19–97 [58]	[104]
Coulter Gen S	0.5–1.8 (1.0)	20–85 (43)	[103]
Coulter General S		16–79 [47.5]	[104]
Sysmex SE 9500 RET	0.5–1.9 (0.9)	23–95 (44)	[103]
		9–72 [44]	[104]
VEGA RETIC / ABX Pentra 120 Retic	0.6–2.6 (1.3)	30–130 (60)	[103]
		16–100 [58]	[104]

Extended matching question (EMQ)

Select the most accurate options for each of the stems. Each option may be used once, more than once or not at all.

EMQ 5.1
Theme: normal ranges
Options
A African ancestry
B Age
C Cigarette smoking
D Excess ethanol intake
E Female gender
F Indian ethnic origin
G Male gender
H Pregnancy

For each combination of features described, select the most likely explanation from the list of options above.

Variable	Matching option
1 Increased white cell count, neutrophil count and lymphocyte count	
2 Lower haemoglobin concentration, higher white cell count, neutrophil count and platelet count, higher erythrocyte sedimentation rate	
3 Lower white cell count, neutrophil count and platelet count	
4 Higher white cell count and MCV, lower haemoglobin concentration, left shift	
5 Higher MCV with stomatocytes	

References

1 Bain BJ. *Blood Cells: a Practical Guide*. Gower, London, 1989.

2 Moe PJ (1967) Umbilical cord blood and capillary blood in the evaluation of anaemia in erythroblastosis foetalis. *Acta Pediatr Scand*, **56**, 391–394.

3 Özbek N, Gürakan B and Kayiran SM (2000) Complete blood cell counts in capillary and venous blood of healthy term newborns. *Acta Haematol*, **103**, 226–228.

4 Yang Z-W, Yang S-H, Chen L, Qu J, Zhu J and Tang Z (2001) Comparison of blood counts in venous, fingertip and arterial blood and their measurement variation. *Clin Lab Haematol*, **23**, 155–159.

5 Bryner MA, Houwen B, Westengard J and Klein O (1997) The spun micro-haematocrit and mean red cell volume are affected by changes in the oxygenation state of red blood cells. *Clin Lab Haematol*, **19**, 99–103.

6 Campbell PJ, Aurelius S, Blowees G and Harvey J (1995) Decrease in CD4 counts with rest; implications for the monitoring of HIV infection. *Br J Haematol*, **89**, 73.

7 Balloch Al and Cauchi MN (1993) Reference ranges for haematology parameters in pregnancy derived from patient populations. *Clin Lab Haematol*, **15**, 7–14.

8 Beutler E and West C (2005) Hematologic differences between African-Americans and whites; the role of iron deficiency and α-thalassaemia on hemoglobin levels and mean corpuscular volume. *Blood*, **106**, 740–745.

9 Beutler E, Felitti V, Gelbart T and Waalen J (2003) Haematological effects of the C282Y *HFE* mutation in homozygous and heterozygous states among subjects of northern and southern European ancestry. *Br J Haematol*, **120**, 887–893.

10 Barton JC, Bertoli LF and Rothenberg BE (2000) Peripheral blood erythrocyte parameters in hemochromatosis: evidence for increased erythrocyte hemoglobin content. *J Lab Clin Med*, **135**, 96–104.

11 Giorno R, Clifford JH, Beverly S and Rossing RG (1980) Hematology reference ranges. Analysis by different statistical technics and variations with age and sex. *Am J Clin Pathol*, **74**, 765–770.

12 Solberg EK. Statistical treatment of collected reference values and determination of reference limits. In: Grasbeck R, Alstrom W, eds. *Reference Values in Laboratory Medicine*. John Wiley, Chichester, 1981.

13 Amador E (1975) Health and normality. *JAMA*, **232**, 953–955.

14 Nilsson-Ehle A, Jagenburg R, Landahl S and Svanborg A (2000) Blood hemoglobin declines in the elderly: implications for reference intervals for 70–88. *Eur J Haematol*, **65**, 297–305.

15 Ruiz-Argüelles GJ, Sanchez-Medal L, Loria A, Piedras J and Córdova MS (1980) Red cell indices in normal adults residing at altitude from sea level to 2670 meters. *Am J Hematol*, **8**, 265–271.

16 Bonfichi M, Balduini A, Arcaini L, Lorenzi A, Marseglia C, Malcovati L *et al.* (2000) Haematological modifications after acute exposure to high altitude: possible applications for detection of recombinant erythropoietin misuse. *Br J Haematol,* **109**, 895–896.

17 Bowen AL, Hudson JG, Navia P, Rios-Dalenz J, Pollard AJ, Williams D and Heath D (1977) The effect of altitude on blood platelet count. *Br J Haematol,* **97**, Suppl 1, 83.

18 Carballo C, Foucar K, Swanson P, Papile LA and Watterberg KL (1992) Effect of high altitude on neutrophil counts in newborn infants. *J Pediatr,* **119**, 464–466.

19 Kristal-Bonch E, Froom P, Harari G, Shapiro Y and Green MS (1993) Seasonal changes in red blood cell parameters. *Br J Haematol,* **85**, 603–607.

20 Kristal-Bonch E, Froom P, Harari G and Ribak J (1997) Seasonal differences in blood cell parameters and the association with cigarette smoking. *Clin Lab Haematol,* **19**, 177–181.

21 Bertouch JV, Roberts-Thomson PJ and Bradley J (1983) Diurnal variation of lymphocyte subsets identified by monoclonal antibodies. *BMJ,* **286**, 1171–1172.

22 Philips D, Rezvani K and Bain BJ (2000) Exercise induced mobilisation of the marginated granulocyte pool in the investigation of ethnic neutropenia. *J Clin Pathol,* **53**, 481–483.

23 Bain BJ, Phillips D, Thomson K, Richardson D and Gabriel I (2000) Investigation of the effect of marathon running on leucocyte counts of subjects of different ethnic origins: relevance to the aetiology of ethnic neutropenia. *Br J Haematol,* **108**, 483–487.

24 Bain BJ (1992) Haematological effects of smoking. *J Smoking Rel Dis,* **3**, 99–108.

25 Milman N, Byg K-E, Mulvad G, Pedersen HS and Bjerregaard P (2001) Haemoglobin concentrations appear to be lower in indigenous Greenlanders than in Danes: assessment of haemoglobin in 234 Greenlanders and in 2804 Danes. *Eur J Haematol,* **67**, 23–29.

26 Wilson CA, Bekele G, Nicolson M, Ravussin E and Pratley RE (1997) Relationship of the white blood cell count to body fat: role of leptin. *Br J Haematol,* **99**, 447–451.

27 Nanji AA and Freeman JB (1985) Relationship between body weight and total leukocyte count in morbid obesity. *Am J Clin Pathol,* **84**, 346–347.

28 Fairbanks VF and Tefferi A (2001) Letter to the Editor. *Eur J Haematol,* **67**, 203–204.

29 Waalen J, Felitti V and Beutler E (2002) Haemoglobin and ferritin concentrations in men and women: cross sectional study. *BMJ,* **325**, 137.

30 Rezvani K, Flanagan AM, Sarma U, Constantinovici N and Bain BJ (2000) Investigation of ethnic neutropenia by assessment of bone marrow colony-forming cells. *Acta Haematol,* **105**, 32–37.

31 Marks J, Gairdner D and Roscoe JD (1955) Blood formation in infancy. Part III. Cord blood. *Arch Dis Child,* **30**, 117–120.

32 Pranke P, Failace RR, Allebrandt WF, Steibel G, Schmidt F and Nardi NB (2001) Hematologic and immunophenotypic characterization of human umbilical cord blood. *Acta Haematol,* **105**, 71–76.

33 Matoth Y, Zaizov R and Varsano I (1971) Postnatal changes in some red cell parameters. *Acta Paediatr Scand,* **60**, 317–323.

34 Lanzkowsky P (1960) Effects of early and late clamping of umbilical cord on infant's haemoglobin level. *BMJ,* **ii**, 1777–1782.

35 www.beckman.com

36 Saarinem UM and Siimes MD (1978) Developmental changes in red blood cell counts and indices of infants after exclusion of iron deficiency by laboratory criteria and continuous iron supplementation. *J Pediatr,* **92**, 412–416.

37 Serjeant GR, Grandison Y, Mason K, Serjeant B, Sewell A and Vaidya V (1980) Hematological indices in normal Negro children: a Jamaican cohort from birth to five years. *Clin Lab Haematol,* **2**, 169–178.

38 Scott-Emuakpor AB, Okolo AA, Omene JA and Ukpe SI (1985) The limits of physiological anaemia in the African neonate. *Acta Haematol,* **74**, 99–103.

39 Gregory J and Hey E (1972) Blood neutrophil response to bacterial infection in the first month of life. *Arch Dis Child,* **47**, 747–753.

40 Weinberg AG, Rosenfeld CR, Manroe BL and Browne R (1985) Neonatal blood cell count in health and disease. II Values for lymphocytes, monocytcs, and eosinophils. *J Pediatr,* **106**, 462–466.

41 Manroe BL, Weinberg AG, Rosenfeld CR and Brown R (1979) The neonatal blood count in health and disease. I. Reference values for neutrophilic cells. *J Pediatr,* **95**, 89–98.

42 Chan PCY, Hayes L and Bain BJ (1985) A comparison of the white cell counts of cord bloods from babies of different ethnic origins. *Ann Trop Paediatr,* **5**, 153–155.

43 Xanthou M (1970) Leucocyte blood picture in full-term and premature babies during neonatal period. *Arch Dis Child*, **45**, 242–249.

44 Cranendonk E, van Gennip AH, Abeling NGGM, Behrendt H and Hart AA (1985) Reference values for automated cytochemical differential count of leukocytes in children 0–16 years old: a comparison with manually obtained counts from Wright-stained smears. *J Clin Chem Clin Biochem*, **23**, 663–667.

45 Dallman PR and Siimes MA (1979) Percentile curves for hemoglobin and red cell volume in infancy and childhood. *J Pediatr*, **94**, 26–31.

46 Playfair JHL, Wolfendale MR and Kay HEM (1963) The leucocytes of peripheral blood in the human foetus. *Br J Haematol*, **9**, 336–344.

47 Millar DS, Davis LR, Rodeck CH, Nicolaides KH and Mibashan RS (1985) Normal blood cell values in the early mid-trimester fetus. *Prenat Diagn*, **5**, 367–373.

48 Forestier F, Daffos F, Galactéros F, Bardakjian J, Rainaut M and Beuzard Y (1986) Haematological values of 163 normal fetuses between 18 and 30 weeks of gestation. *Paediatr Res*, **20**, 342–346.

49 Mari G, Zimmerman R and Oz U (2000) Non-invasive diagnosis of fetal anemia by Doppler ultrasonography. *N Engl J Med*, **343**, 67–68.

50 Hohlfeld P, Forestier F, Kaplan C, Tissot JD and Daffos F (1994) Fetal thrombocytopenia: a retrospective survey of 5,194 fetal blood samplings. *Blood*, **84**, 1851–1856.

51 Forestier F, Hohlfeld P, Vial Y, Olin V, Andreux J-P and Tissot J-D (1996) Blood smears and prenatal diagnosis. *Br J Haematol*, **95**, 278–280.

52 Aneja S, Manchanda R, Patwari A, Sagreiya K and Bhargava SK (1979) Normal hematological values in newborns. *Indian Pediatr*, **16**, 781–786.

53 Ezeilo GC (1978) A comparison of the haematological values of cord bloods of African, European and Asian neonates. *Afr J Med Sci*, **7**, 163–169.

54 Green DW and Mimouni F (1990) Nucleated erythrocytes in healthy infants and in infants of diabetic mothers. *J Pediatr*, **116**, 129–131.

55 Frazier JP, Cleary TG, Pickering LK, Kohl S and Ross PJ (1982) Leukocyte function in healthy neonates following vaginal and cesarean section deliveries. *J Pediatr*, **101**, 269–272.

56 Harrison KL (1979) The effect of maternal smoking on neonatal leucocytes. *Aust NZ J Obstet Gynaecol*, **19**, 166–168.

57 McIntosh N, Kempson C and Tyler RM (1988) Blood counts in extremely low birth weight infants. *Arch Dis Child*, **63**, 74–76.

58 Green DW, Hendon B and Mimouni FB (1995) Nucleated erythrocytes and intraventricular haemorrhage in preterm neonates. *Pediatrics*, **96**, 475–478.

59 Coulombel L, Dehan M, Tchernia G, Hill C and Vial M (1979) The number of polymorphonuclear leucocytes in relation to gestational age in the newborn. *Acta Paediatr Scand*, **68**, 709–711.

60 Zaizov R and Matoth Y (1976) Red cell values on the first postnatal day during the last sixteen weeks of gestation. *Am J Hematol*, **1**, 275–278.

61 Castriota-Scanderberg A, Fedrazzi G, Mercadanti M, Stapane I, Butturini A and Izzi G (1992) Normal values of total reticulocytes and reticulocyte subsets in children and young adults. *Haematologica*, **77**, 363–364.

62 Natvig H and Vellar OD and Andersen J (1967) Studies on hemoglobin value in Norway. VII. Hemoglobin, hematocrit and MCHC values among boys and girls aged 7–20 years in elementary and grammar school. *Acta Med Scand*, **182**, 183–191.

63 Dallman PR, Looker AC, Johnson CL and Carroll M, Influence of age on laboratory criteria for the diagnosis of iron deficiency in infants and children. In: *Iron Nutrition in Health and Disease* Hallberg L and Asp NG (Eds) pp. 65–74, John Libbey, London, 1996, quoted by Wharton BA (1999) Iron deficiency in children: detection and prevention. *Br J Haematol*, **106**, 270–280.

64 Hunter RE and Smith NJ (1972) Hemoglobin and hematocrit values in iron deficiency in infancy. *J Pediatr*, **81**, 710–713.

65 Burman D (1972) Haemoglobin levels in normal infants aged 3 to 24 months, and the effect of iron. *Arch Dis Child*, **47**, 261–271.

66 Emond AM, Hawkins N, Pennock C, Golding J and the ALSPAC children in focus team (1996) Haemoglobin and ferritin concentrations in infants at 8 months of age. *Arch Dis Child*, **74**, 36–69.

67 Sherriff A, Emond A, Hawkins N, Golding J and the ALSPAC Children in Focus Study Team (1999) Haemoglobin and ferritin concentrations in children aged 12 and 18 months. *Arch Dis Child*, **80**, 153–157.

68 Morley R, Abbott R, Fairweather-Tait S, MacFadyen U, Stephenson T and Lucas A (1999) Iron fortified follow on formula from 9 to 18 months improves

iron status but not development or growth: a randomised trial. *Arch Dis Child*, **81**, 247–252.

69 Viteri FE, de Tuna V and Guzmán MA (1972) Normal haematological values in the Central American population. *Br J Haematol*, **23**, 189–204.

70 Taylor MRH, Holland CV, Spencer R, Jackson JF, O'Connor GI and O'Donnell JR (1997) Haematological references ranges for schoolchildren. *Clin Lab Haematol*, **19**, 1–15.

71 Flegar-Měštrić Z, Nazor A and Jagarinic N (1999) Reference intervals for haematological parameters in urban school children. *Clin Lab Haematol*, **21**, 72–74.

72 Bellamy GJ, Hinchliffe RF, Crawshaw KJ, Finn AH and Bell F (2000) Total and differential leucocyte counts in infants at 2, 5 and 13 months of age. *Clin Lab Haematol*, **22**, 81–87.

73 Dallman PR. Blood and blood forming tissues. In Rudolph AM, Hoffman JIE (eds), *Rudolph's Pediatrics*, 19th Edn. Appleton & Lange, New York, 1991.

74 Osgood EE, Brownlee IE, Osgood MW, Ellis DM and Cohen W (1939) Total, differential and absolute leukocyte counts and sedimentation rates of healthy children four to seven years of age. *Am J Dis Child*, **58**, 61–70.

75 Osgood EE, Brownlee IE, Osgood MW, Ellis DM and Cohen W (1939) Total, differential and absolute leukocyte counts and sedimentation rates of healthy children. Standards for children eight to fourteen years of age. *Am J Dis Child*, **58**, 282–294.

76 Lundstrom U, Siimes MA and Dallman PR (1977) At what age does iron supplementation become necessary in low-birth-weight infants. *J Pediatr*, **91**, 878–883.

77 Caramihai E, Karayalcin G, Aballi AJ and Lanzkowsky P (1975) Leukocyte count differences in healthy white and black children 1 to 5 years of age. *J Pediatr*, **86**, 252–254.

78 Sadowitz PD and Oski FA (1983) Differences in polymorphonuclear cell counts between healthy white and black infants: response to meningitis. *Pediatrics*, **72**, 405–407.

79 Williams TN, Maitland K, Ganczakowski M, Peto TEA, Clegg JB, Weatherall DJ and Bowden DK (1996) Red blood cells phenotypes in the α⁺ thalassaemias from early childhood to maturity. *Br J Haematol*, **95**, 266–272.

80 Cruikshank JM (1970) Some variations in the normal haemoglobin concentration. *Br J Haematol*, **18**, 523–529.

81 England JM and Bain BJ (1976) Annotation: total and differential leucocyte count. *Br J Haematol*, **33**, 1–7.

82 Brecher G and Cronkite EP (1950) Morphology and enumeration of human blood platelets. *J Appl Physiol*, **3**, 365–377.

83 Sloan AW (1951) The normal platelet count in man. *J Clin Pathol*, **4**, 37–46.

84 Miale JB. *Laboratory Medicine Hematology*, 6th Edn. CV Mosby, St Louis, 1982.

85 Bain BJ and Forster T (1980) A sex difference in the bleeding time. *Thromb Haemost*, **43**, 131–132.

86 Giles C (1981) The platelet count and mean platelet volume. *Br J Haematol*, **48**, 31–37.

87 Bain BJ and Seed M (1986) Platelet count and platelet size in Africans and West Indians. *Clin Lab Haematol*, **8**, 43–48.

88 Payne BA and Pierre RV (1986) Using the three-part differential. Part 1. Investigating the possibilities. *Lab Med*, **17**, 459–462.

89 Gladwin AM, Trowbridge EA, Slater DN, Reardon D and Martin JF (1990) The size and number of bone marrow megakaryocytes in malignant lymphoma and their relationship to the platelet count. *Am J Hematol*, **35**, 225–231.

90 Brummitt DR and Barker HF (2000) The determination of a reference range for new platelet parameters produced by the Bayer ADVIA™ 120 full blood count analyser. *Clin Lab Haematol*, **22**, 103–107.

91 Giacomini A, Legovini P, Gessoni G, Antico F, Valverde S, Salvadego MM and Manoni F (2001) Platelet count and parameters determined by the Bayer ADVIA™ 120 in reference subjects and patients. *Clin Lab Haematol*, **23**, 181–186.

92 Takamatsu N, Yamamoto H, Onomura Y and Ichikawa N (1992) A study of the hematological reference ranges and changes with age using the automated hematology analyzer K-1000™. *Sysmex J Int*, **2**, 136–145.

93 Essien EM, Usanga EA and Ayeni O (1973) The normal platelet count and platelet factor 3 availability in some Nigerian population groups. *Scand J Haematol*, **10**, 378–383.

94 Gill GV, England A and Marshal C (1979) Low platelet counts in Zambians. *Trans R Soc Trop Med Hyg*, **73**, 111–112.

95 Wilson CA, Bekele G, Nicolson M, Ravussin E and Pralley RE (1997) Relationship of the white blood cell count to role of leptin. *Br J Haematol*, **99**, 447–451.

96 Sell EJ and Corrigan JJ (1973) Platelet counts, fibrinogen concentrations, and factor V and factor VII levels in healthy infants according to gestational age. *J Pediatr*, **82**, 1028–1032.

97 Hinchliffe RF, Bell FG, Vora AJ, Shearstone NN, Martin AA and Finn AHR (1997) The platelet count in children at two, five and thirteen months of age. *Br J Haematol*, **97**, Suppl. 1, 33.

98 Crouch JY and Kaplow LS (1985) Relationship of reticulocyte age to polychromasia, shift cells and shift reticulocytes. *Arch Pathol Lab Med*, **109**, 325–329.

99 Deiss A and Kurth D (1970) Circulating reticulocytes in normal adults as determined by the new methylene blue method. *Am J Clin Pathol*, **53**, 481–484.

100 Lee GR. Normal blood and bone marrow values in men. In: Wintrobe MM, Lee GR, Boggs DR, Bithell TC, Foerster J, Athens JW and Lukens IN (eds) *Clinical Hematology*, 8th Edn. Lea & Febiger, Philadelphia, 1981, p. 1855.

101 Nobes PR and Carter AB (1990) Reticulocyte counting using flow cytometry. *J Clin Pathol*, **43**, 675–678.

102 Chin-Yee I, Keeney M and Lehmann C (1991) Flow cytometric reticulocyte analysis using thiazole orange: clinical experience and technical limitations. *Clin Lab Haematol*, **13**, 177–188.

103 Buttarello M, Bulian P, Farina G, Temporin V, Toffolo L, Trabuio E and Rizzotti P (2000) Flow cytometric reticulocyte counting: parallel evaluation of five fully automated analyzers: an NCCLS-ICSH approach. *Am J Clin Pathol*, **115**, 100–111.

104 Van den Bossche J, Devreese K, Malfait R, van de Vyvere M and Schouwer P (2001) Comparison of the reticulocyte mode of the Abx Pentra 120 Retic, Coulter General-S, Sysmex SE 9500, Abbott CD 4000 and Bayer Advia 120 haematology analysers in a simultaneous evaluation. *Clin Lab Haematol*, **23**, 355–360.

Answers to test questions

Multiple choice questions

MCQ 5.1	FTTTT
MCQ 5.2	TTTFT
MCQ 5.3	FTTTT
MCQ 5.4	TTFFF

Extended matching question

EMQ 5.1

1 C
2 E
3 A
4 H
5 D

6 Quantitative changes in blood cells

This chapter deals with quantitative changes in blood cells, first the causes of increased cell counts for each lineage then the causes of decreased counts. An increase of a cell type usually results either from redistribution of cells or from increased bone marrow output; occasionally an increased count, most noticeably of red cells, can result from a decrease of plasma volume. A decreased count of any cell type can result from diminished bone marrow output, redistribution, or shortened survival in the circulation.

Polycythaemia

The term polycythaemia, strictly speaking, should indicate an increase in the number of red cells in the circulation but, in practice, the term is used for an increase of the haemoglobin concentration (Hb) and packed cell volume/haematocrit (PCV/Hct) above that which is normal for the age and sex of the subject. Usually, the red blood cell count (RBC), Hb and PCV/Hct rise in parallel. Conventionally, the term polycythaemia does not refer to an increased RBC if the Hb is normal as may be seen, for example, in thalassaemia trait. A raised Hb can be due to a decreased plasma volume occurring either acutely or chronically. An acute decrease in plasma volume can

be caused by shock, when there is a loss of fluid from the intravascular compartment, or by dehydration. An intermittent apparent polycythaemia, which can be very striking, occurs in the idiopathic capillary leak syndrome [1]. It can also occur in capillary leak syndromes associated with viral haemorrhagic fevers. A chronic decrease in plasma volume is sometimes due to cigarette smoking but in many cases the cause is unknown. The phenomenon has been referred to as 'stress polycythaemia' but 'pseudopolycythaemia' or 'relative polycythaermia' is a better designation since there is no clear relationship to 'stress'.

Alternatively, a raised Hb can be due to true polycythaemia, i.e. to an increase in the total volume of circulating red cells often referred to, inaccurately, as the 'red cell mass'. True polycythaemia can be primary or secondary. In primary polycythaemia there is an intrinsic bone marrow disorder, either inherited or acquired. Erythropoietin concentration is decreased. In contrast, secondary polycythaemia is generally mediated by increased erythropoietin production, usually occurring either as a physiological response to hypoxia or as a result of inappropriate secretion by a diseased kidney or by a tumour. Causes of polycythaemia are summarized in Table 6.1. The differential diagnosis of polycythaemia rubra vera

Table 6.1 Some causes of polycythaemia.

Primary

Inherited

Erythroid progenitor cells with enhanced sensitivity to erythropoietin [2], sometimes caused by mutation of the erythropoietin receptor gene [3];

Homozygosity for a mutation in the *VHL* gene in mid-Volga (Chuvash) familial polycythaemia (which also occurs in occasional families in Pakistan and Bangladesh and in western Europe) [3–5] and other rare familial polycythaemias [6]—resulting in protection of HIP1α (hypoxia-inducible protein 1α) from degradation and consequent increased synthesis of erythropoietin

Acquired

Polycythaemia rubra vera (polycythaemia vera)
Essential or idiopathic erythrocytosis

Continued p. 218

Table 6.1 *Continued*

Secondary
Caused by tissue hypoxia
Inherited
  Inadequate oxygen-carrying capacity
    Caused by congenital deficiency of NAD-linked or NADH-linked methaemoglobin reductase with consequent
      methaemoglobinaemia
    Haemoglobin M (structurally abnormal haemoglobins with tendency to form methaemoglobin)
  Impaired release of oxygen from haemoglobin
    High affinity haemoglobins including some methaemoglobins and hereditary persistence of fetal haemoglobin
    Oxygen affinity of haemoglobin increased by very low levels of 2,3 DPG (2,3 diphosphoglycerate) resulting from
      deficiency of diphosphoglycerate mutase or, occasionally, deficiency of phosphofructokinase [7]

Acquired
  Hypoxia
    Residence at high altitude. Use of simulated high altitude in athletic training (hypoxic tent or 'high altitude bed')
    Cyanotic heart disease
    Chronic hypoxic lung disease
    Sleep apnoea and other hypoventilation syndromes including morbid obesity (Pickwickian syndrome)
    Hepatic cirrhosis (consequent on pulmonary arteriovenous shunting) [8]
    Pulmonary arteriovenous malformations in hereditary haemorrhagic telangiectasia [9]
  Inadequate oxygen-carrying capacity
    Chronic carbon monoxide poisoning [10] or heavy cigarette smoking
    Chronic methaemoglobinaemia or sulphaemoglobinaemia caused by drugs or chemicals

Consequent on inappropriate synthesis of erythropoietin (proven or presumptive) [11,12] or administration of erythropoietin or androgens
Inherited
  Familial inappropriate increase of erythropoietin synthesis [13,14], sometimes with preceding multiple
    paraganglionomas [15]

Acquired
  Renal lesions including carcinoma (hypernephroma), Wilms' tumour, renal adenoma, renal haemangioma, renal
    sarcoma, renal cysts including polycystic disease of the kidney, renal artery stenosis, renal vein thrombosis, post-
    transplant polycythaemia, hydronephrosis, horseshoe kidney, nephrocalcinosis (including that caused by
    hyperparathyroidism), Bartter's syndrome, perinephric lymphangioma [16]
  Cerebellar haemangioblastoma
  Meningioma
  Hepatic lesions including hepatoma, hepatic hamartoma, hepatic angiosarcoma, hepatic haemangioma
  Uterine leiomyoma (uterine fibroid)
  Tumours of the adrenal gland, ovary, lung, thymus, parathyroid (carcinoma/adenoma)
  Phaeochromocytoma [17]
  Atrial myxoma [18]
  Cushing's syndrome and primary aldosteronism
  Erythropoietin administration (e.g. illicit use in athletes)
  Androgen administration or androgen-secreting tumours in women
  Androgen abuse in males (e.g. in athletes) [19]

'Blood doping'
Illicit homologous transfusion or re-transfusion of autologous blood by athletes

Unknown mechanisms
Inherited
  Some familial cases [20]
Acquired
  Cobalt toxicity [21]
  Monge's disease (excessive erythrocytosis at altitude—possibly related to cobalt toxicity [22])
  Associated with POEMS [23]
  Administration of antivascular endothelial growth factor receptor (SU5416) therapy in von Hippel–Lindau syndrome [24]

NAD, nicotinamide adenine dinucleotide; NADH, reduced nicotinamide adenine dinucleotide; POEMS, **P**olyendocrinopathy,
Organomegaly, **E**ndocrinopathy, **M**-protein, **S**kin changes syndrome.

Table 6.2 Some causes of polycythaemia of particular importance in or peculiar to the neonatal period.

Intrauterine twin-to-twin transfusion
Intrauterine maternal to fetal transfusion
Placental insufficiency and intrauterine hypoxia
   Small-for-dates babies
   Post-mature babies
   Maternal pregnancy-associated hypertension
   Maternal smoking
   Maternal diabetes mellitus
Chromosomal abnormalities
   Down's syndrome
   Trisomy 13 syndrome
   Trisomy 18 syndrome
Neonatal thyrotoxicosis
Neonatal hypothyroidism
Congenital adrenal hyperplasia
Delayed cord clamping
Underwater labour with late cord clamping [25]

Table 6.3 Causes of reticulocytosis.

Common causes
Shortened red cell lifespan (i.e. haemolytic anaemia)
Recent blood loss
Response to therapy in a patient with deficiency of
   vitamin B_{12}, folic acid or iron
Recovery from bone marrow (or erythroid) suppression
   or failure
Administration of erythropoietin
Hypoxia
Diabetes mellitus (possibly representing compensated
   haemolysis) [26]

Rare causes
Delayed maturation of reticulocytes (in myelodysplastic
   syndrome)
Genetic haemochromatosis [27]

(PRV) is discussed on p. 364. Neonates have higher Hbs than adults but the Hb may rise even higher in pathological conditions. Some causes of polycythaemia that are peculiar to the neonatal period are summarized in Table 6.2.

Reticulocytosis

Either the percentage or absolute reticulocyte count or both may be increased. With rare exceptions, an increased reticulocyte percentage indicates an increased proportion of young erythrocytes. Again with rare exceptions, an increased absolute reticulocyte count indicates an increased marrow output of erythrocytes. Often both the percentage and absolute count are increased but a patient with significant anaemia may have an increased percentage of reticulocytes without an increase in the absolute count.

Causes of an increased reticulocyte count are shown in Table 6.3.

Leucocytosis

Leucocytosis is an increase in the total white cell count. It most often results from an increase in neutrophils but sometimes from an increase in lymphocytes and occasionally from an increase in eosinophils or from the presence of abnormal myeloid or lymphoid cells in the blood.

Leucocytosis cannot be interpreted without knowledge of the differential count.

Neutrophil leucocytosis—neutrophilia

Neutrophil leucocytosis or neutrophilia is the elevation of the absolute neutrophil count above that expected in a healthy subject of the same age, gender, ethnic origin and physiological status. Healthy neonates have both a higher neutrophil count than is normal at other stages of life and also a left shift. Similarly, women in the reproductive age range have somewhat higher neutrophil counts than men, the count varying with the menstrual cycle. During pregnancy, a marked rise in the neutrophil count occurs and this is further accentuated during labour and the postpartum period. In addition, pregnancy is associated with a left shift (with myelocytes and even a few promyelocytes appearing in the blood), with 'toxic' granulation and with Döhle bodies.

Neutrophil leucocytosis is usually due to redistribution of white cells or increased bone marrow output. Rarely, there is a prolongation of the period a neutrophil spends in the circulation. Exercise can alter the distribution of white cells within the circulation with cells that were previously marginated (against the endothelium) being mobilized into the circulating blood. Vigorous exercise can double the neutrophil count. The absolute number of lymphocytes, monocytes, eosinophils and basophils also increases but because of the more striking increase in neutrophil numbers the increase of other cell types may go unnoticed. If exercise is both severe and prolonged a left shift can occur, indicating that there is then increased bone marrow output in addition to redistribution. Patients do not usually undergo severe exercise before having a blood sample taken but epinephrine (adrenaline) administration and epileptiform convulsions can mobilize neutrophils similarly and even severe pain can have an effect on the neutrophil count. Corticosteroids also alter neutrophil kinetics. The output from the bone marrow is increased and there is a concomitant decrease in egress to the tissues. Experiments in rabbits suggest that there is also mobilization of neutrophils from the marginated granulocyte pool [28]. A rise in the white blood cell count (WBC) starts within a few hours of intravenous administration or within 1 day of oral administration. WBCs as high as $20 \times 10^9/l$ occur, the elevation being predominantly due to neutrophilia but with some increase also in the absolute monocyte count, and with a fall in the absolute eosinophil and lymphocyte counts. Epinephrine and corticosteroids do not cause toxic granulation, Döhle bodies, left shift or neutrophil vacuolation.

Neutrophilia in pathological conditions is usually consequent on increased output from the bone marrow, which more than compensates for any increased egress to the tissues. The major causes of neutrophilia are shown in Table 6.4 and some causes of particular importance in the neonatal period in Table 6.5.

An increased neutrophil count can be of adverse prognostic significance. This is so for long-term prognosis in sickle cell anaemia and for short-term prognosis in unstable angina and following myocardial infarction.

Eosinophil leucocytosis—eosinophilia

Eosinophil leucocytosis or eosinophilia is the elevation of the eosinophil count above levels observed in healthy subjects of the same age with no history of allergy. Eosinophil counts are higher in neonates than in adults. A slow decline in the eosinophil count occurs in elderly people. Eosinophil counts are the same in men and women. Contrary to earlier reports, counts do not differ between different ethnic groups. High eosinophil counts previously reported in Indians and Africans are attributable to environmental influences.

The absolute eosinophil count is increased with vigorous exercise but not out of proportion to the increase in other leucocytes.

Some of the causes of eosinophilia are shown in Tables 6.6, 6.7 and 6.8, the commonest being allergic diseases (particularly asthma, hay fever and eczema) and, in some parts of the world, parasitic infection. When the eosinophil count is greatly elevated (greater than $10 \times 10^9/l$) the likely causes are far fewer (Table 6.9). Allergic conditions causing eosinophilia are usually readily apparent from the patient's medical history but, in the case of parasitic infections, the laboratory detection of eosinophilia may be the finding that leads to the correct diagnosis. In hospital patients, eosinophilia can be a useful sign of drug allergy. Following bone marrow transplantation, eosinophilia may be a feature of graft-versus-host disease and has been found to be predictive of extensive scleroderma-like changes [119].

The laboratory detection of eosinophilia in patients with lung disease (Table 6.10) is important in indicating relevant diagnostic possibilities and in excluding conditions, such as Wegener's granulomatosis, which are not associated with eosinophilia. In patients with symptoms suggestive of obstructive airways disease, the presence of eosinophilia usually indicates a reversible or asthmatic component, although it does not necessarily indicate allergic rather than other triggering factors [126]. In uncomplicated asthma the eosinophil count is rarely in excess of $2 \times 10^9/l$. Higher counts, often in association with deteriorating pulmonary function, may indicate either allergic aspergillosis or the Churg–Strauss syndrome. The Churg–Strauss syndrome is a variant of polyarteritis nodosa characterized by pulmonary infiltrates and eosinophilia, neither of which is typical of classical polyarteritis nodosa [127]. Patients are also seen with some features of classical polyarteritis nodosa and some of the Churg–Strauss syndrome: this has been referred to as 'chronic necrotizing vasculitis' or 'the overlap syndrome'. Eosinophilia of $1.5 \times 10^9/l$ or more is an important criterion in making the diagnosis of the Churg–Strauss syndrome or the overlap syndrome.

In some patients with eosinophilia and pulmonary

Table 6.4 Some causes of neutrophil leucocytosis.

Inherited

As a direct effect of the condition
Hereditary neutrophilia [29]
Inherited deficiency of CR3 complement receptors [30]
Deficient surface expression of leucocyte adhesion molecules, CD11b or CD15 (leucocyte adhesion deficiencies types I and II) [31–33]
Defective integrin rearrangement in response to chemokines and chemo-attractants [34]

As an indirect effect of the condition
Familial cold urticaria with leucocytosis [35]
Hyperimmunoglobulin D syndrome [36]
Familial Mediterranean fever
TNF receptor-associated periodic syndrome [36]
Inherited metabolic disorders, e.g. ornithine transcarbamylase deficiency [37]

Acquired
Infections
  Many acute and chronic bacterial infections, including miliary tuberculosis and some rickettsial infections, e.g. Rocky Mountain Spotted fever (*Rickettsia rickettsii* infection), *Rickettsia parkeri* infection and some cases of typhus and murine typhus
  Some viral infections, e.g. chicken pox, herpes simplex infection, rabies, poliomyelitis, St Louis encephalitis virus infection, Eastern equine encephalitis virus infection, hantavirus infection including hantavirus pulmonary syndrome (Sin Nombre virus infection) [38,39], Japanese encephalitis [40]
  Some fungal infections, e.g. actinomycosis, coccidioidomycosis, North American blastomycosis, nocardiosis [41], cepacia syndrome (colonization of the lungs by *Burkholderia cepacia* in cystic fibrosis) [42], cryptococcosis [43]
  Some parasitic infections, e.g. liver fluke, hepatic amoebiasis, filariasis, malaria [44], some *Pneumocystis carinii* infections
Tissue damage, e.g. trauma, surgery (particularly splenectomy), burns, acute hepatic necrosis, acute pancreatitis, haemolytic uraemic syndrome
Tissue infarction, e.g. myocardial infarction, pulmonary embolism causing pulmonary infarction, sickle cell crisis, atheroembolic disease
Acute inflammation and severe chronic inflammation, e.g. gout, pseudogout (calcium pyrophosphate crystal deposition disease), rheumatic fever, rheumatoid arthritis, Still's disease, ulcerative colitis, enteritis necroticans ('pigbel'), polyarteritis nodosa, scleroderma
Acute haemorrhage
Acute hypoxia
Heat stress [45]
Metabolic and endocrine disorders, e.g. diabetic ketoacidosis, acute renal failure, Cushing's syndrome, thyrotoxic crisis
Malignant disease (particularly but not only when there is extensive disease or tumour necrosis), e.g. carcinoma, sarcoma, melanoma, Hodgkin's disease
Myeloproliferative and leukaemic disorders, e.g. chronic granulocytic leukaemia, chronic myelomonocytic leukaemia, neutrophilic leukaemia, acute myeloid leukaemia (not commonly), other rare leukaemias, polycythaemia rubra vera, essential thrombocythaemia, idiopathic myelofibrosis (early in the disease process), systemic mastocytosis
Post-neutropenia rebound, e.g. following dialysis-induced neutropenia, recovery from agranulocytosis and cytotoxic chemotherapy, treatment of megaloblastic anaemia
Administration of cytokines such as G-CSF, GM-CSF, IL1, IL2 [46], IL3 [47], IL6 [48], IL10 [49]
Administration of drugs, e.g. epinephrine (adrenaline), corticosteroids, lithium, clozapine [50], desmopressin [51], initiation of rituximab therapy [52]
Poisoning by various chemicals and drugs, e.g. ethylene glycol [53], iron
Hypersensitivity reactions including those due to drugs
Envenomation, e.g. scorpion bite [54], 'killer bee' attack [55], snake bite [56]
Cigarette smoking
Vigorous exercise
Acute pain, epileptic convulsions, electric shock, paroxysmal tachycardia
Eclampsia and pre-eclampsia (pregnancy-associated hypertension)
Kawasaki's disease
Sweet's syndrome [57]
Neuroleptic malignant syndrome [58]
Blood transfusion in critically ill patients [59]
Infusion of cryoprecipitate [60]
Chronic idiopathic neutrophilia [61]

G-CSF, granulocyte colony-stimulating factor; GM-CSF, granulocyte macrophage colony-stimulating factor; IL, interleukin.

Table 6.5 Significant causes of neutrophilia in the neonate.

Maternal factors
Maternal smoking
Maternal fever
Prolonged intrapartum oxytocin administration
Administration of dexamethasone

Fetal factors
Stressful delivery
Birth asphyxia or other hypoxia
Crying
Physiotherapy
Pain, e.g. lumbar puncture
Hypoglycaemia
Seizures
Infection
Haemolysis
Intraventricular haemorrhage
Meconium aspiration syndrome
Hyaline membrane disease with pneumothorax
Thrombocytopenia with absent radii

Table 6.6 Some of the more common causes of eosinophilia.

Allergic diseases, e.g. atopic eczema, asthma, allergic rhinitis (hay fever), acute urticaria, allergic bronchopulmonary aspergillosis and other bronchoallergic fungal infections
Drug hypersensitivity (particularly to gold, sulphonamides, penicillin, nitrofurantoin) including drug-induced Churg–Strauss syndrome or eosinophilia–myalgia syndrome [62,63]
Parasitic infection (particularly when tissue invasion has occurred)—see Table 6.7
Skin diseases, e.g. pemphigus, bullous pemphigoid, herpes gestationalis, eosinophilic pustular folliculitis [64], familial peeling skin syndrome [65]

infiltration no underlying condition can be found. Many such patients have a condition known as eosinophilic pneumonia; its cause is unknown, but chest radiology shows distinctive peripheral infiltration and there is a predictable response to corticosteroid therapy. The combination of the characteristic X-ray appearance with eosinophilia has been considered sufficient to make the diagnosis [128] whereas in the minority of patients lacking eosinophilia a lung biopsy is needed to establish the diagnosis.

Eosinophilia is a rare manifestation of non-haemopoietic malignancy. It is usually associated with widespread malignant disease but rarely may provide a clue to a localized tumour. Eosinophilia may also occur as a reaction to lymphoid malignancy, particularly Hodgkin's disease, T-lineage non-Hodgkin's lymphoma and T-lineage or B-lineage acute lymphoblastic leukaemia. In Hodgkin's disease, isolated eosinophilia has been associated with a better prognosis [129]. Eosinophilia associated with lymphoid malignancy has been observed up to 1 year in advance of other evidence of the disease, and may recur some weeks before relapse can be detected. In some patients with an initially unexplained eosinophilia, an occult T-cell clone can be demonstrated [130].

In a minority of cases, eosinophilia is neoplastic rather than reactive. Eosinophilia is present in more than 90% of cases of chronic granulocytic leukaemia (CGL) and in a lower percentage of other myeloid leukaemias and myeloproliferative disorders. It occurs occasionally in acute myeloid leukaemia (AML) and rarely in the myelodysplastic syndromes. In some patients with leukaemia, differentiation is predominantly to eosinophils and the term 'eosinophilic leukaemia' is then applicable (see p. 432).

An absolute, or even a relative, eosinophilia can be useful in the intensive care ward setting, in alerting clinicians to the possibility of adrenal insufficiency. The presence of more than 3% eosinophils has been suggested as a criterion for further investigation [117,131,132].

There remains a group of patients with persistent, moderate or marked eosinophilia for which no cause can be found despite detailed investigation. This condition is designated the 'idiopathic hypereosinophilic syndrome (HES)' (see p. 407). This diagnosis should only be made when a patient has been fully investigated to exclude identifiable causes.

Basophil leucocytosis—basophilia

Some of the causes of basophilia are shown in Table 6.11. The detection of basophil leucocytosis is useful in making the distinction between a myeloproliferative disorder and a reactive condition since only in myeloproliferative disorders and certain leukaemias is a marked increase in the basophil count at all

Table 6.7 Parasitic infections known to cause eosinophilia.

Disease	Parasite	Usual degree of eosinophilia*
Protozoan		
Dientamoeba fragilis infection [66]	*Dientamoeba fragilis*	Absent or mild [67]
Isospora belli infection [66]	*Isospora belli*	Absent, in immunosuppressed patients, or mild [67]
Blastocystis hominis infection [68]	*Blastocystis hominis*	
Nematode (round worm) infections		
Hookworm infection	*Ancylostoma duodenale* (Old World hookworm) *Necator americanus* (New World hookworm)	Absent in chronic infection, mild or moderate during stage of larval migration through the lung (Löffler's syndrome) [67]
Cutaneous larva migrans	*Ancylostoma braziliense* (dog and cat hookworm) [69] *Ancylostoma caninum* (dog hookworm) [69] *Gnathostoma doloresi* [70]	Rarely associated with eosinophilia
Epidemic eosinophilic enteritis [71]	*Ancylostoma caninum* (dog hookworm)	
Ascariasis	*Ascaris lumbricoides* (large intestinal roundworm)	Absent during adult stage, moderate during stage of larval migration through the lungs (Löffler's syndrome) [67]
Strongyloidiasis	*Strongyloides stercoralis* (threadworm)[†]	Absent, mild or moderate; moderate during stage of larval migration through the lungs (Löffler's syndrome) [67]; usually present in stronglyloides hyperinfection in immunosuppressed subjects
Trichuriasis [69]	*Trichuris trichiuria* (whipworm)	Absent or mild [67]
Trichinellosis, trichinosis [69]	*Trichinella spiralis* (trichina worm)	Moderate or marked during the acute phase [67]
Capillariasis [69,72]	Hepatic infection by *Capillaria hepatica* (*Calodium hepaticum*) a roundworm of rodents)	
Trichostrongyliasis [69,73]	*Trichostrongylus colubriformis* (a roundworm of sheep)	
Anisakiasis [74]	*Anisakis simplex* (herring worm) or *Pseudoterranova osculatum* (another fish roundworm)	
Enterobiasis	*Enterobius vermicularis* (pinworm or threadworm[†])	Rarely causes eosinophilia but may do so when there is enteritis [75]
Filariasis (lymphatic filariasis including tropical pulmonary eosinophilia resulting from occult lymphatic filariasis)	*Wuchereria bancrofti* (Bancroft's filaria) *Brugia malayi* (Malayan filaria) *Brugia timori* (Timorian filariasis)	Mild, moderate or marked, marked in tropical pulmonary eosinophilia [67]
Loiasis [69]	*Loa loa* (eyeworm)	Moderate or marked [67]
Onchocerciasis (river blindness) [69]	*Onchocerca volvulus* (blinding filaria)	Mild, moderate or marked [67]
Mansonellosis [69]	*Mansonella perstans*	
Dirofilariasis (tropical eosinophilia, eosinophilic pneumonia)	*Dirofilaria immitis* (dog heartworm), *Dirofilaria repens* [76] (roundworm of dogs, cats and foxes)	
Dracunculiasis [69]	Subcutaneous infection by *Dracunculus medinensis* (Guinea worm) *Spirurina* type X infection [77]	

Continued p. 224

Table 6.7 *Continued*

Disease	Parasite	Usual degree of eosinophilia*
Angiostrongyloidiasis, eosinophilic meningitis [78,79]	*Angiostrongylus cantonensis* (rat lungworm)	Mild or moderate [67]
Eosinophilic enteritis [69]	*Angiostrongylus costaricensis* (rat roundworm)	
Gnathostomiasis [69] (including eosinophilic meningitis and visceral larva migrans)	*Gnathostoma spinigerum*	Mild, moderate or marked [67]
Visceral larva migrans (including toxocariasis, gnathostomiasis, capillariasis)	*Toxocara canis* or *Toxocara cati* (toxocariasis) *Baylisascaris procyonis* [80] *Gnathostoma* spp [80], e.g. *Gnathostoma doloresi, Gnathostoma spinigerum* ? *Ascaris suum* [80,81] *Capillaria hepatica*	Moderate or marked
Trematode (fluke) infection Clonorchiasis	*Clonorchis sinensis* (Oriental or Chinese liver fluke)	Absent or mild in chronic infection, may be moderate or marked in acute infection
Fascioliasis (liver fluke infection)	*Fasciola hepatica* (sheep liver fluke) [82] *Fasciola gigantica* [69] *Metorchis conjunctus* (North American liver fluke) [83]	Mild, moderate or marked during stage of larval migration [67]
Fasciolopsiasis (intestinal fluke infection)	*Fasciolopsis buski* (large intestinal fluke) [69,73]	Marked eosinophilia
Heterophyiasis or echinostomiasis [69]	*Heterophyes heterophyes* or *Echinostoma* spp (intestinal flukes)	
Opisthorchiasis [69]	*Opisthorchis viverrini* (a South-East Asian liver fluke) or *Opisthorchis felineus* (a Russian liver fluke)	Usually absent or mild, may be moderate or marked in early infection
Paragonimiasis, distomiasis [69]	*Paragonimus westermani* (Oriental lung fluke) [84]	
Schistosomiasis	*Schistosoma mansoni* *Schistosoma haematobium*	Usually absent or mild but may be moderate to high in acute schistosomiasis (Katayama fever) [67]
Cestode (tape worm) infection Cysticercosis	Larval stage of *Taenia solium* (pig tapeworm)	Absent or mild, may be moderate if encysted larvae die and release antigen [67]
Echinococcosis (hydatid cyst)	Larval stage of *Echinococcus granulosus* (dog tapeworm)	Absent or mild, may increase if cysts rupture or leak [67]
Coenurosis [69]	*Coenurus cerebralis* (larval stage of a dog tapeworm, *Taenia multiceps*, which rarely occurs in man)	
Hymenolepsiasis [69]	*Hymenolepis nana* (dwarf tapeworm)	
Sparganosis [69]	*Spirometra* ssp	Absent or mild
Ectoparasite Scabies [85]	*Sarcoptes scabiei*	
Myiasis [86]	Cutaneous larvae of flies	

* Mild = $0.4 - 1.0 \times 10^9/l$; moderate = $1.0 - 3.0 \times 10^9/l$; marked = greater than $3.0 \times 10^9/l$.

† The term 'threadworm' is used for two different parasites.

Table 6.8 Some of the less common and rare causes of eosinophilia.

Hereditary eosinophilia

Myeloid leukaemias, e.g. chronic granulocytic leukaemia and some other chronic myeloid leukaemias, systemic mastocytosis and less often other chronic myeloproliferative disorders, acute myeloid leukaemia (particularly FAB categories M2 and M4), chronic eosinophilic leukaemia including the *FIP1L1-PDGFRA* syndrome [87]

Lymphoproliferative disorders, e.g. acute lymphoblastic leukaemia (B-lineage and T-lineage), non-Hodgkin's lymphoma (particularly T-cell and including angioimmunoblastic T-cell lymphoma [88], mycosis fungoides and Sézary syndrome, enteropathy-associated T-cell lymphoma [89]), angiolymphoid hyperplasia with eosinophilia, multiple myeloma [90], Hodgkin's disease

Presence of an occult T-cell clone secreting cytokines (such as IL3 and IL5) capable of increasing eosinophil production [91]

Autoimmune lymphoproliferative syndrome [92] (uncommonly)

Non-haematological malignant disease, e.g. carcinoma, sarcoma, glioma, mesothelioma, malignant melanoma, hepatoma, metastatic pituitary tumour [93]

Bowel disease, e.g. eosinophilic enteritis, and milk precipitin disease [94], Crohn's disease, ulcerative colitis

Autoimmune and connective tissue disorders, e.g. Churg–Strauss variant of polyarteritis nodosa, systemic necrotizing vasculitis (variant of polyarteritis nodosa), rheumatoid arthritis, eosinophilic fasciitis (some cases caused by L-tryptophan) [95], eosinophilic cellulitis [96], progressive systemic sclerosis [97], systemic lupus erythematosus, chronic active hepatitis [98], sclerosing cholangitis (uncommonly) [99], eosinophilic cystitis [100], chronic eosinophilic pneumonia, ulcerative colitis [94], Crohn's disease [94], idiopathic pulmonary haemosiderosis [101]

Administration of cytokines (e.g. G-CSF [102], GM-CSF, IL2, IL3, IL5) that are capable of increasing eosinophil production or administration of cytokines (e.g. IL2 or IL15) that stimulate T-cell proliferation [103]

Immune deficiency states and other conditions with recurring infections, e.g. Wiskott–Aldrich syndrome, Job's syndrome (hyperimmunoglobulin E syndrome), severe congenital neutropenia, HIV infection [104] particularly if complicated by HTLV-II infection [91]

Cyclical neutropenia

Cyclical eosinophilia with angio-oedema [105]

Miscellaneous, e.g. recovery from some bacterial and viral infections, premature neonates during the first few weeks of life, cytomegalovirus pneumonia of infancy [94], scarlet fever, tuberculosis, coccidioidomycosis, *Pneumocystis carinii* infection, disseminated histoplasmosis [106], cat-scratch disease [94], infectious lymphocytosis [94], propanolol administration, drug abuse including cocaine inhalation [107,108], toxic oil syndrome [109], L-tryptophan toxicity [110], haemodialysis and occasionally peritoneal dialysis [94], atheroembolic disease [111,112], chronic graft-versus-host disease, thrombocytopenia with absent radii syndrome, chronic pancreatitis, Omenn's syndrome [113], hepatitis B vaccination [114], treatment of lymphoid malignancies with nucleoside analogues (fludarabine or cladribine) [115], Kimura's disease [116], adrenal insufficiency [117], arsenic toxicity [118]

Unknown—idiopathic hypereosinophilic syndrome [66]

FAB, French–American–British; G-CSF, granulocyte colony-stimulating factor; GM-CSF, granulocyte macrophage colony-stimulating factor; HIV, human immunodeficiency virus; HTLV-II, human T-cell lymphotropic virus II; IL, interleukin.

Table 6.9 Some causes of marked eosinophilia.

Parasitic infections, e.g. toxocariasis, trichinosis, tissue migration by larvae of ascaris, ankylostoma or strongyloides

Drug hypersensitivity

Churg–Strauss variant of polyarteritis nodosa

Hodgkin's disease

Acute lymphoblastic leukaemia

Eosinophilic leukaemia

Idiopathic hypereosinophilic syndrome

common. A rising basophil count in CGL is of prognostic significance since it often indicates an accelerated phase of the disease and impending blast transformation. The occurrence of basophilia in association with acute lymphoblastic leukaemia (ALL) may indicate that the patient is Philadelphia-positive and in AML may indicate Philadelphia-positivity or the presence of t(6;9)(p23;q34.3), both karyotypic abnormalities being of adverse prognostic significance. Chronic basophilic leukaemia is often Philadelphia-positive and in this case should be regarded as a variant of CGL.

Table 6.10 Some causes of eosinophilia with pulmonary infiltration.

Parasitic infections, e.g. toxocariasis, filariasis, schistosomiasis, larval migration stage of strongyloidiasis, ascariasis, ankylostomiasis
Asthma
Allergic bronchopulmonary aspergillosis
Hypersensitivity reactions to drugs (such as sulindac, fenoprofen, ibuprofen, diclofenac, tenidap [120], amoxicillin, clarithromycin [121]) and chemicals (such as zinc, chromium or beryllium)
Cocaine pneumonitis
Churg–Strauss variant of polyarteritis nodosa and systemic necrotizing vasculitis
Infections
    Tuberculosis (rarely), brucellosis [122], coccidioidomycosis (rarely), histoplasmosis [122], *Pneumocystis carinii* pneumonia (rarely)
Sarcoidosis [122]
Hodgkin's disease [122]
Carcinoma [123]
Cytokine (GM-CSF) administration [124]
Bronchocentric granulomatosis [125]
Chronic idiopathic eosinophilic pneumonia
Idiopathic hypereosinophilic syndrome

GM-CSF, granulocyte macrophage colony-stimulating factor.

Table 6.11 Some causes of basophil leucocytosis.

Myeloproliferative and leukaemic disorders
Chronic granulocytic leukaemia (almost invariably)
Other chronic myeloid leukaemias
Acute myeloid leukaemia (very rarely)
Polycythaemia rubra vera
Essential thrombocythaemia
Idiopathic myelofibrosis
Systemic mastocytosis
Some cases of Ph-positive ALL
Basophilic leukaemia

Reactive basophilia
Myxoedema (hypothyroidism)
Ulcerative colitis
Juvenile rheumatoid arthriris [94]
Immediate hypersensitivity reactions
Oestrogen administration
Hyperlipidaemia
Administration of IL3 [47]
Idiopathic hypereosinophilic syndrome

ALL, acute lymphoblastic leukaemia; IL3, interleukin 3.

Lymphocytosis

Lymphocytosis is an increase in the absolute lymphocyte count above that expected in a healthy subject of the same age. Since the lymphocyte counts of infants and children are considerably higher than those of adults it is particularly important to use age-adjusted reference ranges. There are no gender or ethnic differences in the lymphocyte count. In an adult, a count greater than $3.5 \times 10^9/l$ may be considered abnormal. Some of the causes of lymphocytosis are shown in Table 6.12.

In assessing a lymphocytosis it is important to consider cytology as well as the lymphocyte count and both should be assessed in relation to the age and clinical features of the patient. Children are more prone than adults to both lymphocytosis and reactive changes in lymphocytes and even apparently healthy children may have some lymphocytes showing atypical features.

Lymphocytosis can occur without there being any cytological abnormality. This is usual when lymphocytosis is due to redistribution of lymphocytes (e.g. following exercise or epinephrine (adrenaline) injection or as an acute response to severe stress), in endocrine abnormalities and in 'acute infectious lymphocytosis' (see Table 6.12). Cytological abnormalities are also uncommon in whooping cough but sometimes there are cleft cells resembling those of follicular lymphoma [160]. In other viral and bacterial infections there are often minor changes in lymphocytes, such as a visible nucleolus or increased cytoplasmic basophilia, which are often referred to as 'reactive changes'. Infectious mononucleosis and to a lesser extent other conditions are associated

Table 6.12 Some causes of lymphocytosis.

Constitutional
Defective integrin rearrangement in response to chemokines and chemo-attractants [34]
DiGeorge's syndrome (polyclonal B lymphocytosis can occur) [133]

Acquired
Viral infections including measles (rubeola), German measles (rubella), mumps, chickenpox (varicella), influenza,
  infectious hepatitis (hepatitis A), infectious mononucleosis (EBV infection), CMV infection, infectious lymphocytosis
  (caused by infection by certain Coxsackie viruses, adenovirus types 1, 2 and 5, and echovirus 7) [134–138], HIV
  infection, infection by the human lymphotropic viruses (HTLV-I and HTLV-II) [139]
Certain bacterial infections including whooping cough (pertussis, infection by *Bordetella pertussis*), brucellosis,
  tuberculosis, syphilis, plague (*Yersinia pestis* infection) [140], Lyme disease [141], human monocytic ehrlichiosis
  (recovery phase) [142], human granulocytic ehrlichiosis (recovery phase) [143]; rickettsial infections including scrub
  typhus (*Rickettsia tsutsugamushi*—now known as *Orientia tsutsugamushi*) and murine typhus (*Rickettsia typhi*) [144,145],
  toxic shock syndrome [146] and bacterial infections in infants and young children
Malaria [44], hyper-reactive malarial splenomegaly [147] and the acute phase of Chagas' disease [148]
Transient stress-related lymphocytosis, e.g. associated with myocardial infarction, cardiac arrest, trauma, obstetric
  complications, sickle cell crisis [149,150]
Epinephrine (adrenaline) administration
Vigorous muscular contraction, e.g. vigorous exercise, status epilepticus
Cigarette smoking causing either T-lymphocytosis (common) or persistent polyclonal B-lymphocytosis (uncommon) [151]
Administration of cytokines, e.g. IL3 [47] or G-CSF [152]
Allergic reactions to drugs
Serum sickness
Splenectomy
Endocrine disorders, e.g. Addison's disease, hypopituitarism, hyperthyroidism [153]
β thalassaemia intermedia [154]
Gaucher's disease [155]
Thymoma [156]
Autoimmune lymphoproliferative syndrome [157]
Associated with rituximab-induced autoimmune neutropenia [158]
Lymphoid leukaemias and other lymphoproliferative disorders, e.g. chronic lymphocytic leukaemia, non-Hodgkin's
  lymphoma, Hodgkin's disease (rarely) [159], adult T-cell leukaemia/lymphoma, hairy cell leukaemia and hairy cell
  variant leukaemia, Waldenström's macroglobulinaemia, heavy chain disease, mycosis fungoides and Sézary syndrome,
  large granular lymphocyte leukaemia

CMV, cytomegalovirus; EBV, Epstein–Barr virus; G-CSF, granulocyte colony-stimulating factor; HIV, human immunodeficiency virus;
HTLV-I and HTLV-II, human T-cell lymphotropic viruses I and II; IL3, interleukin 3.

with much more striking reactive changes, the abnormal cells being referred to as 'atypical lymphocytes' or 'atypical mononuclear cells' (see p. 400). Post-splenectomy lymphocytosis is usually mild with only minor atypical features. However, it is important to realize that post-splenectomy counts can be in excess of $10 \times 10^9/l$ and misdiagnosis as a lymphoproliferative disorder has occurred. Large granular lymphocytes are often prominent in post-splenectomy lymphocytosis. Many heavy cigarette smokers have a mild lymphocytosis without cytological abnormalities. A minority of smokers, mainly women, have a persistent polyclonal B-cell lymphocytosis (see p. 405). An increase of large granular

lymphocytes can occur as a reactive change, e.g. in human immunodeficiency virus (HIV) infection [161] and chronic hepatitis B or Epstein–Barr virus (EBV) infection, sometimes without an increase in the total lymphocyte count.

In lymphoproliferative disorders, lymphocytosis is usually caused by the presence of considerable numbers of lymphoma cells in the peripheral blood. However, occasionally, e.g. in Hodgkin's disease, there is a lymphoma-associated polyclonal reactive lymphocytosis [159]. Neoplastic lymphocytes almost always show cytological abnormalities. The exception is large granular lymphocyte leukaemia in which the neoplastic cells are usually cytologically indistinguishable from normal cells. It is often said that in chronic lymphocytic leukaemia (CLL) there is an increase in apparently normal, mature lymphocytes but in fact subtle abnormalities are present. The specific cytological features of this and other lymphoproliferative disorders are described in Chapter 9. In general, lymphoproliferative disorders have distinctive cytological features and can thus be readily distinguished from reactive changes in lymphocytes. An exception may occur in some low-grade non-Hodgkin's lymphomas, particularly mantle cell lymphoma, some cases of which have neoplastic cells that can be confused with reactive lymphocytes. For this reason the term 'reactive changes' should be used with circumspection.

Monocytosis

Monocytosis is an increase of the monocyte count above that expected in a healthy subject of the same age. The absolute monocyte count is higher in neonates than at other stages of life. A rise occurs in pregnancy in parallel with the rise in the neutrophil count. Some of the common causes of monocytosis are shown in Table 6.13.

In examining a film of a patient with an unexplained monocytosis, evidence of chronic infection or myelodysplasia should be sought. The presence of promonocytes and blasts suggest AML with monocytic differentiation.

Plasmacytosis

Plasmacytosis is the appearance in the blood of appreciable numbers of plasma cells. These may be reactive or neoplastic. Some of the causes of plasmacytosis are shown in Table 6.14.

In reactive plasmacytosis, the number of circulating plasma cells is usually low but occasionally quite considerable numbers are present. A case of serum sickness due to tetanus antitoxin, for example, was found to have $3.2 \times 10^9/l$ plasma cells [172]. In reactive plasmacytosis the plasma cells are usually mature but occasionally plasmablasts are present. Plasma cells may contain vacuoles or, occasionally, crystals. Atypical lymphocytes and plasmacytoid lymphocytes may also be present and cells of other lineages may show reactive changes.

Table 6.13 Some causes of monocytosis [162].

Chronic infection including miliary tuberculosis [163] and congenital syphilis [164]
Rocky Mountain spotted fever [94]
Malaria [44] and babesiosis [165]
Chronic inflammatory conditions including Crohn's disease, ulcerative colitis, rheumatoid arthritis and systemic lupus erythematosus
Carcinoma [166]
Administration of cytokines including G-CSF, GM-CSF, M-CSF, IL3, IL10 and FLT ligand [47,167–169]
Administration of desmopressin [51]
Myeloproliferative and leukaemic conditions including CMML, atypical CML, JMML, CGL*, MDS, systemic mastocytosis, AML
Neutropenia and immune deficiency syndromes of various causes, e.g. cyclical neutropenia, severe congenital neutropenia, chronic idiopathic neutropenia, autoimmune neutropenia
Long-term haemodialysis [170]
Lymphomatoid granulomatosis [171]

AML, acute myeloid leukaemia; CGL, chronic granulocytic leukaemia; CML, chronic myeloid leukaemia; CMML, chronic myelomonocytic leukaemia; G-CSF, granulocyte colony-stimulating factor; GM-CSF, granulocyte macrophage colony-stimulating factor; IL, interleukin; JMML, juvenile myelomonocytic leukaemia; M-CSF, macrophage colony-stimulating factor; MDS, myelodysplastic syndrome.
* Absolute but not relative monocytosis.

Neoplastic plasma cells usually show more cytological abnormality than those produced in reactive states. The haematological features of plasma cell leukaemia and multiple myeloma and their differential diagnosis are discussed on p. 448.

Table 6.14 Some causes of peripheral blood plasmacytosis.

Reactive
Bacterial and viral infections and immunizations
Hypersensitivity reactions to drugs
Streptokinase administration
Serum sickness
Systemic lupus erythematosus
Angioimmunoblastic lymphadenopathy

Neoplastic
Multiple myeloma and plasma cell leukaemia
Gamma heavy chain disease
Waldenström's macroglobulinaemia (rarely)

Thrombocytosis

Thrombocytosis is an increase of the platelet count above that expected in a healthy subject of the same age and sex. Use of the term 'thrombocythaemia' is usually restricted to a thrombocytosis occurring as the consequence of a myeloproliferative disorder; the term 'essential thrombocytosis' is synonymous but is little used. Thrombocytosis is usually consequent on increased marrow production of platelets, either autonomous or reactive. Following splenectomy and in hyposplenism, thrombocytosis is due to redistribution of platelets. Some of the causes of thrombocytosis are shown in Table 6.15 and the

Table 6.15 Some causes of thrombocytosis.

Primary
Inherited
Familial thrombocytosis (sometimes caused by a mutation in the thrombopoietin gene with autosomal dominant inheritance [173], sometimes unlinked to thrombopoietin and showing either dominant [174] or recessive, possibly X-linked recessive, inheritance [175], sometimes resulting from a mutation in the *MPL* gene [176])

Acquired
Essential thrombocythaemia (all cases)
Chronic granulocytic leukaemia (most cases)
Idiopathic myelofibrosis (early in the disease course)
Polycythaemia rubra vera (many cases)
Myelodysplastic syndromes (a minority of cases, e.g. in the 5q- syndrome and in some cases of refractory anaemia with ring sideroblasts)
Myelodysplastic-myeloproliferative disorders (some cases), e.g. thrombocytosis with sideroblastic erythropoiesis
Acute myeloid leukaemia (a minority of cases, particularly acute megakaryoblastic leukaemia including transient abnormal myelopoiesis in neonates with Down's syndrome, some cases with inv(3)(q21q26) and acute hypergranular promyelocytic leukaemia during all-*trans* retinoic acid therapy [177])

Secondary
Infection (including some patients with miliary tuberculosis) [178]
Inflammation
Haemorrhage
Surgery and trauma
Malignant disease
Kawasaki's disease [179]
Iron deficiency
Rebound after cytotoxic chemotherapy
Rebound after alcohol withdrawal
Following treatment of severe megaloblastic anaemia
Severe haemolytic anaemia, particularly after unsuccessful splenectomy
Multicentric angiofollicular hyperplasia [180], Castleman's disease [181] and POEMS [181]
Chronic eosinophilic pneumonia [182]
Epinephrine (adrenaline) administration
Vinca alkaloid (e.g. vincristine) administration
Administration of recombinant thrombopoietin or PEG-rHuMGDF [183]
Administration of IL3 [47], IL6 [184], IL11 [185]
Administration of erythropoietin [186] or vitamin E to premature infants [187]
Infantile cortical hyperostosis [188]
In infants of drug-abusing mothers [189]
Erdheim–Chester disease [190]
Type Ib glycogen storage disease [191]
Severe congenital neutropenia (Kostmann's syndrome) [192]
Enzyme replacement in Gaucher's disease [193]

Redistributional
Splenectomy and hyposplenism

Unknown mechanism
Premature infants at 4–6 weeks of age [194]
Tidal platelet dysgenesis

IL, interleukin; PEG-rHuMGDF, pegylated recombinant human megakaryocyte growth and development factor; POEMS, **P**olyendocrinopathy, **O**rganomegaly, **E**ndocrinopathy, **M**-protein, **S**kin changes syndrome.

Table 6.16 Some causes of markedly elevated platelet counts.

Platelet count	> 1000 × 10⁹/l [195]	> 900 × 10⁹/l [196]	> 1000 × 10⁹/l [197]	> 500 × 10⁹/l [198]
Patients (n)	102	526	280	777
Cause	Cases attributable (%)			
Malignant disease	45	27	11.5	5.9
Splenectomy or hyposplenism	40	20	16	1.9
Myeloproliferative disorder	28	26	14	3.4
Infection or inflammation	30	19	26	35
Connective tissue disorder	2	9		
Iron deficiency	4			
Trauma or other tissue damage			11.5	17.9
Blood loss			5	
Rebound			2.5	19.4

causes of a marked increase in the platelet count in Table 6.16. It should be noted that as more and more routine platelet counts are performed on very sick patients the percentage of even very high platelet counts that are reactive is increasing and myeloproliferative disorders are now responsible for only 10–15% of counts greater than 1000×10^9/l.

Blood film and count

Increased platelet size, platelet anisocytosis, the presence of poorly granulated platelets, circulating megakaryocyte nuclei or micromegakaryocytes and an increased basophil count are all suggestive of a primary bone marrow disease rather than a reactive thrombocytosis. Large platelets are also seen in hyposplenism whereas in reactive thrombocytosis platelets are generally small and normally granulated. The blood film may also show abnormalities of other lineages, which indicate the correct diagnosis. The features of hyposplenism should be specifically sought.

The degree of elevation of the platelet count is of some use in the differential diagnosis. Counts of greater than 1500×10^9/l are usually indicative of a myeloproliferative disorder but reactive thrombocytosis with counts as high as 2000×10^9/l [197] and even 6000×10^9/l [199] have been reported. In primary thrombocytosis the automated blood count may show an increased mean platelet volume (MPV) and platelet distribution width (PDW), indicative of increased platelet size and platelet anisocytosis,

respectively. In secondary or reactive thrombocytosis the MPV and PDW are more often normal.

Further tests

The cause of reactive thrombocytosis is usually readily apparent from the clinical history. When the cause is not apparent a bone marrow aspirate, trephine biopsy and cytogenetic analysis are indicated. Indirect evidence favouring a reactive thrombocytosis includes increased erythrocyte sedimentation rate (ESR) and concentration of C-reactive protein, fibrinogen, factor VIII and von Willebrand's factor. It can sometimes be difficult to distinguish iron deficiency with a marked reactive thrombocytosis from PRV with complicating iron deficiency and in these circumstances a judicious trial of iron therapy may be needed.

Anaemia

Anaemia is a reduction in the haemoglobin concentration in the peripheral blood below that expected for a healthy person of the same age, gender and physiological status (pregnant or not). It can be due to: (i) defective production of red cells; (ii) reduced red cell survival in the circulation due to haemolysis or blood loss; (iii) increased pooling of essentially normal red cells in a large spleen; or (iv) sequestration of abnormal red cells such as those in sickle cell anaemia or sickle cell/haemoglobin C disease, in the spleen or, less often, in the liver. Anaemia may be an isolated abnormality or there may be pancytopenia (see p. 243).

Blood film and count

The blood film and count commonly give a clue to the cause of the anaemia by showing microcytosis, macrocytosis or a specific type of poikilocyte. Red cell disorders associated with these features are discussed in Chapter 8. The presence of polychromasia suggests an adequate bone marrow response to anaemia and indicates that anaemia may have been caused by haemolysis or haemorrhage. The differential diagnosis of a normocytic, normochromic anaemia and the peripheral blood features that may be helpful in suggesting the diagnosis are summarized in Table 6.17. Various other rare and curious causes of anaemia exist, e.g. that due to therapy with leeches, which sometimes necessitates blood transfusion [210]. Causes of pure red cell aplasia are detailed in Table 6.18. In some anaemic patients the blood film is leucoerythroblastic, i.e. granulocyte precursors and nucleated red blood cells (NRBC) are present. In these cases the differential diagnosis is more limited, as summarized in Table 6.19. A leucoerythroblastic blood film is normal in the neonatal period and pregnant women occasionally have NRBC in addition to the more usual granulocyte precursors. Otherwise a leucoerythroblastic blood film, other than during an acute illness, is likely to indicate serious underlying disease.

In the perinatal period, the conditions responsible for anaemia differ somewhat from those operating later in life (Table 6.20). Other rare causes include anaemia associated with cystic hygroma or chorioangioma and anaemia resulting from fetal haematuria caused by congenital mesoblastic nephroma [228]. Occasional neonates are anaemic as a result of haemoglobin H disease, Blackfan–Diamond syndrome, Pearson's syndrome, cartilage-hair hypoplasia, congenital sideroblastic anaemia or osteopetrosis [228]. In the fetus and neonate, haemolytic anaemia may be consequent on transplacental passage of antibodies (alloantibodies or, less often, maternal autoantibodies) or on intrauterine infections by micro-organisms that in later life do not usually cause anaemia (e.g. cytomegalovirus infection, toxoplasmosis, syphilis and rubella) [237]. The consequences of anaemia also differ from those at other periods of life. Severe anaemia in the fetus can lead to hydrops fetalis, a condition characterized by gross oedema of the fetus and placenta, often leading to intrauterine death. In the neonate, because of the immaturity of the liver, severe haemolysis can lead to marked hyperbilirubinaemia with consequent brain damage. The identification of anaemia, particularly haemolytic anaemia, in the fetus and neonate is therefore of considerable importance.

Further tests

When the cause of anaemia is not apparent from the clinical history or the blood film and count other tests are needed. Those most likely to be useful are: (i) a reticulocyte count; (ii) assay of serum ferritin or of serum iron and transferrin concentrations; (iii) serum B_{12} and red cell folate assays; and (iv) tests of renal, thyroid and hepatic function. If these investigations do not reveal the cause of the anaemia a bone marrow aspirate is usually indicated. When there is an unexplained leucoerythroblastic anaemia, other than during an acute illness, a bone marrow aspirate and trephine biopsy is indicated without delay.

In the neonate, serological tests on mother and baby, a Kleihauer test to detect fetomaternal haemorrhage, haematological assessment of both parents and a glucose-6-phosphate dehydrogenase (G6PD) assay may be useful.

Reticulocytopenia

Reticulocytopenia means that there is a reduction in the absolute reticulocyte count below that expected in a healthy subject of the same age. Usually the reticulocyte percentage is also reduced. In assessing the reticulocyte count it is important not only to consider whether the value falls within the reference range but also whether it is appropriate to the degree of anaemia and to any shortening of red cell lifespan. Thus a patient with a haemolytic anaemia should have a reticulocyte count above the normal range; lack of reticulocytosis in such a patient may indicate pure red cell aplasia or folic acid deficiency.

Causes of reticulocytopenia are shown in Table 6.21.

Table 6.17 Some causes of normocytic normochromic anaemia (other than conditions which usually cause pancytopenia, these being listed in Table 6.30).

Causative conditions	Peripheral blood features that may be useful in diagnosis
Early iron deficiency*	A few hypochromic cells may be present, RDW increased
Anaemia of chronic disease*	Increased rouleaux and ESR, occasionally increased platelet count or WBC, RDW often normal
Lead poisoning*[†]	Basophilic stippling, some cases have polychromasia
Double deficiency of iron and vitamin B_{12} or folic acid*	Hypersegmented neutrophils, increased RDW
Blood loss	If blood loss is severe and acute, anaemia is leucoerythroblastic; polychromasia, reticulocytosis and increased RDW develop within a few days
Non-spherocytic haemolytic anaemia*	Occasional poikilocytes, polychromasia, increased reticulocyte count, RDW increased (see p. 338)
Some congenital dyserythropoietic anaemias[†]	Striking anisocytosis and poikilocytosis (see p. 358)
Paroxysmal nocturnal haemoglobinuria	Sometimes other cytopenias—particularly a low WBC, low neutrophil alkaline phosphatase score, polychromasia in some cases
Myelodysplastic syndromes[†]	Other features of myelodysplastic syndromes (see p. 42)
Renal failure	Sometimes keratocytes or schistocytes
Liver failure[†]	Target cells, stomatocytes, acanthocytes, other cytopenias
Hypothyroidism[†]	Sometimes acanthocytes
Addison's disease and hypopituitarism	Lymphocytosis, eosinophilia, neutropenia, monocytopenia
Androgen ablation therapy, e.g. for carcinoma of the prostate	Nil
Hyperparathyroidism	Nil
Anorexia nervosa	Other cytopenia, acanthocytes, poikilocytosis, basophilic stippling
Pure red cell aplasia[†]	Normal RDW, reticulocyte count very low or reticulocytes absent
Pearson's syndrome (mitochondrial cytopathy)[†] [200]	Nil
Administration of IL2, IL6 [201], IL11 [202] or IL12 [203]	Other features of cytokine administration
Bortezomib therapy	
Autonomic failure [204] including dopamine-β-hydroxylase deficiency [205]	Nil
Vitamin D intoxication [206]	Nil
Hypervitaminosis A [207]	Platelet count also reduced
Arsenic poisoning	There may be basophilic stippling, neutropenia and thrombocytopenia [208]
Graft-versus-host disease [209]	Clinical features of graft-versus-host disease
Alemtuzumab (anti-CD52) therapy	Nil

ESR, erythrocyte sedimentation rate; RDW, red cell distribution width; WBC, white blood cell count; IL, interleukin.
* Can also be microcytic.
[†] Can also be macrocytic.

Table 6.18 Some causes of pure red cell aplasia.

Transient
Parvovirus B19-induced
Drug-induced [211], e.g. antibiotics, antithyroid drugs, anticonvulsants, azathioprine, tacrolimus [212], allopurinol [213], phenytoin, isoniazid, ribavirin [214]
Transient erythroblastopenia of childhood

Chronic
Constitutional
Diamond–Blackfan syndrome
Hereditary transcobalamin II deficiency [215]

Acquired
Associated with chronic lymphocytic leukaemia, large granular lymphocyte leukaemia (T or NK cell), Hodgkin's disease, thymoma or autoimmune disease such as systemic lupus erythematosus, rheumatoid arthritis or autoimmune polyglandular syndrome
Tumour-associated [216]
Pregnancy-associated [217]
Chronic parvovirus B19 infection (in individuals with impaired immunity)
ABO-incompatible stem cell transplantation [218], particularly but not only with non-myelo-ablative conditioning [219]
Development of antibodies to erythropoietin after recombinant erythropoietin therapy [220]
Myelodysplastic syndrome and other myeloid neoplasm (e.g. refractory anaemia)

Table 6.19 Some causes of leucoerythroblastic anaemia.

Bone marrow infiltration in carcinoma, lymphoma (Hodgkin's disease, non-Hodgkin's lymphoma), chronic lymphocytic leukaemia, multiple myeloma, acute lymphoblastic leukaemia or other malignant disease
Myeloproliferative disorders, particularly idiopathic myelofibrosis and chronic granulocytic leukaemia
Acute myeloid leukaemia and the myelodysplastic syndromes
Bone marrow granulomas, e.g. in miliary tuberculosis
Storage diseases (e.g. Gaucher's disease)
Acute haemolysis (including erythroblastosis fetalis)
Shock, e.g. due to severe haemorrhage
Severe infection
Rebound following bone marrow failure or suppression
Crises of sickle cell anaemia
Bone marrow infarction
Thalassaemia major
Severe megaloblastic anaemia
Systemic lupus erythematosus [221]
Severe nutritional rickets [222]
Marble bone disease (osteopetrosis)

Leucopenia

Leucopenia is a reduction of the total white cell count below that expected in a healthy subject of the same age, gender, physiological status and ethnic origin. It can result from a decrease in the neutrophil count, the lymphocyte count or both and cannot be interpreted without knowledge of the differential count. There are, however, certain infections that are associated with leucopenia rather than leucocytosis and the presence of leucopenia in a febrile patient can therefore be of some diagnostic use. They include dengue fever, rickettsial infections, typhoid fever and leishmaniasis.

Neutropenia

Neutropenia is a reduction of the absolute neutrophil count below that expected in a subject of the same age, gender, physiological status and ethnic origin. It is particularly important to use an appropriate reference range in individuals with African ancestry, to avoid a misdiagnosis of neutropenia, since Africans and, to a lesser extent, Afro-Americans and Afro-Caribbeans, have neutrophil counts much lower than those of Caucasians. Neutropenia may be an isolated phenomenon or part of a pancytopenia. Mechanisms of neutropenia include: (i) inadequate production by the bone marrow because of reduced stem cell numbers, bone marrow replacement or ineffective granulopoiesis; (ii) destruction by bone marrow macrophages and other reticuloendothelial cells in haemophagocytic syndromes; (iii) defective release from the bone marrow as in myelokathexis; (iv) redistribution within the vasculature as occurs early during haemodialysis; (v) pooling in the spleen; (vi) shortened intravascular lifespan as in immune neutropenias; and (vii) rapid egress to the tissues when the bone marrow output cannot increase adequately, as in neonates with sepsis.

An unexpected apparent neutropenia on an automated counter should always be confirmed on a blood film since it may be factitious (see Chapter 4). The detection of unexpected neutropenia by the laboratory can be of vital importance, since

Table 6.20 Some causes of anaemia of importance in the fetus and neonate.

Fetus and neonate

Severe inherited haemolytic anaemias (G6PD deficiency (sometimes following maternal ingestion of oxidants), triose phosphate isomerase deficiency, glucose phosphate isomerase deficiency, pyruvate kinase deficiency [223], hexokinase deficiency [224], hereditary xerocytosis [225], homozygosity for hereditary spherocytosis caused by band 3 Coimbra [226], homozygosity for haemoglobin Taybe [227])

Haemoglobin F-Poole [228]

Haemoglobin Bart's hydrops fetalis

εγδβ thalassaemia [229]

Congenital dyserythropoietic anaemia [230]

Diamond–Blackfan syndrome [231]

Congenital hypotransferrinaemia [232]

Haemolysis due to transplacental passage of alloantibodies, e.g. Rh or Kell antibodies, rarely ABO [233]

Pure red cell aplasia caused by transplacental passage of maternal anti-Kell or anti-M antibodies [234]

Parvovirus B19 infection

Cytomegalovirus infection

Malaria

Congenital leukaemia [235]

Transient abnormal myelopoiesis of Down's syndrome

Feto-maternal haemorrhage (including following external cephalic version, amniocentesis, antepartum haemorrhage and abdominal trauma)

Twin-to-twin haemorrhage

Haemorrhage resulting from amniocentesis or cordocentesis

Neonate

Haemorrhage from the cord or the placenta or internal haemorrhage (e.g. cephalohaematoma, intracranial haemorrhage, ruptured liver or spleen), during or as a consequence of birth

Twin–twin transfusion during birth

Haemolytic disease of the newborn (e.g. ABO haemolytic disease of the newborn)

Transient severe haemolysis in hereditary elliptocytosis

Haemolysis associated with disseminated intravascular coagulation caused by sepsis

Congenital infections, e.g. rubella, adenovirus infection [228]

Prematurity

Vitamin E deficiency [236]

Removal of inappropriately large amounts of blood for laboratory testing

Table 6.21 Some causes of reticulocytopenia.

Deficiency of vitamin B_{12}, iron or folic acid
Anaemia of chronic disease
Bone marrow suppression by cytotoxic chemotherapy or other bone marrow-damaging drugs
Aplastic anaemia
Pure red cell aplasia
Acute leukaemia
Myelodysplastic syndromes (most cases)

drug-induced agranulocytosis can be rapidly fatal. In many clinical circumstances the likely cause of neutropenia will be readily apparent from the patient's medical history, including the history of drug intake. When the history and examination of the blood film do not reveal the cause, bone marrow investigation is usually necessary. The causes of neutropenia are summarized in Tables 6.22 and 6.23.

Eosinopenia

Eosinopenia is a reduction of the eosinophil count below that expected in a healthy subject of the same age. Eosinopenia is rarely noted on a routine blood film and cannot be detected on a routine 100-cell differential cell count since the eosinophil is a relatively infrequent cell and the reference limits include zero. Since the introduction of automated differential counts, eosinopenia is far more often noted. However, it is a common non-specific abnormality so its detection is not of much clinical significance.

Table 6.22 Some inherited disorders causing neutropenia.

Reticular agenesis or dysgenesis (severe granulocytopenia, monocytopenia and lymphocytopenia with hypoplasia of thymus and lymph nodes and impaired cellular and humoral immunity)

Neutropenia with pancreatic exocrine deficiency and dyschondroplasia—neutropenia may be intermittent (Shwachman or Shwachman–Diamond syndrome, resulting from mutations in the *SBDS* gene)

Neutropenia with pancreatic exocrine deficiency and sideroblastic erythropoiesis (Pearson's syndrome, an inherited mitochondrial disorder) [200]

Familial benign neutropenia

Familial severe neutropenia (previously known as infantile genetic agranulocytosis (Kostmann's syndrome) (autosomal recessive, autosomal dominant or X-linked, some cases due to mutations in *ELA2* (elastase) gene; less often results from mutation in the gene encoding the G-CSF [238] receptor or activating mutations of the *WASp* gene [239,240])

Familial cyclical neutropenia[†] (autosomal dominant) [241]; may result from mutation of the *ELA2* gene

Congenital dysgranulopoietic neutropenia [242]

Myelokathexis, also known as the WHIM (warts, hypogammaglobulinaemia, infections and myelokathexis) syndrome [243]

Lazy leucocyte syndrome (may actually represent childhood autoimmune neutropenia rather than being inherited) [94]

Chédiak–Higashi syndrome

Dyskeratosis congenita

Associated with X-linked agammaglobulinaemia (occurring in a third of cases)

Associated with hyper-immunoglobulin M syndrome [244]

Associated with cartilage-hair hypoplasia

Cohen's syndrome [245]

Bloom's syndrome [246]

Diamond–Blackfan syndrome, during the course of the disease [247]

Griscelli's syndrome [248]

Barth syndrome (cardiomyopathy, growth retardation and congenital neutropenia) [249]

Hermansky–Pudlak syndrome due to mutation of *ADTB3A* gene (Hermansky–Pudlak syndrome 2) [250]

Glutathione synthase deficiency [94]

Associated with certain inborn errors of metabolism (idiopathic hyperglycinaemia, isovaleric acidaemia, methylmalonic acidaemia, type Ib glycogen storage disease [251], carnitine deficiency [252], methylglutaconic aciduria [253], propionic acidaemia [254], hyperzincaemia with hypercalprotectinaemia [255], tyrosinaemia [94])

Table 6.23 Some acquired disorders causing neutropenia.

Infections

Viral infections, e.g. measles, mumps, rubella including intrauterine rubella infection [256], MMR (measles, mumps and rubella) vaccination, influenza, avian influenza A [257], infectious hepatitis, infectious mononucleosis, cytomegalovirus infection including intrauterine cytomegalovirus infection [256], human herpesvirus 6 infection [258,259], parvovirus B19 infection (occasionally) [260], yellow fever, dengue fever, Colorado tick fever, Venezuelan haemorrhagic fever [261], Crimean–Congo haemorrhagic fever [262], lymphocytic choriomeningitis virus infection [263], corona virus-associated severe acute respiratory distress syndrome (SARS) (occasionally) [264], advanced HIV infection (AIDS)

Bacterial infections, e.g. typhoid, paratyphoid, brucellosis, tularaemia [265], some cases of miliary tuberculosis [162], some Gram-negative infections (early in the disease process), overwhelming bacterial infection—particularly but not only Gram-negative infection, bacterial infection in neonates, rickettsial infections including scrub typhus [266], rickettsial pox [267], *Rickettsia africae* infection [268] and some cases of typhus, granulocytic and monocytic ehrlichiosis [269]

Protozoal infection, e.g. malaria, visceral leishmaniasis (kala azar), trypanosomiasis

Fungal infections, e.g. histoplasmosis [270]

Drugs, e.g. alkylating agents and other anticancer and related drugs (including azathioprine and zidovudine and including, rarely, neutropenia in infancy following perinatal exposure to zidovudine [271]; including methotrexate used for rheumatological and skin conditions), idiosyncratic reaction to drugs (most often with antithyroid drugs, sulphonamides, chlorpromazine, gold), interferon, alemtuzumab (anti-CD52), rituximab (probably autoimmune) [272], bortezomib [273], sirolimus, imatinib [274]

Continued p. 236

Table 6.23 *Continued*

Mustard gas exposure [275]
Administration of IL12 [203]
Irradiation
Bone marrow replacement, e.g. in ALL, multiple myeloma or carcinoma
Idiopathic and secondary myelofibrosis
Ineffective granulopoiesis, e.g. in most cases of AML and most MDS
Megaloblastic anaemia
Aplastic anaemia
Paroxysmal nocturnal haemoglobinuria
Acute anaphylaxis
Hypersplenism
Haemophagocytic syndromes
Immune neutropenia
    Alloimmune neutropenia, following blood transfusion [276] or in neonates, as a result of transplacental passage of
        maternal alloantibody
    Immune neutropenia in neonates, as a result of transplacental passage of maternal autoantibody [277]
    Autoimmune neutropenia [278] including isolated autoimmune neutropenia and autoimmune neutropenia associated
        with autoimmune haemolytic anaemia, autoimmune thrombocytopenia, autoimmune lymphoproliferative
        syndrome, systemic lupus erythematosus, rheumatoid arthritis (Felty's syndrome), scleroderma, hyperthyroidism,
        chronic active hepatitis, polyarteritis nodosa, primary biliary cirrhosis, thymoma, Hodgkin's disease, non-Hodgkin's
        lymphoma, angioimmunoblastic lymphadenopathy, large granular lymphocyte leukaemia (both T cell and NK cell)
        and increased activated T lymphocytes [279], viral infection (e.g. chronic parvovirus infection [280], HIV infection,
        infectious mononucleosis), Castleman's disease, Sjögren's syndrome, mannosidosis and hypogammaglobulinaemia
    Autoimmune panleucopenia [281]
    Autoimmune pure white cell aplasia [282]
    Graft-versus-host disease [209]
    Administration of anti-Rh D for the treatment of autoimmune thrombocytopenic purpura [283]
Severe combined immunodeficiency, possibly due to graft-versus-host disease induced by maternal T lymphocytes [284]
Cyclical neutropenia, including adult onset cyclical neutropenia associated with large granular lymphocyte leukaemia
    (see above)
Haemodialysis and filtration leukapheresis (early during the procedures)
Tranfusion-associated lung injury ('TRALI') [285]
Peripheral blood stem cell apheresis [286]
Endocrine disorders, e.g. hypopituitarism, Addison's disease, hyperthyroidism [153]
Alcoholism [287]
Kawasaki's disease
Kikuchi's disease (necrotizing lymphadenitis) [288]
Copper deficiency [289,290]
Arsenic poisoning [208]
Hypercarotenaemia [291]
Placental insufficiency—babies with intrauterine growth retardation and babies born to hypertensive and diabetic
    mothers [292,293]
Babies with asphyxia neonatorum [293]
Rh haemolytic disease of the newborn [292]
Extracorporeal membrane oxygenation in neonates [294]
Administration of erythropoietin to premature babies [186]
Associated with transient erythroblastopenia of childhood [295]
Intravenous immunoglobulin infusion in infants [292]
Therapy with anti-CD52 monoclonal antibodies [296]

AIDS, acquired immune deficiency syndrome; ALL, acute lymphoblastic leukaemia; AML, acute myeloid leukaemia; HIV, human immunodeficiency virus; IL, interleukin; MDS, myelodysplastic syndrome.

Table 6.24 Some causes of eosinopenia.

Acute stress including trauma, surgery, burns,
  epileptiform convulsions, acute infections, acute
  inflammation, myocardial infarction, anoxia and
  exposure to cold
Cushing's syndrome
Administration of various drugs including corticosteroids
  and ACTH, epinephrine (adrenaline) and other β
  agonists, histamine and aminophylline
Haemodialysis (during procedure)

ACTH, adrenocorticotropic hormone.

Table 6.25 Some causes of basopenia.

Acute stress including infection and haemorrhage
Cushing's syndrome and administration of ACTH
Administration of prednisone in healthy subjects [301]
Anaphylaxis, acute urticaria and other acute allergic
  reactions
Chronic urticaria (increased by prednisolone therapy)
  [301]
Hyperthyroidism
Progesterone administration

ACTH, adrenocorticotropic hormone.

A physiological fall in the eosinophil count occurs during pregnancy and there is a further fall during labour. Common causes of a low eosinophil count are shown in Table 6.24. The eosinophil count has been reported to be reduced in Down's syndrome [297]. Rare causes that have been reported include thymoma, pure eosinophil aplasia [298], and apparent autoimmune destruction of eosinophils and basophils [299]. The eosinophil count is reduced in human T-cell lymphotropic virus I (HTLV-I) carriers [300].

Basopenia

Basopenia is a reduction in the basophil count below that which would be expected in a healthy subject. Some of the causes are shown in Table 6.25. Basophils are so infrequent in normal blood that their reduction is not likely to be noticed on inspection of the film or on a routine 100-cell or even 500-cell differential count. In theory, basopenia can be detected on automated differential counters since they have reference ranges for basophils that do not include zero. However, in practice, automated basophil counts are not very accurate and the observation of basopenia has not yet been found to be of any great importance in diagnosis.

Monocytopenia

Monocytopenia is the reduction of the monocyte count below that expected in a healthy subject of the same age. It may accompany other cytopenias, e.g. in reticular agenesis and aplastic anaemia. The monocyte counts falls after administration of corticosteroids and in acute infections associated with endotoxaemia [94]. Monocyte numbers are conspicuously reduced in hairy cell leukaemia. The monocyte count falls, together with the neutrophil count, in transfusion-associated acute lung injury ('TRALI') [285].

Lymphocytopenia (lymphopenia)

Lymphopenia or, more correctly, lymphocytopenia, is a reduction of the lymphocyte count below what would be expected in a healthy subject of the same age. It is important in assessing babies with suspected immunodeficiency to use an appropriate reference range; counts below $2.8 \times 10^9/l$ in a baby with infection raise the possibility of severe combined immunodeficiency [302].

Lymphocytopenia is extremely common as part of the acute response to stress although it is often overshadowed by the coexisting changes in neutrophils. It is more likely to be noticed when an automated differential count is performed and counts are expressed in absolute numbers. With the increasing importance of the diagnosis of the acquired immune deficiency syndrome (AIDS), characterized by increasingly severe lymphopenia with disease progression, it is important to realize how common this abnormality is in acutely ill patients, regardless of the nature of the underlying illness. In one study of patients with bacteraemia, lymphopenia was observed more consistently than neutrophilia [303]. In Hodgkin's disease, a lymphocyte count of less than $0.6 \times 10^9/l$ is of prognostic significance [304]. Causes of lymphocytopenia are summarized in Table 6.26.

Table 6.26 Some causes of lymphocytopenia.

Inherited

Certain rare congenital immune deficiency syndromes including reticular dysgenesis, severe combined immunodeficiency, Swiss type agammaglobulinaemia, some case of thymic hypoplasia (diGeorge's syndrome) and ataxia telangiectasia

Congenital dyserythropoietic anaemia, type I [305]

Acquired

Acute stress including trauma, surgery, burns, acute infection, fulminant hepatic failure

Acute and chronic renal failure and (including patients on dialysis)

Cushing's syndrome and the administration of corticosteroids or ACTH

Carcinoma (particularly with advanced disease)

Hodgkin's disease (particularly with advanced disease)

Some non-Hodgkin's lymphomas

Angioimmunoblastic lymphadenopathy

Acquired immune deficiency syndrome (AIDS)

Cytotoxic and immunosuppressive therapy, particularly nucleoside analogue therapy, and also use of antilymphocyte and antithymocyte globulin and monoclonal antibody therapy directed at lymphocytes (e.g. alemtuzumab—anti-CD52)

Clozapine therapy [58]

Quinine hypersensitivity [306]

Erythropoietin therapy [307]

IL12 administration [203]

Influenza vaccination [308]

Irradiation

Alcoholism [287]

Rheumatoid arthritis [309] and systemic lupus erythematosus [310]

Sarcoidosis [311]

Aplastic anaemia and agranulocytosis

Megaloblastic anaemia

The myelodysplastic syndromes [312]

Anorexia nervosa [313]

Intestinal lymphangiectasia and Whipple's disease

Peripheral blood stem cell apheresis [286]

Iron deficiency anaemia [314]

Chronic platelet apheresis [315]

Graft-versus-host disease

Administration of 'Lorenzo's oil' [316]

Thymoma [317]

ACTH, adrenocorticotropic hormone; IL12, interleukin 12.

Thrombocytopenia

Thrombocytopenia is a reduction of the platelet count below the level expected in a healthy subject of the same age and gender. Ethnic origin may also be relevant since lower platelet counts have been observed in Africans and Afro-Caribbeans. Thrombocytopenia may be congenital or acquired and due to reduced production or to increased destruction, consumption or extravascular loss. The causes are summarized in Table 6.27. Information on drugs recognized as causing thrombocytopenia is available on a web site, which is updated annually [397]. Some causes of thrombocytopenia of particular importance in the fetus and the neonate are summarized in Tables 6.28 and 6.29. In fetuses with intrauterine growth retardation, thrombocytopenia is indicative of a worse prognosis [398]. The most common cause of severe thrombocytopenia in neonates is alloimmune thrombocytopenia.

Blood film and count

In unexplained congenital thrombocytopenia both

Table 6.27 Some causes of thrombocytopenia (excluding conditions which usually cause pancytopenia).

Failure of platelet production
Congenital (inherited or resulting from intrauterine events)
    May–Hegglin anomaly, Sebastian's syndrome, Epstein's syndrome, Fechtner's syndrome (all resulting form a *MYH9*
        mutation)
    Bernard–Soulier syndrome
    Other inherited thrombocytopenias, some with large platelets and some with platelets of normal size (see Table 8.13)
    Megakaryocytic hypoplasia, inherited or due to intrauterine events (including some mutations of the gene encoding
        mpl (the thrombopoietin receptor), some cases of trisomy 13, trisomy 18 and trisomy 21 syndromes,
        thrombocytopenia with absent radii, thrombocytopenia with radio-ulnar synostosis (*HOXA11* mutation),
        thrombocytopenia with normal radii but with other physical abnormalities in 40% of cases and having an autosomal
        recessive or X-linked recessive inheritance [318]), amegakaryocytic thrombocytopenia with Noonan's syndrome [319]
    Reticular agenesis (variable thrombocytopenia)
    Placental insufficiency—associated with fetal hypoxia/intrauterine growth retardation/babies of hypertensive or
        diabetic mothers [292,320]
    Haemolytic disease of the newborn (Rh and, particularly, Kell) [321,322]
    Transplacental passage of maternal anti-platelet antibodies inhibiting megakaryocytopoiesis, e.g. anti-HPA-2b [323]

Inherited but not present at birth
    Fanconi's anaemia

Acquired
    Following bone marrow damage by some of the drugs which can cause aplastic anaemia or as the first manifestation of
        aplastic anaemia or as a feature of mustard gas exposure [324]
    Thiazide administration
    Valproic acid administration [325]
    Myelodysplastic syndromes
    Severe iron deficiency (rarely)
    Parvovirus infection (rarely) [326]
    Human herpesvirus 6 infection [259]
    Chronic hepatitis C virus infection (probably) [327]
    Interferon therapy
    Paroxysmal nocturnal haemoglobinuria
    Alcohol abuse [328]
    Autoimmune acquired amegakaryocytic thrombocytopenia [328] including amegakaryocytic thrombocytopenia
        associated with large granular lymphocyte leukaemia and sometimes causing cyclical thrombocytopenia [329]
    Graft-versus-host disease [209]
    Chronic renal failure on haemodialysis and, to a lesser extent, on peritoneal dialysis [330]
    Development of antibodies to thrombopoietin after administration of pegylated recombinant thrombopoietin [331]
    Hypervitaminosis A [207]
    Copper deficiency [290]
    Arsenic poisoning [208]
    Imatinib (rarely) [274]

Increased platelet consumption, destruction or removal
Immune mechanisms
Congenital
    Alloimmune thrombocytopenia
    Transplacental transfer of maternal autoantibody
    Transplacental transfer of maternal anti GpIIb/IIIa (in the case of a mother with Glanzmann's thrombasthenia) [323]
    Transplacental transfer of maternal anti-CD36 isoantibodies from CD36-deficient mothers [333]
    Transplacental transfer of maternal HLA antibodies (uncommon) [322]
    Transplacental transfer of maternal ABO antibodies (rare) [323]
    Maternal drug hypersensitivity

Continued p. 240

Table 6.27 *Continued*

Acquired

Autoimmune thrombocytopenic purpura as an isolated abnormality or associated with other autoimmune disease (systemic lupus erythematosus, primary antiphospholipid syndrome, rheumatoid arthritis, autoimmune haemolytic anaemia (Evans syndrome), autoimmune lymphoproliferative syndrome), with a lymphoproliferative disease (chronic lymphocytic leukaemia, non-Hodgkin's lymphoma, Hodgkin's disease, large granular lymphocyte leukaemia), sarcoidosis [333], common variable immune deficiency [334] or angioimmunoblastic lymphadenopathy

Alloimmune, e.g. caused by transfer of donor lymphocytes during stem cell transplantation [335], infusion of plasma containing platelet alloantibodies [336]

Drug-induced immune thrombocytopenia including heparin-induced thrombocytopenia and thrombocytopenia induced by anti-platelet monoclonal antibodies such as abciximab* (anti-platelet glycoprotein IIb/IIIa) [337] and other drugs interfering with binding of fibrinogen to platelet glycoprotein IIb/IIIa—eptifibatide, orbofiban, roxifiban, tirofiban and xemilofiban [338], rituximab [339]

Food-associated immune thrombocytopenia [340]

Immune thrombocytopenia associated with HIV infection

Immune thrombocytopenia associated with cytomegalovirus infection [341], HHV6 infection [342], hepatitis C infection [343], *Mycoplasma pneumoniae* infection [344], scarlet fever (β haemolytic streptococcal infection) [345], tuberculosis [346,347], brucellosis [348], toxoplasmosis [348], *Helicobacter pylori* infection [349]

Post-infection thrombocytopenia, particularly after rubella but also after chicken pox (varicella), infectious mononucleosis, other viral infections and vaccinations

Post-transfusion purpura

Cocaine abuse [350]

Anaphylaxis

Onyalai [351]

Rituximab administration [352]

Non-immune mechanisms

Congenital

Schulman–Upshaw syndrome [253,354]

Hereditary phytosterolaemia [355]

Kaposiform haemangioendothelioma [356] or tufted haemangioma (Kasabach–Merritt syndrome)

Intrahepatic infantile haemangioma [356]

Type IIB von Willebrand's disease, particularly after DDAVP therapy, and platelet-type (pseudo) von Willebrand's disease (inherited defect of platelet GpIb)

Acquired

Disseminated intravascular coagulation (including that associated with heat stroke, IL2 administration [357,358] and trypanosomiasis [359])

Thrombotic microangiopathy (thrombotic thrombocytopenic purpura and related conditions, see Table 8.8)

Post-transplant hepatic veno-occlusive disease [360]

Venous thrombo-embolism [361]

Viral haemorrhagic fevers—arenavirus infection (Lassa fever and Argentinian, Bolivian, Venezuelan and Brazilian haemorrhagic fevers), Bunyaviridae infections (Rift Valley fever, Crimean Congo haemorrhagic fever, haemorrhagic fever with renal syndrome due to Hantaan, Seoul, Puumala and other viruses and hantavirus pulmonary syndrome due to Sin Nombre virus [39], Black Creek Canal and other viruses), Filoviridae infections (Marburg and Ebola haemorrhagic fevers), Flaviviridae infections (yellow fever [362], dengue, Kyasanur Forest disease and Omsk haemorrhagic fever)—and certain other viral infections, e.g. Colorado tick fever (coltivirus infection), acute HIV infection, Cache valley virus infection [363], lymphocytic choriomeningitis virus infection [263], Nipah virus encephalitis [364], corona-virus associated severe acute respiratory distress syndrome (SARS) [263], avian influenza A infection [257]

Rickettsial infections, e.g. Rocky Mountain spotted fever, malignant Mediterranean spotted fever, Queensland tick typhus [365], scrub typhus [366], murine typhus [367]

Certain bacterial infections, e.g. Brazilian haemorrhagic fever (*Haemophilus aegypticus* infection), relapsing fever (*Borrelia recurrentis* infection), human monocytic ehrlichiosis (*Ehrlichia chaffeensis* infection), human granulocytic ehrlichiosis (*Anaplasma phagocytophilum* infection) and infection by *Ehrlichia ewingii*, *Bartonella quintana* infection (trench fever) [368], inhalational anthrax [369], brucellosis [370], typhoid fever [371], leptospirosis [372]

Certain protozoal infections, e.g. malaria and babesiosis

Extracorporeal circulation

Use of intra-aortic balloon pump [373]

Peripheral blood stem cell apheresis [286]

Continued

Table 6.27 *Continued*

Massive transfusion
Kaposi's sarcoma [374]
'Histiocytic sarcoma' of the spleen [375]
Administration of M-CSF [376]
Snake bite [56]
Envenomation by bees [377]
Acquired phytosterolaemia associated with soy-based parenteral nutrition [378]

Redistribution of platelets
Congenital
Hypersplenism

Acquired
Hypersplenism (including acute sequestration in sickle cell disease)
Administration of Lorenzo's oil [316,379]
Hypothermia [380]

Uncertain or complex mechanisms
Congenital
Wiskott–Aldrich syndrome
The grey platelet syndrome
Chédiak–Higashi anomaly
Griscelli's syndrome [248]
Cyclical thrombocytopenia and tidal platelet dysgenesis
Mediterranean macrothrombocytosis
Jacobsen's syndrome (Paris–Trousseau thrombocytopenia, terminal deletion of 11q with q21–q24 breakpoint)
Congenital infections (toxoplasmosis, cytomegalovirus infection, rubella, syphilis, listeriosis, coxsackie B infection, herpes simplex virus infection, relapsing fever (*Borrelia hermsii* infection) [381])
Associated with certain inborn errors of metabolism (idiopathic hyperglycinaemia [382], methylmalonic acidaemia [382], isovaleric acidaemia [382], propionic acidaemia [254]; hyperzincaemia with hypercalprotectinaemia [255]; holocarboxylase synthetase deficiency
Mitochondrial cytopathy [383]
Associated with factor V Quebec [384]
Extreme prematurity

Acquired
Phototherapy in the neonate [385]
Respiratory distress syndrome and mechanical ventilation in the neonate [386,387]
Neonatal herpes simplex infection
Associated with cyanotic congenital heart disease
Neonatal hyperthyroidism [388]
Miliary tuberculosis [178]
Graves' disease [389]
Hypothyroidism [390]
Pregnancy-associated thrombocytopenia
Monge's disease (inappropriate altitude-related polycythaemia) [391]
Paracetamol (acetaminophen) overdose [392]
Thrombocytopenia with exanthem in Japanese neonates [393]
Wilson's disease [394]
IL12 therapy [203]
Alemtuzumab (anti-CD52) therapy
Omalizumab (anti-immunoglobulin E) therapy [395]
Bortezomib therapy [273]
Sirolimus therapy
Use of Jui (traditional Chinese herbal medicine) [396]
Oroya fever [138]

DDAVP, 1-deamino-8-D-arginine vasopressin; HIV, human immunodeficiency virus; HHV6, human herpesvirus 6, IL, interleukin; HLA, human histocompatibility antigen; M-CSF, macrophage colony-stimulating factor.
* But note that abciximab can also cause factitious thrombocytopenia as a result of platelet aggregation.

Table 6.28 Some causes of fetal thrombocytopenia (platelet count less than $150 \times 10^9/l$) [398]; the prevalence among fetuses with certain specified abnormalities is shown in brackets.

Category	Frequency among instances of thrombocytopenia	Cause and % of cases of condition in which it was found
Intrauterine infection	28%	Toxoplasmosis (26%), cytomegalovirus infection (36%), rubella (20%)
Immune	18%	Alloimmune thrombocytopenia, maternal autoimmune thrombocytopenia
Chromosomal abnormalities	17%	Trisomy 13 (54%), trisomy 18 (86%), trisomy 21 (6%), Turner's syndromes (31%), triploidy (3/4)
Unknown and presumably heterogeneous mechanisms	12%	Associated with multiple congenital abnormalities without a chromosomal abnormality
Intrauterine growth retardation	6%	
Unknown mechanism	4%	Rh haemolytic disease

platelet size and granularity and white cell morphology should be assessed. A number of inherited conditions have thrombocytopenia associated with morphological abnormalities of platelets or neutrophils (see p. 367). In acquired thrombocytopenia, platelet size is also relevant since increased platelet consumption or destruction with increased bone marrow output is associated with increased platelet size whereas bone marrow failure is associated with small or normal sized platelets. Red cells should be assessed for any evidence of a microangiopathic haemolytic anaemia, which may be associated with thrombocytopenia caused by a thrombotic micro-angiopathy. The blood film should also be examined for abnormal lymphocytes (indicative of viral infection or lymphoproliferative disorder), blast cells, immature granulocytes or NRBC (indicative of leukaemia or bone marrow infiltration) and dysplastic features (indicative of a myelodysplastic syndrome or AML). Children with amegakaryocytic thrombocytopenia may have macrocytosis [319].

The automated blood count shows an increased MPV and PDW when there is increased platelet consumption or destruction and a low MPV when there is failure of bone marrow output. The count of 'reticulated platelets' is increased when there is increased

Table 6.29 Some causes of thrombocytopenia of particular importance in the neonate (for mechanisms and other rare causes see Table 6.27).

Maternal antiplatelet antibodies (autoantibodies, alloantibodies or drug-dependent antibodies)
Intrauterine infection
    Viral infection (cytomegalovirus infection, congenital rubella, human immunodeficiency virus (HIV) infection, herpes simplex infection, varicella-zoster infection, coxsackie B infection)
    Congenital syphilis
    Listeriosis
    Congenital toxoplasmosis
Intrauterine growth retardation as a result of placental insufficiency
Congenital leukaemia including transient abnormal myelopoiesis of Down's syndrome
Disseminated intravascular coagulation (e.g. resulting from bacterial sepsis, acute asphyxia, respiratory distress syndrome, pulmonary hypertension, necrotizing enterocolitis) [194]
Exchange transfusion
Hyperbilirubinaemia and phototherapy [194]

platelet turnover and decreased when there is a failure of production.

Other tests

In congenital thrombocytopenia, the patient should be assessed for evidence of associated congenital defects and other family members should be assessed for platelet number and morphology and other evidence of inherited abnormalities. Children with amegakaryocytic thrombocytopenia may have an increased percentage of haemoglobin F and increased i expression [319].

In acquired thrombocytopenia not readily explained by the clinical circumstances, a bone marrow aspiration, tests for autoantibodies (antinuclear factor, anti-DNA antibodies and the lupus anticoagulant) and coagulation tests to exclude disseminated intravascular coagulation can be useful. Testing for HIV antibodies should be considered.

Pancytopenia

Pancytopenia is a combination of anaemia (with reduction of the RBC), leucopenia and thrombocytopenia. Leucopenia is usually mainly due to a reduction in the neutrophil count although the numbers of other granulocytes, monocytes and lymphocytes are often also reduced.

Pancytopenia is usually caused by bone marrow replacement or failure but it sometimes results from splenic pooling or peripheral destruction of mature cells. Cyclical pancytopenia, probably cytokine-induced, is an unusual manifestation of Hodgkin's disease [399]. Some of the causes of pancytopenia are shown in Table 6.30. In hospital practice, pancytopenia is most often the result of cytotoxic or immunosuppressive drug therapy.

Blood film and count

When the aetiology is not readily apparent from the clinical history the blood film should be carefully examined for blast cells, dysplastic features in any cell lineage, lymphoma cells, hairy cells, myeloma cells, increased rouleaux formation, macrocytes, hypersegmented neutrophils, NRBC and immature granulocytes. Blast cells should be specifically sought along the edges of the film. Blast cells and hairy cells may be very infrequent but the presence of even small numbers is significant. In aplastic anaemia the red cells may be normocytic or macrocytic, polychromasia is absent and the platelets are usually small and uniform in size; occasionally poikilocytosis is quite marked.

Differential diagnosis

The presence of dysplastic features in the absence of administration of cytotoxic drugs and toxic chemicals suggests either HIV infection or a myelodysplastic syndrome (MDS) or AML. Macrocytosis may be present in liver disease and alcohol abuse, megaloblastic anaemia and hypoplastic and aplastic anaemias, MDS and following cytotoxic chemotherapy. Poikilocytic red cells and a leucoerythroblastic blood film (see Table 6.19) suggest bone marrow infiltration or idiopathic myelofibrosis. A low reticulocyte count indicates failure of bone marrow output whereas an elevated reticulocyte count suggests peripheral destruction, e.g. paroxysmal nocturnal haemoglobinuria or immune destruction of cells.

The full blood count (FBC) may show an elevated mean cell volume (MCV) and elevated red cell distribution width (RDW). An appropriately increased MPV and 'reticulated platelet' count suggest peripheral platelet destruction whereas a reduced MPV and a low 'reticulated platelet' count despite thrombocytopenia suggest failure of bone marrow output.

Further tests

A reticulocyte count is indicated and a bone marrow aspirate is usually necessary. Unless a cellular aspirate is obtained, a trephine biopsy is also required. Bone marrow aspiration is needed urgently if the clinical history suggests the possibility of a haemophagocytic syndrome, acute infection or the rapid onset of megaloblastic anaemia. In the latter condition macrocytes and hypersegmented neutrophils may be infrequent or absent and only the bone marrow aspirate reveals the diagnosis. The other tests that are needed will be determined by the results of these initial investigations and by the specific diagnosis that is suspected.

Table 6.30 Some causes of pancytopenia.

Inherited disorders

Inherited conditions causing aplastic anaemia: Fanconi's anaemia, dyskeratosis congenita, WT syndrome of radioulnar hypoplasia, hypoplastic anaemia and susceptibility to leukaemia [400], xeroderma pigmentosa, late stages of Shwachman–Diamond syndrome, aplastic anaemia following congenital amegakaryocytic thrombocytopenia [318] including some patients with amegakaryocytic thrombocytopenia as a result of a defective thrombopoietin receptor [401], ataxia-pancytopenia syndrome [402]; Jacobsen's syndrome (terminal deletion of 11q with q21–q24 breakpoint), Dubowitz' syndrome (microcephaly and other developmental defects with aplastic anaemia) [319], Seckel's syndrome (microcephaly, and dwarfism with aplastic anaemia) [319]

Marble bone disease (osteopetrosis)

Inherited metabolic disorders: mannosidosis, Gaucher's disease, adult Niemann–Pick disease, methylmalonic aciduria, oxalosis, isovaleric acidaemia, alpha methyl beta hydroxybutyric aciduria, propionic acidaemia, oxalosis [403–406]

Other rare inherited conditions: some cases of Pearson's syndrome [200], cobalamin C deficiency [407], pancytopenia associated with necrotizing encephalopathy [408], Griscelli's syndrome [409], thiamine-responsive anaemia [410], Wolfram's syndrome (DIDMOAD—**D**iabetes **I**nsipidus **D**iabetes **M**ellitus **O**ptic **A**tropy **D**eafness syndrome), methylmalonicaciduria

Acquired disorders

Aplastic and hypoplastic anaemias including: idiopathic, virus-induced, drug-induced and chemical-induced aplastic anaemia; hypopituitarism [411]; bone marrow aplasia preceding ALL; bone marrow aplasia associated with thymoma and large granular lymphocyte leukaemia; graft-versus-host disease including transfusion-associated graft-versus-host disease; irradiation; use of alkylating agents and other anticancer and related drugs, alemtuzumab (anti-CD52) therapy, development of anti-thrombopoietin antibodies [412]

Bone marrow infiltration, with or without associated fibrosis, including ALL, AML (ineffective haemopoiesis also contributes), multiple myeloma, carcinoma, non-Hodgkin's lymphoma, hairy cell leukaemia and hairy cell variant leukaemia

Hodgkin's disease (cytokine-induced) [399]

Clonal disorders of haemopoiesis: the myelodysplastic syndromes, paroxysmal nocturnal haemoglobinuria, acute myelofibrosis, advanced idiopathic myelofibrosis

Ineffective haemopoiesis: acute or severe megaloblastic anaemia

Arsenic poisoning [413]

Acute infections: some cases of acute HIV infection [414], parvovirus [415], ehrlichiosis [416], brucellosis [417] miliary tuberculosis, cytomegalovirus infection in bone marrow transplant recipients [418], human herpesvirus 6 infection [419], Legionnaires' disease [420]

Some chronic infections, especially visceral leishmaniasis (kala azar), when it is due to hypersplenism; rarely chronic parvovirus infection [421], miliary tuberculosis (a minority of patients) [178]

Haemophagocytic syndromes (including familial and infection-related)

Acquired immune deficiency syndrome (AIDS)

Fusariosis [422]

Systemic lupus erythematosus

Combined immunocytopenia [423]

Autoimmune lymphoproliferative syndrome [424]

Severe or chronic graft-versus host disease [425]

Drug-induced immune pancytopenia (e.g. caused by phenacetin, para-amino salicylic acid, sulphonamides, rifampicin and quinine)

Hypersplenism (e.g. kala azar and *Schistisoma mansoni* infection)

Acquired sea-blue histiocytosis during prolonged parenteral nutrition (the mechanism is probably hypersplenism) [426]

Wilson's disease [427]

Hyperthyroidism (rarely) [428]

Alcohol toxicity [287]

Copper deficiency [428]

Hypothermia [429]

Paget's disease [430]

AIDS, acquired immune deficiency syndrome; ALL, acute lymphoblastic leukaemia; AML, acute myeloid leukaemia; HIV, human immunodeficiency virus.

Test your knowledge

Multiple choice questions (MCQs)

(1–5 answers may be correct)

MCQ 6.1 Lymphocytosis may be a feature of
(a) Bordetella pertussis infection
(b) Addison's disease
(c) An acute response to stress
(d) Hyposplenism
(e) Corticosteroid administration

MCQ 6.2 Polycythaemia may result from
(a) The presence of a low oxygen affinity haemoglobin
(b) Cyanotic heart disease
(c) Cigarette smoking
(d) Uterine fibroids
(e) Hypothyroidism

MCQ 6.3 Pure red cell aplasia is or may be a feature of
(a) Myelodysplastic syndrome
(b) Large granular lymphocyte leukaemia
(c) Parvovirus B19 infection
(d) Fanconi's anaemia
(e) Diamond–Blackfan syndrome

MCQ 6.4 Eosinophilia can be a feature of
(a) Cushing's syndrome
(b) T-cell lymphoma
(c) Hodgkin's disease
(d) Acute stress
(e) Hookworm infection

MCQ 6.5 A leucoerythroblastic blood film may result from
(a) Severe infection
(b) Bone marrow infiltration
(c) Haemorrhagic shock
(d) Aplastic anaemia
(e) Idiopathic myelofibrosis

MCQ 6.6 Splenectomy can cause
(a) Neutrophilia
(b) Lymphocytosis
(c) Eosinophilia
(d) Basophilia
(e) Thrombocytosis

Extended matching question (EMQ)

Select the most accurate options for each of the stems. Each option may be used once, more than once or not at all. Only one answer is correct.
Options
A Leucocytosis with increased neutrophils and monocytes
B Leucopenia
C Neutrophilia
D Neutropenia
E Increased haemoglobin concentration with high erythropoietin concentration
F Increased haemoglobin concentration with low erythropoietin concentration
G Thrombocytosis
H Leucoerythroblastic anaemia
I Anaemia with reticulocytosis
J Anaemia with reticulocytopenia and an otherwise normal blood count and film
K Leucocytosis with increased neutrophils, eosinophils, basophils and their precursors

For each diagnosis select the option that indicates the most important diagnostic feature of the disease.

Diagnosis	Matching option
1 Polycythaemia rubra vera	
2 Chronic granulocytic leukaemia	
3 Essential thrombocythaemia	
4 Idiopathic myelofibrosis	
5 Chronic myelomonocytic leukaemia	

References

1 Doubek M, Brychtova Y, Tomiska M and Mayer J (2005) Idiopathic systemic capillary leak syndrome misdiagnosed and treated as polycythemia vera. *Acta Haematol*, **113**, 150–151.
2 Juvonen E, Ikkala E, Fyhrquist F and Ruutu T (1991) Autosomal dominant erythrocytosis caused by increased sensitivity to erythropoietin. *Blood*, **78**, 3066–3069.

3 Prchal JT and Sokol L (1996) 'Benign erythrocytosis' and other familial and congenital polycythemias. *Eur J Haematol*, **57**, 263–268.

4 Ang SO, Chan H, Stockton DW, Sergueeva A, Gordeuk WF, Prchal JT (2001) Von Hippel–Lindau protein, Chuvash polycythemia and oxygen sensing. *Blood*, **98**, 748a.

5 Percy MJ, McMullin MF, Jowitt SN, Potter M, Treacy M, Watson WH and Lappin TRJ (2003) Chuvash-type congenital polycythaemia in 4 families of Asian and Western European ancestry. *Blood*, **102**, 1097–1099.

6 Ang SO, Guan Y, Pastore YD, Jelinek J, Krishnamurti L and Prchal JT (2001) Polycythemia in a family with a VHL mutation. *Blood*, **98**, 570a.

7 Tanaka KR and Zerez CR (1990) Red cell enzymopathies of the glycolytic pathway. *Semin Hematol*, **27**, 165–185.

8 Hutchinson DCS, Sapru RP, Sumerling MD, Donaldson GWK and Richmond J (1968) Cirrhosis, cyanosis and polycythemia: multiple pulmonary arteriovenous anastomoses. *Am J Med*, **45**, 139–151.

9 Gajra A and Grethlein SJ (1999) Hereditary haemorrhagic telangiectasia—an unusual cause of polycythemia in pregnancy. *Blood*, **94**, Suppl. 1, 14b.

10 di Marco AT (1989) Carbon monoxide poisoning presenting as polycythemia. *N Engl J Med*, **319**, 874.

11 Hammond D and Winnick S (1974) Paraneoplastic erythrocytosis and ectopic erythropoietins. *Ann N Y Acad Sci*, **230**, 219–227.

12 Souid AK, Dubanshy AS, Richman P and Sadowitz PD (1993) Polycythemia: a review article and a case report of erythrocytosis secondary to Wilms' tumor. *Pediatr Hematol Oncol*, **10**, 215–221.

13 Distelhorst CW, Wagner DS, Goldwasser E and Adamson JW (1981) Autosomal dominant familial erythrocytosis due to anomalous erythropoietin production. *Blood*, **58**, 1155–1158.

14 Manglani MV, DeGroff CG, Dukes PP and Ettinger LJ (1998) Congenital erythrocytosis with elevated erythropoietin level: an incorrectly set 'erythrostat'? *J Pediatr Hematol Oncol*, **20**, 560–562.

15 Guan Y, Wu JK, Jastaniah W, Moss LG, Digman C, Mostacci S *et al.* (2004) A new polycythaemia syndrome: congenital polycythemia with high erythropoietin and propensity for malignant hypertension due to paraganglionoma. *Blood*, **104**, 171b.

16 Shaheen M, Hilgarth KA, Antony AC, Hawes D and Badve S (2003) A Mexican man with 'too much blood'. *Lancet*, **362**, 806.

17 Jacobs P and Wood L (1994) Recurrent benign erythropoietin-secreting pheochromocytomas. *Am J Med*, **97**, 307–308.

18 Reynen K (1995) Cardiac myxomas. *N Engl J Med*, **333**, 1610–1617.

19 Dickerman RD, Pertusi R, Miller J and Zachariah NY (1999) Androgen-induced erythrocytosis: is it erythropoietin? *Am J Hematol*, **61**, 154–155.

20 Emanuel PD, Eaves CJ, Broody C, Papayannopoulo T, Moore MR, D'Andrea AD *et al.* (1992) Familial and congenital polycythemia in three unrelated families. *Blood*, **79**, 3019–3030.

21 Norberg G (1994) Assessment of risk in occupational cobalt exposures. *Sci Total Environ*, **150**, 201–207.

22 Jefferson JA, Escudero E, Hurtado M-E, Pando J, Tapia R, Swenson ER *et al.* (2002) Excessive erythrocytosis, chronic mountain sickness, and serum cobalt levels. *Lancet*, **359**, 407–408.

23 Nakanishi T, Sobue I, Tokokura Y, Nishitani H, Kuroiwa Y, Satayoshi L *et al.* (1984) The Crow–Fukase syndrome: a study of 102 cases in Japan. *Neurology*, **34**, 712–20.

24 Richard S, Croisille L, Yvart J, Casadeval N, Eschwège P, Aghakhani N *et al.* (2002) Paradoxical secondary polycythemia in von Hippel–Lindau patients treated with anti-vascular endothelial growth factor receptor therapy. *Blood*, **99**, 3851–3853.

25 Austin T, Bridges N, Markiewicz M and Abrahamson E (1997) Severe neonatal polycythaemia after third stage labour underwater. *Lancet*, **350**, 1445.

26 Hudson PR, Tandy SC, Child DF, Williams CP and Cavill I (2001) Compensated haemolysis: a consistent features of diabetes mellitus. *Br J Haematol*, **113**, Suppl. 1, 47.

27 Worwood M, Carter K, Jackson HA, Hutton RD and Cavill I (2001) Erythropoiesis and iron status in asymptomatic subjects homozygous for HFE C282Y. *Br J Haematol*, **113**, Suppl. 1, 63.

28 Nakagawa M, Terashima T, D'yachkova Y, Bondy GP, Hogg JC and van Eeden SF (1998) Glucocorticoid-induced granulocytosis: contribution of marrow release and demargination of intravascular granulocytes. *Circulation*, **98**, 2307–2313.

29 Herring WB, Smith LG, Walker RI and Herion JC (1974) Hereditary neutrophilia. *Am J Med*, **56**, 729–734.

30 Malech HL and Gallin JI (1987) Current concepts: immunology, neutrophils in human disease. *N Engl J Med*, **317**, 687–694.

31 Arnaout MA (1990) Structure and function of the leukocyte adhesion molecules CD11/CD18. *Blood*, **75**, 1037–1050.

32 Etzione A, Frydman M, Pollack S, Avidor I, Phillips ML, Paulson JC and Gershoni-Baruch R (1992) Recurrent severe infections caused by a novel leukocyte adhesion deficiency. *N Engl J Med*, **327**, 1789–1792.

33 Etzioni A, Doerschuk CM and Harlan JM (1999) Of man and mouse: leukocyte and endothelial adhesion molecule deficiencies. *Blood*, **94**, 3281–3288.

34 Alon R, Aker M, Feigelson S, Sokolovsky-Eisenberg M, Staunton DE, Cinamon G *et al.* (2003) A novel genetic leukocyte adhesion deficiency in subsecond triggering of integrin avidity by endothelial chemokines results in impaired leukocyte arrest on vascular endothelium under shear flow. *Blood*, **101**, 4437–4445.

35 Tindall JP, Beeker SK and Rose WF (1969) Familial cold urticaria: a generalized reaction involving leucocytosis. *Arch Intern Med*, **124**, 129–134.

36 Drenth J and van der Meer JWM (2001) Hereditary periodic fever. *N Engl J Med*, **345**, 1748–1757.

37 Blans MJ, Vos PE, Faber HJ and Boers GH (2001) Coma in a young anorexic woman. *Lancet*, **357**, 1944.

38 Duchin JC, Koster FT, Peters CJ, Simpson GL, Tempest B, Zaki SR *et al.* (1994) Hantavirus pulmonary syndrome. *N Engl J Med*, **330**, 949–955.

39 Khan AS, Ksiazek TG and Peters CJ (1996) Hantavirus pulmonary syndrome. *Lancet*, **347**, 739–741.

40 Phoncharoensri D, Witoonpanich R, Tunlayadechanont S and Laothamatas J (2004) Confusion and paraparesis. *Lancet*, **363**, 1954.

41 Case Records of the Massachusetts General Hospital (2000) Case 29-2000: A 69-year-old renal transplant recipient with low-grade fever and multiple pulmonary nodules. *N Engl J Med*, **343**, 870–877.

42 Dobbin CJ, Soni R, Jelihovsky T and Bye PTP (2000) Cepacia syndrome occurring following prolonged colonisation with *Burkholderia cepacia*. *Aust NZ J Med*, **30**, 288–289.

43 Case Records of the Massachusetts General Hospital (2002) A 46-year-old woman with extensive pulmonary infiltrates. *N Engl J Med*, **347**, 517–524.

44 Ladhani S, Lowe B, Cole AO, Kowuondo K and Newton CRJC (2003) Changes in white blood cells and platelets in children with falciparum malaria: relationship to disease outcome. *Br J Haematol*, **119**, 839–847.

45 Keatinge WR, Coleshaw SRK, Easton JC, Coller F, Mattock MB and Chelliah R (1986) Increased platelet and red cell counts, blood viscosity, and plasma cholesterol levels during heat stress, and mortality from coronary and cerebral thrombosis. *Am J Med*, **81**, 795–800.

46 Locker GJ, Kapiotis S, Veitl M, Mader RM, Stoiser B, Kofler J *et al.* (1999) Activation of endothelium by immunotherapy with interleukin-2 in patients with malignant disorders. *Br J Haematol*, **105**, 912–919.

47 Ganser A, Lindemann A, Siepelt G, Ottman OG, Herrmann F, Eder M *et al.* (1990) Effects of recombinant human interleukin-3 in patients with normal haematopoiesis and in patients with bone marrow failure. *Blood*, **76**, 666–676.

48 Asano S, Okano A, Ozawa K, Nakahata T, Ishibashi T, Koike K *et al.* (1990) *In vivo* effects of recombinant human interleukin-6 in primates: stimulated production of platelets. *Blood*, **75**, 1602–1605.

49 Huhn RD, Radwanski E, O'Connell SM, Sturgill MG, Clarke L, Cody RP *et al.* (1996) Pharmacokinetics and immunomodulatory properties of intravenously administered recombinant human interleukin-10 in healthy volunteers. *Blood*, **87**, 699–705.

50 Gershon SL (1993) Clozapine—deciphering the risks. *N Engl J Med*, **329**, 204–205.

51 Harrison P, Cardigan R, Harrison C, Addison I, Chavda N, Chitolie A and Machin SJ (1996) Delayed effect of desmopressin on circulating neutrophils and monocytes. *Br J Haematol*, **95**, 570–571.

52 Bienvenu J, Chvetzoff R, Salles G, Balter C, Tilly H, Herbrecht R *et al.* (2001) Tumour necrosis factor α release is a major biological event associated with rituximab treatment. *Hematol J*, **2**, 378–384.

53 Sahoo S (2005) Pathologic Quiz Case: A 44-year-old man with acute renal failure. *Arch Pathol Lab Med*, **129**, e81–83.

54 Berg RA and Tarantino MD (1991) Envenomation by scorpion *Centruroides exilicauda* (*C. sculpturatus*): severe and unusual manifestations. *Pediatrics*, **87**, 930–933.

55 Franca FOS, Benvenuti LA, Fan HW, Dos Santos DR, Hain SH, Picchi-Martins FR *et al.* (1994) Severe and fatal mass attack by 'killer' bees (Africanized

honey bee—*Apis mellifera scutellata*) in Brazil: clinicopathological studies with measurement of serum venom concentrations. *Q J Med*, **87**, 269–282.

56 Warrell DA (1998) Antivenoms and treatment of snake-bite. *Prescribers J*, **38**, 10–18.

57 Cooper PH, Innes DJ and Greer KE (1983) Acute febrile neutrophilic dermatosis (Sweet's syndrome) and myeloproliferative disorders. *Cancer*, **51**, 1518–1526.

58 Rosenberg MR and Green M (1989) Neuroleptic malignant syndrome: review of response to therapy. *Arch Intern Med*, **149**, 1927–1931.

59 Fenwick JC, Cameron M, Naiman SC, Haley LP, Ronco JJ, Wiggs BR and Tweeddale MG (1994) Blood transfusion as a cause of leucocytosis in critically ill patients. *Lancet*, **344**, 855–856.

60 Mayne EE, Fitzpatrick J and Nelson SD (1970) Leucocytosis following administration of cryoprecipitate. *Acta Haematol*, **44**, 155–160.

61 Ward H and Reinhard D (1971) Chronic idiopathic leukocytosis. *Ann Intern Med*, **75**, 193–198.

62 Hübner C, Dietz A, Stremmel W, Stiehl A and Andrassy K (1997) Macrolide-induced Churg–Strauss syndrome in a patient with atopy. *Lancet*, **350**, 563.

63 Kränke B and Arberer W (1997) Macrolide-induced Churg–Strauss syndrome in patient with atopy. *Lancet*, **350**, 1551–1552.

64 Darmstadt GL, Tunnessen WW and Sweren RJ (1992) Eosinophilic pustular folliculitis. *Pediatrics*, **89**, 1095–1098.

65 Janin A, Copin MC, Dubos JP, Rouland V, Delaporte E and Blanchet-Bardon C (1996) Familial peeling skin syndrome with eosinophilia: clinical, histologic, and ultrastructural study of three cases. *Arch Pathol Lab Med*, **120**, 662–665.

66 Weller PF and Bubley GJ (1994) The idiopathic hypereosinophilic syndrome. *Blood*, **83**, 2759–2779.

67 Ryan ET, Wilson ME and Kain KC (2002) Illness after international travel. *N Engl J Med*, **347**, 505–516.

68 Sheehan DJ, Rancher BG and McKitrick JC (1986) Association of *Blastocystis hominis* with signs and symptoms of human disease. *J Clin Microbiol*, **24**, 548–550.

69 Leder K and Weller PF (2000) Eosinophilia and helminth infections. *Baillière's Clin Haematol*, **13**, 301–317.

70 Diaz Camacho SP, Zazueta Ramos M, Ponce Torrecillas E, Osuna Ramirez I, Castro Velazquez R, Flores Gaxiola A *et al.* (1998) Clinical manifestations and immunodiagnosis of gnathostomiasis in Culiacan, Mexico. *Am J Trop Med Hyg*, **59**, 908–915.

71 Prociv P and Croese J (1990) Epidemic eosinophilic enteritis in north Queensland caused by common dog hookworm, *Ancylostoma caninum*. *Aust NZ J Med*, **20**, 439.

72 Yfanti G, Andreadis E, Spiliadou C and Diamantopoulos EJ (1996) A woman with fever and a jejunal stricture. *Lancet*, **347**, 802.

73 Petithory J-C (1998) Les éosinophilies familiales: apports de la parasitologie à leur diagnostic. *Bull Acad Natl Med*, **182**, 1823–1835.

74 Gomez B, Tabar AI, Tunon T, Larrinaga B, Alvarez MJ, Garcia BE and Olaguibel JM (1998) Eosinophilic gastroenteritis and Anisakis. *Allergy*, **53**, 1148–1154.

75 Surmont I and Liu LX (1995) Enteritis, eosinophilia, and Enterobius vermicularis. *Lancet*, **346**, 1167.

76 Marty P (1997) Human dirofilariasis due to Dirofilaria repens in France. A review of reported cases. *Parassitologia*, **39**, 383–386.

77 Goto Y, Tamura A, Ishikawa O, Miyachi Y, Ishii T and Akao N (1998) Creeping eruption caused by a larva of the suborder Spirurina type X. *Br J Dermatol*, **139**, 315–318.

78 Paine M, Davis S and Brown G (1994) Severe forms of infection with *Angiostrongylus cantonensis* acquired in Australia and Fiji. *Aust NZ J Med*, **24**, 415–416.

79 Slom TJ, Cortese MM, Gerber SI, Jones RC, Holtz TH, Lopez AS *et al.* (2002) An outbreak of eosinophilic meningitis caused by *Angiostrongylus cantonensis* in travellers returning from the Caribbean. *N Engl J Med*, **346**, 668–675.

80 Petithory JC (1996) Can *Ascaris suum* cause visceral larva migrans? *Lancet*, **348**, 689.

81 Maruyama H, Nawa Y, Noda S, Mimori T, and Choi WY (1996) An outbreak of visceral larva migrans due to *Ascaris suum* in Kyushu, Japan. *Lancet*, **347**, 1766–1767.

82 el-Karaksy H, Hassanein B, Okasha S, Behairy B and Gadallah I (1999) Human fascioliasis in Egyptian children: successful treatment with triclabendazole. *J Trop Pediatr*, **45**, 135–138.

83 MacLean JD, Arthur JR, Ward BJ, Gyorkos TW, Curtis MA and Kokoskin E (1996) Common-source outbreak of acute infection due to the North American liver fluke *Metorchis conjunctus*. *Lancet*, **347**, 154–158.

84 Burton K, Yogev R, London N, Boyer K and Shulman ST (1982) Pulmonary paragonimiasis in Laotian refugee children. *Pediatrics*, **70**, 246–248.

85 Seymour JF (1997) Splenomegaly, eosinophilia, and pruritis: Hodgkin's disease, or . . . ? *Blood*, **90**, 1719–1720.

86 Navajas A, Cardenal I, Pinan MA, Ortiz A, Astigarraga I and Fdez-Teijeiro A (1998) Hypereosinophilia due to myiasis. *Acta Haematol*, **99**, 27–30.

87 Cools J, DeAngelo DJ, Gotlib J, Stover EH, Legare RD, Cortes J et al. (2003) A tyrosine kinase created by the fusion of the PDGFRA and FIP1L1 genes as a therapeutic target of imatinib in idiopathic hypereosinophilic syndrome. *N Engl J Med*, **348**, 1201–1214.

88 Cullen MH, Stansfield AG, Oliver RTD, Lister TA and Malpas JS (1979) Angio-immunoblastic lymphadenopathy: report of ten cases and review of the literature. *Q J Med*, **48**, 151–177.

89 Jayakar V, Goldin RD and Bain BJ (2006) Teaching cases from the Royal Marsden and St Mary's Hospitals: Eosinophilia and Pruritus. *Leuk Lymphoma*, in press.

90 Glantz L, Rintels P, Samoszuk M and Medeiros LJ (1995) Plasma cell myeloma associated with eosinophilia. *Am J Clin Pathol*, **103**, 583–587.

91 Kaplan MH, Hall WW, Susin M, Pahwa S, Salahuddin SZ, Heilman C et al. (1991) Syndrome of severe skin disease, eosinophilia, and dermato-pathic lymphadenopathy in patients with HTLV-II complicating human immunodeficiency virus infection. *Am J Med*, **91**, 300–309.

92 Aspinall AI, Pinto A, Auer IA, Bridges P, Luider J, Dimnik L et al. (2001) Identification of new fas mutations in a patient with autoimmune lympho-proliferative syndrome (ALPS) and eosinophilia. *Blood Cells Mol Dis*, **25**, 227–238.

93 Lowe D, Jorizzo J and Hutt MSR (1981) Tumour-associated eosinophilia: a review. *J Clin Pathol*, **34**, 1343–1348.

94 Dinauer MC. The phagocytic system and dis-orders of granulopoiesis and granulocyte function. In: Nathan DG, Orkin SH, Ginsburg D and Look AT, *Nathan and Oski's Hematology of Infancy and Childhood*, 6th Edn. Saunders, Philadelphia, 2003.

95 Case records of the Massachusetts General Hospital (1992) Case 18-1992. *N Engl J Med*, **326**, 1204–1212.

96 Wells GC and Smith NP (1979) Eosinophilic cel-lulitis. *Br J Dermatol*, **100**, 101–109.

97 Don IJ, Khettry U and Canoso JJ (1978) Progressive systemic sclerosis with eosinophilia and a fulmi-nant course. *Am J Med*, **65**, 346–348.

98 Panush RS, Wilkinson LS and Fagin RR (1973) Chronic active hepatitis associated with Coombs-positive hemolytic anemia. *Gastroenterology*, **64**, 1015–1019.

99 Neeman A and Kadish U (1987) Marked eosinophilia in a patient with primary sclerosing cholangitis. *Am J Med*, **83**, 378–379.

100 Case Records of the Massachusetts General Hospital (1998) A 10-year-old girl with urinary retention and a filling defect in the bladder. *N Engl J Med*, **339**, 616–622.

101 Ezekowitz RAB and Stockman JA. Hematologic manifestations of systemic diseases. In: Nathan DG, Orkin SH, Ginsburg D and Look AT, *Nathan and Oski's Hematology of Infancy and Childhood*, 6th Edn. Saunders, Philadelphia, 2003.

102 Karawajczyk M, Höglund M, Ericsson J and Venge P (1997) Administration of G-CSF to healthy subjects: the effects on eosinophil counts and mobilization of eosinophil granule proteins. *Br J Haematol*, **96**, 259–265.

103 Means-Markwell M, Burgess T, de Keratry D, O'Neil K, Mascola J, Fleisher T and Lucey D (2000) Eosinophilia with aberrant T cells and elevated serum levels of interleukin-2 and interleukin-15. *N Engl J Med*, **342**, 1568–1571.

104 van der Graaf W and Borleffs JCC (1994) Eosinophilia in patients with HIV infection. *Eur J Haematol*, **52**, 246–247.

105 Gleich GJ, Schroeter AL, Marcoux P, Sachs MI, O'Connell EJ and, Kohler PF (1984) Episodic angioedema associated with eosinophilia. *N Engl J Med*, **310**, 1621–1626.

106 Bullock WE, Artz RP, Bhathena D and Tung KSK (1979) Histoplasmosis: association with circulating immune complexes, eosinophilia, and mesangio-capillary glomerulonephritis. *Arch Intern Med*, **139**, 700–702.

107 Mayron LW, Alling S and Kaplan E (1972) Eosinophilia and drug abuse. *Ann Allergy*, **30**, 632–637.

108 Rubin RB and Neugarten J (1990) Cocaine-associated asthma. *Am J Med*, **88**, 438–439.

109 Gabriel LC, Escribano LM, Villa E, Leiva C and Valdes MD (1968) Ultrastructural studies of blood cells in toxic oil syndrome. *Acta Haematol*. **75**, 165–170.

110 Kilbourne EM, Swygert LA, Philen RM, Sun RK, Auerbach SB, Miller L et al. (1990) Interim guid-ance on the eosinophilia-myalgia syndrome. *Ann Intern Med*, **112**, 85–87.

111 Carvajal JA, Anderson R, Weiss L, Grismer J and Berman R (1967) Atheroembolism. An etiologic factor in renal insufficiency, gastrointestinal haemorrhages, and peripheral vascular diseases. *Arch Intern Med*, **119**, 593–599.

112 Cogan E, Schandene L, Papadopoulos T, Crusiaux A and Goldman M (1995) Interleukin-5 production by T lymphocytes in atheroembolic disease with hypereosinophilia. *Allergy Clin Immunol*, **96**, 427–429.

113 Omenn GS (1965) Familial reticuloendotheliosis with eosinophilia. *N Engl J Med*, **273**, 427–432.

114 Nagafuchi S, Tokiyama K, Kashiwagi S, Yayashi S, Imayama S and Niho Y (1993) Eosinophilia after intradermal hepatitis B vaccination. *Lancet*, **342**, 998.

115 Lärfars G, Uden-Blohmë AM and Samuelsson J (1996) Fludarabine, as well as 2-chlorodeoxyadenosine, can induce eosinophilia during treatment of lymphoid malignancies. *Br J Haematol*, **94**, 709–712.

116 Weiden PL, Bauermeister DE and Fatta EA (1998) An Asian man with enlarged glands. *Lancet*, **351**, 1098.

117 Angelis M, Yu M, Takanishi D, Hasaniya NWMA and Brown MR (1996) Eosinophilia as a marker of adrenal insufficiency in the surgical intensive care unit. *J Am Coll Surg*, **183**, 589–596.

118 Feussner JR, Shelburne JD, Bredhoeft S and Cohen HJ (1978) Arsenic-induced bone marrow toxicity: ultrastructural and electron-probe analysis. *Blood*, **53**, 820–827.

119 Hildebrandt GC, Hahn J, Erdmann A, Grube M, Andreesen R and Holler E (2000) Eosinophilia after bone marrow transplantation as a predictor of extensive and sclerodermatous chronic graft versus host disease. *Blood*, **96**, 194a.

120 Martinez BM and Domingo P (1997) Acute eosinophilic pneumonia associated with tenidap. *BMJ*, **314**, 349.

121 Terzano C and Petroianni A (2003) Clarithromycin and pulmonary infiltration with eosinophilia. *BMJ*, **326**, 1377–1378.

122 Crofton JW, Livingstone IL, Oswald NC and Roberts ATM (1952) Pulmonary eosinophilia. *Thorax*, **7**, 1–35.

123 Horie S, Okubo Y, Suzuki J and Isobe M (1996) An emaciated man with eosinophilic pneumonia. *Lancet*, **348**, 166.

124 Donhuijsen K, Haedicke C, Hattenberger C and Freund M (1992) Granulocyte-macrophage colony-stimulating factor-related eosinophilia and Loeffler's endocarditis. *Blood*, **79**, 2798.

125 Allen JN and Davis WB (1994) Eosinophilic lung disease. *Am J Respir Crit Care Med*, **150**, 1423–1438.

126 Schatz M, Wasserman S and Patterson R (1982) The eosinophil and the lung. *Arch Intern Med*, **142**, 1515–1519.

127 Fauci AS, Harley JB, Roberts WC, Ferrans VJ, Gralnick HR and Bjornson BH (1982) NIH Conference. The idiopathic hypereosinophilic syndrome. *Ann Intern Med*, **97**, 78–92.

128 Dines DE (1978) Chronic eosinophilic pneumonia. *Mayo Clin Proc*, **53**, 129–130.

129 Vaughan Hudson B, Linch DC, Macintyre EA, Bennett MH, MacLennan KA, Vaughan Hudson G and Jelliffe AM (1987) Selective peripheral blood eosinophilia associated with survival advantage in Hodgkin's disease (BNLI Report No 31). British National Lymphoma Investigation. *J Clin Pathol*, **40**, 247–250.

130 Simon HU, Plötz SG, Dummer R and Blaser K (1999) Abnormal clones of interleukin-5-producing T cells in idiopathic eosinophilia. *N Engl J Med*, **341**, 1112–1120.

131 Beishuizen A, Vermes I, Hylkema BS and Haanen C (1999) Relative eosinophilia and functional adrenal insufficiency in critically ill patients. *Lancet*, **353**, 1675–1676.

132 Loughlin KR (2000) Hypereosinophilic syndrome. *N Engl J Med*, **342**, 442.

133 Davies JK, Telfer P, Cavenagh JD, Foot N and Neat M (2003) Case Report. Autoimmune cytopenias in the 22q11.2 deletion syndrome. *Clin Lab Haematol*, **25**, 195–197.

134 Olson LC, Miller G and Hanshaw JB (1964) Acute infectious lymphocytosis presenting as a pertussis-like illness: its association with adenovirus type 12. *Lancet*, **i**, 200–201.

135 Anonymous (1968) Lymphocytopoietic viruses. *N Engl J Med*, **279**, 432–433.

136 Mandal BK and Stokes KJ (1973) Acute infectious lymphocytosis and enteroviruses. *Lancet*, **ii**, 1392–1393.

137 Nkrumah FK and Addy PAK (1973) Acute infectious lymphocytosis. *Lancet*, **i**, 1257–1258.

138 Horwitz CA, Henle W, Henle G, Polesky H, Balfour HH, Siem RA *et al.* (1977) Heterophile-negative infectious mononucleosis and mononucleosis-like illnesses. *Am J Med*, **63**, 947–957.

139 Rosenblatt JD, Plaeger-Marshall S, Giorgi JV, Swanson P, Chen ISY, Chin E *et al.* (1990) A clinical, hematologic, and immunologic analysis of 21 HTLV-I infected intravenous drug users. *Blood*, **76**, 409–417.

140 Rogers L (1905) The blood changes in plague. *J Pathol*, **10**, 291–295.

141 Kvasnicka HM, Thiele J and Ahmadi T (2003) Bone marrow manifestation of Lyme disease (Lyme Borreliosis). *Br J Haematol*, **120**, 723.

142 Caldwell CW and Lacombe F, Evaluation of peripheral blood lymphocytosis. Academic Information Systems, 2000, pp. 113–119.

143 Heller HM, Telford SR and Branda JA (2005) Case records from the Massachusetts general hospital: case 10-2005: a 73-year-old man with weakness and pain in the legs. *N Engl J Med*, **352**, 1358–1364.

144 McDonald JC, MacLean JD and McDade JE (1988) Imported rickettsial disease: clinical and epidemiologic features. *Am J Med*, **85**, 799–805.

145 Wilson ME, Brush AD and Meany MC (1989) Murine typhus acquired during short-term urban travel. *Am J Med*, **57**, 233–234.

146 Carulli G, Lagomarsini G, Azzarà A, Testi R, Riccioni R and Petrini M (2004) Expansion of TcRαβ+CD3+CD4–CD8–(CD4/CD8 double-negative) T lymphocytes in a case of staphylococcal toxic shock syndrome. *Acta Haematol*, **111**, 163–167.

147 Bates I, Bedu-Addo G, Bevan DH and Rutherford TR (1991) Use of immunoglobulin gene rearrangements to show clonal lymphoproliferation in hyper-reactive malarial splenomegaly. *Lancet*, **337**, 505–507.

148 Weatherall D and Kwiatkowski D. Hematologic manifestations of systemic diseases in children in developing countries. In: Nathan DG, Orkin SH, Ginsburg D and Look AT, *Nathan and Oski's Hematology of Infancy and Childhood*, 6th Edn. Saunders, Philadelphia, 2003.

149 Groom DA, Kunkel LA, Brynes RK, Parker JW, Johnson CS and Endres D (1990) Transient stress lymphocytosis during crisis of sickle cell anaemia and emergency trauma and medical conditions. *Arch Pathol Lab Med*, **114**, 570–576.

150 Wentworth P, Salonen V and Pomeroy J (1991) Transient stress lymphocytosis during crisis of sickle cell anaemia. *Arch Pathol Lab Med*, **115**, 211.

151 Chow K-C, Nacilla JQ, Witzig TE and Li C-Y (1992) Is persistent polyclonal B lymphocytosis caused by Epstein–Barr virus? A study with polymerase chain reaction and *in situ* hybridization. *Am J Hematol*, **41**, 270–275.

152 Kerrigan DP, Castillo A, Foucar K, Townsend K and Neidhart J (1989) Peripheral blood morphologic changes after high-dose antineoplastic chemotherapy and recombinant human granulocyte colony-stimulating factor administration. *Am J Clin Pathol*, **92**, 280–285.

153 Lascari AD. *Hematologic Manifestations of Childhood Diseases*. Theme-Stratton, New York, 1984.

154 Kapadia A, de Sousa M, Markenson AL, Miller DR, Good RA and Gupta S (1980) Lymphoid cell sets and scrum immunoglobulins in patients with thalassaemia intermedia: relationship to scrum iron and splenectomy. *Br J Haematol*, **45**, 405–416.

155 Marti GE, Ryan ET, Papadopoulos NM, Filling-Katz M, Barton N, Fleischer TA *et al.* (1988) Polyclonal B-cell lymphocytosis and hypergammaglobulinaemia in patients with Gaucher's disease. *Am J Hematol*, **29**, 189–194.

156 Medeiros LJ, Bhagat SK, Naylor P, Fowler D, Jaffe E and Stetler-Stevenson M (1993) Malignant thymoma associated with T-cell lymphocytosis. *Arch Pathol Lab Med*, **117**, 279–283.

157 Sneller MC, Wang J, Dale JK, Strober W, Middelton LA, Choi Y *et al.* (1997) Clinical, immunologic, and genetic features of an autoimmune lymphoproliferative syndrome associated with abnormal lymphocyte apoptosis. *Blood*, **15**, 1341–1348.

158 Papadaki T, Stamatopoulos K, Stavroyianni N, Paterakis G, Phisphis M and Stefanoudaki-Sofianatou K (2002) Evidence for T-large granular lymphocyte-mediated neutropenia in Rituximab-treated lymphoma patients: report of two cases. *Leuk Research*, **26**, 597–600.

159 Mariette X, Tsapis A, Oksenhendlcr E, Daniel M-T, d'Agay M-F, Berger R and Brouet J-C (1993) Nodular lymphocyte predominance Hodgkin's disease featuring blood atypical polyclonal B-cell lymphocytosis. *Br J Haematol*, **85**, 813–815.

160 Cook PD, Osborn CD, Helbert BJ and Rappaport ES (1991) Cleaved lymphocytes in pertussis. *Am J Clin Pathol*, **96**, 428.

161 Milne TM, Cavenagh JD, Macey MG, Dale C, Howes D, Wilkes S and Newland AC (1998) Large granular lymphocyte (LGL) expansion in 20 HIV infected patients: analysis of immunophenotype and clonality. *Br J Haematol*, **101**, Suppl. 1, 107.

162 Maldonado J and Hanlon DG (1965) Monocytosis: a current appraisal. *Mayo Clin Proc*, **40**, 248–259.

163 Glaser RM, Walker RI and Herion JC (1970) The significance of hematologic abnormalities in patients with tuberculosis. *Arch Intern Med*, **125**, 691–695.

164 Dorfman DH and Glader JH (1990) Congenital syphilis presenting in infants after the newborn period. *N Engl J Med*, **323**, 1299–1302.

165 Gutman JD, Kotton CN and Kratz A (2003) Case Records of the Massachusetts General Hospital, Case 29-2003: a 60-year-old man with fever, rigors, and sweats. *N Engl J Med*, **349**, 1168–1175.

166 Barrett O'N (1970) Monocytosis in malignant disease. *Ann Intern Med*, **73**, 991–992.

167 Schmitz LL, McClure JS, Letz CE, Dayton V, Weisdorf DJ, Parkin IL and Brunning RD (1994) Morphologic and quantitative changes in blood and marrow cells following growth factor therapy. *Am J Clin Pathol*, **101**, 67–75.

168 Huhn RD, Radwanski E, O'Connell SM, Sturgill MG, Clarke L, Cody RP *et al.* (1996) Pharmacokinetics and immunomodulatory properties of intravenously administered recombinant human interleukin-10 in healthy volunteers. *Blood*, **87**, 699–705.

169 Lebsack ME, McKenna HJ, Hoek JA, Hanna R, Feng A, Marashovsky E and Hayes FA (1997) Safety of FLT3 ligand in healthy volunteers. *Blood*, **90**, Suppl. 1, 170a.

170 Raska K, Raskova J, Shea SM, Frankel RM, Wood RH, Lifter J *et al.* (1983) T cell subsets and cellular immunity in end-stage renal disease. *Am J Med*, **75**, 734–740.

171 Pisani RJ, Witzig TE, Li CY, Morris MA and Thibodeau SN (1990) Confirmation of lymphomatous pulmonary involvement by immunophenotypic and gene rearrangement analysis of bronchoalveolar lavage fluid. *Mayo Clin Proc*, **65**, 651–656.

172 Moake IL, Landry PR, Oren ME, Sayer BL and Heffner LT (1974) Transient peripheral plasmacytosis. *Am J Clin Pathol*, **62**, 8–15.

173 Ghilardi N, Wiestner A, Kikuchi M, Ohsaka A and Skoda RC (1999) Hereditary thrombocythaemia in a Japanese family is caused by a novel point mutation in the thrombopoietin gene. *Br J Haematol*, **107**, 310–316.

174 Fujiwara T, Hariqae H, Kameoka J, Yokoyama H, Takahashi S, Tomiya Y *et al.* (2004) A case of familial thrombocytosis: possible role of altered thrombopoietin production. *Am J Hematol*, **76**, 395–397.

175 Sturhmann M, Bashawri L, Ahmed MA, Al-Awamy BH, Kühnau W, Schmidtke J and El-Harith EA (2001) Familial thrombocytosis as a recessive, possibly X-linked trait in an Arab family. *Br J Haematol*, **112**, 616–620.

176 Ding J, Komatsu H, Wakita A, Kato-Uranishi M, Ito M, Satoh A *et al.* (2004) Familial essential thrombocythaemia associated with a dominant-positive activating mutation of the *c-MPL* gene, which encodes for the receptor for thrombopoietin. *Blood*, **103**, 4198–4200.

177 Losada R, Espinosa E, Hernández C, Dorticos E and Hernández P (1996) Thrombocytosis in patients with acute promyelocytic leukaemia during all-*trans* retinoic acid treatment. *Br J Haematol*, **95**, 704–705.

178 Maartens G, Willcox PA and Benatar SR (1990) Miliary tuberculosis: rapid diagnosis, hematologic abnormalities, and outcome in 109 treated adults. *Am J Med*, **89**, 291–296.

179 Meade RH and Brandt L (1982) Manifestations of Kawasaki disease in New England outbreak of 1980. *J Pediatr*, **100**, 558–562.

180 Feigert JM, Sweet DL, Coleman M, Variakojis D, Wisch N, Schulman J and Markowitz MH (1990) Multicentric angiofollicular lymph node hyperplasia with peripheral neuropathy, pseudotumor cerebri, IgA dysproteinaemia, and thrombocytosis in women: a distinct syndrome. *Ann Intern Med*, **113**, 362–367.

181 Gherardi RK, Maleport D and Degos J-D (1991) Castleman disease-POEMS syndrome overlap. *Ann Intern Med*, **114**, 520–521.

182 Brezis M and Lafair J (1979) Thrombocytosis in chronic eosinophilic pneumonia. *Chest*, **76**, 231–232.

183 Harker LA, Roskos LK, Marzec UM, Carter RA, Cherry JK, Sundell B *et al.* (2000) Effects of megakaryocyte growth development factor on platelet production, platelet life span, and platelet function in healthy volunteers. *Blood*, **95**, 2514–2533.

184 Weber J, Yang IC, Topalian SL, Parkinson DR, Schwartzentruber DS, Ettinghausen SE *et al.* (1993) Phase I trial of subcutaneous interleukin-6 in patients with advanced malignancies. *J Clin Oncol*, **11**, 499–506.

185 Kaushansky K (1996) The thrombocytopenia of cancer. Prospects for effective cytokine therapy. *Hematol Oncol Clin North Am*, **10**, 431–455.

186 Halpérin DS, Wacker P, Lacourt G, Félix M, Babel J-F, Aapro M and Wyss M (1990) Effects of recombinant human erythropoietin in infants with anemia of prematurity: a pilot study. *J Pediatr*, **116**, 779.

187 Ritchie JH, Fish MB, McMasters V and Grossman M (1968) Edema and hemolytic anemia in premature infants. A vitamin E deficiency syndrome. *N Engl J Med*, **279**, 1185–1190.

188 Pickering D and Cuddigan B (1969) Infantile cortical hyperostosis associated with thrombocythaemia. *Lancet*, **ii**, 464–465.

189 Bornstein Y, Rausen AR and Peterson CM (1982) Duration of thrombocytosis in infants of polydrug (including methadone) users. *J Pediatr*, **100**, 506.

190 Case Records of the Massachusetts General Hospital (2000) A 41-year-old man with multiple bony lesions and adjacent soft tissue masses. *N Engl J Med*, **342**, 875–884.

191 Kuijpers TW, Maianaski NA, Tool ATJ, Smit PA, Rake JP, Roos D and Visser G (2003) Apoptotic neutrophils in the circulation of patients with glycogen storage disease type Ib (GSD1b). *Blood*, **101**, 5021–5024.

192 Dale DC, Person RE, Bolyard AA, Aprikyan AG, Bos C, Bonilla MA *et al.* (2000) Mutation in the gene encoding neutrophil elastase in congenital and cyclical neutropenia. *Blood*, **96**, 2317–2322.

193 Dweck A, Blickstein D, Elstein D and Zimran A (2002) Thrombocytosis associated with enzyme replacement therapy in Gaucher disease. *Acta Haematol*, **108**, 94–96.

194 Monagle P and Andrew M. Developmental hemostasis: relevance to newborns and infants. In: Nathan DG, Orkin SH, Ginsburg D and Look AT, *Nathan and Oski's Hematology of Infancy and Childhood*, 6th Edn. Saunders, Philadelphia, 2003.

195 Schilling RF (1980) Platelet millionaires. *Lancet*, **ii**, 372–373.

196 Jones MI and Pierre RV (1981) The causes of extreme thrombocytosis. *Am J Clin Pathol*, **76**, 349.

197 Buss DH, Cashell AW, O'Connor ML, Richards F and Case LD (1994) Occurrence, etiology, and clinical significance of extreme thrombocytosis: a study of 280 cases. *Am J Med*, **96**, 247–253.

198 Santhosh-Kumar CR, Yohannan MD, Higgy KE and al-Mashhadani SA (1991) Thrombocytosis in adults: analysis of 777 patients. *J Intern Med*, **229**, 493–495.

199 Spigel SC and Mooney LR (1977) Extreme thrombocytosis associated with malignancy. *Cancer*, **39**, 339–341.

200 Pearson HA, Lobel JS, Kocoshis SA, Naiman IL, Windmiller J, Lammi AT *et al.* (1979) A new syndrome of refractory sideroblastic anemia with vacuolation of marrow precursors and exocrine pancreatic dysfunction. *J Pediatr*, **95**, 976–984.

201 Nieken J, Mulder NH, Buter J, Vellenga E, Limburg PC, Piers DA and de Vries EG (1995) Recombinant human interleukin-6 induces a rapid and reversible anemia in cancer patients. *Blood*, **86**, 900–905.

202 Bussel JB, Mukherjee R and Stone AJ (2001) A pilot study of rhuIL-11 treatment of refractory ITP. *Am J Hematol*, **66**, 172–177.

203 Gołab J, Zagożdżon R, Stokłosa T, Lasek W, Jakóbisiak M, Pojda Z and Machaj E (1998) Erythropoietin prevents the development of interleukin-12-induced anemia and thrombocytopenia but does not decrease its antitumor activity in mice. *Blood*, **91**, 4387–4388.

204 Biaggioni I, Robertson D, Krantz S, Jones M and Haile V (1994) The anemia of primary autonomic failure and its reversal with recombinant erythropoietin. *Ann Intern Med*, **121**, 181–186.

205 Gomes MER, Deinum J, Timmers HJLNM and Lenders JWM (2003) Occam's razor; anaemia and orthostatic hypotension. *Lancet*, **363**, 1282.

206 Puig J, Corcoy R and Rodriguez-Espinosa J (1998) Anemia secondary to vitamin D intoxication. *Ann Intern Med*, **128**, 602–603.

207 Perrotta S, Nobili B, Rossi F, Criscuolo M, Iolascon A, Di Pinto D *et al.* (2002) Infant hypervitaminosis A causes severe anemia and thrombocytopenia: evidence of a retinol-dependent bone marrow growth inhibition. *Blood*, **99**, 2017–2022.

208 Hammett-Stabler CA, Broussard LA, Winecker RE and Ropero-Miller JD (2002) New insights into an old poison, arsenic. *Lab Med*, **33**, 437–447.

209 Arai S and Vogelsang GB (2000) Management of graft-versus-host disease. *CME Bulletin Haematology*, **14**, 190–204.

210 Steer A, Daley AJ and Curtis N (2005) Suppurative sequelae of symbiosis. *Lancet*, **365**, 188.

211 Fisch P, Handgretinger R and Schaefer H-E (2000) Pure red cell aplasia. *Br J Haematol*, **111**, 1010–1022.

212 Winkler M, Schulze F, Jost U, Ringe B and Pichlmayr R (1993) Anaemia associated with Fk-506 immunosuppression. *Lancet*, **341**, 1035–1036.

213 Lin Y-W, Okazaki S, Hamahata K, Watanabe K-i, Asami I, Yoshibayashi M *et al.* (1999) Acute pure

red cell aplasia associated with allopurinol therapy. *Am J Hematol*, **61**, 209–211.

214 Tanaka N, Ishada F and Tanaka E (2004) Ribavirin-induced red-cell aplasia during treatment of hepatitis C. *N Engl J Med*, **350**, 1264–1265.

215 Niebrugge DJ, Benjamin DR, Christie D and Scott CR (1982) Hereditary transcobalamin II deficiency presenting as red cell hypoplasia. *J Pediatr*, **101**, 732–735.

216 Tauchi T, Iwama H, Kaku H, Kimura Y and Ohyashiki K (1999) Remission of pure-red-cell aplasia associated with operative cure of lung cancer. *Am J Hematol*, **61**, 157–158.

217 Baker RI, Manoharan A, de Luca E and Begley CG (1993) Pure red cell aplasia of pregnancy: a distinct clinical entity. *Br J Haematol*, **85**, 619–622.

218 Volin L and Ruutu T (1990) Pure red-cell aplasia of long duration after major ABO-incompatible bone marrow transplantation. *Acta Haematol*, **84**, 195–197.

219 Bolan CD, Leitman SF, Griffith LM, Wesley RA, Procter Jl, Stroncek DF *et al.* (2001) Delayed donor red cell chimerism and pure red cell aplasia following major ABO-incompatible nonmyeloablative hematopoietic stem cell transplantation. *Blood*, **98**, 1687–1694.

220 Casadevall N, Nataf J, Viron B, Kolta A, Kiladjian J-J, Martin-Dupont P *et al.* (2002) Pure red cell aplasia and antierythropoietin antibodies in patients treated with recombinant erythropoietin. *N Engl J Med*, **346**, 469–475.

221 Lau KS and White JC (1969) Myelosclerosis associated with systemic lupus erythematosus in patients in West Malaysia. *J Clin Pathol*, **22**, 433–438.

222 Yetgin S and Ozsoylu S (1982) Myeloid metaplasia in vitamin D deficiency rickets. *Scand J Haematol*, **28**, 180–185.

223 Ravindranath Y, Paglia DE, Warrier I, Valentine W, Nakatani M and Brockway RA (1987) Glucose phosphate isomerase deficiency as a cause of hydrops fetalis. *N Engl J Med*, **316**, 258–261.

224 Kanno H, Ishikawa K, Fujii H and Miwa S (1997) Severe hexokinase deficiency as a cause of hemolytic anemia, periventricular leucomalacia and intrauterine death of the fetus. *Blood*, **90**, Suppl. 1, 8a.

225 Rodriguez V, Godwin JE, Ogburn PL, Smithson WEA and Fairbanks VF (1997) Severe anemia and hydrops fetalis in hereditary xerocytosis. *Blood*, **90**, Suppl. 1, 18b.

226 Ribeiro ML, Alloisio N, Almeida H, Gomez C, Texier P, Lemos C *et al.* (2000) Severe hereditary spherocytosis and distal renal tubular acidosis associated with total absence of band 3. *Blood*, **96**, 1602–1604.

227 Arnon S, Tamary H, Dgany O, Litmanovitz I, Regev R, Bauer R *et al.* (2004) Hydrops fetalis associated with homozygosity for hemoglobin Taybe (α 38/39 THR deletion) in newborn triplets. *Am J Hematol*, **76**, 263–266.

228 Brugnara C and Platt OS, The neonatal erythrocyte and its disorders. In: Nathan DG, Orkin SH, Ginsburg D and Look AT, *Nathan and Oski's Hematology of Infancy and Childhood*, 6th Edn. Saunders, Philadelphia, 2003.

229 Game L, Bergounioux J, Close JP, Marzouka BE and Thein SL (2003) A novel deletion causing (εγδβ)⁰ thalassaemia in a Chilean family. *Br J Haematol*, **123**, 154–159.

230 Parez N, Dommergues M, Zupan V, Chambost H, Fieschi JB, Delaunay J *et al.* (2000) Severe congenital dyserythropoietic anaemia type I: prenatal management, transfusion support and alpha-interferon therapy. *Br J Haematol*, **110**, 420–421.

231 Van Hook JW, Gill P, Cyr D and Kapur RP (1995) Diamond–Blackfan anemia as an unusual cause of nonimmune hydrops fetalis: a case report. *J Reprod Med*, **40**, 850–854.

232 Goldwurm S, Casati C, Venturi N, Strada S, Santambrighio P, Indraccolo S *et al.* (2000) Biochemical and genetic defects underlying human congenital hypotransferrinemia. *Hematol J*, **1**, 390–398.

233 McDonnell M, Hannam S and Devane SP (1998) Hydrops fetalis due to ABO incompatibility. *Arch Dis Child Fetal Neonatal Ed*, **78**, F220–221.

234 Nolan B, Hinchliffe R and Vora A (2000) Neonatal pure red cell aplasia due to maternal anti-M. *Blood*, **96**, 8a.

235 Gray ES, Balch NJ, Kohler H, Thompson WD and Simson JG (1986) Congenital leukaemia: an unusual cause of stillbirth. *Arch Dis Child*, **61**, 1001–1006.

236 Swann IL and Kendra JR (1998) Anaemia, vitamin E deficiency and failure to thrive in an infant. *Clin Lab Haematol*, **20**, 61–63.

237 Lasky EA, Polycythaemia in the newborn infant. In: Hann IM, Gibson BES, Lasky EA, (eds). *Fetal and Neonatal Haematology*. Baillière Tindall, London, 1991.

238 Sinha S, Watkins S and Corey SJ (2001) Genetic and biochemical characterization of a deletional

mutation of the extra-cellular domain of the human G-CSF receptor in a child with severe congenital neutropenia unresponsive to Neupogen. *Blood*, **98**, 440a.

239 Ancliff PJ, Blundell MP, Gale RE, Liesner R, Hann IM, Thrasher AJ and Linch DC (2001) Activating mutations in the Wiskott Aldrich Syndrome protein may define a subgroup of severe congenital neutropenia (SCN) with specific and unusual laboratory features. *Blood*, **98**, 439a.

240 Ancliff PJ (2003) Congenital neutropenia. *Blood Rev*, **17**, 209–216.

241 Sieff CA, Nisbet-Brown E and Nathan DG (2000) Congenital bone marrow failure syndromes. *Br J Haematol*, **111**, 30–42.

242 Parmley RT, Crist WM, Ragab AH, Boxer LA, Malluh A, Liu VK and Darby CP (1980) Congenital dysgranulopoietic neutropenia: clinical, serologic, ultrastructural and *in vitro* proliferative characteristics. *Blood*, **56**, 465–475.

243 Wetzler M, Talpaz M, Kleinerman ES, King A, Huh YO, Gutterman JU and Kurzrock R (1990) A new familial immunodeficiency disorder characterized by severe neutropenia, a defective marrow release mechanism, and hypogammaglobulinemia. *Am J Med*, **89**, 663–672.

244 Hadžić N, Pagliuca A, Rela M, Portmann B, Jones A, Veys P *et al.* (2000) Correction of the hyper-IgM syndrome after liver and bone marrow transplantation. *N Engl J Med*, **342**, 320–324.

245 Pitcher LA, Taylor KM, Bartold PM, Seow K, Tong YH and Fanning S (1996) Filgrastim used successfully for asymptomatic neutropenia in Cohen's syndrome. *Aust NZ J Med*, **26**, 258.

246 van den Tweel JG (1997) Preleukaemic disorders in children: hereditary disorders and myelodysplastic syndromes. *Current Diagnostic Pathol*, **4**, 45–50.

247 Casadevall N, Croisille L, Auffray I, Tchernia G and Coulombel L (1994) Age-related alterations in erythroid and granulopoietic progenitors in Diamond Blackfan anaemia. *Br J Haematol*, **87**, 369–375.

248 Aksu G, Kütükçüler N, Genel F, Vergin C and Omowaire B (2003) Griscelli syndrome without hemophagocytosis in an eleven-year-old girl: Expanding the phenotypic spectrum of *Rab27A* mutations in humans. *Am J Med Genet*, **116A**, 329–333.

249 Kuijpers TW, Maianski NA, Tool ATJ, Becker K, Plecko B, Valianpour F *et al.* (2004) Neutrophils in Barth syndrome (BTHS) avidly bind annexin-V in the absence of apoptosis. *Blood*, **103**, 3915–3923.

250 Corral J, Gonzalez-Conejero R, Pujol-Moix N, Domenech P and Vicente V (2004) Mutation analysis of HPS1, the gene mutated in Hermansky–Pudlak syndrome, in patients with isolated platelet dense-granule deficiency. *Haematologica*, **89**, 325–329.

251 Roe TF, Coates TD, Thomas DW, Miller JH and Gilsanz V (1992) Treatment of chronic inflammatory bowel disease in glycogen storage disease type Ib with colony-stimulating factors. *N Engl J Med*, **326**, 1666–1669.

252 Ino T, Sherwood G, Cutz E, Benson LN, Rose IV and Freedman RM (1988) Dilated cardiomyopathy with neutropenia, short stature and abnormal carnitine metabolism. *J Pediatr*, **113**, 511–514.

253 Ronghe M, Cantlay AM, Chasty RC, Allen JT, Pennock CA, Oakhill A and Steward CG (1998) Exclusion of organic acid disorders in children with chronic idiopathic neutropenia. *Br J Haematol*, **101**, Suppl. 1, 74.

254 Susa JS, Bennett MJ and Jones PM (2003) Lethargy, failure to thrive, and vomiting in a neonate. *Lab Med*, **34**, 775–778.

255 Sampson B, Fagerhol MK, Sunderkötter C, Golden BE, Richmond P, Klein N *et al.* (2003) Hyperzincaemia with hypercalprotectinaemia: a new disorder of zinc metabolism. *Lancet*, **360**, 1742–1745.

256 Al Mulla ZS and Christensen RD (1995) Neutropenia in the neonate. *Clin Perinatol*, **22**, 711–739.

257 Hien TT, Liem NT, Dung NT, San LT, Mai PP, Chau NN van V *et al.* (2004) Avian influenza A (H5N1) in 10 patients in Vietnam. *N Engl J Med*, **350**, 1179–1188.

258 Penchansky L and Jordan JA (1997) Transient erythroblastopenia of childhood associated with human herpesvirus type 6, variant B. *Am J Clin Pathol*, **108**, 127–132.

259 Hashimoto H, Maruyama H, Fujimoto K, Sakakura T, Seishu S and Okuda N (2002) The hematologic findings associated with thrombocytopenia during the acute phase of exanthem subitum confirmed by primary human herpesvirus-6 infection. *J Pediatr Hematol Oncol*, **24**, 211–214.

260 Pont J, Puchhammer-Stockl E, Chott A, Popow-Kraupp T, Kienzer H, Postner G and Honetz N (1992) Recurrent granulocytic aplasia as clinical presentation of a persistent parvovirus B19 infection. *Br J Haematol*, **80**, 160–165.

261 Salas R, de Manzione N, Tesh RB, Rico-Hesse R, Shope RE, Betancourt A *et al.* (1991) Venezuelan haemorrhagic fever. *Lancet*, **338**, 1033–1036.

262 Fisher-Hoch SP, Khan JA, Rehman S, Mirza S, Khurshid M and McCormick JB (1995) Crimean Congo-haemorrhagic fever treated with oral ribavirin. *Lancet*, **346**, 472–475.

263 Schanen A, Gallou G, Hincky JM and Saron MF (1998) A rash, circulating anticoagulant, then meningitis. *Lancet*, **351**, 1856.

264 Lee N, Hui D, Wu A, Chan P, Cameron P, Joynt GM *et al.* (2003) A major outbreak of severe acute respiratory syndrome in Hong Kong. *N Engl J Med*, **348**, 1986–1994.

265 Pullen RL and Stuart BM (1945) Tularemia. *JAMA*, **129**, 495–500.

266 Sheehy TW, Hazlett D and Turk RE (1973) Scrub typhus: a comparison of chloramphenicol and tetracycline in its treatment. *Arch Intern Med*, **132**, 77–80.

267 Brettman LR, Lewin S, Holzman RS, Goldman WD, Marr JS, Kechijian P and Schinella R (1981) Rickettsial pox: report of an outbreak and a contemporary review. *Medicine*, **60**, 363–372.

268 Parola P, Jourdan J and Raoult D (1998) Tick-borne infection caused by *Rickettsia africae* in the West Indies. *N Engl J Med*, **338**, 1391.

269 Goodman JL, Nelson C, Vitale B, Madigan JE, Dumler JS, Kurtti TJ and Munderloh UG (1996) Direct cultivation of the causative agent of human granulocytic ehrlichiosis. *N Engl J Med*, **334**, 209–215.

270 Goodwin RA, Shapiro JL, Thurman GH, Thurman SS and des Prez RM (1980) Disseminated histoplasmosis: clinical and pathological correlations. *Medicine*, **59**, 1–33.

271 Blanche S, Tardieu M, Rustin P, Slama A, Barret B, Firtion G *et al.* (1999) Persistent mitochondrial dysfunction and perinatal exposure to antiretroviral nucleoside analogues. *Lancet*, **354**, 1084–1089.

272 Voog E, Morschhauser F and Solal-Céligny P (2003) Neutropenia in patients treated with rituximab. *N Engl J Med*, **348**, 2691–2694.

273 Richardson PG, Barlogie B, Berenson J, Singhal S, Jagannath S, Irwin D *et al.* (2003) A phase 2 study of bortezomib in relapsed refractory myeloma. *N Engl J Med*, **348**, 2609–2617.

274 Demetri GD, von Mehren M, Blanke CD, Van den Abbeele AD, Eisenberg B, Roberts PJ *et al.* (2002) Efficacy and safety of imatinib mesylate in advanced gastrointestinal stromal tumours. *N Engl J Med*, **347**, 472–480.

275 Eisenmenger W, Drasch G, von Clarmann M, Kretschmer E and Roider G (1991) Clinical and morphological findings on mustard gas [bis(2-chloroethyl)sulfide] poisoning. *J Forensic Sci*, **36**, 1688–1698.

276 Wallis JP, Haynes S, Stark G, Green FA, Lucas GF and Chapman CD (2002) Transfusion-related alloimmune neutropenia: an undescribed complication of blood transfusion. *Lancet*, **360**, 1073–1074.

277 Kameoka J, Funato T, Miura T, Harigae H, Saito J, Yokoyama H *et al.* (2001) Autoimmune neutropenia in pregnant women causing neonatal neutropenia. *Br J Haematol*, **114**, 198–200.

278 Bux J and Mueller-Eckhardt C (1992) Autoimmune neutropenia. *Semin Hematol*, **29**, 45–53.

279 Papadaki HA, Stamatopoulos K, Damianaki A, Anagnostopoulos A, Papadaki T, Eliopoulos AG and Eliopoulos GD (2005) Activated T-lymphocytes with myelosuppressive properties in patients with chronic idiopathic neutropenia. *Br J Haematol*, **128**, 863–876.

280 McClain K, Estrov Z, Chen H and Mahoney DH (1993) Chronic neutropenia of childhood: frequent association with parvovirus infection and correlations with bone marrow culture studies. *Br J Haematol*, **85**, 57–62.

281 Cline MI, Opelz G, Saxon A, Fahey JL and Golde DW (1976) Autoimmune panleukopenia. *N Engl J Med*, **295**, 1489–1493.

282 Levitt LJ, Ries CA and Greenberg PL (1983) Pure white cell aplasia: antibody-mediated autoimmune inhibition of granulopoiesis. *N Engl J Med*, **308**, 1141–1146.

283 Longhurst HJ, O'Grady C, Evans G, De Lord C, Hughes A, Cavenagh J and Helbert MR (2002) Anti-D immunoglobulin treatment for thrombocytopenia associated with primary antibody deficiency. *J Clin Pathol*, **55**, 64–66.

284 Niehues T, Schwarz K, Schneider M, Schroten H, Schroder E, Stephan V and Wahn V (1996) Severe combined immunodeficiency (SCID) associated neutropenia: a lesson from monozygotic twins. *Arch Dis Child*, **74**, 340–342.

285 Marques MB, Tuncer HH, Divers SG, Baker AC and Harrison DK (2005) Acute transient leucopenia as a sign of TRALI. *Am J Hematol*, **80**, 90–91.

286 Anderlini P, Przepiorka D, Champlin R and Körbling M (1996) Peripheral blood stem cell

apheresis in normal donors: the neglected side. *Blood*, **88**, 3663–3664.

287 Liu YK (1973) Leukopenia in alcoholics. *Am J Med*, **54**, 605–610.

288 Kubota M, Tsukamoto R, Kurokawa K, Imai T and Furusho K (1996) Elevated serum interferon gamma and interleukin-6 in patients with necrotizing lymphadenitis (Kikuchi's disease). *Br J Haematol*, **95**, 613–615.

289 Cordano A, Placko RP and Graham GG (1966) Hypocupremia and neutropenia in copper deficiency. *Blood*, **28**, 280–283.

290 Miyoshi I, Saito T and Iwahara Y (2004) Copper deficiency anaemia. *Br J Haematol*, **125**, 106.

291 Shoenfeld Y, Shaklai M, Ben-Baruch N, Hirschorn M and Pinkhas J (1982) Neutropenia induced by hypercarotenaemia. *Lancet*, **i**, 1245.

292 Koenig IM and Christensen RD (1989) Incidence, neutrophil kinetics, and natural history of neonatal neutropenia associated with maternal hypertension. *N Engl J Med*, **321**, 557–562.

293 Engle WD and Rosenfeld CR (1984) Neutropenia in high-risk neonates. *J Pediatr*, **105**, 982–986.

294 Zach TL, Steinhorn RH, Georgieff MK, Mills MM and Green TP (1990) Leukopenia associated with extracorporeal membrane oxygenation in newborn infants. *J Pediatr*, **116**, 440–443.

295 Rogers ZR, Bergstrom SK, Amylon MD, Buchanan GR and Glader BE (1989) Reduced neutrophil counts in children with transient erythroblastopenia of childhood. *J Pediatr*, **115**, 746–8.

296 Lundin J, Kimby E, Björkholm M, Broliden P-A, Gelsing F, Hjalmar V et al. (2002) Phase II trial of subcutaneous anti-CD53 monoclonal antibody alemtuzumab (Campath 1H) in the first-line treatment of chronic lymphocytic leukemia (B-CLL). *Blood*, **100**, 768–773.

297 Archer RK, Engisch HJC, Gaha T and Ruxton J (1971) The eosinophil leucocytes in the blood and bone marrow of patients with Down's anomaly. *Br J Haematol*, **21**, 271–276.

298 Nakahatc T, Spicer SS, Leary AG, Ogawa M, Franklin W and Goetzl EJ (1984) Circulating eosinophil colony-forming cells in pure eosinophil aplasia. *Ann Intern Med*, **101**, 321–324.

299 Juhlin LL and Michaelsson G (1977) A new syndrome characterized by absence of eosinophils and basophils. *Lancet*, **i**, 1233–1235.

300 Welles SL, Mueller N, Tachibana N, Shishime E, Okayama A, Murai K and Tsuda K (1991) Decreased eosinophil numbers in HTLV-I carriers. *Lancet*, **337**, 987.

301 Grattan CEH, Dawn G, Gibbs S and Francis DM (2003) Blood basophil numbers in chronic ordinary urticaria and healthy controls: diurnal variation, influence of loratadine and prednisolone and relationship to disease activity. *Clin Exp Immunol*, **33**, 337–341.

302 Gossage DL and Buckley RH (1990) Prevalence of lymphocytopenia in severe combined immunodeficiency. *N Engl J Med*, **323**, 1422–1423.

303 Wyllie DH, Bowler ICJW and Peto TEA (2004) Relation between lymphopenia and bacteraemia in UK adults with medical emergencies. *J Clin Pathol*, **57**, 950–955.

304 Hasenclever D and Diehl V (1998) A prognostic score for advanced Hodgkin's disease. International Prognostic Factors Project on Advanced Hodgkin's Disease. *N Engl J Med*, **339**, 1506–1514.

305 Wickramasinghe SN (1998) Congenital dyserythropoietic anaemias: clinical features, haematological morphology and new biochemical data. *Blood Rev*, **12**, 178–200.

306 Hou M, Horney E, Stockelberg D, Jacobsson S, Kutti J and Wadenvik H (1997) Multiple quinine-dependent antibodies in a patient with episodic thrombocytopenia, neutropenia, lymphocytopenia, and granulomatous hepatitis. *Blood*, **90**, 4806–4811.

307 Berglund B and Ekblom B (1991) Effect of recombinant human erythropoietin treatment on blood pressure and some haematological parameters in healthy men. *J Intern Med*, **229**, 125–130.

308 Cummins D, Wilson ME, Foulgar KJ, Dawson D and Hogarth AM (1995) Effects of influenza vaccination on the blood counts of people aged over 65: case report and prospective study. *Br J Haematol*, **101**, Suppl. 1, 54.

309 Symmons DPM, Farr M, Salmon M and Bacon PA (1989) Lymphopenia in rheumatoid arthritis. *J R Soc Med*, **82**, 462–463.

310 Budman DR and Steinberg AD (1977) Hematologic aspects of systemic lupus erythematosus. *Ann Intern Med*, **86**, 220–229.

311 Daniele RP and Rowlands DT (1976) Lymphocyte subpopulations in sarcoidosis: correlation with disease activity and duration. *Ann Intern Med*, **85**, 593–600.

312 Bynoe AG, Scott CS, Ford P and Roberts BE (1983) Decreased T helper cells in the myelodysplastic syndromes. *Br J Haematol*, **54**, 97–102.

313 Bowers TK and Eckert E (1978) Leukopenia in anorexia nervosa: lack of an increased risk of infection. *Arch Intern Med*, **138**, 1520–1523.

314 Santos PC and Falcao RP (1990) Decreased lymphocyte subsets and K-cell activity in iron deficiency anemia. *Acta Haematol*, **84**, 118–121.

315 Robbins G and Brozovic B (1985) Lymphocytopenia in regular platelet apheresis donors. *Br J Haematol*, **61**, 558–559.

316 Unkrig CJ, Schroder R and Scharf RE (1994) Lorenzo's oil and thrombocytopenia. *N Engl J Med*, **330**, 577.

317 Masci AM, Palmieri G, Vitiello L, Montella L, Perna F, Orlandi P *et al.* (2003) Clonal expansion of CD8+ BV8 T lymphocytes in bone marrow characterizes thymoma-associated B lymphopenia. *Blood*, **101**, 3106–3108.

318 Lackner A, Basu O, Bierings M, Lassay L, Schaefer UW, Révész T *et al.* (2000) Haematopoietic stem cell transplantation for amegakaryocytic thrombocytopenia. *Br J Haematol*, **109**, 773–775.

319 Alter B. Inherited bone marrow failure syndromes. In: Nathan DG, Orkin SH, Ginsburg D and Look AT, *Nathan and Oski's Hematology of Infancy and Childhood*, 6th Edn. Saunders, Philadelphia, 2003.

320 Roberts IA and Murray NA (1999) Management of thrombocytopenia in neonates. *Br J Haematol*, **105**, 864–870.

321 Koenig JM and Christensen RD (1989) Neutropenia and thrombocytopenia in infants with Rh hemolytic disease. *J Pediatr*, **114**, 625–631.

322 Wagner T, Bernaschek G and Geissler G (2000) Inhibition of megakaryopoiesis by Kell-related antibodies. *N Engl J Med*, **343**, 72.

323 Blanchette VS, Johnson J and Rand M (2000) The management of alloimmune neonatal thrombocytopenia. *Baillière's Clin Haematol*, **13**, 365–390.

324 Abelman W and Virchis A (2005) An unusual cause of thrombocytopenia. *Clin Lab Haematol*, **27**, 215–216.

325 Acharya S and Bussel JB (2000) Hematologic toxicity of sodium valproate. *J Pediatr Hematol Oncol*, **22**, 62–65.

326 Bhattacharyya J, Kumar R, Tyagi S, Kishore J, Mahapatra M and Choudhry VP (2005) Human parvovirus B19-induced acquired pure amegakaryocytic thrombocytopenia. *Br J Haematol*, **128**, 128–129.

327 Garcia-Suárez J, Burgaleta C, Hernanz N, Albarran F, Tobaruela P and Alvarez-Mon M (2000) HCV-associated thrombocytopenia: clinical characteristics and platelet response after recombinant α2b-interferon therapy. *Br J Haematol*, **110**, 98–103.

328 Hoffman R (1991) Acquired pure amegakaryocytic thrombocytopenic purpura. *Semin Hematol*, **28**, 303–312.

329 Fogarty PF, Stetler-Stevenson M, Pereira A and Dunbar CE (2005) Large granular lymphocytic proliferation-associated cyclic thrombocytopenia. *Am J Hematol*, **79**, 334–336.

330 Ando M, Iwamoto Y, Suda A, Tsuchiya K and Nihei H (2001) New insights into the thrombopoietic status of patient on dialysis through the evaluation of megakaryocytopoiesis in bone marrow and of endogenous thrombopoietin levels. *Blood*, **97**, 915–921.

331 Li J, Yang C, Xia Y, Bertino A, Glaspy J, Roberts M and Kuter DJ (2001) Thrombocytopenia caused by the development of antibodies to thrombopoietin. *Blood*, **98**, 3241–3248.

332 Curtis BR, Ali S, Aitman TJ, Ebert DD, Lenes BA and Aster RH (2001) Maternal isoimmunization against CD36 (GPIV) should be considered in unresolved cases of apparent immune neonatal thrombocytopenia. *Blood*, **98**, 710a.

333 Dickerman JD, Holbrook PR and Zinkham WH (1972) Etiology and therapy of thrombocytopenia associated with sarcoidosis. *J Pediatr*, **81**, 758–764.

334 Parameswaran R, Cavenagh JD, Davies JK and Newland AC (1999) Immune cytopenias as the presenting feature of common variable immune deficiency. *Br J Haematol*, **105**, Suppl. 1, 51.

335 West KA, Anderson DR, McAlister VC, Hewlett TJ, Belitsky P, Smith JW and Kelton JG (1999) Alloimmune thrombocytopenia after organ transplantation. *N Engl J Med*, **341**, 1504–1507.

336 Solenthaler M, Krauss JK, Boehlen F, Koller R, Hug M and Lammle B (1999) Fatal fresh frozen plasma infusion containing HPA-1a alloantibodies. *Br J Haematol*, **106**, 258–259.

337 Jubelirer SJ, Koenig BA and Bates MC (1999) Acute profound thrombocytopenia following C7E3 Fab (Abciximab) therapy: case reports, review of the literature and implications for therapy. *Am J Hematol*, **62**, 205–208.

338 Bougie DW, Wilker PR, Wuitschick ED, Curtis BR, Malik M, Levine S *et al.* (2002) Acute thrombocytopenia after treatment with tirofiban or eptifibatide is associated with antibodies specific for ligand-occupies GPIIb/IIIa. *Blood*, **100**, 2071–2076.

339 Pamuk GE, Donmez S, Turgut B, Demir M and Vural O (2005) Rituximab-induced acute thrombocytopenia in a patient with prolymphocytic leukemia. *Am J Hematol*, **78**, 81.

340 Arnold J, Ouwehand WH, Smith GA and Cohen H (1998) A young woman with petechiae. *Lancet*, **351**, 618.

341 Wright JG (1992) Severe thrombocytopenia secondary to asymptomatic cytomegalovirus infection in an immunocompetent host. *J Clin Pathol*, **45**, 1037–1038.

342 Kitamura K, Ohta H, Ihara T, Kamiya H, Ochiai H, Yamanishi K and Tanaka K (1994) Idiopathic thrombocytopenic purpura after human herpesvirus 6 infection. *Lancet*, **344**, 830.

343 Bauduer F, Marty F, Larrouy M and Ducout L (1998) Immunologic thrombocytopenic purpura as presenting symptom of hepatitis C infection. *Am J Hematol*, **57**, 338–340.

344 Beanie RM (1993) Mycoplasma and thrombocytopenia. *Arch Dis Child*, **68**, 250.

345 Castagnola E, Dufour C, Timitilli A and Giacchino R (1994) Idiopathic thrombocytopenic purpura associated with scarlet fever. *Arch Dis Child*, **70**, 164.

346 al-Majed SA, al-Momen AK, al-Kassimi FA, al-Zeer A, Kambal AM and Baaqil H (1995) Tuberculosis presenting as immune thrombocytopenic purpura. *Acta Haematol*, **94**, 135–138.

347 Spedini P (2002) Tuberculosis presenting as immune thrombocytopenic purpura. *Haematologica*, **87**, ELTO9.

348 Gürkan E, Başlamişli F, Güvenç B, Bozkurt B and Ünsal Ç (2003) Immune thrombocytopenic purpura associated with *Brucella* and *Toxoplasma* infections. *Am J Hematol*, **74**, 52–54.

349 Franchini M and Veneri D (2003) *Helicobacter pylori* infection and immune thrombocytopenic purpura. *Haematologica*, **88**, 1087–1091.

350 Leissinger CA (1990) Severe thrombocytopenia associated with cocaine abuse. *Ann Intern Med*, **112**, 708–710.

351 Hesseling PB (1992) Onyalai. *Bailliere's Clin Haematol*, **5**, 457–473.

352 Shah C and Grethlein SJ (2004) Case report of rituximab-induced thrombocytopenia. *Am J Hematol*, **75**, 263.

353 Schulman I, Pierce M, Lukens A and Currimbhoy Z (1960) Studies on thrombopoiesis I. A factor in normal human plasma required for platelet production; chronic thrombocytopenia due to its deficiency. *Blood*, **16**, 943–957.

354 Upshaw JD (1978) Congenital deficiency of a factor in normal plasma that reverses microangiopathic hemolysis and thrombocytopenia. *N Engl J Med*, **298**, 1350–1352.

355 Rees DC, Iolascon A, Carella M, O'Marcaigh AS, Kendra JR, Jowitt SN et al. (2005) Stomatocytic haemolysis and macrothrombocytopenia (Mediterranean stomatocytosis/macrothrombocytopenia) is the haematological presentation of phytosterolaemia. *Br J Haematol*, **130**, 297–309.

356 Mulliken JB, Anupindi S, Ezekowitz RAB and Mihm MC (2004) Case records of the Massachusetts General Hospital, Case 13-2004: a newborn girl with a large cutaneous lesion, thrombocytopenia, and anemia. *N Engl J Med*, **350**, 1764–1775.

357 Paciucci PA, Mandeli J, Oleksowicz L, Ameglio F and Holland JF (1990) Thrombocytopenia during immunotherapy with interleukin-2 by constant infusion. *Am J Med*, **89**, 308–312.

358 Locker GJ, Kapiotis S, Veitl M, Mader RM, Stoiser B, Kofler J et al. (1999) Activation of endothelium by immunotherapy with interleukin-2 in patients with malignant disorders. *Br J Haematol*, **105**, 912–919.

359 Maddocks S and O'Brien R (2000) African trypanosomiasis in Australia. *N Engl J Med*, **342**, 1254.

360 McDonald GB, Sharma P, Matthews DE, Shulman HM and Thomas ED (1984) Venocclusive disease of the liver after bone marrow transplantation: diagnosis, incidence, and predisposing factors. *Hepatology*, **4**, 116–122.

361 Kitchens CS (2004) Thrombocytopenia due to acute venous thromboembolism and its role in expanding the differential diagnosis of heparin-induced thrombocytopenia. *Am J Hematol*, **76**, 69–73.

362 Van der Stuyft P, Gianella A, Pirard M, Cespedes J, Lora J, Peredo C et al. (1999) Urbanisation of yellow fever in Santa Cruz, Bolivia. *Lancet*, **354**, 1559–1562.

363 Sexton DJ, Rollin PE, Breitschwerdt EB, Corey GR, Myers SA, Dumais MR et al. (1997) Life-threatening Cache Valley virus infection. *N Engl J Med*, **336**, 547–549.

364 Goh KJ, Tan CT, Chew NK, Tan PSK, Kamarulzaman A, Sarji SA et al. (2000) Clinical features of Nipah virus encephalitis among pig farmers in Malaysia. *N Engl J Med*, **342**, 1229–1235.

365 Pinn TG and Sowden D (1998) Queensland tick typhus. *Aust NZ J Med*, **28**, 824–826.

366 Thiebaut MM, Bricaire F and Raoult D (1997) Scrub typhus after a trip to Vietnam. *N Engl J Med*, **336**, 1613–1614.

367 Roberts SA and Ellis-Pegler RB (1997) Murine typhus in the Kaukapakapa area again. *Aust NZ J Med*, **27**, 446–447.

368 Brouqui P, Lascola B, Roux V and Raoult D (1999) Chronic *Bartonella quintana* bacteremia in homeless patients. *N Engl J Med*, **340**, 184–189.

369 Bush LM, Abrams BH, Beall A and Johnson CC (2001) Index case of fatal inhalational anthrax due to bioterrorism in the United States. *N Engl J Med*, **345**, 1607–1610.

370 Sevinc A, Kutlu NO, Kuku I, Ozgen U, Aydogdu I and Soylu H (2000) Severe epistaxis in brucellosis-induced isolated thrombocytopenia: a report of two cases. *Clin Lab Haematol*, **22**, 373–375.

371 Serefhanoglu K, Kaya E, Sevinc A, Aydogdu I, Kuku I and Ersoy Y (2003) Isolated thrombocytopenia: the presenting feature of typhoid fever. *Clin Lab Haematol*, **25**, 63–65.

372 Tunbridge AJ, Dockrell DH, Channer KS and McKendrick MW (2002) A breathless triathlete. *Lancet*, **359**, 130.

373 Vonderheide RH, Thadhani R and Kuter DJ (1996) Association of thrombocytopenia and the use of intra-aortic balloon pump. *Blood*, **88**, Suppl. 1, 63b.

374 Turnbull A and Almeyda J (1970) Idiopathic thrombocytopenic purpura and Kaposi's sarcoma. *Proc R Soc Med*, **63**, 603–605.

375 Kimura H, Nasu K, Sakai C, Shiga Y, Miyamoto E, Shintaku M *et al.* (1998) Histiocytic sarcoma of the spleen associated with hypoalbuminemia, hypoγ-globulinemia and thrombocytopenia as a possibly unique clinical entity—report of three cases. *Leuk Lymphoma*, **31**, 217–224.

376 Baker GR and Levin J (1998) Transient thrombocytopenia produced by administration of macrophage colony-stimulating factor: investigations of the mechanism. *Blood*, **91**, 89–99.

377 Diaz-Sánchez CL, Lifshitz-Guinzberg A, Ignacio-Ibarra G, Halabe-Cherem J and Quinones-Galvan A (1998) Survival after massive (> 2000) Africanized honeybee stings. *Arch Intern Med*, **158**, 925–927.

378 Clayton PT, Bowron A, Mills KA, Massoud A, Casteels M and Milla PJ (1993) Phytosterolaemia in children with parenteral nutrition-associated cholestatic liver disease. *Gastroenterology*, **105**, 1806–1813.

379 Auborg P (1994) Lorenzo's oil and thrombocytopenia. *N Engl J Med*, **330**, 577.

380 O'Brien H, Amess JAL and Mollin JD (1982) Recurrent thrombocytopenia, erythroid hypoplasia and sideroblastic anaemia associated with hypothermia. *Br J Haematol*, **51**, 451–456.

381 Dittman WA (2000) Congenital relapsing fever (*Borrelia hermsii* infection) *Blood*, **96**, 3333.

382 Willoughby MLN. *Paediatric Haematology*. Churchill Livingstone, Edinburgh, 1977.

383 Bader-Meunier B, Breton-Gorius B, Cramer E, Mielot F, Rötig A, Dommergues JP and Tchernia G (1997) Hematology: a clue to the diagnosis of mitochondrial cytopathies. *Blood*, **96**, Suppl. 1, 9b.

384 Hayward CP, Rivard GE, Kane WH, Drouin J, Zheng S, Moore JC and Kelton JG (1996) An autosomal dominant, qualitative platelet disorder associated with multimerin deficiency, abnormalities in platelet factor V, thrombospondin, von Willebrand factor, and fibrinogen and an epinephrine aggregation defect. *Blood*, **87**, 4967–4978.

385 Maurer HM, Fratkin M, McWilliams NB, Kirkpatrick D, Draper DW, Haggins JC and Hunter CR (1976) Effects of phototherapy on platelet counts in lowbirthweight infants and on platelet production and life span in rabbits. *Pediatrics*, **57**, 506–512.

386 Ballin A, Korea G, Kohelet D, Burger R, Greenwald M, Bryan AC and Zipursky A (1987) Reduction in platelet counts induced by mechanical ventilation in the newborn infants. *J Pediatr*, **111**, 445–449.

387 Yang J, Lee C-H, Yang M, Li K, Ng P-C, Yuen M-P and Fok T-F (2001) Association between thrombocytopenia and mechanical ventilation in infants with respiratory distress syndrome. *Blood*, **98**, 37a.

388 Carroll DN, Kamath P and Stewart L (2005) Congenital viral infection? *Lancet*, **365**, 1110.

389 Kurata Y, Nishioeda Y, Tsubakio T and Kitani T (1980) Thrombocytopenia in Graves' disease: effect of T_3 on platelet kinetics. *Acta Haematol*, **63**, 185–190.

390 Bowles KM, Turner GE and Wimperis JZ (2004) Resolution of chronic severe refractory thrombocytopenia after treatment of hypothyroidism. *J Clin Pathol*, **57**, 995–996.

391 Pei SX, Chen XJ, Si Ren BZ, Liu YH, Cheng XS, Harris EM *et al.* (1989) Chronic mountain sickness in Tibet. *Q J Med*, **71**, 555–574.

392 Fischereder M and Jaffe JP (1994) Thrombocytopenia following acute acetaminophen overdose. *Am J Hematol*, **45**, 258–259.

393 Takahashi N and Nishida H (1997) New exanthematous disease with thrombocytopenia in neonates. *Arch Dis Child Fetal Neonatal Ed*, **77**, F79.

394 Prella M, Baccalà R, Horisberger J-D, Belin D, di Raimondo F, Invernizzi R *et al.* (2001) Haemolytic onset of Wilson's disease in a patient with homozygous truncation of ATP7B at ARG1319. *Br J Haematol*, **114**, 230–232.

395 Smith KA, Nelson PN, Warren P, Astley SJ, Murray PG and Greenman J (2004) Demystified . . . recombinant antibodies. *J Clin Pathol*, **57**, 912–917.

396 Azuno Y, Yaga K, Sasayama T and Kimoto K (1999) Thrombocytopenia induced by Jui, a traditional Chinese herbal medicine. *Lancet*, **354**, 304–305.

397 http//:moon.ouhsc.edu/george

398 Hohlfeld P, Forestier F, Kaplan C, Tissot JD and Daffos F (1994) Fetal thrombocytopenia: a retrospective survey of 5,194 fetal blood samplings. *Blood*, **84**, 1851–1856.

399 Chng WJ and Howard MR (2001) Pel–Ebstein fever with cyclical pancytopenia. *J R Soc Med*, **94**, 84–85.

400 Gonzalez CH, Durkin-Stamm MV, Geimer NF, Shahidi NT, Schilling RF, Rubira F and Opitz JM (1977) The WT syndrome—a 'new' autosomal dominant pleiotropic trait of radial/ulnar hypoplasia with high risk of bone marrow failure and/or leukemia. *Birth Defects Orig Artic Ser*, **13(3B)**, 31–38.

401 Ihara K, Ishii I, Eguchi M, Takada H, Suminoe A, Good RA and Hara T (1999) Identification of mutations in the c-mpl gene in congenital amegakaryocytic thrombocytopenia. *Proc Natl Acad Sci USA*, **96**, 3132–3136.

402 González-del Angel A, Cervera M, Gómez L, Pérez-Vera P, Orozco L, Carnevale A, Del Castillo V (2000) Ataxia-pancytopenia syndrome. *Am J Med Genet*, **90**, 252–254.

403 Press OW, Fingert H, Lott IT and Dickersin R (1983) Pancytopenia in mannosidosis. *Arch Intern Med*, **143**, 1266–1268.

404 Hricik DE and Hussain R (1984) Pancytopenia and hepatosplenomegaly in oxalosis. *Arch Intern Med*, **144**, 167–168.

405 Kelleher JF, Yudkoff M, Hutchinson R, August CS and Cohn RM (1980) The pancytopenia of isovaleric acidemia. *Pediatrics*, **65**, 1023–1027.

406 Walter MJ and Dang CV (1998) Pancytopenia secondary to oxalosis in a 23-year-old woman. *Blood*, **91**, 4394.

407 Kind T, Levy J, Lee M, Kaicker S, Nicholson J and Kane SA (2002) Cobalamin C disease presenting as hemolytic-uremic syndrome in the neonatal period. *J Pediatr Hematol Oncol*, **24**, 327–329.

408 Blatt J, Katerji A, Barmada M, Wenger SL and Penchansky L (1994) Pancytopenia and vacuolation of marrow precursors associated with necrotizing encephalopathy. *Br J Haematol*, **86**, 207–209.

409 Çetin M, Hiçsönmez G and Gögüs S (1998) Myelodysplastic syndrome associated with Griscelli syndrome. *Leuk Res*, **22**, 859–862.

410 Bazarbachi A, Muakkit S, Ayas M, Taher A, Salem Z, Solh H and Haidar JH (1998) Thiamine-responsive myelodysplasia. *Br J Haematol*, **102**, 1098–1100.

411 Ferrari E, Ascari E, Bossolo PA and Barosi G (1976) Sheehan's syndrome with complete bone marrow aplasia: long-term results of substitution therapy with hormones. *Br J Haematol*, **33**, 575–582.

412 Basser RL, O'Flaherty E, Green M, Edmonds M, Nichol J, Menchaca DM, Cohen B and Begley CG (2002) Development of pancytopenia with neutralizing antibodies to thrombopoietin after multicycle chemotherapy supported by megakaryocyte growth and development factor. *Blood*, **99**, 2599–2602.

413 Resuke WH, Anderson C, Pastuszak WT, Conway SR and Firshein SI (1991) Arsenic intoxication presenting as a myelodysplastic syndrome: a case report. *Am J Hematol*, **36**, 291–293.

414 Case records of the Massachusetts General Hospital (1989) Case 33–1989. *N Engl J Med*, **321**, 454–463.

415 Millá F, Feliu E, Ribera JM, Junta J, Flores A, Vidal J *et al.* (1993) Electron microscopic identification of parvovirus virions in erythroid and granulocytic-line cells in a patient with human parvovirus B19 induced pancytopenia. *Leuk Lymphoma*, **10**, 483–487.

416 Harkess JR (1993) Ehrlichiosis: a cause of bone marrow hypoplasia in humans. *Am J Hematol*, **30**, 265–266.

417 Al-Eissa YA, Assuhaimi SA, Al-Fawaz IM, Higgy KE, Al-Nasser MN and Al-Mobaireck KF (1993) Pancytopenia in children with brucellosis: clinical manifestations and bone marrow findings. *Acta Haematol*, **89**, 132–136.

418 Bilgrami S, Almeida GD, Quinn JJ, Tuck D, Bergstrom S, Dainiak N *et al.* (1994) Pancytopenia

in allogeneic marrow transplant recipients: role of cytomegalovirus. *Br J Haematol*, **87**, 357–362.

419 Gompels UA, Luxton J, Knox KK and Carrigan DR (1994) Chronic bone marrow suppression in immunocompetent adult by human herpesvirus 6. *Lancet*, **343**, 735–736.

420 Martinez E, Domingo P and Ruiz D (1991) Transient aplastic anaemia associated with legionnaires' disease. *Lancet*, **338**, 264.

421 Hasle H, Kerndrup G, Jacobsen BB, Heegaard ED, Hornsleth A and Lillevang ST (1994) Chronic parvovirus infection mimicking myelodysplastic syndrome in a child with subclinical immunodeficiency. *Am J Pediatr Hematol Oncol*, **16**, 329–333.

422 Hoagland HC and Goldstein NP (1978) Hematologic (cytopenic) manifestations of Wilson's disease (hepatolenticular degeneration). *Mayo Clin Proc*, **53**, 498–500.

423 Wiesneth M, Pflieger H, Frickhofen N and Heimpel H (1985) Idiopathic combined immunocytopenia. *Br J Haematol*, **61**, 339–348.

424 van der Werff ten Bosch J, Delabie J, Böhler T, Verschuere J and Thielemans K (1999) Revision of the diagnosis of T-zone lymphoma in the father of a patient with autoimmune lymphoproliferative syndrome type II. *Br J Haematol*, **106**, 1045–1048.

425 Barrett AJ (1987) Graft-versus-host disease: a review. *J R Soc Med*, **80**, 368–373.

426 Bigorgne C, Le Tourneau A, Messing B, Rio B, Giraud V, Molina T *et al.* (1996) Sea-blue histiocyte syndrome in bone marrow secondary to total parenteral nutrition including fat-emulsion sources: a clinicopathologic study of seven cases. *Br J Haematol*, **95**, 258–262.

427 Talansky AL, Schulman P, Vinciguerra VP, Margouleff D, Budman DR and Degman TJ (1981) Pancytopenia complicating Graves' disease and drug-induced hypothyroidism (sic). *Arch Intern Med*, **141**, 544–545.

428 Ruocco L, Baldi N, Ceccone A, Marini A, Azzara A, Ambrogi F and Grassi B (1986) Severe pancytopenia due to copper deficiency. *Acta Haematol*, **76**, 224–226.

429 Lo L, Singer S and Vichinsky E (2002) Pancytopenia induced by hypothermia. *J Pediatr Hematol Oncol*, **24**, 681–684.

430 Murrin RJA and Harrison P (2004) Abnormal osteoclasts and bone marrow fibrosis in Paget's disease of bone. *Br J Haematol*, **124**, 3.

Answers to questions

Multiple choice questions

MCQ 6.1	TTTTF
MCQ 6.2	FTTTF
MCQ 6.3	TTTFT
MCQ 6.4	FTTFT
MCQ 6.5	TTTFT
MCQ 6.6	TTFFT

Extended matching question

EMQ 7.1

1 F
2 K
3 G
4 H
5 A

7 Important supplementary tests

Peripheral blood cells can be used for many other tests which supplement the full blood count (FBC) and May-Grünwald–Giemsa (MGG)-stained blood film. These include cytochemical tests, immunophenotyping, cytogenetic analysis, molecular genetic analysis and ultrastructural examination. Only those techniques that involve counting or examining cells will be dealt with in any detail in this chapter.

Cytochemical techniques

Some recommended techniques for cytochemical stains are given in Table 7.1. Reticulocyte counting and staining are dealt with in Chapter 2. The application of other cytochemical stains will be discussed in this chapter.

Heinz bodies

Heinz bodies are red cell inclusions composed of denatured haemoglobin. They can be seen as refractile bodies in dry unstained films viewed with the condenser lowered. They can be stained by a number of vital dyes including methyl violet, cresyl violet, 'new methylene blue', brilliant cresyl blue, brilliant green and rhodanile blue. Their characteristic shape and size (Fig. 7.1), see also Table 2.3, aid in their identification. Heinz bodies are not seen in normal subjects since they are removed by the splenic macrophages in a process often known as 'pitting'. Small numbers are seen in the blood of splenectomized subjects. Larger numbers are found following exposure to oxidant drugs, particularly in

Table 7.1 Some recommended methods for cytochemical stains.

Procedure	Recommended method
Heinz body preparation	Rhodanile blue with 2 minutes incubation [1] or methyl violet
Haemoglobin H preparation	Brilliant cresyl blue with 2 hours incubation [1]
Haemoglobin F-containing cells	Acid elution [1]
Perls' reaction for iron	Potassium ferrocyanide [1]
Myeloperoxidase	p-Phenylenediamine + catechol + H_2O_2 [2]*
Sudan black B	Sudan black B [1]*
Naphthol AS-D chloroacetate esterase (chloroacetate esterase)	Naphthol AS-D chloroacetate + hexazotized fuchsin [3] or fast blue BB [4] or Corinth V*
α Naphthyl acetate esterase	α Naphthyl acetate + hexazotized pararosaniline [3] or fast blue RR*
Neutrophil alkaline phosphatase	Naphthol AS-MX phosphate + fast blue RR*
Periodic acid–Schiff (PAS)	Periodic acid + Schiff's reagent [1]
Acid phosphatase and tartrate-resistant acid phosphatase	Naphthol AS-BI phosphate + fast garnet GBC, with and without tartaric acid [5]

Reagents suitable for these methods can be purchased from Sigma Diagnostics.

Fig. 7.1 A methyl violet preparation showing Heinz bodies in a patient exposed to the oxidant drug, dapsone. Courtesy of Dr D Swirsky, Leeds and Mr D. Roper, London.

subjects who are glucose-6-phosphate dehydrogenase (G6PD) deficient or who have been splenectomized. They may also be seen post-splenectomy in patients with an unstable haemoglobin. Patients with an unstable haemoglobin who have not been splenectomized sometimes, but not always, show Heinz bodies; in some patients they form *in vitro* during prolonged incubation.

A stain for Heinz bodies is indicated when Heinz body-haemolytic anaemia is suspected. However, sometimes this diagnosis is readily evident from the clinical history and the MGG-stained film and the test is then redundant.

Haemoglobin H inclusions

Haemoglobin H (an abnormal haemoglobin with no α chains but with a β chain tetramer) is denatured and stained by the same vital dyes that stain reticulocytes. The characteristic regular 'golf ball' inclusions (Fig. 7.2a) take longer to appear than the reticulum of a reticulocyte. An incubation period of 2 hours is recommended. It is important that either new methylene blue or brilliant cresyl blue is used to demonstrate the characteristic inclusions. Methylene blue (which has been sold by manufacturers wrongly identified as new methylene blue) does not give the typical appearance [6]. Patients with haemoglobin H disease who have not been splenectomized show the characteristic golf-ball appearance whereas post-splenectomy patients have, in

addition, Heinz bodies that represent preformed inclusions of haemoglobin H (Fig. 7.2b). Cells containing haemoglobin H are readily detected in patients with haemoglobin H disease, in whom they may form the majority of cells. In patients with α thalassaemia trait, their frequency is of the order of one in 1000 cells (when two of the four α genes are missing) or less (when one of the four α genes is missing); even when a prolonged search is made, they are not always detectable, particularly in individuals who lack only a single α gene. Haemoglobin H inclusions are not found in the red cells of haematologically normal subjects; apparently similar cells may be seen, however, in very occasional cells in normal subjects so that a control normal sample should be incubated in parallel with the patient's sample.

The identification of occasional haemoglobin H-containing cells may be useful in the diagnosis of haemoglobin H disease. However, the search for infrequent inclusion-containing cells is very time-consuming and, when the diagnosis is important, e.g. for genetic counselling, definitive confirmation by DNA analysis is required.

Haemoglobin F-containing cells

Haemoglobin F-containing cells are identified cytochemically by their resistance to haemoglobin elution in acid conditions (Fig. 7.3); the procedure is commonly referred to as a Kleihauer test from its originator, although Kleihauer's method is often modified. The test is useful for detecting fetal cells in the maternal circulation and thus for detecting and quantitating fetomaternal haemorrhage; it is indicated for the detection of fetomaternal haemorrhage in unexplained neonatal anaemia and for quantifying fetomaternal haemorrhage from a Rh D-positive fetus to an Rh D-negative mother. The Kleihauer test will also detect autologous cells containing appreciable quantities of haemoglobin F, such as may be seen in hereditary persistence of fetal haemoglobin and β thalassaemia, and in some patients with thalassaemia major, δβ thalassaemia trait, sickle cell disease, juvenile chronic myelomonocytic leukaemia, myelodysplastic syndromes (MDS) and various other conditions. The distribution of haemoglobin F in adult cells may be homogeneous (in

(a)

Fig. 7.2 Haemoglobin H
preparations showing:
(a) haemoglobin H-containing cells
(containing multiple small pale blue
inclusions) and reticulocytes (with a
purple reticular network) in a patient
with haemoglobin H disease); and
(b) haemoglobin H-containing cells,
a reticulocyte and Heinz bodies
(large peripherally placed blue
inclusions) in the blood of a patient
with haemoglobin H disease who
had been splenectomized.

(b)

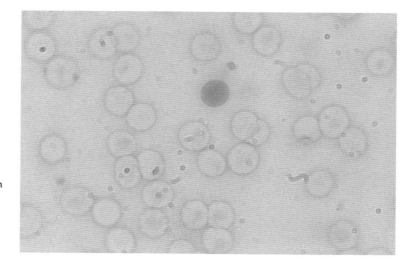

Fig. 7.3 Acid elution technique
(Kleihauer test) for haemoglobin F-
containing cells; the blood specimen
was taken from a postpartum woman
and shows that a fetomaternal
haemorrhage had occurred. A single
stained fetal cell is seen against a
background of ghosts of maternal
cells.

some types of hereditary persistence of fetal haemoglobin) or heterogeneous (in other types of hereditary persistence of fetal haemoglobin and in other conditions). Both a positive and a negative control should be tested in parallel with the sample under investigation. A positive control can be prepared by mixing together adult and fetal cells.

It should be noted that a Kleihauer test cannot be used for detection of fetal cells in the maternal circulation if the mother already has a positive Kleihaeur test as a result of a high level of haemoglobin F.

Perls' reaction for iron

Perls' stain is based on a reaction between acid ferrocyanide and the ferric ion (Fe^{3+}) of haemosiderin to form ferric ferrocyanide, which has an intense blue colour (Prussian blue). Ferritin, which is soluble, does not give a positive reaction. Perls' stain is most often performed on the bone marrow but it can be used to stain peripheral blood cells in order to detect sideroblasts and siderocytes.

On a Romanowsky-stained blood film, haemosiderin appears as small blue granules, designated Pappenheimer bodies (see p. 87). On a Perls' stain they are referred to as siderotic granules and the cells containing them are known as siderocytes (Fig. 7.4a). Siderocytes are rarely detected in the blood of normal subjects; siderotic granules are present in reticulocytes newly released from the bone marrow, but disappear during maturation of the reticulocyte in the spleen, probably because the haemosiderin is utilized for further haemoglobin synthesis. When haematologically normal subjects are splenectomized, small numbers of siderocytes are seen in the blood. When red cells containing abnormally large or numerous siderotic granules are released from the bone marrow, as in sideroblastic anaemia or in thalassaemia major, many of the abnormal inclusions are 'pitted' by the spleen. Some remain detectable in the peripheral blood, both in reticulocytes and in mature red cells. If a patient with a defect of iron incorporation has been splenectomized or is hyposplenic for any reason, very numerous siderocytes are seen.

A sideroblast is a nucleated red blood cell that contains siderotic granules. Sideroblasts are normally present in the bone marrow, but since nucleated red

(a)

(b)

Fig. 7.4 Perls' stain showing: (a) siderocytes (cells containing fine blue dots) in the blood of a patient with thalassaemia major; and (b) a ring sideroblast in the blood of a patient with sideroblastic anaemia.

blood cells (NRBC) do not normally circulate, it is unusual to see them in the peripheral blood. When they do appear, they may be morphologically normal, containing only one or a few fine granules, or abnormal with the granules being increased in number, size or both. Abnormal sideroblasts include ring sideroblasts in which a siderotic granules are present in a ring immediately adjacent to the nuclear membrane (Fig. 7.4b). When NRBC are present in the peripheral blood they can be stained with a Perls' stain to allow any siderotic granules present to be identified reliably. Abnormal sideroblasts may be detected in the peripheral blood in sideroblastic anaemia, megaloblastic anaemia and thalassaemia major. They are seen in larger numbers when the spleen is absent or hypofunctional. Sideroblastic anaemia is usually diagnosed by bone marrow aspiration but strong support for the diagnosis is obtained if ring sideroblasts are detected in the peripheral blood, if necessary in a buffy coat preparation in which any NRBCs are concentrated.

Glucose-6-phosphate dehydrogenase

A cytochemical stain for glucose-6-phosphate dehydrogenase (G6PD) is useful in detecting females who are heterozygous for G6PD deficiency [7]. Although the G6PD assay may be normal, a cytochemical stain shows that there is a population of normal cells and a population of deficient cells.

Cytochemical stains used in the diagnosis and classification of leukaemias

Cytochemical stains used in the diagnosis and classification of leukaemias can be applied to both the bone marrow and peripheral blood. Studies of peripheral blood cells are needed when bone marrow aspiration is difficult or impossible. In other circumstances, studies of peripheral blood and bone marrow are complementary. Cytochemical stains for neutrophil alkaline phosphatase are performed on the peripheral blood.

Neutrophil alkaline phosphatase

Mature neutrophils, but not eosinophils, have alkaline phosphatase in specific cytoplasmic organelles [8], which have been called secretory vesicles or phosphosomes. Neutrophil alkaline phosphatase (NAP) has sometimes been referred to as leucocyte alkaline phosphatase (LAP) but the former designation is more accurate since it is the neutrophils that are assessed. A number of cytochemical stains can be used for demonstrating NAP activity. One suitable stain is that recommended by Ackerman [9], which permits grading of alkaline phosphatase activity as shown in Table 7.2 and Fig. 7.5 to give a NAP score that falls between 0 and 400. The normal range is dependent on the substrate used. With the above method it is of the order of 30–180. It is preferable for NAP scores to be determined on either native or heparinized blood. The cytochemical reaction should be carried out within 8 hours of obtaining the blood specimen but, if this is not possible, the films can be fixed and stored, in the dark, at room temperature. Ethylenediaminetetra-acetic acid (EDTA)-anticoagulated blood is not ideal as enzyme activity is inhibited; if it is used, the films should be made within 10–20 minutes of obtaining the blood, but even then there is some loss of activity. Low, normal and high controls should be stained in parallel with the patient's sample. A low control can be obtained from a patient with chronic granulocytic leukaemia (CGL), or can be prepared by immersing an appropriately fixed film of normal blood in boiling water for 1 minute. A high control can be

Table 7.2 Scoring neutrophil alkaline phosphatase (NAP) activity (after Kaplow [10]) one hundred neutrophils are scored as shown.

Score of cell	Percentage of cytoplasm occupied by precipitated dye	Size of granules	Intensity of staining	Cytoplasmic background
0	None	–	None	Colourless
1	50	Small	Faint to moderate	Colourless to very pale blue
2	50–80	Small	Moderate to strong	Colourless to pale blue
3	80–100	Medium to large	Strong	Colourless to blue
4	100	Medium and large	Very strong	Not visible

Following the scoring of individual neutrophils, the scores are summed to produce the final NAP score. This is most easily done by multiplying each score by the number of cells having that score and adding the results together.

(a)

(b)

(c)

(d)

Fig. 7.5 Neutrophil alkaline phosphatase (NAP) reaction (method of Ackerman [9]) showing cells with reactions graded 0–4: (a) neutrophil with a score of 0 plus a lymphocyte which is also negative; (b) two band cells with a score of 1; (c) two neutrophils with a score of 2 and one with a score of 3; and (d) two neutrophils with a score of 4 and one with a score of 2.

obtained from a patient with infection or from a pregnant or postpartum woman or from a woman taking oral contraceptives. Positive and negative control films, which have been appropriately fixed and wrapped in Parafilm, can be stored at –70°C for at least 1 year.

Some of the causes of high and low NAP scores are shown in Table 7.3. Synthesis of NAP mRNA is stimulated by granulocyte colony-stimulating factor (G-CSF) but inhibited by granulocyte-macrophage colony-stimulating factor (GM-CSF), interleukin 3 (IL3) and interferon. The low NAP score sometimes seen in viral infections may reflect the effect of interferon. Neonates have very high NAP scores, usually exceeding 200. A fall to levels more typical of childhood occurs between 5 and 10 months of age [15]. Premature and low birth-weight babies have lower scores than full-term babies. Children have higher NAP scores than adults with a gradual fall to adult levels occurring before puberty [16]. Women in the reproductive age range have higher NAP scores than men with the score varying with the menstrual

Table 7.3 Some causes of high and low neutrophil alkaline phosphatase (NAP) scores [4,10].

High NAP	Low NAP
Inherited conditions	
Down's syndrome	Inherited hypophosphatasia (NAP absent)
	Lactoferrin deficiency [11]
	Isolated primary NAP deficiency [12]
	Grey platelet syndrome (some families) [13]
Physiological effects	
Cord blood and neonate	
Mid-cycle in menstruating females	
Oral contraceptive intake	
Pregnancy and the postpartum period	
Reactive changes	
Bacterial infection	Some cases of infectious mononucleosis and other viral infections
Inflammation	
Surgery and trauma, tissue infarction, burns and other tissue damage	
Corticosteroids and ACTH administration and acute stress	
Leukaemoid reactions including those due to ectopic secretion of G-CSF, e.g. in multiple myeloma [14]	
Administration of G-CSF	
Carcinomatosis	
Acute lymphoblastic leukaemia	
Most cases of aplastic anaemia	Some cases of aplastic anaemia
Hairy cell leukaemia	
Some cases of chronic lymphocytic leukaemia	
Some cases of monoclonal gammopathy of undetermined significance	
Hodgkin's disease	
Hepatic cirrhosis (particularly when decompensated)	
Myeloid neoplasms	
Neutrophilic leukaemia	Chronic granulocytic leukaemia
Some cases of atypical chronic myeloid leukaemia	Most cases of atypical chronic myeloid leukaemia
Some cases of AML, particularly acute monoblastic leukaemia	Some cases of AML, particularly when there is differentiation
Most cases of idiopathic myelofibrosis	Some cases of idiopathic myelofibrosis
Some cases of MDS	Some cases of MDS
Some cases of JMML	Some cases of JMML
Some cases of essential thrombocythaemia	Paroxysmal nocturnal haemoglobinuria
Most cases of polycythaemia rubra vera	

ACTH, adrenocorticotropic hormone; AML, acute myeloid leukaemia; G-CSF, granulocyte colony-stimulating factor; JMML, juvenile myelomonocytic leukaemia; MDS, myelodysplastic syndrome.

cycle (Fig. 7.6). After the menopause, NAP scores of women approach those of men (Fig. 7.7) [16,17].

The NAP score is low in 95% of patients with CGL. The test is useful in distinguishing between CGL and other chronic myeloproliferative disorders, which usually have a normal or elevated NAP score, and between CGL and reactive neutrophilia, since the latter almost invariably has a high score. Patients with CGL may have a normal or elevated NAP during pregnancy, postoperatively (particularly following splenectomy), during bacterial infection, when the bone marrow is rendered hypoplastic by chemotherapy, and following the onset of transformation. It should be noted that, when cytogenetic

Fig. 7.6 Changes in neutrophil alkaline phosphatase (NAP) score during the menstrual cycle.

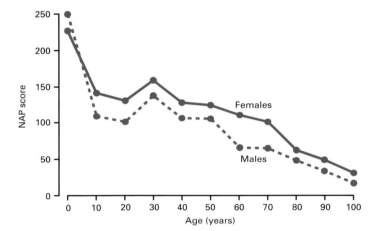

Fig. 7.7 Changes in neutrophil alkaline phosphatase (NAP) score with age in men and women. Data from Stavridis *et al.* [17].

and molecular genetic analyses are available, the NAP score is redundant in the investigation of suspected CGL.

The NAP score may be of use in distinguishing between polycythaemia rubra vera (PRV), which usually has an elevated score, and secondary polycythaemia, in which the score is more likely to be normal. In multiple myeloma, the increased NAP score correlates with disease activity.

Myeloperoxidase

Peroxidases are enzymes that catalyse the oxidation of substrates by hydrogen peroxide. The granules of neutrophils and eosinophils contain peroxidases, which are designated leucocyte peroxidase or mye-

loperoxidase (MPO). The demonstration of myeloperoxidase activity is useful in establishing and confirming the diagnosis of acute myeloid leukaemia (AML), since lymphoblasts are uniformly negative. Myeloperoxidase was initially demonstrated with benzidine or one of its derivatives as a substrate. A suitable non-carcinogenic substrate used in the method of Hanker *et al.* [2] is p-phenylene diamine, which produces a brownish-black reaction product. Myeloperoxidase is demonstrated in neutrophils and their precursors (Fig. 7.8), eosinophils and their precursors and the precursors of basophils. In neutrophils and eosinophils the primary granules have peroxidase activity and in eosinophils this is also true of secondary granules. Neutrophil and eosinophil peroxidases differ from each other, e.g. in their

Fig. 7.8 Leukaemic blast cells stained by the Hanker technique [2] for myeloperoxidase showing a brownish-black deposit in the cytoplasm. This was a case of acute myeloid leukaemia of FAB M2 category.

pH optima and in their sensitivity to inhibition by cyanide. The peroxidase activity of eosinophils is stronger than that of neutrophils. Auer rods are peroxidase-positive. In the monocyte lineage, peroxidase activity is detectable at the promonocyte stage. Monocytes and promonocytes have fewer peroxidase-positive granules than neutrophils and their precursors. Inherited deficiency of neutrophil peroxidase is quite common. Deficiencies of eosinophil peroxidase and monocyte peroxidase also occur.

An acquired peroxidase deficiency may be seen in AML and MDS. Although it cannot be excluded that a patient has acute lymphoblastic leukaemia (ALL) and a coincidental congenital peroxidase deficiency, the demonstration of peroxidase-deficient mature cells nevertheless provides indirect evidence that an apparently undifferentiated leukaemia is actually AML of M0 category.

It should be noted that when a laboratory uses an automated haematology analyser employing peroxidase cytochemistry, such as the Bayer H.1 series and Advia 120, the instrument scatterplots can be useful for detecting both peroxidase activity in blast cells and peroxidase-deficient neutrophils.

Sudan black B

Sudan black B (SBB) (Fig. 7.9) has an affinity for polymorphonuclear and monocyte granules. In general, the intensity of a positive staining reaction parallels myeloperoxidase activity. SBB staining is slightly more sensitive than myeloperoxidase activity in the detection of myeloblasts. SBB stains the granules of neutrophils (both the primary and the specific granules) and the specific granules of eosinophils and, to a variable extent, the specific granules of basophils. The staining of eosinophil granules may be peripheral with the central core remaining unstained. Auer rods are stained. Monoblasts are either negative or show a few small SBB-positive granules. Promonocytes and monocytes have a variable number of fine positively staining granules. In hereditary neutrophil, eosinophil and monocyte peroxidase deficiencies, the granules of cells of the deficient lineages are SBB-negative. Lymphoblasts can have occasional fine positive dots, which may represent mitochondria [4]. Very rarely a stronger reaction is seen in the lymphoblasts of ALL [18] or in lymphoma cells of T or B lineage [19].

Naphthol AS-D chloroacetate esterase

Naphthol AS-D chloroacetate esterase ('chloroacetate esterase', CAE) activity is found in neutrophils and their precursors (Fig. 7.10) and in mast cells. Auer rods are sometimes positive but this stain is much less useful than the SBB and MPO reactions for the detection of Auer rods. Normal eosinophils and basophils are negative but the eosinophils of certain types of eosinophil leukaemia may be positive.

Fig. 7.9 Leukaemic blast cells stained with Sudan black B. One large blast cell contains both granules and Auer rods. Several other blasts contain granules. The cells of this case, which was acute myeloid leukaemia of FAB M1 category, had very few granules and only rare Auer rods visible on a May-Grünwald–Giemsa (MGG)-stained film.

Fig. 7.10 Leukaemic blast cells stained for chloroacetate esterase (CAE) activity, using Corinth V as the dye. This was a case of acute myeloid leukaemia of FAB M2 category.

Monocytes are usually negative, but may show a weak reactivity. CAE is generally less sensitive than either MPO or SBB in the detection of myeloblasts, although occasional cases have been noted to be positive for CAE despite being MPO-negative [3,4].

Non-specific esterases

Esterase activity is common in haemopoietic cells. Nine isoenzymes have been demonstrated of which four are found in neutrophils and are responsible for their CAE activity. Five are found in monocytes and a variety of other cells and the esterase activity of these cells has been designated 'non-specific' esterase [4,20]. Different isoenzymes are preferentially detected by different substrates and at different pHs. The most useful cytochemical reaction to detect the esterase activity of monocytes is α-naphthyl acetate esterase (ANAE) activity at acid pH (Fig. 7.11). α-Naphthyl butyrate esterase (ANBE) activity is quite similar. With ANAE, strongly positive reactions are given by monocytes and their precursors and by megakaryocytes and platelets. Weaker reactions are given by plasma cells. ANBE is more often negative with megakaryocytes and platelets than is ANAE. Monocyte and megakaryocyte non-specific esterase activity can also be detected as naphthol AS-D acetate esterase (NASDA esterase) activity or the very similar naphthol AS acetate esterase (NASA esterase). NASDA esterase is weakly positive in neutrophils and their precursors. It is therefore less suitable than ANAE for differentiating between the monocyte lineage and the neutrophil lineage; the specificity of the test can be improved by carrying out the reaction with and without fluoride since the monocyte and megakaryocyte enzymes are inhibited by fluoride whereas the neutrophil enzyme is fluoride-resistant. The ANAE activity of monocytes and megakaryocytes is also fluoride-sensitive, but ANAE permits a clearer distinction between monocytes and

Fig. 7.11 Leukaemic blast cells stained for α-naphthyl acetate esterase (ANAE) activity using fast RR as the dye. This was a case of acute myeloid leukaemia of FAB M5 category.

Fig. 7.12 Periodic acid–Schiff (PAS) reaction showing block positivity in the blast cells of a case of B-lineage acute lymphoblastic leukaemia of FAB L1 category. Courtesy of Dr A. Eden, Southend-on-Sea.

neutrophils and the addition of fluoride is not necessary. Non-specific esterase activity is often demonstrable in normal T lymphocytes and also in acute and chronic leukaemias of T lineage. With ANAE, a characteristic dot positivity is often demonstrable in T-lineage ALL and T-prolymphocytic leukaemia; ANAE is superior to NASDA esterase in this regard [15] but this use of esterase cytochemistry is largely redundant since immunophenotyping is now widely available. The abnormal erythroblasts of erythroleukaemia or megaloblastic anaemia may also have non-specific esterase activity.

Combined esterase

A combined reaction for ANAE and CAE activities permits both reactions to be studied on the one blood film and is useful in characterizing acute leukaemias. The monocytic and granulocytic differentiation of French–American–British (FAB) M4 category (acute myelomonocytic leukaemia) is clearly seen. The demonstration of an increased percentage (more than 3%) of cells staining for both chloroacetate esterase and non-specific esterase can provide evidence of MDS and in one reported patient provided evidence that an apparently undifferentiated leukaemia was actually myeloid, of FAB M0 category [21].

Periodic acid–Schiff reaction

The periodic acid–Schiff (PAS) reaction stains a variety of carbohydrates including the glycogen that is often found in haemopoietic cells. The main clinical application of the stain is in the differential diagnosis of the acute leukaemias but its role has diminished considerably with the increasing use of immunophenotyping. Lymphoblasts of ALL are PAS-positive in the great majority of cases, this positivity often being in the form of coarse granules or large blocks on a clear background (Fig. 7.12). A negative PAS reaction is more often seen in T-lineage than in B-lineage ALL. Myeloblasts and monoblasts may be PAS-negative or may have faint diffuse or granular positivity. Block positivity is rare in AML but it has been observed in basophil precursors, monoblasts, megakaryoblasts and erythroblasts.

Many other haemopoietic cells are PAS-positive but the reaction is rarely of diagnostic importance. The reaction has a limited application in the diagnosis of erythroleukaemias, megakaryoblastic leukaemia and acute promyelocytic leukaemia. Platelets, megakaryocytes and the more mature megakaryoblasts are positive. Megakaryoblasts may have PAS-positive granules within cytoplasmic blebs. Normal erythroblasts are PAS-negative. Strong diffuse or block

PAS positivity may be seen in erythroleukaemia. However, quite strong reactions, either diffuse or granular, may also be seen in thalassaemia major and iron deficiency, and weaker reactions in sideroblastic anaemia, severe haemolytic anaemia and a number of other disorders of erythropoiesis. Acute promyelocytic leukaemia has moderately strong diffuse cytoplasmic positivity, appearing as a 'cytoplasmic blush'. Mature neutrophils have fine positive granules, which appear to pack the cytoplasm whereas eosinophils and basophils have a positive cytoplasmic reaction contrasting with the negative granules. Most normal lymphocytes are PAS-negative. Lymphocytes containing PAS-positive granules become more numerous in reactive conditions, such as infectious mononucleosis and other viral infections, and in lymphoproliferative disorders such as chronic lymphocytic leukaemia (CLL) and non-Hodgkin's lymphoma. A circlet of PAS-positive granules surrounding the nucleus, likened to rosary beads, may be found in Sézary cells.

A PAS stain can be performed on a film which has been stained previously with a Romanowsky stain.

Acid phosphatase

Acid phosphatase activity is demonstrated by a variety of haemopoietic cells. The two main applications of this reaction are in the diagnosis of hairy cell leukaemia and in the diagnosis of T-lineage leukaemias, particularly T-lineage ALL.

Acid phosphatase activity is usually stronger in acute and chronic leukaemias of T lineage than in those of B lineage where it is often negative. T-lineage ALL often demonstrates focal positivity (Fig. 7.13), which is of some use in confirming this diagnosis. However, with the availability of immunophenotyping, its importance has declined greatly. Acid phosphatase activity is also demonstrable in granulocytes and their precursors, in the monocyte lineage, and in platelets, megakaryocytes and the more mature megakaryoblasts. Auer rods are positive.

A number of isoenzymes of acid phosphatase are found in haemopoietic cells. That of hairy cells is characteristically tartrate-resistant whereas that of other cells is sensitive to inhibition by tartrate. The demonstration of tartrate-resistant acid phosphatase (TRAP) activity remains useful in the diagnosis of

Fig. 7.13 Acid phosphatase stain by the method of Janckila *et al.* [5] showing focal positivity in the blast cells of a patient with T-lineage acute lymphoblastic leukaemia.

hairy cell leukaemia. It is present in the great majority of cases and is uncommon in other lymphoproliferative disorders; however TRAP positivity has also been reported in occasional cases of infectious mononucleosis, CLL, prolymphocytic leukaemia (PLL), non-Hodgkin's lymphoma and the Sézary syndrome. The monocytes of patients with Gaucher's disease are also TRAP-positive but normal monocytes are not [22].

Immunophenotyping

Immunophenotyping is now of major importance in the diagnosis of leukaemia and lymphoma. It is essential for confirmation of the diagnoses of ALL and acute biphenotypic leukaemia. When acute leukaemia is obviously myeloid, immunophenotyping is unnecessary for diagnosis but, in the case of AML with no cytochemical evidence of myeloid differentiation (M0 AML) and acute megakaryoblastic leukaemia (M7 AML), it is essential. Even when not essential for diagnosis, immunophenotyping may be required for patients being entered into leukaemia trials and it can also be useful to establish the immunophenotype of the leukaemic cells so that immunophenotyping can be used for monitoring of minimal residual disease.

Immunophenotyping is often very important to avoid diagnostic errors in the chronic lymphoproliferative disorders.

An important but more specialized application of immunophenotyping is when expression of an antigen is used for the enumeration of cells of a specific type, e.g. CD4-positive T cells in the blood of human immunodeficiency virus (HIV)-positive patients, CD34-positive stem cells when a stem cell harvest is being performed for transplantation purposes or Rh D-positive cells in the maternal circulation of a Rh D-negative mother with an Rh D-positive baby. The demonstration of fetal cells in the maternal circulation can also be useful in investigating unexplained anaemia in a fetus or neonate. These and other less common applications of immunophenotyping are summarized in Table 7.4.

Immunophenotyping of the neoplastic cells in leukaemia and lymphoma is carried out with a panel of antibodies, mainly monoclonal antibodies, which detect antigens on the surface membrane or, if the cell is lightly fixed or 'permeabilized', cytoplasmic or nuclear antigens [28,29]. With such panels, cells can be assigned to T-cell, B-cell or myeloid lineages. Certain specific antibodies can identify cells of erythroid, megakaryocyte and natural killer (NK) lineages. The use of secondary panels of antibodies permits the establishment of characteristic profiles that are very useful in the identification of specific types of lymphoproliferative disorder. Typical immunophenotypic findings in haematological neoplasms are shown in Tables 9.6 and 9.15–9.17. For a more detailed analysis of the role of immunophenotyping in haematological neoplasms the reader is referred to reference [30].

Immunophenotyping by flow cytometry

Immunophenotyping is now usually performed by flow cytometry, using antibodies directly labelled

Table 7.4 Applications of immunophenotyping of peripheral blood cells*.

Applications	Specific details
Immunophenotyping of abnormal cells in suspected leukaemia or lymphoma—for diagnosis and classification and establishing phenotype to permit monitoring of minimal residual disease	See Chapter 9
Confirmation that stem cells are increased in peripheral blood, permitting harvesting for autologous transplantation	Counting of CD34-positive cells with weak expression of CD45 and low forward and side light scatter
Detection of circulating non-haemopoietic tumour cells for diagnosis or staging	Detection of circulating neuroblastoma cells by their CD81-positive, CD56-positive, CD45-negative immunophenotype
Exclusion of the presence of contaminating carcinoma cells, leukaemic cells or lymphoma cells in a peripheral blood stem cell harvest	Detection of cells expressing cytokeratin or aberrant antigen expression characteristic of cells of leukaemia or lymphoma
Diagnosis of paroxysmal nocturnal haemoglobinuria	Detection of lack of expression of CD55 and CD59 by peripheral blood cells (erythrocytes, granulocytes, platelets)
Diagnosis of hereditary spherocytosis	Reduced binding of eosin-5-maleimide, which binds specifically to band 3 of the erythrocyte membrane†
Detecting and quantification of fetomaternal haemorrhage [23]	Enumeration of Rh D-positive cells in pregnant women in whom a high haemoglobin F invalidates a Kleihauer test; an alternative to a Kleihauer test in other women Detection of fetal cells by an anti-haemoglobin F antibody, the distinction from elevation of haemoglobin F in maternal cells being on the basis of the strength of the signal

Continued p. 276

Table 7.4 *Continued*

Applications	Specific details
	Detection of fetal cells by dual colour flow cytometry, using an antibody to haemoglobin F and an antibody to the i antigen; the expression of the i antigen on fetal cells permits the distinction of fetal cells containing haemoglobin F from maternal cells containing haemoglobin F; similarly an antibody to carbonic anhydrase can be used together with an antibody to haemoglobin F, carbonic anhydrase being strongly expressed in maternal cells containing haemoglobin F but quite weakly expressed in fetal cells
Diagnosis of inherited platelet defects with reduction or absence of specific glycoproteins, e.g. Glanzmann's thrombasthenia, Bernard–Soulier homozygotes and heterozygotes, Wiskott–Aldrich syndrome and X-linked thrombocytopenia	Lack of expression of platelet glycoproteins, e.g. lack of expression of glycoprotein IIb/IIIa in Glanzmann's thrombasthenia, lack of expression of glycoprotein Ib/IX/V in Bernard–Soulier syndrome and lack of expression of the WAS protein in Wiskott–Aldrich and related syndromes [24]
Detection of acquired platelet abnormalities, e.g. in MDS	Abnormal expression of platelet antigens or antigens do not show an appropriately increased or decreased expression in response to platelet agonists
Tracking of transfused platelets	Two-colour immunofluorescence can be used to determine the survival of transfused platelets [25]
Diagnosis and monitoring of immunodeficiency (congenital or acquired)	Enumeration of T, B and NK lymphocytes and subset analysis, as appropriate, in suspected congenital or acquired immunodeficiency—detection of lack of expression of HLA-DR in 'bare lymphocyte syndrome'; detection of lymphocyte activation and increased expression of TCR-γδ in Omenn's syndrome and severe combined immunodeficiency with maternofetal engraftment; lack of expression of Bruton's tyrosine kinase (Btk) on some platelets in carrier females of X-linked agammaglobulinaemia; enumeration of CD4-positive cells in initial assessment and follow-up of the acquired immune deficiency syndromes (AIDS)
Diagnosis of auto-immune lymphoproliferative syndrome	Distinctive immunophenotype with increased CD8-positive T cells, increased CD8-positive CD57-positive T cells, increased αβ-positive CD4-negative CD8-negative cells, increased γδ-positive CD4-negative CD8-negative cells, increased CD3-positive HLA-DR-positive T cells, decreased CD3-positive CD25-positive T cells and increased B cells including CD5-positive B cells [26]
Diagnosis of familial haemophagocytic lymphohistiocytosis type 2	Lack of expression of perforin by CD8-positive and CD56-positive lymphocytes [27]
Detection of HLA-B27 histocompatibility antigens	Useful in supporting the diagnosis of ankylosing spondylitis, Reiter's syndrome, psoriatic arthropathy and inflammatory bowel disease
T-cell monitoring and detection of T-cells sensitized to an antigen	Monitoring of T-cell subsets following transplantation or immunosuppressive treatment; detection of antigen-specific T cells by their expression of the activation marker CD69 following exposure to the antigen

MDS, myelodysplastic syndrome; NK, natural killer.

* The role of immunophenotyping is greater when bone marrow cells are also available for study, e.g. for monitoring of minimal residual disease, for establishing clonality of plasma cells with anti-κ and anti-λ antibodies or for confirming a diagnosis of mastocytosis by demonstration of CD117-positive mast cells that express CD2 and CD25.

† This test does not use an antibody but nevertheless permits recognition of a specific antigenic structure on the red cell membrane.

Fig. 7.14 Immunophenotyping by flow cytometry in a case of follicular lymphoma. The lower plot demonstrates clonality, cells being κ (kappa)-negative and λ (lambda)-positive, and shows that surface membrane immunoglobulin is strongly expressed. The upper plot demonstrates that the lymphoma cells are CD19 positive and CD5 negative thus differing both from CLL and from mantle cell lymphoma. Courtesy of Mr R. Morilla, London.

with a fluorochrome (Fig. 7.14). This is efficient when large numbers of specimens are being processed and permits simultaneous analysis of the expression of two, three or four antigens together with an assessment of the strength of antigen expression. Flow cytometry immunophenotyping is used mainly for characterizing neoplastic cells in leukaemia and lymphoma but there are multiple other applications (see Table 7.4).

Immunophenotyping by immunocytochemistry

Immunophenotyping can also be carried out on fixed cells in blood films or on cytospin preparations, using antibodies that are detected by either an immunoperoxidase (Fig. 7.15) or an alkaline phosphatase–anti-alkaline phosphatase (APAAP) technique (Fig. 7.16). Using these techniques, surface membrane, cytoplasmic and nuclear antigens are readily detected. These techniques have some advantages over flow cytometry since the cytological features of positive cells can be appreciated but they are labour-intensive and thus are less suitable for routine use.

Cytogenetic analysis

The peripheral blood can be used for cytogenetic analysis for the identification of constitutional disorders and for the investigation of leukaemia and lymphoma.

When investigating suspected constitutional abnormalities, e.g. Down's syndrome, peripheral blood lymphocytes can be stimulated with phytohaemagglutinin (PHA) to induce mitosis and provide analysable metaphases. Cytogenetic techniques can also be applied to the diagnosis of Fanconi's anaemia, susceptibility to clastogenic agents being shown.

In investigating leukaemias and lymphomas, the bone marrow is usually a more suitable tissue for analysis but successful results are sometimes possible with peripheral blood cytogenetic analysis, in the case of acute leukaemias, when there are a large number of circulating immature cells, or in the case of mature B-lineage and T-lineage lymphoproliferative disorders, when B-cell and T-cell mitogens respectively are employed.

For a detailed analysis of the role of cytogenetic analysis in haematological neoplasms the reader is referred to reference [30].

Fluorescence *in situ* hybridization

Fluorescence *in situ* hybridization (FISH) can be performed on peripheral blood cells. Applications include the detection of abnormalities typical of haematological neoplasms, e.g. trisomy 12 in chronic

Fig. 7.15 Immunophenotyping using a monoclonal antibody to CD13 and the immunoperoxidase technique. The blast cells of this case gave negative reactions with myeloperoxidase (MPO), Sudan black B (SBB) and chloroacetate esterase (CAE) but were identified as myeloid (FAB M0 category) by the positivity with CD13 and negativity with monoclonal antibodies directed at lymphoid antigens. Courtesy of Professor D. Catovsky, London.

Fig. 7.16 Immunophenotyping using a monoclonal antibody to CD42 (antiplatelet glycoprotein Ib) and the alkaline phosphatase–anti-alkaline phosphatase (APAAP) technique. Positive reactions are given by two platelets, by a lymphocyte-sized micromegakaryocyte and by a larger mononuclear megakaryocyte.

lymphocytic leukaemia, and the rapid detection of constitutional chromosome abnormalities, such as trisomy 18 [31] or trisomy 21.

Molecular genetic analysis

Peripheral blood cells are used for molecular genetic analysis with three main aims. Firstly, such studies are used to show clonality (and, by implication, neoplasia) by demonstration of clonal rearrangement of T-cell receptor or immunoglobulin genes. Secondly, they are used to demonstrate the presence of various oncogene rearrangements that are strongly associated with specific haematological neoplasms. Thirdly, they can demonstrate inherited abnormalities of genes, e.g. α and β globin genes, that cause haematological abnormalities.

Molecular diagnostic techniques that may be employed include Southern blot analysis and the polymerase chain reaction (PCR), for the analysis of DNA, and reverse-transcriptase-PCR (RT-PCR) for the investigation of RNA. For further details on the principles and applications of these techniques the reader is referred to references [30,32,33].

Fig. 7.17 Ultrastructural examination in Sézary syndrome showing a Sézary cell with a highly irregular nuclear outline. Courtesy of Dr Estella Matutes, London.

Ultrastructural examination

Ultrastructural examination of peripheral blood cells by electron microscopy is labour intensive and therefore is not often employed in routine diagnostic haematology. Scanning electron microscopy has been useful in increasing understanding of the actual shapes of the various abnormal erythrocytes seen in fixed and stained blood films (see Chapter 3). Transmission electron microscopy has been used for the demonstration of the lineage of neoplastic cells (e.g. megakaryoblasts or myeloblasts) and for the detection of Sézary cells by demonstration of their characteristic nuclear form (Fig. 7.17). Transmission electron microscopy can also be useful in distinguishing the various congenital thrombocytopenia syndromes resulting from mutation of the *MYH9* gene (see p. 368).

Test your knowledge

Multiple choice questions (MCQs)

(1–5 statements may be correct)

MCQ 7.1 A reticulocyte count of 8% is consistent with
(a) Untreated megaloblastic anaemia
(b) Onset of parvovirus B19 infection
(c) Lead poisoning
(d) Sickle cell disease
(e) Fanconi's anaemia

MCQ 7.2 Haemoglobin H inclusions may be detected in
(a) Sickle cell trait
(b) β Thalassaemia trait
(c) α^0 Thalassaemia trait
(d) Haemoglobin H disease
(e) β Thalassaemia major

MCQ 7.3 Heinz bodies may be a feature of
(a) Sideroblastic anaemia
(b) Acute oxidant-induced haemolysis
(c) Hereditary persistence of fetal haemoglobin
(d) Acute haemolysis in glucose-6-phosphate dehydrogenase (G6PD) deficiency
(e) Unstable haemoglobin, post-splenectomy

MCQ 7.4 CD5 is likely to be expressed in
(a) T-lineage acute lymphoblastic leukaemia
(b) B-lineage chronic lymphocytic leukaemia
(c) Follicular lymphoma
(d) Mantle cell lymphoma
(e) A subset of normal B cells

MCQ 7.5 Immunophenotyping is essential for the diagnosis of
(a) Acute myeloid leukaemia without maturation (M0 AML)
(b) Acute myeloid leukaemia with granulocytic differentiation (M1 or M2 AML)
(c) Acute promyelocytic leukaemia (M3 AML)
(d) Acute biphenotypic leukaemia
(e) Acute lymphoblastic leukaemia

MCQ 7.6 A reduced neutrophil alkaline phosphatase score is expected
(a) During pregnancy
(b) During bacterial infection
(c) In women taking the oral contraceptive
(d) In most patients with chronic granulocytic leukaemia
(e) In some patients with paroxysmal nocturnal haemoglobinuria

MCQ 7.7 In B-lineage chronic lymphocytic leukaemia strong positive reactions are expected with
(a) Surface membrane immunoglobulin
(b) CD23
(c) CD79a
(d) CD79b
(e) Terminal dexynucleotidyl transferase (TdT)

Extended matching questions (EMQs)

Select the most accurate options for each of the stems. Each option may be used once, more than once or not at all. Only one answer is correct.

EMQ 7.1
Theme: leukaemia diagnosis
Options
A Perls' reaction
B Tartrate-resistant acid phosphatase
C Naphthol AS-D chloroacetate esterase (chloroacetate esterase)
D α-Naphthyl acetate esterase
E Combined esterase (naphthol AS-D chloroacetate esterase and alpha naphthyl acetate esterase)
F Periodic acid–Schiff (PAS) reaction, block positivity
G Myeloperoxidase or Sudan black B
H Acid phosphatase, strong focal positivity

For each suspected diagnosis select the cytochemical reaction most likely to be useful in confirming or supporting the diagnosis.

Suspected diagnosis	Matching option
1 Acute myeloid leukaemia with granulocytic differentiation (FAB M1 AML)	
2 B-lineage acute lymphoblastic leukaemia	
3 Acute myelomonocytic leukaemia (M4 AML)	
4 Acute monocytic leukaemia (M5 AML)	
5 Hairy cell leukaemia	

EMQ 7.2
Theme: immunophenotyping
Options
A Cytoplasmic CD3
B CD19
C CD34
D CD61
E CD117
F Perforin
G Glycophorin

For each suspected diagnosis, lineage or cell, select the antigen, from the options listed above, that is most likely to give a positive result.

Suspected diagnosis	Matching option(s)
1 Myeloid lineage	
2 Haemopoietic stem cell	
3 T-lineage acute lymphoblastic leukaemia	
4 Hairy cell leukaemia	
5 Acute megakaryoblastic leukaemia	

References

1 Swirsky D and Bain BJ, Erythrocyte and leucocyte cytochemistry. In: Lewis SM, Bain BJ and Bates I. *Dacie and Lewis Practical Haematology*, 10th Edn. Churchill Livingstone, Philadelphia, 2006.
2 Hanker JS, Yates PE, Metz CB and Rustioni A (1977) A new, specific, sensitive and non-carcinogenic reagent for the demonstration of horseradish peroxidase. *Histochem J*, **9**, 789–792.
3 Yam LT, Li CY and Crosby WH (1971) Cytochemical identification of monocytes and granulocytes. *Am J Clin Pathol*, **55**, 283–290.

4 Hayhoe FGJ and Quaglino D. *Haematological Cytochemistry*. Churchill Livingstone, Edinburgh, 1980.

5 Janckila A, Li C-Y, Lam K-W and Yam LT (1978) The cytochemistry of tartrate-resistant acid phosphatase technical considerations. *Am J Clin Pathol*, **70**, 45–55.

6 Gadson D, Hughes M, Dean A and Wickramasinghe SN (1986) Morphology of redox-dye-treated HbH-containing red cells: confusion caused by wrongly identified dyes. *Clin Lab Haematol*, **8**, 365–366.

7 Roper D and Layton M, Investigation of the hereditary haemolytic anaemias: membrane and enzyme abnormalities. In: Lewis SM, Bain BJ and Bates I. *Dacie and Lewis Practical Haematology*, 10th Edn. Churchill Livingstone, Philadelphia, 2006.

8 Rustin GJS, Wilson PD and Peters TJ (1979) Studies on the subcellular localization of human neutrophil alkaline phosphatase. *J Cell Sci*, **36**, 401–412.

9 Ackerman GA (1962) Substituted naphthol AS phosphate derivatives for the localization of leukocyte alkaline phosphatase activity. *Lab Invest*, **11**, 563–567.

10 Kaplow LS (1968) Leukocyte alkaline phosphatase cytochemistry: applications and methods. *Ann NY Acad Sci*, **155**, 911–947.

11 Breton-Gorius J, Mason DY, Buriot D, Vilde J-L and Griscelli C (1980) Lactoferrin deficiency as a consequence of a lack of specific granules in neutrophils from patient with recurrent infections. *Am J Pathol*, **99**, 413–419.

12 Repine JE, Clawson CC and Brunning D (1976) Primary leucocyte alkaline phosphatase deficiency in an adult with repeated infections. *Br J Haematol*, **34**, 87–94.

13 Drouin A, Favier R, Massé J-M, Debili N, Schmitt A, Elbin C *et al.* (2001) Newly recognized cellular abnormalities in the gray platelet syndrome. *Blood*, **98**, 1382–1391.

14 Kohmura K, Miyakawa Y, Kameyama K, Kizaki M and Ikeda Y (2004) Granulocyte colony stimulating factor-producing multiple myeloma associated with neutrophilia. *Leuk Lymphoma*, **45**, 1475–1479.

15 O'Kell RT (1968) Leukocyte alkaline phosphatase activity in the infant. *Ann NY Acad Sci*, **155**, 980–982.

16 Rosner F, Lee SL, Schultz FS and Gorfien PC (1968) The regulation of leukocyte alkaline phosphatase. *Ann NY Acad Sci*, **155**, 902–910.

17 Stavridis J, Creatsas G, Lolis D, Traga G, Antonopoulos M and Kaskarelis D (1981) Relationships between leucocyte alkaline phosphatase and nitroblue tetrazolium reduction activities in the peripheral blood polymorphonuclear leucocytes in normal individuals. *Br J Haematol*, **47**, 157–159.

18 Stein P, Peiper S, Butler D, Melvin S, Williams D and Stass S (1983) Granular acute lymphoblastic leukaemia. *Am J Clin Pathol*, **79**, 426–430.

19 Savage RA, Fishleder J and Tubbs SRR (1983) Confirming myeloid differentiation. *Am J Clin Pathol*, **80**, 412.

20 Catovsky D. Leucocyte enzymes in leukaemia. In: S Roath, ed. *Topical Reviews in Haematology*, Vol. 1. John Wright, Bristol, 1980.

21 Elghetany MT (1999) Double esterase staining of the bone marrow contributes to lineage identification in a case of minimally differentiated acute myeloid leukaemia (AML M0). *Clin Lab Haematol*, **21**, 293–295.

22 Beutler E (1988) Gaucher disease. *Blood Rev*, **2**, 59–70.

23 Gómez-Arbonés X, Pinacho A, Ortiz P, Maciá J, Gallart M, Araguás C *et al.* (2002) Quantification of foetomaternal haemorrhage. An analysis of two cytometric techniques and a semi-quantitative gel agglutination test. *Clin Lab Haematol*, **24**, 47–53.

24 Balduini CL, Cattaneo M, Fabris F, Gresele P, Iolascon A, Pulcinelli FM and Savoia A (2003) Inherited thrombocytopenias: a proposed diagnostic algorithm from the Italian Gruppo di Studio delle Piastrine. *Haematologica*, **89**, 325–329.

25 Hughes DL, Evans G, Metcalfe P, Goodall AH and Williamson LM (2005) Tracking and characterisation of transfused platelets by two colour, whole blood flow cytometry. *Br J Haematol*, **130**, 791–794.

26 Bleesing JJH, Brown MR, Straus SE, Dale JK, Siegel RM, Johnson M *et al.* (2001) Immunophenotypic profiles in families with autoimmune lymphoproliferative syndrome. *Blood*, **98**, 2466–2473.

27 Suga N, Takada H, Nomura A, Ohga S, Ishii E, Ihara K *et al.* (2002) Perforin defects of primary haemophagocytic lymphohistiocytosis in Japan. *Br J Haematol*, **116**, 346–349.

28 General Haematology Task Force of BCSH (1994) Immunophenotyping in the diagnosis of the acute leukaemias. *J Clin Pathol*, **47**, 777–781.

29 General Haematology Task Force of BCSH (1994) Immunophenotyping in the diagnosis of the chronic lymphoproliferative disorders. *J Clin Pathol*, **47**, 871–875.

30 Bain BJ. *Leukaemia Diagnosis*, 3rd Edn. Blackwell Publishing, Oxford, 2003.

31 McKeown CME, Waters JJ, Stacey M, Newman BF, Cardy DLN and Hultén M (1992) Rapid interphase FISH diagnosis of trisomy 18 in blood smears. *Lancet*, **340**, 495.

32 Bain BJ, Clarke DAC, Lampert IA and Wilkins BS. *Bone Marrow Pathology*, 3rd Edn. Blackwell Science, Oxford, 2001.

33 Bain BJ. *Haemoglobinopathy Diagnosis*. 2nd Edn. Blackwell Publishing, Oxford, 2005.

Answers to questions

Multiple choice questions

MCQ 7.1 FFTTF
MCQ 7.2 FFTTF
MCQ 7.3 FTFTT
MCQ 7.4 TTFTT
MCQ 7.5 TFFTT
MCQ 7.6 FFFTT
MCQ 7.7 FTTFF

Extended matching questions

EMQ 7.1
1 G
2 F
3 E
4 D
5 B

EMQ 7.2
1 E
2 C
3 A
4 B
5 D

8 Disorders of red cells and platelets

DISORDERS OF RED CELLS

Disorders of red cells are most often divided into three broad categories, depending on whether the erythrocytes are: (i) microcytic and hypochromic; (ii) normocytic and normochromic; or (iii) macrocytic. Red cell disorders can also be classified as congenital or acquired. Anaemia can be further categorized according to the mechanism, whether due predominantly to a failure of production or to shortened red cell survival, and if the latter whether it is caused by an intrinsic defect of the red cell or by extrinsic factors. In this chapter red cell disorders will be discussed in groups that relate mainly to the morphological features of the cells including their size and degree of haemoglobinization.

Hypochromic and microcytic anaemias and thalassaemias

Disorders resulting from a defect in haem synthesis

Iron deficiency anaemia

Iron deficiency develops when: (i) iron intake is inadequate for needs (e.g. during growth spurts or during pregnancy); (ii) there is malabsorption of iron; (iii) there is increased loss of iron, usually consequent on gastrointestinal or uterine blood loss; (iv) there is renal loss of haemosiderin, as a result of chronic intravascular haemolysis; (v) there is a combination of these factors; or, rarely, (vi) there is sequestration of iron at an inaccessible site, as in idiopathic pulmonary haemosiderosis. In countries where *Schistosoma haematobium* infection occurs, urinary loss of blood may also be causative. Anaemia occurs when a lack of reticuloendothelial storage iron and an inadequate rate of delivery of iron to developing erythroid cells in the marrow leads to reduced synthesis of haem and therefore reduced production of haemoglobin and red blood cells. Clinical features include those attributable to anaemia, such as fatigue, pallor and exertional dyspnoea. More specific features of iron deficiency, apparent only when iron deficiency is severe, include koilonychia (spoon-shaped nails), angular cheilosis (cracks in the skin at the corners of the mouth) and glossitis (inflammation of the tongue).

Blood film and count

In iron deficiency, a normocytic normochromic anaemia with anisocytosis precedes the development of anisochromasia, hypochromia and microcytosis. Morphological changes are not usually marked until haemoglobin concentration (Hb) falls below 10–11 g/dl when characteristic features appear (Fig. 8.1). Poikilocytes include elliptocytes, particularly very narrow elliptocytes, which are often referred to as pencil cells. Occasional target cells can be present but they are not usually numerous, except in patients with haemoglobin C or S trait who sometimes develop target cells only when they become iron deficient. Basophilic stippling is infrequent. Polychromasia is sometimes present.

With most automated full blood counters the earliest evidence of iron deficiency is an increase in the red cell distribution width (RDW). This is indicative of the anisocytosis that precedes anaemia. The next change observed is a fall in the Hb, red blood cell count (RBC) and packed cell volume/haematocrit (PCV/Hct) followed by a fall in the mean cell volume (MCV) and mean cell haemoglobin (MCH). In a study using one of two impedance counters (Sysmex K4500 or Coulter S890) an MCH of less than 26 pg was found to be a more sensitive indicator of iron deficiency than an MCV of less than 80 fl;

Fig. 8.1 The blood film of a patient with iron deficiency anaemia showing anisocytosis, poikilocytosis (including elliptocytes), hypochromia and microcytosis. The blood count (Coulter S Plus IV) was: RBC 4.22×10^{12}/l, Hb 7 g/dl, Hct 0.29, MCV 67 fl, MCH 16.6 pg, MCHC 24.5 g/dl.

sensitivity to a reduced serum ferritin was 97% and 85% respectively [1]. In early iron deficiency anaemia, the RBC is occasionally elevated rather than decreased, particularly in children. With Bayer H.1 series and Advia 120 automated counters the appearance of a population of hypochromic cells and an increase in the haemoglobin distribution width (HDW) is the earliest change detected; a fall in the MCH and mean cell haemoglobin concentration (MCHC) precedes any fall in the MCV [2]. A low MCHC is a sensitive indicator of iron deficiency when it is calculated from a microhaematocrit and the Hb or when it is measured by current Bayer instruments. When measured by impedance-based instruments (such as Coulter or Sysmex instruments) it is insensitive but more specific for iron deficiency. The reticulocyte percentage may be normal or elevated in iron deficiency anaemia, while the absolute reticulocyte count is normal or reduced.

Patients with iron deficiency not infrequently have an increased platelet count, which may be consequent on the iron deficiency itself, on blood loss or on an underlying malignant disease. In severe iron deficiency the platelet count is sometimes low. Leucopenia and thrombocytopenia occur in up to 10% of patients. Hypersegmented neutrophils are sometimes present and are not necessarily indicative of coexisting vitamin B_{12} or folate deficiency. In geographical regions where hookworm occurs, the observation of eosinophilia may suggest that this is the cause of the iron deficiency.

Differential diagnosis

The important differential diagnoses of iron deficiency anaemia are thalassaemia trait and the anaemia of chronic disease. The blood film and count are of some use in distinguishing these disorders but specific tests are needed for a precise diagnosis. Prominent target cells and basophilic stippling favour thalassaemia trait whereas anisochromasia and pencil cells favour iron deficiency; increased rouleaux formation, background staining and other signs of inflammation suggest the anaemia of chronic disease. A high RBC and a low MCV despite a normal Hb are characteristic of thalassaemia trait but very similar red cell indices occur in patients with polycythaemia rubra vera (PRV) who are iron deficient. The RDW is usually elevated in iron deficiency and most often normal in thalassaemia trait [3]. A low MCHC on the less sensitive impedance counters is strongly suggestive of iron deficiency since it is usually normal in thalassaemia trait and in the anaemia of chronic disease. Copper deficiency, a rare cause of a microcytic anaemia, is associated with a low serum iron, normal transferrin concentration and normal ferritin [4]. The equally rare acaeruloplasminaemia is associated with a microcytic anaemia, low serum iron, normal transferrin concentration and moderately elevated serum ferritin. Other rare conditions that can cause a microcytic anaemia are listed in Table 3.1.

Further tests

In uncomplicated iron deficiency anaemia, the diagnosis can be confirmed by either: (i) a low serum ferritin; or (ii) a low serum iron coexisting with an increased transferrin concentration or serum iron binding capacity. It should be noted that a low serum iron by itself gives little useful information since it is found in both iron deficiency and anaemia of chronic disease. When iron deficiency and chronic inflammation coexist there may be no elevation in transferrin concentration and iron binding capacity, and serum ferritin may be in the lower part of the normal range rather than reduced. Whereas a serum ferritin of 20 μg/l is useful for the diagnosis of iron deficiency anaemia when there are no complicating factors, a cut-off of 50 μg/l has been suggested in patients with liver disease [5] and of 70 μg/l in patients with chronic inflammation [6].

An elevated free erythrocyte protoporphyrin or zinc protoporphyrin concentration is found in iron deficiency anaemia, in the anaemia of chronic disease and in lead poisoning but is less often found in thalassaemia trait. It is useful for supporting the diagnosis of iron deficiency in clinical situations where uncomplicated iron deficiency is common, e.g. in children or obstetric patients, and since it can be measured on a very small volume of blood can be useful in field surveys.

Soluble transferrin receptor in serum is increased in iron deficiency and not in the anaemia of chronic disease. However, the usefulness of this test is reduced by the fact that the concentration is also increased whenever erythropoiesis is expanded, e.g. in megaloblastic anaemia, haemolytic anaemias, thalassaemia trait and myelodysplastic syndromes. The soluble transferrin receptor/log serum ferritin gives improved discrimination between iron deficiency and other conditions; this ratio is increased in iron deficiency but not in anaemia of chronic disease [7], in β thalassaemia trait [8] or when erythropoiesis is expanded because of a myelodysplastic syndrome (MDS) [8]. Another ratio, the log[soluble transferrin receptor/serum ferritin] shows a linear relationship with body iron stores [9] and also gives improved separation of iron deficiency (with or without chronic inflammation) from other conditions. If measurement of soluble transferrin receptor is not available, it is possible to identify most iron-deficient patients accurately by means of a graph of serum ferritin plotted against the erythrocyte sedimentation rate (ESR) [10]. In complicated cases the definitive test is the demonstration of absent bone marrow iron.

Biochemical abnormalities of iron deficiency anaemia are summarized in Table 8.1.

There is a very significant incidence of unsuspected coeliac disease (around 10%) in unselected UK adults presenting with iron deficiency anaemia. Screening for coeliac disease may therefore be justifiable, particularly if there is no obvious cause for iron deficiency [11].

Anaemia of chronic disease

'Anaemia of chronic disease' is a term used to describe anaemia that is the result of chronic infection or inflammation or, less often, of malignant disease and that is characterized by: (i) low serum iron concentration and defective incorporation of iron into haemoglobin despite adequate bone marrow stores of iron; (ii) a blunted erythropoietin response to anaemia; and (iii) some shortening of red cell survival [12]. Clinical features are attributable to the primary disease, the effects of anaemia or both.

Blood film and count

Anaemia of chronic disease, when mild, is normocytic and normochromic, but as it becomes more severe hypochromia and microcytosis develop (Fig. 8.2). In severe chronic inflammation, the degree of microcytosis may be just as marked as in iron deficiency. The RDW has been reported to be normal in anaemia of chronic disease [3] but this has not been a consistent observation [13]. The absolute reticulocyte count is reduced. Associated features indicative of chronic inflammation may be present, e.g. neutrophilia, thrombocytosis, increased rouleaux formation and increased background staining.

Table 8.1 A comparison of laboratory tests in iron deficiency, and the anaemia of chronic disease and thalassaemia trait.

	Iron deficiency anaemia	Anaemia of chronic disease	Anaemia of chronic disease and iron deficiency	Thalassaemia trait
Serum iron	Reduced	Reduced	Reduced	Normal
Serum transferrin/serum iron binding capacity	Increased	Normal or reduced	Reduced	Normal
Transferrin saturation	Reduced, sometimes markedly	Reduced	Reduced	Normal
Serum ferritin	Reduced, less than 20 μg/l	Normal or increased	Normal or reduced, generally less than 70 μg/l	Normal
Red cell zinc protoporphyrin	Increased	Increased	Increased	Normal or somewhat increased
Soluble transferrin receptor	Increased	Normal or reduced	Normal or increased	Increased
Soluble transferrin receptor/log serum ferritin	Increased	Normal	Probably increased	Normal
Log[soluble transferrin receptor/serum ferritin]	Increased	Normal	Increased	Normal
Bone marrow iron	Absent	Present, often increased	Absent	Present

Fig. 8.2 The blood film of a patient with the anaemia of chronic disease consequent on a lymphoma, showing mild anisocytosis, poikilocytosis and hypochromia. The blood count (Coulter S Plus IV) was: RBC 3.10×10^{12}/l, Hb 7.4 g/dl, Hct 0.23, MCV 75.6 fl, MCH 23.8 pg, MCHC 31.5 g/dl.

Differential diagnosis

The differential diagnosis is iron deficiency anaemia (see above) and other causes of normochromic normocytic and hypochromic microcytic anaemia.

Further tests

Serum iron and serum transferrin (or iron binding capacity) are reduced. Serum ferritin is increased, consequent on synthesis of apoferritin by inflammatory or neoplastic cells. Associated features indicative of chronic inflammation are useful in making the diagnosis. In addition to blood film features, these commonly include elevated plasma viscosity, ESR and C-reactive protein, a reduced serum albumin concentration and an increased concentration of fibrinogen, α_2 macroglobulin and γ globulins. Red cell free protoporphyrin or zinc protoporphyrin is increased so that this test is not useful in distinguishing between iron deficiency and the anaemia of chronic disease. Soluble serum transferrin receptor is generally reduced or normal.

It is not uncommon for a patient with anaemia of chronic disease due to malignancy or chronic inflammation to develop iron deficiency, usually as a consequence of gastrointestinal blood loss. The usual results of laboratory tests in anaemia of chronic disease, in iron deficiency anaemia and when both conditions are present, are shown in Table 8.1. However, it may not always be possible recognize the combination of iron deficiency and anaemia of chronic disease on the basis of the blood film and biochemical tests. A bone marrow aspiration will allow a correct appraisal.

Congenital sideroblastic anaemia

Congenital sideroblastic anaemia is a rare inherited condition. In most families, it has an X-linked inheritance and is therefore largely confined to males. Rarely it occurs in women as a result of skewed X-chromosome inactivation and onset may then be delayed till old age [14]. X-linked sideroblastic anaemia usually results from a defect in haem synthesis as a result of mutation in the erythroid specific 5-amino laevulinic acid synthase gene, *ALAS2*, but occasionally results from a mutation in *ABC7*, a gene encoding a mitochondrial transporter protein [15,16]. Sideroblastic anaemia usually occurs as an isolated anomaly but when due to an *ABC7* mutation it is associated with spinocerebellar ataxia [16]. Otherwise the clinical features are those of anaemia. Usually there is hypochromia and microcytosis but in Pearson's syndrome, resulting from mutation in a mitochondrial gene, there is normocytic or macrocytic anaemia rather than microcytic anaemia [17]. Similarly, in two other rare inherited syndromes there is macrocytosis associated with erythropoiesis which is both sideroblastic and megaloblastic; these syndromes are thiamine-responsive megaloblastic anaemia with diabetes mellitus and sensorineural deafness, due to a mutation in the *SLC19A2* gene, and the **D**iabetes **I**nsipidus, **D**iabetes **M**ellitus **O**ptic **A**trophy and **D**eafness (DIDMOAD) syndrome (also known as Wolfram's syndrome), due to a mutation in the *WFS1* gene [18].

Blood film and count

The Hb ranges from 3–4 g/dl to almost normal. The blood film (Fig. 8.3) may be dimorphic or show uniform hypochromia and microcytosis. Occasionally,

Fig. 8.3 A dimorphic blood film from a patient with congenital sideroblastic anaemia. There is a minor population of cells that are hypochromic and microcytic with a tendency to target cell formation; there is also poikilocytosis. The patient had previously responded to pyridoxine with a rise of Hb and was taking pyridoxine when this blood specimen was obtained.

Fig. 8.4 Blood film obtained from a non-anaemic carrier of congenital sideroblastic anaemia, the daughter of a patient with moderately severe microcytic anaemia. The film is dimorphic, showing a minor population of hypochromic microcytes.

target cells and basophilic stippling are present. Poikilocytosis is sometimes marked and Pappenheimer bodies may be detectable. In older subjects, hypersplenism due to iron overload may cause mild leucopenia and thrombocytopenia.

The MCV and MCH are reduced and the MCHC is sometimes reduced. Red cell histograms and cytograms may show two populations of red cells.

Female carriers of X-linked sideroblastic anaemia resulting from an *ALAS2* mutation who are not themselves anaemic may have a minor population of hypochromic microcytic cells (Fig. 8.4). Rarely, females have a hypochromic microcytic anaemia similar to that observed in males, as a result of skewed X-chromosome inactivation. Carriers of the *ABC7* mutation may also have a population of hypochromic macrocytes [16].

In Pearson's syndrome there is not only a normocytic or macrocytic anaemia but, in about a quarter of patients, neutropenia or thrombocytopenia [17].

Differential diagnosis

The differential diagnosis of X-linked sideroblastic anaemia includes iron deficiency anaemia and thalassaemia trait. Serum iron and ferritin are normal or elevated, haemoglobin electrophoresis is normal and haemoglobin A_2 concentration is not increased. There is usually no difficulty distinguishing between congenital and acquired sideroblastic anaemia since

the latter is usually characterized by predominantly normocytic or macrocytic cells with only a small population of hypochromic microcytes.

The differential diagnosis of Pearson's syndrome includes congenital bone marrow failure syndromes. The differential diagnosis of thiamine-responsive megaloblastic anaemia and Wolfram's syndrome includes other causes of megaloblastic anaemia.

Further tests

Diagnosis is by bone marrow aspiration; a Perls' stain demonstrates ring sideroblasts. Biochemical assays of enzymes involved in haem synthesis will help to categorize cases further. Pearson's syndrome shows, in addition to ring sideroblasts, erythroid hypoplasia with vacuolation of erythroid and granulocytic precursors.

Lead poisoning

Excess lead interferes with haem synthesis and also causes haemolysis. Patients with significant haematological effects often have other symptoms and signs of lead poisoning such as abdominal pain, constipation and a lead line on the gums. The clinical history and physical examination can thus be helpful in making the diagnosis. The source may be lead-glazed pottery, cosmetics or 'herbal' and other alternative remedies.

Fig. 8.5 The blood film of a patient with lead poisoning showing anisocytosis, hypochromia and prominent basophilic stippling. The blood count (Coulter S Plus IV) was: RBC $2.99 \times 10^{12}/l$, Hb 8.3 g/dl, Hct 0.25, MCV 85 fl, MCH 27.8 pg, MCHC 32.7 g/dl. The reticulocyte count was $281 \times 10^{9}/l$.

Blood film and count

Anaemia is usually mild or moderate in severity. The blood film may show hypochromia and microcytosis or normocytic normochromic red cells with some polychromasia. Basophilic stippling is often prominent (Fig. 8.5). Pappenheimer bodies may also be present since lead causes sideroblastic erythropoiesis. The reticulocyte percentage and absolute count may be elevated.

Red cell indices may be normal or there may be a reduction in the MCV, MCH and MCHC.

Differential diagnosis

The differential diagnosis includes other causes of hypochromic microcytic anaemia and also haemolytic anaemias, particularly that due to inherited pyrimidine 5′ nucleotidase deficiency in which basophilic stippling is also prominent. It should be noted that lead poisoning and iron deficiency often coexist.

Further tests

An appropriately elevated serum lead concentration is confirmatory. Erythrocyte free protoporphyrin or zinc protoporphyrin is increased, since ferrochelatase is inhibited by lead, but this test is not useful in making a distinction from iron deficiency. When there is a haemolytic element there is likely to be increased serum transferrin receptor so this test is also not helpful in making a distinction from iron deficiency.

Disorders resulting from a defect in β globin chain synthesis

β Thalassaemia trait

β Thalassaemia trait refers to heterozygosity for β thalassaemia, an inherited condition in which a mutation in a β globin gene or, less often, the deletion of a β globin gene leads to a reduced rate of synthesis of β globin chains. There is consequently a reduced rate of synthesis of haemoglobin. Compensatory erythroid hyperplasia leads to the production of increased numbers of red cells of reduced size and haemoglobin content. The mutations giving rise to β thalassaemia are very numerous and very heterogeneous. In some cases the abnormal gene leads to no β chain production (β° thalassaemia) whereas in others the abnormal gene permits β chain synthesis at a reduced rate (β⁺ thalassaemia). Different mutations producing defects of varying severity are prevalent in different parts of the world.

β Thalassaemia trait occurs in virtually all ethnic groups although in northern European Caucasians it is very infrequent. It is common in Greece and Italy where the prevalence in some regions reaches

15–20%. There is a similar prevalence in Cyprus among both Greek and Turkish Cypriots. The prevalence in some parts of India, Thailand and other parts of South-East Asia reaches 5–10%. In Black Americans the prevalence is about 0.5% and in Afro-Caribbeans it is about 1%.

Heterozygosity for β thalassaemia is usually clinically inapparent and for this reason the term 'thalassaemia minor' is sometimes used to describe it. Occasional patients have mild splenomegaly or signs or symptoms of anaemia.

An acquired deficiency of pyrimidine 5′ nucleotidase has been found to be common in β thalas-saemia heterozygosity, possibly resulting from oxidant damage to the enzyme [19].

Blood film and count

The majority of subjects with β thalassaemia trait have a normal Hb; a minority are mildly anaemic, particularly during pregnancy or intercurrent infections. Anaemia is more common among Greeks and Italians than among those with African ancestry. Despite the lack of anaemia, microcytosis is usually marked. The blood film (Figs 8.6 & 8.7) may or may not show hypochromia in addition to microcytosis.

Fig. 8.6 The blood film of a healthy subject with β thalassaemia trait showing minimal morphological abnormalities—microcytosis and mild poikilocytosis. The diagnosis could easily be missed without the red cell indices. The blood count (Coulter S Plus IV) was RBC 7.3×10^{12}/l, Hb 14.3 g/dl, Hct 0.43, MCV 59 fl, MCH 19.7 pg, MCHC 32.8 g/dl.

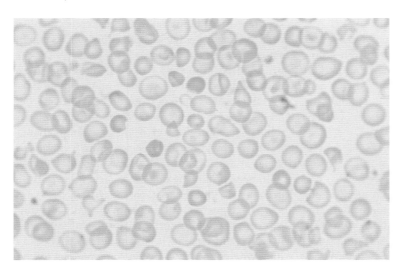

Fig. 8.7 The blood film of a healthy subject with β thalassaemia trait showing more marked morphological abnormalities— anisocytosis, poikilocytosis, hypochromia, microcytosis, occasional target cells and several irregularly contracted cells. The blood count (Coulter S Plus IV) was: RBC 5.78×10^{12}/l, Hb 10.5 g/dl, Hct 0.32, MCV 56 fl, MCH 18.2 pg, MCHC 32.3 g/dl.

The haemoglobin concentration of cells may appear very uniform, in contrast to the anisochromasia that is usual in iron deficiency. Poikilocytosis varies from trivial to marked. Target cells may be prominent but in some patients they are infrequent or absent. A few irregularly contracted cells are seen in some patients. Occasional patients have marked elliptocytosis but, in general, elliptocytes are not a feature. Basophilic stippling is quite common in Mediterranean subjects with β thalassaemia trait but is less often seen in those of African or Chinese/South-East Asian ancestry. Acquired deficiency of pyrimidine 5′ nucleotidase (see above) provides a possible explanation of the frequency of basophilic stippling. The reticulocyte percentage and absolute count are often somewhat elevated [20]. In uncomplicated cases the white cell and platelet counts are normal.

The red cell indices of β thalassaemia trait are very characteristic and it is often easier to make a correct provisional diagnosis from the red cell indices than from the blood film. The Hb and Hct are normal or close to normal while the MCV and MCH are usually markedly reduced. The MCHC is usually normal when measured by impedance counters such as Sysmex and Coulter instruments but is often somewhat reduced when measured by Bayer H.1 series instruments and the Advia 120. When the numbers of hypochromic cells and microcytic cells are measured independently, the percentage of microcytes usually exceeds the percentage of hypochromic cells in thalassaemia trait whereas the reverse is found in iron deficiency [21]. The red cell cytogram characteristically has a 'comma' shape (Fig. 8.8). In contrast to iron deficiency, the RDW is usually normal [3] but when a patient with β thalassaemia trait becomes anaemic the RDW tends to rise [3] so that this measurement is least useful when most needed. Other observers have often found the RDW to be elevated even in non-anaemic patients [13].

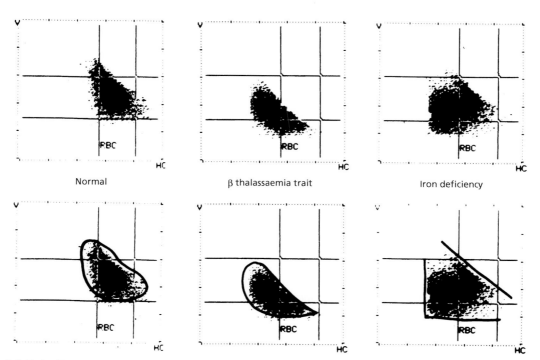

Fig. 8.8 Red cell cytograms from a Bayer H.2 counter showing the relationship between haemoglobinization (*x*-axis) and volume (*y*-axis) of individual red cells in a normal subject (left) and patients with β thalassaemia trait (centre) and iron deficiency (right). The 'comma' shape of β thalassaemia trait is apparent and has been emphasized by the sketched outlines of the cytograms in the lower series of scatter plots.

The diagnosis of thalassaemia trait is more difficult in pregnant patients for two reasons. Firstly, the red cell indices are less characteristic since haemodilution, which is a physiological effect of pregnancy, lowers the Hb, RBC and Hct; the Hb may fall as low as 5–6 g/dl [22]. The rise in MCV that occurs in pregnancy also contributes to the red cell indices being less characteristic than in a non-pregnant subject. Secondly, iron deficiency anaemia has an increased prevalence during pregnancy and when the two conditions coexist diagnosis is more complicated.

Differential diagnosis

The important differential diagnoses of β thalassaemia trait are α thalassaemia trait and iron deficiency anaemia. Various formulae have been devised in an attempt to separate iron deficiency from β thalassaemia trait [23–30]. Although such formulae may be useful in separating uncomplicated cases into the two diagnostic groups, they are not generally applicable to pregnant women [31] or children and are not useful in patients who have both iron deficiency *and* thalassaemia trait, a not uncommon situation with patients from the Indian subcontinent. Although these formulae are useful in suggesting the most likely diagnosis, there is little choice but to carry out specific diagnostic tests in circumstances where the diagnosis of thalassaemia trait is important, e.g. for antenatal or pre-conceptual genetic counselling. In this situation either the MCV or the MCH can be used as a screening test with all patients whose test results fall below an arbitrary limit having haemoglobin electrophoresis or an equivalent test performed. Occasional patients with mild variants of β thalassaemia trait have only a very trivial reduction of the MCV and MCH and if such cases are to be identified it is necessary to test all patients whose results fall below the lower limit of the reference range. Even this will not detect all cases since in some mild thalassaemic variants there is no apparent haematological defect in heterozygotes; such cases cannot be diagnosed from the blood film and indices. However, except when genetic counselling is being carried out in high incidence areas, it is generally necessary to have a cut-off point for further investigation that is at or below the lower limit of the reference range in order to avoid having a very high percentage of negative tests with a very low yield of positive diagnoses.

It is not possible on the basis of the blood film and count to distinguish β thalassaemia trait from δβ or εγδβ thalassaemia trait or from cases of α thalassaemia trait in which two of the four α genes are deleted. Cases of α thalassaemia trait in which only one of the four α genes is deleted have only minor haematological abnormalities and are less likely to be confused with β thalassaemia trait. Occasional patients with a blood film and red cell indices suggestive of thalassaemia trait have either a highly unstable globin chain or an abnormal haemoglobin that is synthesized at a reduced rate. The commonest of the latter group is haemoglobin Lepore, consequent on a formation of a δβ fusion gene. Haemoglobin E is also synthesized at a reduced rate and both heterozygosity and homozygosity for this abnormal haemoglobin can produce indices suggestive of thalassaemia trait. Sickle cell trait and haemoglobin C trait are also not infrequently associated with microcytosis, although this may be only because of associated α thalassaemia trait.

The red cell indices in iron deficient polycythaemia may be indistinguishable from those of thalassaemia trait but the RDW is more likely to be elevated and there may be associated features that are useful in the differential diagnosis such as neutrophilia, basophilia, thrombocytosis and the presence of giant platelets. The characteristic indices of thalassaemia can also be simulated by iron deficiency anaemia undergoing treatment. A marked elevation of the RDW (and HDW) or the detection of two cell populations on a blood film or on the graphical output of an automated counter suggests that the correct diagnosis is iron deficiency.

Anaemia of chronic disease can usually be readily distinguished from β thalassaemia because of the greater degree of anaemia and retention of a normal MCV until significant anaemia has developed.

Further tests

Haemoglobin electrophoresis and demonstration of an increased percentage of haemoglobin A_2 are necessary for the definitive diagnosis of β thalassaemia trait. Alternatively, high performance liquid chromatography (HPLC) both permits quantification of haemoglobin A_2 and excludes the presence of a variant haemoglobin. Haemoglobin F is elevated in one-third to half of patients but is less specific than an increased percentage of haemoglobin A_2. δβ or $^A\gamma\delta\beta^0$ thalassaemia trait is diagnosed when there are thalassaemic indices with a normal or low haemoglobin A_2 and an elevated haemoglobin F. Diagnosis of the rare cases of εγδβ thalassaemia (also known as γδβ thalassaemia) trait requires DNA analysis. Haemoglobin Lepore trait is diagnosed when there are thalassaemic indices with a normal or reduced haemoglobin A_2 and with a minor abnormal haemoglobin having the same mobility as haemoglobin S at alkaline pH, the same mobility as haemoglobin A at acid pH and a retention time on HPLC that is similar to that of haemoglobin A_2. Haemoglobins E, C and S will also be detected on electrophoresis.

Because iron deficiency causes a reduction of the haemoglobin A_2 percentage, some cases of mild β thalassaemia trait may be missed if tests are done when the patient has a coexisting iron deficiency. Except in pregnant patients, when immediate diagnosis is needed, it is better not to carry out electrophoresis in patients who appear to have uncomplicated iron deficiency, but rather to check that the full blood count (FBC) returns to normal after treatment.

Most of the tests used to confirm a diagnosis of iron deficiency are normal in β thalassaemia trait (see Table 8.1). However zinc protoporphyrin is somewhat increased and soluble transferrin receptor is increased to similar levels to those seen in iron deficiency [8].

β Thalassaemia major

β Thalassaemia major is an inherited disease resulting from homozygosity or compound heterozygosity for β thalassaemia that leads to a severe reduction or total lack of synthesis of β globin chains. Consequently, there is a marked reduction or total failure to synthesize haemoglobin A. There is marked erythroid hyperplasia and ineffective haemopoiesis consequent on damage to developing erythroblasts by excess free α chains. Clinical features are severe anaemia, hepatomegaly, splenomegaly and expansion of marrow-containing bones leading to frontal bossing of the skull and deformity of the jaw bones. There is significant growth retardation. Treatment of β thalassaemia major by blood transfusion ameliorates many of the clinicopathological features seen in the untreated patient but, in the absence of effective chelation therapy, leads to iron overload, resultant organ damage and premature death.

Blood film and count

Anaemia is severe with the Hb sometimes being as low as 2–3 g/dl. The blood film (Fig. 8.9) shows very marked anisocytosis and poikilocytosis with the

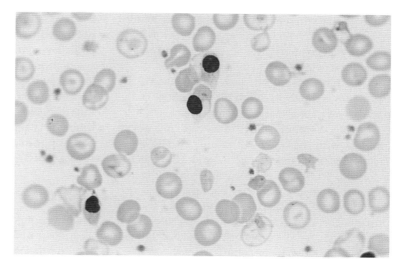

Fig. 8.9 The blood film of a patient with β thalassaemia major who has been splenectomized and is receiving intermittent blood transfusions. The blood film is dimorphic with about two-thirds of the erythrocytes being donor cells. The patient's own red cells show marked anisocytosis, poikilocytosis and hypochromia. There are several target cells and three nucleated red blood cells (NRBC). Some cells contain Pappenheimer bodies and in two cells (a very hypochromic cell and an NRBC) there are inclusions that represent precipitated α chains.

poikilocytes including target cells, teardrop cells, elliptocytes, fragments and many cells of bizarre shape. Hypochromia is very striking but microcytosis is not always so obvious on the blood film since the cells are very flat and red cell diameter is thus greater than would be expected from the red cell size. Basophilic stippling and Pappenheimer bodies are present. Sometimes a minority of cells have inclusions with the same staining characteristics as haemoglobin; these represent precipitates of excess α chains and are much more readily identified on a Heinz body preparation. Nucleated red blood cells (NRBC) are frequent. The circulating erythroblasts are micronormoblastic and show dyserythropoietic features, defective haemoglobinization and the presence of Pappenheimer bodies. There is often leucocytosis, resulting from neutrophilia and, in younger children, lymphocytosis. The platelet count may be normal or increased. In advanced disease with marked splenomegaly, the platelet count falls.

Following splenectomy (which may be performed because of discomfort from splenomegaly or to reduce transfusion requirement), the total nucleated cell count (TNCC), white blood cell count (WBC) and platelet count rise; the blood film is even more strikingly abnormal with many abnormal NRBC and numerous target cells, Pappenheimer bodies and Howell–Jolly bodies. Post-splenectomy, Heinz body preparations show ragged inclusions in 10–20% of cells; these represent α chain precipitates and differ from the Heinz bodies consequent on oxidant stress in that they are not attached to the red cell membrane and are present in NRBC as well as mature erythrocytes [32]. Following splenectomy, there is often an exaggerated lymphocytosis or neutrophilia in response to intercurrent infections.

When patients are adequately transfused, the blood film is dimorphic with the percentage of the patient's own abnormal cells being low.

The blood count shows a severe microcytic anaemia with the MCV, MCH and MCHC being greatly reduced and the RDW and HDW being increased. The TNCC, as measured on automated counters, is greatly increased because of the presence of many NRBC; a true leucocytosis is also often present. The TNCC may be erroneous since, with some automated instruments, some but not all NRBC are included in the count.

Differential diagnosis

Thalassaemia intermedia is distinguished from thalassaemia major on clinical rather than haematological grounds. It is a genetically heterogeneous condition but most often results from homozygosity or compound heterozygosity for mild β^+ thalassaemia. The Hb is usually above 7–8 g/dl and other peripheral blood features are also intermediate between those of thalassaemia major and thalassaemia minor. The compound heterozygous state for β thalassaemia and haemoglobin E can also have haematological features that resemble those of thalassaemia major.

Further tests

Diagnosis requires haemoglobin electrophoresis or HPLC which show only haemoglobins F and A_2 when the genotype is β°/β° and haemoglobins F and A_2 with a variable amount of haemoglobin A when the genotype is β°/β^+ or β^+/β^+. Some cases of thalassaemia intermedia have a relatively high percentage of haemoglobin A while others have almost exclusively haemoglobin F. Patients with severe disease as a result of compound heterozygosity for haemoglobin E and β thalassaemia are distinguished from thalassaemia major by haemoglobin electrophoresis or HPLC.

β Thalassaemia intermedia

β Thalassaemia intermedia refers to a clinical phenotype with diverse genetic explanations [30]. The patient is symptomatic from anaemia, often has splenomegaly and sometimes has bony deformities. However, in contrast to β thalassaemia major, the patient is not transfusion-dependent. β thalassaemia intermedia varies in severity, from a disabling condition in which survival without transfusion is barely possible to a condition only slightly more severe than β thalassaemia minor.

Blood film and count

There is a moderately severe microcytic anaemia. The blood film shows features similar to those of typical β thalassaemia trait but the abnormalities are

Fig. 8.10 The blood film of a patient with β thalassaemia intermedia caused by homozygosity for a mild β thalassaemia variant.

more severe (Fig. 8.10). Polychromasia and circulating NRBC may be present.

Differential diagnosis

The differential diagnosis is β thalassaemia minor and β thalassaemia major. Diagnosis depends more on clinical than on laboratory features.

Other tests

Haemoglobin electrophoresis or HPLC show the presence of considerable amounts of haemoglobin F. The proportion of haemoglobin A_2 is increased. In some patients there is also some haemoglobin A.

Disorders resulting from a defect in α globin chain synthesis

α Thalassaemia trait

Haematologically normal subjects have four α genes. α Thalassaemia trait is consequent on deletion of either one or two of the four α genes. The genotype $-\alpha/\alpha\alpha$ is designated α^+ thalassaemia. The genotype $--/\alpha\alpha$ is designated α° thalassaemia. Homozygosity for α^+ thalassaemia, i.e. $-\alpha/-\alpha$, or heterozygosity for the much less common non-deletional α thalassaemia trait, $\alpha^T\alpha/\alpha\alpha$ or $\alpha\alpha^T/\alpha\alpha$, produce a phenotype similar to that of α° thalassaemia trait. α thalassaemia is

common among many ethnic groups. A high incidence is found among various South-East Asian populations, particularly among Thais and Chinese, who have both the $-\alpha/\alpha\alpha$ and the $--/\alpha\alpha$ genotypes. Among Black Americans 25–30% have $-\alpha/\alpha\alpha$ and 1–2% have $-\alpha/-\alpha$ [33]. In Jamaicans the prevalence is approximately 30% and 3%, respectively [34]. In Nigerians the prevalence is even higher with 35% having $-\alpha/\alpha\alpha$ and 8% $-\alpha/-\alpha$ [35]. $-\alpha/\alpha\alpha$ occurs in about 7% of Greeks [36] and is common in Cyprus and in some regions of Italy. On some Pacific islands the prevalence of $-\alpha/\alpha\alpha$ is as high as 85%.

α Thalassaemia trait produces no clinically evident effects but can be of genetic significance.

Blood film and count

α° Thalassaemia heterozygosity and α^+ thalassaemia homozygosity produce haematological features similar to those of β thalassaemia trait although basophilic stippling and target cells are often not prominent (Fig. 8.11). α^+ Thalassaemia heterozygosity produces a lesser abnormality and often there is no discernible abnormality in the blood film.

The red cell indices of individuals with only two α genes are similar to those of β thalassaemia trait. The indices in individuals with three rather than four α genes may be either normal or abnormal, in the latter case overlapping the values seen in those with only two α genes.

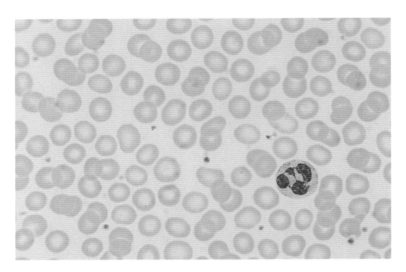

Fig. 8.11 The blood film of a healthy subject with α thalassaemia trait showing microcytosis and mild hypochromia. The blood count (Coulter S) was: RBC 6.24×10^{12}/l, Hb 14.1 g/dl, Hct 0.45, MCV 72 fl, MCH 23 pg, MCHC 31.3 g/dl.

Differential diagnosis

The differential diagnosis of α thalassaemia trait is β thalassaemia trait and iron deficiency. A similar haematological phenotype is also produced by several α chain variant haemoglobins that are synthesized at a greatly reduced rate; the commonest of these is haemoglobin Constant Spring, which is not uncommon in South-East Asia and is also found in the Caribbean area, around the Mediterranean, in the Middle East and in the Indian subcontinent. The blood film in haemoglobin Constant Spring trait often shows prominent basophilic stippling.

An α thalassaemia phenotype can also result from certain rare, highly unstable α chains variants that are largely degraded before haemoglobin can be formed.

Further tests

Haemoglobin electrophoresis and HPLC are normal in α thalassaemia trait, except during the neonatal period when a low percentage of haemoglobin Bart's (γ_4) and haemoglobin H (β_4) may be detected. Haemoglobin Constant Spring can be detected electrophoretically and by HPLC, although sometimes with difficulty since the percentage of the abnormal haemoglobin is usually low. In adults the diagnosis of α thalassaemia trait should be suspected when a subject of an appropriate ethnic group who is not iron deficient has indices suggestive of thalassaemia trait with normal electrophoresis and a normal or low haemoglobin A_2 percentage. The demonstration of haemoglobin H inclusions in a very small percentage of red cells supports the diagnosis but this test is quite time-consuming and it may be negative, particularly in heterozygotes, and to a lesser extent homozygotes, for α^+ thalassaemia. When diagnosis is important, as when genetic counselling is required in a patient of South-East Asian, Greek, Turkish or Cypriot ethnic origin, DNA analysis is necessary.

Haemoglobin H disease

The lack of three of the four α genes (genotype $--/-\alpha$) or a functionally similar disorder [22] causes haemoglobin H disease. This most often occurs in subjects of South-East Asian origin including Thais, Chinese and Indonesians but it is also seen in Greeks and Cypriots and less often in a variety of other ethnic groups. Clinical features are of a chronic haemolytic anaemia with splenomegaly and sometimes hepatomegaly. In patients with more severe disease there is sometimes bony deformity similar to that seen in β thalassaemia major.

Blood film and count

The diagnosis of haemoglobin H disease can usually be suspected from the blood film and red cell indices. There is anaemia of moderate degree; the Hb is typically 6–10 g/dl but it is lower during pregnancy,

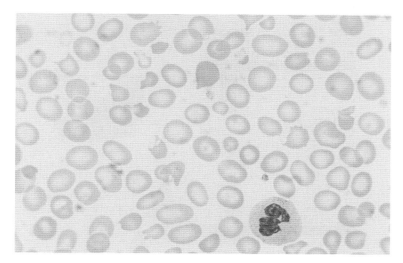

Fig. 8.12 The blood film of a patient with haemoglobin H disease showing anisocytosis, marked poikilocytosis, microcytosis and hypochromia. The blood count (Coulter S Plus IV) was: RBC 4.95×10^{12}/l, Hb 9.6 g/dl, Hct 0.30, MCV 60.5 fl, MCH 19.4 pg, MCHC 32.1 g/dl, RDW 25.7. The corresponding haemoglobin H preparation is shown in Fig. 7.2a.

during intercurrent infections and following exposure to oxidant drugs. The blood film (Fig. 8.12) shows marked hypochromia, microcytosis and poikilocytosis, often including target cells, teardrop cells and fragments. Basophilic stippling and polychromasia are present. The reticulocyte percentage and absolute count are elevated.

The red cell indices show marked reduction of the MCV and MCH and reduction of the MCHC, which are demonstrated by the red cell cytogram (Fig. 8.13). The RDW and HDW are elevated.

Differential diagnosis

The differential diagnosis of haemoglobin H disease is β thalassaemia and other haemolytic and dyserythropoietic anaemias. The blood film and red cell indices are much more abnormal than in most β thalassaemia heterozygotes but may be similar to those in β thalassaemia intermedia; the elevated reticulocyte count and the usual lack of NRBC in haemoglobin H disease are useful in making the distinction from β thalassaemia intermedia. The MCHC is reduced, irrespective of the method of measurement, whereas in β thalassaemia trait it is not reduced when measured by impedance counters but is reduced when measured by Bayer H.1 series and Advia 120 instruments. Congenital dyserythropoietic anaemias and hereditary pyropoikilocytosis can show a similar degree of poikilocytosis to haemoglobin H disease but the former group of disorders have normocytic or macrocytic red cells and no reticulocytosis while

the blood film in the latter condition shows specific types of poikilocyte such as microspherocytes, elliptocytes and red cells with bud-like projections. Acquired haemoglobin H disease, which can be a manifestation of a myelodysplastic syndrome, should also be mentioned in the differential diagnosis of the inherited condition; it is differentiated by the age of onset, the lack of a relevant family history and the demonstration of other features of myelodysplasia (Fig. 8.14).

Further tests

The diagnosis is confirmed by the demonstration of haemoglobin H inclusions in red cells (see Fig. 7.2) and by haemoglobin electrophoresis or HPLC which show 2–40% of haemoglobin H. Haemoglobin electrophoresis will also identify cases with both haemoglobin Constant Spring and haemoglobin H; such cases have the genotype $\alpha^{CS}\alpha$/–– which produces clinical and haematological features similar to haemoglobin H disease although often somewhat more severe.

Haemoglobin Bart's hydrops fetalis

Haemoglobin Bart's hydrops fetalis is a syndrome resulting from an absence of all four α genes (α genotype ––/––) and a consequent total lack of α globin chain synthesis. The result is severe anaemia and hypoalbuminaemia causing stillbirth or early neonatal death of a hydropic fetus.

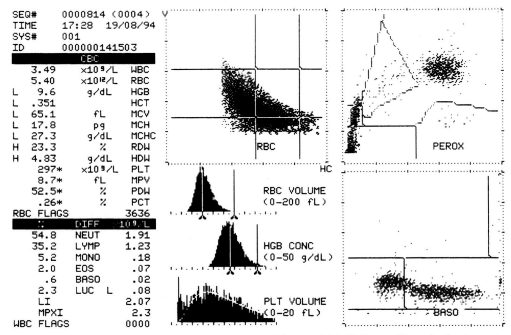

```
SEQ#      0000814 (0004)
TIME      17:28  19/08/94
SYS#      001
ID        000000141503
          CBC
     3.49    ×10⁹/L    WBC
     5.40    ×10¹²/L   RBC
L    9.6     g/dL      HGB
L    .351              HCT
L    65.1    fL        MCV
L    17.8    pg        MCH
L    27.3    g/dL      MCHC
H    23.3    %         RDW
H    4.83    g/dL      HDW
     297*    ×10⁹/L    PLT
     8.7*    fL        MPV
     52.5*   %         PDW
     .26*    %         PCT
RBC FLAGS              3636
          DIFF    10⁹/L
     54.8    NEUT      1.91
     35.2    LYMP      1.23
     5.2     MONO      .18
     2.0     EOS       .07
     .6      BASO      .02
     2.3     LUC   L   .08
     LI                2.07
     MPXI              2.3
WBC FLAGS             0000
```

Fig. 8.13 Bayer H.2 scatter plots and histograms of a patient with haemoglobin H disease. The red cell cytogram and histograms show severe hypochromia and microcytosis. The white cell scatter plots are normal.

Fig. 8.14 The blood film of a patient with acquired haemoglobin H disease as part of a myelodysplastic syndrome showing anisocytosis, poikilocytosis, microcytosis and some hypochromic cells and target cells. One of the hypochromic cells contains Pappenheimer bodies. The blood count was: WBC 9.2×10^9/l, Hb 10.2 g/dl, MCV 66 fl and platelet count 53×10^9/l. Courtesy of Dr A. Hendrick, South Shields.

Blood film and count

There is severe anaemia and the blood film (Fig. 8.15) shows striking hypochromia, microcytosis, poikilocytosis and the presence of NRBC.

Differential diagnosis

The differential diagnosis includes other causes of severe anaemia in the fetus (see Table 6.20) and other causes of hydrops fetalis.

Fig. 8.15 The blood film of neonate with haemoglobin Bart's hydrops fetalis showing anisocytosis, poikilocytosis and numerous nucleated red blood cells (NRBC). Courtesy of Dr Mary Frances McMullin, Belfast.

Further tests

The diagnosis is confirmed by demonstration of α° thalassaemia trait in both parents and by haemoglobin electrophoresis or HPLC, which show only haemoglobins Bart's, H and Portland. Diagnosis in early pregnancy, permitting early termination of an affected pregnancy, can be achieved by molecular analysis of fetal cells obtained by chorionic villus sampling.

Haemoglobinopathies

Haemoglobinopathies are inherited abnormalities of globin chain synthesis. Some haematologists use this term broadly to cover all such abnormalities, including the thalassaemias. Others classify disorders of globin chain synthesis as 'haemoglobinopathies' when there is a structural abnormality and as 'thalassaemias' when the principal abnormality is a reduced rate of synthesis of one of the globin chains. There is necessarily some overlap between 'haemoglobinopathies' and 'thalassaemias' since some abnormal haemoglobins (e.g. haemoglobin E) are synthesized at a reduced rate. Abnormal haemoglobins may also be formed in thalassaemias as a consequence of unbalanced chain synthesis (e.g. haemoglobin Bart's and haemoglobin H in various α thalassaemia syndromes). The most convenient

approach is probably to regard thalassaemia as a subtype of haemoglobinopathy. Haemoglobinopathies (including thalassaemias) result from mutations in the genes encoding the α, β, γ and δ chains of haemoglobin. Mutations of α genes produce abnormalities affecting haemoglobins A, A_2 and F. Mutations in β genes affect haemoglobin A, mutations in γ genes haemoglobin F and mutations in δ genes haemoglobin A_2. Only mutations affecting α and β genes are important in adult life.

Sickle cell anaemia

Sickle cell anaemia is the disease caused by homozygosity for the β chain variant haemoglobin, haemoglobin S or sickle cell haemoglobin. The genotype is $\beta^S \beta^S$. The term 'sickle cell disease' is used more broadly than 'sickle cell anaemia' to include also other conditions that lead to red cell sickling such as sickle cell/β thalassaemia.

Haemoglobin S is prone to polymerize in conditions of low oxygen tension causing the red cell to become sickle shaped and less deformable. There are associated changes in the red cell membrane and in endothelial cells. The resulting obstruction of small blood vessels leads to tissue infarction which underlies the dominant clinical feature of the disease, the recurrent painful crises affecting fingers and toes (in young children), limbs, abdomen and chest. Other

Fig. 8.16 The blood film of a patient with sickle cell anaemia showing anisocytosis, poikilocytosis, one sickle cell, several boat-shaped cells and a cell containing a Howell–Jolly body.

clinical features are anaemia, which is partly caused by shortened red cell lifespan, and splenomegaly, which is present only during childhood.

The β^S gene and therefore sickle cell anaemia have their greatest frequency in individuals with African ancestry but the gene also occurs in Indian, Greek, Italian, Turkish, Cypriot, Spanish, Arab, North African and Central and South American populations.

Blood film and count

In sickle cell anaemia [37] the Hb is usually of the order of 7–8 g/dl, but with a range of 4–11 g/dl or even wider. Higher Hb levels are characteristic of Arabs with sickle cell anaemia. A typical blood film (Fig. 8.16) shows anisocytosis, anisochromasia, sickle cells, boat-shaped cells (pointed at both ends but not crescent shaped), target cells, polychromasia, basophilic stippling, NRBC and sometimes occasional irregularly contracted cells or spherocytes. Scanning electron micrography shows the characteristic form of the sickle cell (see Fig. 3.48). There may be linear fragments of sickle cells (see Fig. 3.42). Once infancy is past, the features of hyposplenism—Howell–Jolly bodies, Pappenheimer bodies and more numerous target cells—are also present. Acanthocytes, which are usually present in hyposplenic states, are not a feature of hyposplenism caused by sickle cell disease. The reticulocyte count is usually 10–20%. The WBC, neutrophil, lymphocyte, monocyte and platelet counts are higher than in control subjects of the

same ethnic group; counts tend to rise with age [38]. Occasional monocytes and neutrophils contain phagocytosed red cells.

At birth, when only a small amount of haemoglobin S is present, the Hb, red cell indices and blood count are normal. The blood film is usually normal but occasionally sickle cells are seen, even in neonates. Haematological abnormalities usually become apparent during the first year of life [39,40]. The Hb falls below the normal range at 1–6 months of age. A few sickle cells and other features of sickle cell anaemia appear at 4–6 months of age; features of hyposplenism usually appear at 9–12 months of age but sometimes as early as 6 months. The features of hyposplenism appear at about the time that splenomegaly is detected. In early infancy hyposplenism can be reversed by blood transfusion but later it cannot. Circulating NRBC only become common after 12 months of age.

Some subjects, although homozygous for β^S, have a normal or near normal Hb and very few signs or symptoms of sickle cell anaemia; they are mainly Arabs with an unusually high percentage of haemoglobin F, which ameliorates the condition. In such subjects the morphological abnormalities may also be slight. When α thalassaemia trait coexists with sickle cell anaemia there are subtle differences in the red cell indices, but only when groups of patients are considered. Individuals cannot be distinguished on haematological grounds. In a group with coexisting α thalassaemia trait, the mean Hb and RBC are higher, whereas the mean MCV, MCH, MCHC, reticulocyte count and degree of polychromasia and number of sickle cells are less. Treatment with hydroxycarbamide (previously hydroxyurea) causes a rise in the MCV and MCH.

During painful crises there is leucocytosis (with the WBC sometimes as high as $40–50 \times 10^9/l$), neutrophilia, a minor fall in the Hb, increasing polychromasia and a rise in the number of NRBC and the reticulocyte count. There is an increase in the number of sickle cells in the blood film but recognition of this requires careful counting and a knowledge of the baseline values for an individual patient. Irregularly contracted cells become much more numerous during pulmonary infarction with hypoxia.

Because of the shortened red cell survival, patients with sickle cell anaemia are prone to acute worsening of the anaemia when complicating conditions develop. The blood film and count may give some clues as to the cause of this. In acute splenic sequestration, which is largely confined to infants, there is a very acute fall of the Hb and the platelet count also falls. Subsequently, there are increased numbers of NRBC, increasing polychromasia and an elevation of the reticulocyte count. In older subjects, acute sequestration may involve the liver rather than the spleen. In bone marrow infarction the WBC and platelet count may fall, there are prominent leucoerythroblastic features and some circulating megakaryocytes may be seen. In parvovirus B19 infection, white cells and platelets are rarely affected; there is a disappearance of NRBC and polychromasia and the reticulocyte count is very low. During the recovery phase there is an outpouring of NRBC and a rise in the WBC, neutrophil count and reticulocyte count. The suppression of reticulocyte production is usually less when other infections lead to the development of anaemia, which has the characteristics of the anaemia of chronic disease. In megaloblastic anaemia due to folate deficiency, some circulating megaloblasts, macrocytes and hypersegmented neutrophils may be seen. The reticulocyte count falls.

The blood count in sickle cell anaemia shows the Hb, RBC and Hct to be reduced. The MCV is normal or elevated but is not increased to a degree commensurate with the increase in the reticulocyte count [41]; this may be regarded as a relative microcytosis. The RDW and HDW are increased. Bayer H.1 series red cell cytograms (Fig. 8.17) show a population of dense cells representing irreversibly sickled cells and a population of hypodense cells representing reticulocytes. Although hyperdense cells are detected, their percentage may be underestimated because irreversibly sickled cells are incapable of undergoing the sphering that should occur before measurement of red cell variables by these instruments [42,33]. Impedance counters fail to detect the increased MCHC of the most dense cells [42]. Further changes in red cell indices occur during, and sometimes 1–3 days before, painful crises [43]. The slight fall in the Hb and rise in the reticulocyte count are accompanied by further increases in the RDW and HDW. There is an increase in the MCHC and the percentage of abnormally dense cells.

Differential diagnosis

The differential diagnosis of sickle cell anaemia is mainly sickle cell/haemoglobin C disease (see p. 304) and sickle cell/β thalassaemia. Sickle cell/β° thalassaemia cannot be distinguished from sickle cell anaemia on haemoglobin electrophoresis or HPLC since there is no haemoglobin A in either condition. The distinction is made on the basis of family studies and the lower MCV and MCH in the compound heterozygous state. Sickle cell/β+ thalassaemia may show a less abnormal blood count and blood film than sickle cell anaemia, depending on the amount of haemoglobin A that is present; haemoglobin electrophoresis is diagnostic. Compound heterozygosity for haemoglobin S and hereditary persistence of fetal haemoglobin can be distinguished by the milder clinical and haematological phenotype, family studies and haemoglobin electrophoresis or HPLC. Sickle cell trait should not be confused with sickle cell anaemia since the Hb is normal and there are no sickle cells in the blood film but heterozygotes for several rare variants, e.g. Hb S-Antilles, may have sickle cells on routine blood films [44].

Further tests

Diagnosis is based on a sickle solubility test and either haemoglobin electrophoresis or HPLC, although it should be noted that if there are obvious sickle cells in a blood film the sickle solubility test could be

Fig. 8.17 Bayer H.1 red cell scatter plots and histograms of a patient with sickle cell anaemia; the presence of cells with an increased haemoglobin content is apparent on both the red cell cytogram and on the histogram of haemoglobin concentration.

considered redundant. Haemoglobin S predominates with smaller amounts of haemoglobins F and A$_2$ and no haemoglobin A. Haemoglobin F varies from 2% to around 15% and haemoglobin A$_2$ may be minimally elevated. If haemoglobin electrophoresis is the primary analytical method, is necessary for this to be performed at acid as well as alkaline pH to distinguish compound heterozygous states such as S/D-Punjab (S/D-Los Angeles) and S/Lepore from sickle cell anaemia; D-Punjab/Los Angeles and Lepore both move with S at alkaline pH but at acid pH move with haemoglobin A. If the primary analytical method is HPLC then these two variant haemoglobins are not confused with haemoglobin S. In infants, the percentage of haemoglobin S may be too low for the sickle solubility test to be positive and diagnosis then rests on electrophoresis at acid and alkaline pH or HPLC with confirmation by electrophoresis or isoelectric focusing.

Diagnostic tests for sickle cell anaemia and other forms of sickle cell disease are recommended in all neonates of appropriate ethnic origin since early

parenteral education and prophylactic penicillin therapy significantly reduce mortality.

Sickle cell trait

Sickle cell trait indicates heterozygosity for β^S so that both haemoglobin S and haemoglobin A are present. The genotype is $\beta\beta^S$. Sickle cell trait is almost always asymptomatic but is of genetic significance and is relevant if a patient is likely to become hypoxic.

Blood film and count

The blood film may be normal or show microcytosis or target cell formation. Although classical sickle cells are not seen there may be small numbers of plump cells that are pointed at both ends [45]; such cells are observed in about 96% of individuals with sickle cell trait in comparison with 4% of normal subjects. Very rarely true sickle cells are seen. This has been reported in a patient with acute lymphoblastic leukaemia with a very high WBC and was attributed to *in vitro* consumption of oxygen by the leukaemic cells [46]. The blood count is either normal or shows reduction of the MCV and MCH. Reduction of the MCV is more common in those with sickle cell trait than in other Black people [47]. This appears to be due to the slightly higher incidence of α thalassaemia trait in subjects with sickle cell trait [48], since no difference in red cell indices is observed between those with and without sickle cell trait when individuals with iron deficiency or α thalassaemia trait are excluded from the analysis [49].

Differential diagnosis

The main differential diagnosis is other conditions that cause microcytosis (see Table 3.1) and other causes of target cell formation (see Table 3.7).

Further tests

The blood film and count must not be relied on for diagnosis. Diagnosis requires both haemoglobin electrophoresis (which shows A and S but with the percentage of A being greater than the percentage of S) and a sickle solubility test (which shows that the abnormal haemoglobin is haemoglobin S rather than another abnormal haemoglobin with the same mobility). Haemoglobin S is usually 25–45% of total haemoglobin. The diagnosis of sickle cell trait should not be excluded on the basis of a negative sickle solubility test alone; if this is done in an emergency, e.g. before anaesthesia, it must be followed by haemoglobin electrophoresis or HPLC to confirm the negative test. Diagnosis in the first 6 months of life, when the haemoglobin S percentage may be too low for a positive sickle solubility test, requires the use of two independent methods to confirm the nature of the variant haemoglobin: e.g. (i) HPLC, supplemented by isoelectric focusing or electrophoresis, or (ii) electrophoresis at both acid and alkaline pH.

Sickle cell/β thalassaemia

Patients who are heterozygous for haemoglobin S and either β° or β+ thalassaemia cannot be distinguished reliably from sickle cell anaemia on the basis of clinical features although those with βSβ+ thalassaemia tend to have milder disease and splenomegaly is more likely to persist beyond early childhood.

Blood film and count

The blood films and counts of compound heterozygotes for haemoglobin S and β thalassaemia cannot be reliably distinguished from sickle cell anaemia, particularly sickle cell anaemia with coexisting α thalassaemia trait but, as a group, some differences are apparent. Those with βSβ° thalassaemia show more microcytosis and hypochromia than is usual in sickle cell anaemia and Pappenheimer bodies may be more prominent (Fig. 8.18). Otherwise blood

Fig. 8.18 The blood film of a patient with sickle cell/β⁰ thalassaemia compound heterozygosity showing anisocytosis, poikilocytosis, one sickle cell, one boat-shaped cell and one NRBC. Many of the red cells contain Pappenheimer bodies.

films are similar. The blood films of compound heterozygotes with $\beta^S\beta^+$ thalassaemia generally show less marked abnormalities, depending on the levels of haemoglobin A and haemoglobin F; target cells are numerous but sickle cells are less frequent. When there is persistent splenomegaly, leucopenia and thrombocytopenia can occur as a consequence of hypersplenism.

The blood counts in compound heterozygotes, particularly those with $\beta^S\beta^+$ thalassaemia, as a group show a higher Hb, RBC and Hct than patients with sickle cell anaemia and a lower MCV, MCH, MCHC, reticulocyte percentage and reticulocyte absolute count [50,51].

Differential diagnosis

The differential diagnosis is sickle cell anaemia and sickle cell/haemoglobin C disease.

Further tests

The diagnosis of $\beta^S\beta^+$ thalassaemia can be confirmed by haemoglobin electrophoresis or HPLC, which demonstrate haemoglobins S and A but, in contrast to sickle cell trait, the S percentage is higher than the A percentage. Haemoglobin F may also be increased but does not usually exceed 10–15%. $\beta^S\beta^0$ Thalassaemia cannot be distinguished readily from sickle cell anaemia by haemoglobin electrophoresis or HPLC, since in neither condition is there any haemoglobin A. Diagnosis of cases with microcytosis and haemoglobins S and F requires family studies and, if necessary, DNA analysis.

Haemoglobin S/hereditary persistence of fetal haemoglobin (HPFH) compound heterozygosity

Patients with compound heterozygosity for haemoglobin S and deletional HPFH, β^SHPFH genotype, have a mild clinical condition in which painful crises are infrequent or absent.

Blood film and count

The haemoglobin is normal. Cells are normocytic and normochromic and features of hyposplenism are usually absent. There is anisocytosis, target cells are present and there are infrequent sickle cells.

The blood count is normal or shows very minor abnormalities.

Differential diagnosis

The differential diagnosis is sickle cell anaemia and sickle cell/β thalassaemia. The blood film shows much less abnormality than in either of the other conditions.

Further tests

Haemoglobin electrophoresis or HPLC shows haemoglobin S and haemoglobin F. F constitutes 20–30% of total haemoglobin. The F percentage is generally higher than in S/β thalassaemia compound heterozygotes who usually have a haemoglobin F of less than 15%. The F percentage is also generally higher than in sickle cell anaemia in which levels of 0.5–15% are usual; however it should be noted that some Arab patients with sickle cell anaemia have higher levels of haemoglobin F as do patients under treatment with hydroxycarbamide.

Sickle cell/haemoglobin C disease

Haemoglobin C is a β chain variant that originated in West Africa, west of the Niger River, and is also present in some Afro-Caribbeans and Afro-Americans and, less commonly, in other ethnic groups such as North Africans, Sicilians, Italians and Spaniards. Compound heterozygotes for haemoglobin S and haemoglobin C, genotype $\beta^S\beta^C$, have a sickling disorder of very variable severity, ranging from virtually asymptomatic to a severity comparable with that of sickle cell anaemia. Splenomegaly is present in childhood and may persist into adult life. Retinal abnormalities and ischaemic necrosis of major bones is more common than in sickle cell anaemia.

Blood film and count

In sickle cell/haemoglobin C disease the Hb is higher than in sickle cell anaemia with little overlap, levels of 8–14 g/dl being seen in women and 8–17 g/dl in men [50]. Sickle cell/haemoglobin C disease can

Fig. 8.19 The blood film of a patient with sickle cell/haemoglobin C compound heterozygosity showing numerous specific SC poikilocytes.

usually be distinguished from sickle cell anaemia on the basis of the blood film (Fig. 8.19) although it may not always be possible to distinguish it from haemoglobin C disease [52]. There are few sickle cells and, in comparison with sickle cell anaemia, fewer NRBC, less polychromasia and less evidence of hyposplenism which tends to develop later in life. Target cells and boat-shaped cells are numerous. Irregularly contracted cells are more prominent and many patients have unusual poikilocytes that are specific to sickle cell/haemoglobin C disease; these resemble sickle cells in being dense and having some degree of curvature but they differ in that they have some straight edges or are angulated or branched [52,53]. Specific SC poikilocytes are sometimes present in large numbers but more often they are infrequent. Rare cells containing haemoglobin C crystals can also be found in a significant minority of patients.

In patients who are heterozygous for $\alpha^{G\,Philadelphia}$ as well as for β^S and β^C morphological features differ [54]. Haemoglobin C crystals are longer and once the cell membrane has ruptured the crystal acquires a scalloped appearance, which has been likened to sugar cane.

A sudden fall in Hb may be due to superimposed megaloblastic anaemia, bone marrow necrosis or parvovirus-induced pure red cell aplasia. Megaloblastic anaemia and bone marrow necrosis are particularly likely during pregnancy. When

these conditions are suspected as a complication of sickle cell/haemoglobin C disease, the same features should be sought as were described under sickle cell anaemia.

The Hb, RBC and Hct are higher than in sickle cell anaemia. The MCV is generally lower and may be below the normal range, even in those who do not have coexisting α thalassaemia trait [55]. The MCHC is higher than in sickle cell disease, often falling above the normal range, and red cell cytograms identify a population of hyperdense cells. The RDW and HDW are increased. The reticulocyte count is lower, averaging 3% in contrast to 10% in sickle cell anaemia [37].

The WBC and neutrophil and monocyte counts are higher than in Black controls [38].

Haemoglobin C disease

Homozygotes for haemoglobin C, genotype $\beta^C\beta^C$, have chronic haemolysis and usually haemolytic anaemia. The spleen is enlarged and the incidence of gallstones is increased.

Blood film and count

There is usually a mild to moderate anaemia. The blood film generally shows large numbers of both target cells and irregularly contracted cells (Fig. 8.20). The latter cells resemble spherocytes but closer

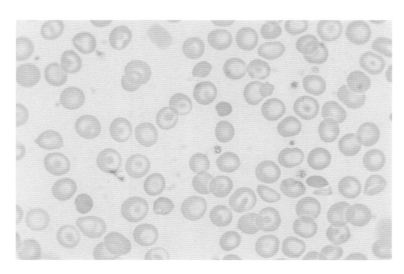

Fig. 8.20 The blood film of a patient with haemoglobin C disease showing a mixture of irregularly contracted cells and target cells.

inspection shows that the majority are irregular in shape. Polychromasia and some NRBC may be noted. Some patients have hypochromia and microcytosis. Haemoglobin C crystals are uncommon but when present are sufficiently distinctive to confirm the presence of this haemoglobin. They are rhomboidal with parallel sides and triangular or obliquely sloping ends (see below). They are usually contained in a cell that appears to be otherwise empty of haemoglobin. A minority of patients have a lesser degree of blood film abnormality with smaller numbers of target cells and irregularly contracted cells.

The Hb, RBC and Hct are normal or mildly to moderately reduced. A marked reduction of MCV and MCH is common with the MCHC being increased [55]. The low MCV and MCH occur even in the absence of coexisting a thalassaemia trait. The RDW and HDW are increased and red cell cytograms show a population of hyperdense cells. The reticulocyte count is increased.

Differential diagnosis

The differential diagnosis is sickle cell/haemoglobin C disease and haemoglobin C/β thalassaemia compound heterozygosity. The blood film of haemoglobin C trait is also occasionally sufficiently abnormal to resemble that of milder cases of haemoglobin C disease.

Further tests

The diagnosis can usually be strongly suspected from the blood film but confirmation requires a sickle solubility test and haemoglobin electrophoresis or HPLC. The haemoglobins present are C, A_2 (which cannot be easily distinguished from C) and small amounts of haemoglobin F. In microcytic cases, family studies or molecular genetic analysis are needed to make the distinction from compound heterozygosity for haemoglobin C and $\beta°$ thalassaemia.

Haemoglobin C trait

Haemoglobin C trait, genotype $\beta\beta^C$, is an asymptomatic abnormality of no significance apart from the possibility of more severe disease in offspring.

Blood film and count

The haemoglobin is normal. The blood film (Fig. 8.21) may be normal or may show target cells, varying from occasional to frequent, or occasional irregularly contracted cells. Red cells are often hypochromic and microcytic, even in the absence of coexisting α thalassaemia trait [55]. The reticulocyte count is normal. The blood count is either normal or shows a reduced MCV and MCH.

Fig. 8.21 The blood film of a patient with haemoglobin C trait showing several target cells.

Fig. 8.22 The blood film of a patient with haemoglobin C/β^0 compound heterozygosity showing crystals of haemoglobin C within cells that otherwise appear empty of haemoglobin.

Differential diagnosis

The differential diagnosis includes other causes of target cells (see Table 3.7) and sometimes other causes of irregularly contracted cells (see Table 3.4).

Further tests

Since the blood film and blood count may be normal, haemoglobin electrophoresis or HPLC is required to confirm or exclude haemoglobin C trait. One of these tests is therefore indicated if genetic counselling is required in West Africans, Afro-Caribbeans or Black Americans, even when a negative sickle solubility test has excluded the presence of haemoglobin S.

Haemoglobin C/β thalassaemia

The compound heterozygous state for haemoglobin C and β^0 or β^+ thalassaemia may cause symptomatic anaemia.

Blood film and count

There is a moderate anaemia. The blood film (Fig. 8.22) shows microcytosis, hypochromia, target cells and irregularly contracted cells. Haemoglobin

C crystals may be present. The blood count shows reduction of the Hb, RBC, Hct, MCV and MCH.

Differential diagnosis

The differential diagnosis is haemoglobin C disease and various thalassaemic conditions.

Further tests

The diagnosis is dependent on haemoglobin electrophoresis or HPLC, if necessary supplemented by family studies or molecular genetic analysis to distinguish haemoglobin C disease from haemoglobin C/$\beta°$ thalassaemia.

Haemoglobin E disease

Haemoglobin E is a β chain variant that is common in Thailand, Burma, Laos, Cambodia, Vietnam and Malaysia and to a lesser extent in other countries in South-East Asia stretching from Indonesia to Nepal. It has a very low frequency in northern European Caucasians and individuals of African origin although occasional cases are observed in West Indians. Haemoglobin E disease, genotype $\beta^E\beta^E$, is usually asymptomatic [56].

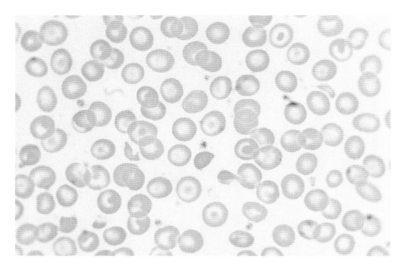

Fig. 8.23 The blood film of a patient with haemoglobin E homozygosity showing hypochromia, microcytosis, target cells and occasional irregularly contracted cells and other poikilocytes. The blood count (Coulter S) was: RBC $6.84 \times 10^{12}/l$, Hb 11.9 g/dl, Hct 0.37, MCV 54 fl, MCH 17.4 pg, MCHC 26.7 g/dl.

Blood film and count

There is a mild anaemia or a normal haemoglobin concentration. The blood film (Fig. 8.23) shows hypochromia and microcytosis, a variable number of target cells and sometimes irregularly contracted cells. The reticulocyte count is usually normal. The blood count is often similar to that of β thalassaemia trait with a mild anaemia or a normal Hb, elevated RBC and reduced MCV and MCH.

Differential diagnosis

The differential diagnosis is haemoglobin E/β thalassaemia compound heterozygosity, β thalassaemia trait and iron deficiency. Haemoglobin C disease would also be included in the differential diagnosis were it not for the fact that there is very little overlap between the ethnic groups in which these two haemoglobinopathies occur. Haemoglobin Eβ° thalassaemia often has a greater degree of anaemia and microcytosis than does haemoglobin E disease and also more NRBC. Haemoglobin Eβ⁺ thalassaemia and the other conditions included in the differential diagnosis are excluded by haemoglobin electrophoresis.

Further tests

Diagnosis requires haemoglobin electrophoresis or HPLC which shows mainly haemoglobin E with up to 5–10% haemoglobin F. Haemoglobin E has the same mobility as haemoglobin C at alkaline pH and the same mobility as haemoglobin A at acid pH. Haemoglobin E can be distinguished from haemoglobins A and C by HPLC, although it may have the same retention time as haemoglobin A_2.

Haemoglobin E trait

Haemoglobin E trait, genotype ββ^E, is a completely asymptomatic condition which is only of importance because of its potential genetic significance.

Blood film and count

The blood film (Fig. 8.24) may be normal or show microcytosis or a few target cells or irregularly contracted cells.

The blood count is normal in a minority of patients. In the majority (about 90%) it shows a minor reduction of MCV and MCH with the Hb usually being normal.

Differential diagnosis

The differential diagnosis includes mild iron deficiency and β thalassaemia trait.

Further tests

Diagnosis is dependent on haemoglobin electrophoresis or HPLC, which show haemoglobin E and haemoglobin A but with haemoglobin E being only

Fig. 8.24 The blood film of a patient with haemoglobin E trait showing hypochromia, microcytosis and occasional irregularly contracted cells. The blood count (Coulter S Plus IV) was: RBC 4.39×10^{12}/l, Hb 11 g/dl, Hct 0.32, MCV 74 fl, MCH 25.1 pg, MCHC 33.2 g/dl.

about one-third of total haemoglobin because of its diminished rate of synthesis.

Haemoglobin E/β thalassaemia

Haemoglobin E/β thalassaemia compound heterozygosity, genotype $\beta^E\beta^\circ$ or $\beta^E\beta^+$ thalassaemia, is in general considerably more severe than haemoglobin E disease. It occurs in South-East Asia and in India and, following migration, in Europe and North America. Severity varies from a mild anaemia to a condition resembling thalassaemia intermedia or thalassaemia major with hepatomegaly, splenomegaly, anaemia and often transfusion-dependence.

Blood film and count

Anaemia is usually moderate with an Hb of 7–9 g/dl although it varies from 2 to 13 g/dl [57]. Marked hypochromia and microcytosis are usual (Fig. 8.25). Red cells of some cases show basophilic stippling, anisocytosis and poikilocytosis. Poikilocytes may include target cells, keratocytes, teardrop cells, fragments and irregularly contracted cells. The reticulocyte percentage is increased and some NRBC may be present. The Hb, RBC, Hct, MCV and MCH are all reduced and often also the MCHC.

Complicating conditions that may affect the blood film and count are aplastic crisis, megaloblastic anaemia and hypersplenism.

Differential diagnosis

The differential diagnosis includes haemoglobin E disease and various thalassaemic conditions.

Further tests

Diagnosis is dependent on haemoglobin electrophoresis or HPLC, which may need to be

Fig. 8.25 The blood film of a patient with haemoglobin E/β thalassaemia compound heterozygosity.

supplemented by family studies or molecular genetic analysis. In haemoglobin Eβ^0 thalassaemia, haemoglobins E and F are present with haemoglobin F levels varying from less than 10% to well over 50%. In haemoglobin E/β^+ thalassaemia there is also haemoglobin A, usually constituting around 30% of total haemoglobin.

Unstable haemoglobins

Heterozygosity for an unstable haemoglobin produces mild, moderate or severe haemolytic anaemia, depending on the severity of the molecular defect. Haemolysis may be chronic or precipitated or aggravated by infection or exposure to oxidant drugs. The spleen is sometimes enlarged and patients may pass dark urine after episodes of haemolysis. Some unstable haemoglobins also have a high oxygen affinity and can therefore cause polycythaemia. If the dominant clinical effect is usually polycythaemia rather than haemolysis the variant haemoglobin is conventionally designated a high affinity haemoglobin rather than an unstable haemoglobin.

Blood film and count

The Hb varies from normal to markedly reduced, in cases with normal oxygen affinity, whereas the less common cases with a high affinity unstable haemoglobin may have a normal Hb. In some patients the blood film is normal or shows only macrocytosis associated with an elevated reticulocyte count. In others there is anisocytosis, poikilocytosis, hypochromia, variable numbers of irregularly contracted cells (Fig. 8.26), 'bite cells', basophilic stippling or polychromasia. During haemolytic crises, features of hyposplenism may appear. Non-splenectomized subjects may be thrombocytopenic, sometimes to a degree that seems out of proportion to the expected degree of hypersplenism.

The FBC shows a reduced Hb, elevated MCV and RDW, and often reduced MCH and MCHC, the latter abnormalities as a consequence of removal of Heinz bodies by the spleen. In some cases a discrepancy has been noted between lowered MCH and MCHC and a lack of hypochromia in the blood film. This has been attributed to the fact that an unstable haemoglobin may lose some of its haem groups; the staining of red cells is attributable to their globin content whereas the biochemical measurement of Hb requires the presence of haem [58]. The reticulocyte count is elevated, sometimes out of proportion to the degree of anaemia. This occurs if an unstable haemoglobin also has an increased oxygen affinity since this will aggravate the tissue hypoxia and stimulate erythropoiesis.

Differential diagnosis

The differential diagnosis includes other causes of irregularly contracted cells and other causes of haemolytic anaemia.

Fig. 8.26 The blood film of a patient who was heterozygous for haemoglobin Köln showing several irregularly contracted cells including one in which the haemoglobin appears to be retracted from the red cell margin. The blood count (Coulter S Plus IV) was: RBC 4.04×10^{12}/l, Hb 11.9 g/dl, Hct 0.40, MCV 100 fl, MCH 29.5 pg, MCHC 29.4 g/dl.

Further tests

Heinz bodies are detected following splenec-tomy and during haemolytic crises in some non-splenectomized patients. The definitive test is a test for an unstable haemoglobin such as a heat or isopropanol instability test. Haemoglobin elec-trophoresis or HPLC should also be performed although HPLC is occasionally normal and elec-trophoresis is not infrequently normal.

Macrocytic anaemias

Macrocytic anaemias result from abnormal erythro-poiesis which may be either megaloblastic or macronormoblastic. Megaloblastic erythropoiesis is characterized by dyserythropoiesis, increased size of erythroid precursors and asynchronous matura-tion of nucleus and cytoplasm so that cytoplasmic maturation is in advance of nuclear maturation. Macronormoblastic anaemia is characterized by increased size of erythroid precursors with or with-out other features of dyserythropoiesis. The com-monest causes of macrocytic anaemia are excess alcohol intake, liver disease, megaloblastic anaemia and the myelodysplastic syndromes.

Megaloblastic anaemia

Megaloblastic anaemia usually results from defi-ciency of vitamin B_{12} or folic acid or the administra-tion of drugs that interfere with DNA synthesis (see Table 3.2). Some causes are particularly important in infancy and childhood [59] (Table 8.2). Excess alcohol intake may be complicated by dietary folic acid deficiency but alcohol can produce macrocyto-sis even in the absence of folate deficiency; in these cases erythropoiesis may be macronormoblastic or mildly megaloblastic. Megaloblastic erythropoiesis can also occur in the myelodysplastic syndromes (see p. 421) and in erythroleukaemia but in these conditions macronormoblastic erythropoiesis is more usual.

The clinical features observed in patients with deficiency of vitamin B_{12} or folic acid include the usual features of anaemia but, in addition, there may be glossitis, mild splenomegaly and jaundice, the latter being the result of ineffective haemopoie-sis. Patients with vitamin B_{12} deficiency may suffer, in addition, from optic atrophy, dementia, periph-eral neuropathy and subacute combined degenera-tion of the spinal cord (causing spastic paraparesis and reduced proprioception). In some patients with

Table 8.2 Some causes of megaloblastic anaemia of particular importance in infants and young children.

Nature of defect	Causes
Vitamin B_{12} deficiency	Maternal vitamin B_{12} deficiency, particularly if baby is breast-fed Absent or non-functional intrinsic factor Imerslund–Gräsbeck syndrome Absent or non-functional transcobalamin II
Inborn errors in vitamin B_{12} metabolism	Methylmalonicaciduria due to combined deficiency of adenosylcobalamin and methylcobalamin Methionine synthase deficiency
Folate deficiency	Premature babies, particularly with coexisting haemolytic anaemia Babies weaned onto goat's milk
Inborn errors of folate metabolism	Hereditary folate malabsorption Glutamate formiminotransferase deficiency
Other inborn errors of metabolism	Thiamine-responsive megaloblastic anaemia Diabetes Insipidus, Diabetes Mellitus Optic Atrophy and Deafness (DIDMOAD) syndrome (Wolfram's syndrome) Lesch–Nyhan syndrome [60]

Fig. 8.27 The blood film of an elderly woman with both malabsorption of vitamin B_{12} and dietary deficiency of folic acid showing marked anisocytosis, macrocytosis, several oval macrocytes, a teardrop poikilocyte and a hypersegmented neutrophil. The blood count (Coulter S Plus IV) was: WBC 4.2×10^9/l, RBC 0.76×10^{12}/l, Hb 3.6 g/dl, Hct 0.10, MCV 133 fl, MCH 47.4 pg, MCHC 35.6 g/dl, platelet count 50×10^9/l.

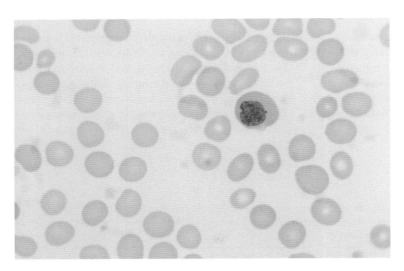

Fig. 8.28 The blood film of a patient with pernicious anaemia showing macrocytosis and a circulating megaloblast.

megaloblastic anaemia as a consequence of vitamin deficiency there are no symptoms and the diagnosis is made incidentally when a blood count is performed for another reason.

Blood film and count

The haematological features of vitamin B_{12} and folate deficiency are indistinguishable. Characteristic blood film features (Figs 8.27 and 8.28) are anaemia, macrocytosis, anisocytosis, poikilocytosis (including the presence of oval macrocytes and teardrop cells) and neutrophil hypersegmentation.

Neutrophil hypersegmentation is not invariable present but, in its absence, a chromatin pattern that is more open than normal may be noted. The macrocytes have increased thickness as well as diameter and central pallor is therefore lacking. There may also be occasional hypersegmented eosinophils, macropolycytes and basophilic stippling. As anaemia becomes more severe there is increasing anisocytosis and poikilocytosis with the appearance of microcytes and fragments. There may be hypochromic microcytes and hypochromic fragments—as a feature of dyserythropoiesis rather than being indicative of coexisting iron deficiency. Small numbers of

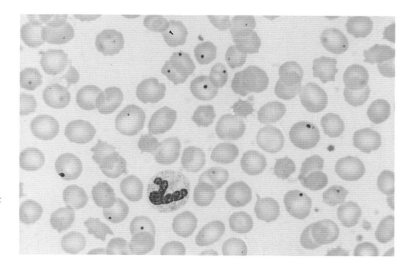

Fig. 8.29 The blood film of a splenectomized post-renal transplant patient with megaloblastic anaemia caused by azathioprine therapy showing macrocytosis, acanthocytes and prominent Howell–Jolly bodies.

Howell–Jolly bodies and circulating megaloblasts and granulocyte precursors may appear. The WBC and platelet count fall with the development of moderate neutropenia and mild lymphopenia. There is usually no polychromasia despite severe anaemia and the reticulocyte count is low. When megaloblastic anaemia develops acutely there may be a sudden failure of bone marrow output of cells. There is pancytopenia with a normal MCV and with few or no macrocytes or hypersegmented neutrophils. Polychromasia is absent and the reticulocyte count is very low. Such 'megaloblastic arrest' is seen in acutely ill patients, often in association with pregnancy, surgery or sepsis. In patients with minimal haematological features of vitamin B_{12} or folic acid deficiency, e.g. some patients presenting with the neurological complications of vitamin B_{12} deficiency, the only haematological features may be occasional round or oval macrocytes and occasional hypersegmented neutrophils. Sometimes macrocytosis is associated with prominent features of hyposplenism, particularly with the presence of Pappenheimer bodies and with large and numerous Howell–Jolly bodies (Fig. 8.29); in a patient who has not had a splenectomy this suggests underlying coeliac disease with splenic atrophy as the cause of vitamin B_{12} or, more often, folate deficiency.

Megaloblastic anaemia resulting from folic acid antagonists such as methotrexate is indistinguishable from that due to vitamin B_{12} or folate deficiency but there are subtle differences when megaloblastosis is caused by other drugs that interfere more directly with DNA synthesis. When these are administered over a long period of time there may be striking macrocytosis with or without anaemia. Sometimes there is also stomatocytosis. Hypersegmented neutrophils are much less common than in the deficiency states.

When iron deficiency coexists with deficiency of either vitamin B_{12} or folic acid, blood film features are variable. There may be hypochromic microcytes in addition to macrocytes or the blood film features of iron deficiency may dominate with only the presence of hypersegmented neutrophils suggesting a possible double deficiency. Hypersegmented neutrophils may, however, be seen in uncomplicated iron deficiency and for other reasons (see p. 91). Iron deficiency is sometimes unmasked when vitamin B_{12} or folic acid treatment is given to a patient with megaloblastic anaemia whose iron stores are inadequate. Following an initial rise of Hb and the production of well-haemoglobinized cells, iron stores are exhausted, hypochromic microcytes are produced and the blood film becomes dimorphic. Thalassaemia trait, like iron deficiency, can prevent the development of macrocytosis in megaloblastic anaemia. The MCV may rise into the normal range rather than above it.

When effective treatment is given to a patient with megaloblastic anaemia there is a lag phase of a few

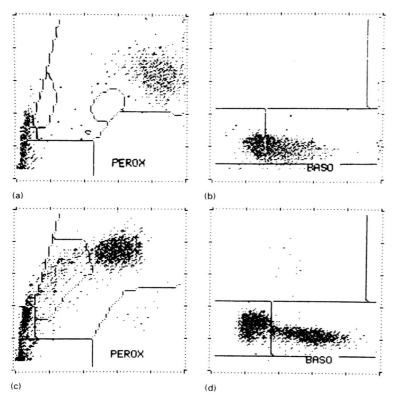

(a) (b) (c) (d)

Fig. 8.30 Bayer H.1 scatter plots of the peroxidase channel and basophil/lobularity channels in a patient with megaloblastic anaemia (a,b) and a normal subject (c,d). In the peroxidase channel the neutrophil cluster is displaced to the right indicating a high peroxidase activity, which is reflected in a high mean peroxidase index (MPXI). In the basophil lobularity channel the abnormal chromatin structure of the neutrophils has led to a loss of the normal valley between the mononuclear cluster (left) and the granulocyte cluster (right), which is reflected in a low 'lobularity index'.

days and then a rise in the WBC and platelet count, followed by the production of polychromatic macrocytes and then a rise in Hb. If the patient has been pancytopenic there may be a rebound thrombocytosis, often associated with left shift or a leucoerythroblastic blood film. Hypersegmented neutrophils persist in the peripheral blood for 5–7 days or even longer and in those who were cytopenic they may actually increase.

The blood count in megaloblastic anaemia shows reduction in the Hb, Hct and RBC. There is a parallel increase in the MCV and MCH. The MCHC is normal and the RDW increased. The increase in RDW precedes a rise in the MCV. As anaemia becomes more severe the presence of severe poikilocytosis with red cell fragmentation may lead to a paradoxical decrease of the MCV; the RDW is then very high. On current Bayer H.1 series and Advia instruments, megaloblastic anaemia is associated with an increased HDW, an increased mean peroxidase index (MPXI)

(indicating an increased mean peroxidase activity of neutrophils) and a reduction of the lobularity index (indicating an immature structure of nuclear chromatin) [61] (Fig. 8.30). On impedance counters the mean platelet volume (MPV) remains relatively low when thrombocytopenia is caused by megaloblastic anaemia whereas it is increased when thrombocytopenia results from decreased platelet lifespan [62].

The various methods of assessing neutrophil hypersegmentation are discussed on p. 91. In a study comparing B_{12} or folate deficient patients who had megaloblastic erythropoiesis with patients who were not vitamin deficient, the index proposed by Edwin was found to be the most sensitive indicator of megaloblastosis [61]. Next most sensitive was the percentage of neutrophils with at least five lobes. In equal third place were the mean lobe count (Arneth score), the presence of neutrophils with at least six lobes and an elevated MPXI on the Bayer H.1 counter.

Differential diagnosis

The differential diagnosis includes other causes of macrocytosis (see Table 3.2) and, in severe cases with rapid onset, other causes of bone marrow failure. An increased RDW [3] and increased MPXI [63] have been found of some use in separating megaloblastic anaemia from other causes of macrocytosis in which these parameters are less often abnormal. Blood film features are also useful. In macrocytosis due to liver disease and chronic alcohol abuse, macrocytes are round rather than oval, hypersegmented neutrophils are absent and there may be other abnormalities (see below). In macrocytosis due to MDS (see p. 421) there may be dysplastic neutrophils (hypogranular or hypolobated) or a population of hypochromic microcytes consequent on sideroblastic erythropoiesis; in a minority there is thrombocytosis. In chronic haemolytic anaemia macrocytosis may be marked but polychromasia is usually apparent. The blood film features are very important in the identification of congenital dyserythropoietic anaemia as a cause of macrocytosis (see p. 358).

Further tests

The peripheral blood features of severe megaloblastic anaemia are so characteristic that the diagnosis is often obvious from the blood film and count. A bone marrow aspiration is confirmatory but is often not necessary. Tests that are useful in distinguishing between vitamin B_{12} and folic acid deficiency are serum B_{12} and red cell folate assays and a test of B_{12} absorption (Schilling test). The serum vitamin B_{12} concentration is reduced in about 97% of patients with clinical evidence of vitamin B_{12} deficiency [64]. Assay of serum holotranscobalamin (i.e. of cobalamin bound to transcobalamin—previously known as transcobalamin II) may detect some further patients with vitamin B_{12} deficiency in whom the concentration of total serum B_{12} is normal. Serum folate assay is a more sensitive indicator of negative folate balance than red cell folate but red cell folate assay is more specific for significant tissue deficiency. Increased plasma homocysteine concentration is a sensitive indicator of vitamin B_{12} deficiency [64] (sensitivity of 96%) [65] but increased levels may

also be found in folic acid deficiency, alcohol abuse and renal insufficiency; the need for rapid processing of the blood sample lessens the clinical usefulness. Serum methylmalonic acid concentration is at least as sensitive as a homocysteine assay (sensitivity 98%) [65] and is more specific for vitamin B_{12} rather than folate deficiency; however, concentration is also increased in renal insufficiency and the assay is more difficult.

Tests for intrinsic factor antibodies are useful in confirming the diagnosis of pernicious anaemia, the commonest cause of vitamin B_{12} deficiency, and may obviate the need for a Schilling test. It should be noted that false positive results may occur if the serum B_{12} is high so assays should not be performed within 24 hours of a vitamin B_{12} injection [66]. Parietal cell antibodies are also usually present in pernicious anaemia but are less specific than intrinsic factor antibodies. A Schilling test with and without intrinsic factor is important if it is not clear whether the patient has a gastric or intestinal cause of vitamin B_{12} malabsorption. If coeliac disease is suspected as a cause of folic acid deficiency or, less often, vitamin B_{12} deficiency, the most useful serological test is for antibody to endomysium; it is usual to test for IgA anti-endomysial antibodies and in patients with coexisting IgA deficiency (increased in frequency in patients with coeliac disease) this test will therefore be negative. If the test is negative it is therefore essential to be sure that the patient is not IgA deficient. The definitive test for coeliac disease is a small bowel biopsy.

In thiamine-responsive megaloblastic anaemia and Wolfram's syndrome, bone marrow aspiration shows erythropoiesis to be sideroblastic as well as megaloblastic.

Macrocytic anaemia associated with excess alcohol intake and liver disease

Both excess alcohol intake and chronic liver disease can cause macrocytic anaemia. The two aetiologies often coexist. Associated leucopenia and thrombocytopenia are common, caused either by the effect of alcohol on the bone marrow or by hypersplenism associated with chronic liver disease. Patients may suffer from bruising or symptoms of anaemia but often the other effects of alcohol excess or liver disease are more evident than the haematological effects.

Blood film and count

The blood film shows macrocytosis with the macrocytes being predominantly round rather than oval. Anisocytosis and poikilocytosis are less marked than in megaloblastic anaemia and there may be associated target cells and stomatocytes. There may be leucopenia and thrombocytopenia but hypersegmented neutrophils are not a feature. In chronic liver disease, rouleaux formation is increased as a result of increased concentration of immunoglobulins. Patients with acute alcoholic liver disease may also suffer from haemolytic anaemia with spherocytes (or, more likely, irregularly contracted cells) and associated hyperlipidaemia (Zieve's syndrome). Patients with advanced liver failure from any cause may suffer 'spur cell haemolytic anaemia', characterized by acanthocytosis.

The Hb, RBC and Hct are reduced. The MCV and MCH are increased. The MCHC is normal and the RDW is often normal.

Differential diagnosis

The major differential diagnosis is megaloblastic anaemia, particularly that due to dietary folate deficiency in 'Skid Row' alcoholics.

Other tests

Red cell folate is normal or low. Serum vitamin B_{12} concentration is increased as a consequence of release of transcobalamin II from the damaged liver. A prothrombin time and liver function tests, including γ glutamyl transpeptidase assay, are useful. A normal bone marrow deoxyuridine suppression test is useful for excluding significant deficiency of vitamin B_{12} or folic acid in alcoholics with macrocytosis.

Congenital haemolytic anaemias

Congenital haemolytic anaemias usually result from inherited abnormalities of the red cell membrane, haemoglobin or red cell enzymes. Enzyme deficiencies are mainly those of the glycolytic pathway, which are concerned with the energy requirements of the cell, and those of the pentose shunt, which protect the cell from oxidant damage. Congenital haemolytic anaemias of these types persist throughout life. Congenital haemolytic anaemia can also be acquired *in utero*, e.g. haemolytic disease of the newborn caused by ABO or Rh incompatibility, in which case it is a transient disorder. Haemolysis associated with abnormal haemoglobins has been discussed above (see pp. 296 and 305). Red cell membrane and enzyme abnormalities will be discussed here. The structure of the normal red cell membrane, which is a lipid bilayer supported by a cytoskeleton, is illustrated in Fig. 8.31.

Hereditary spherocytosis and variants

Hereditary spherocytosis

The condition designated hereditary spherocytosis is actually a heterogeneous group of disorders [67]. Hereditary spherocytosis occurs in various ethnic groups including white, North African, Indian subcontinent and Japanese subjects and rarely in those of sub-Saharan African ethnic origin. The prevalence in northern European Caucasians is at least one in 2000 [68]. About three-quarters of cases show an autosomal dominant inheritance, the remainder either being sporadic new mutations or showing an autosomal recessive inheritance [68]. Of the cases not showing dominant inheritance, the majority result from new mutations and the minority from recessively inherited disease [69]. The underlying genetic defect in the common autosomal dominant form of the disease is a mutation in the ankyrin (*ANK1*) gene in about 50% of cases, in the β spectrin (*SPTB*) gene in about 30%, in the gene for the red cell membrane protein, band 3 (*SLC4A1* or *EPB3*), in 15–20% [68] and in the α spectrin gene (*SPTA*) or the protein 4.2 gene (*EPB4.2*) in a small minority. The rate of synthesis of α spectrin is usually three to four times greater than the rate of synthesis of β spectrin so that hereditary spherocytosis is likely to be associated only with homozygosity or compound heterozygosity for *SPTA* mutations but with heterozygosity for *SPTB* mutations. Mutations in the band

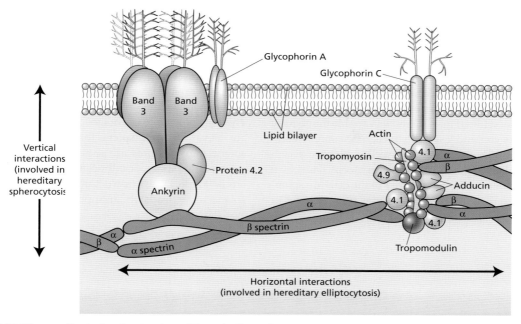

Fig. 8.31 Diagram illustrating the structure of the red cell membrane.

3 gene that can cause hereditary spherocytosis either lead to a reduced synthesis of band 3 or to synthesis of a protein that is unstable or that shows reduced binding to protein 4.2 or ankyrin [70]. The uncommon autosomal recessive forms of hereditary spherocytosis have been associated particularly with compound heterozygosity or homozygosity for α spectrin (*SPTA*) mutations [71] but also with mutations of the band 3 [70], β spectrin and protein 4.2 or palladin (*EPB4.2*) genes [72,73]. Mutations of *EPB4.2* have been reported mainly in Japanese individuals [72]. Rarely mutations in the *SLC4A1* gene resulting in a complete absence of band 3 cause distal renal tubular acidosis and hereditary spherocytosis but in other kindreds mutation leads to the occurrence of one or other condition [67]. The mechanism of spherocytosis in most cases of hereditary spherocytosis is that a deficiency of spectrin, either primary or secondary to an abnormality of ankyrin, leads to reduced density of the cytoskeleton, lack of binding of the cytoskeleton to band 3 and consequent instability of unsupported areas of the lipid bilayer. There is then loss of lipid, as vesicles, from the destabilized membrane, *in vitro* and probably *in*

vivo, leading to spherocytosis. A reduction in band 3 protein has a similar effect. It appears likely that in protein 4.2 deficiency there is impairment of binding of spectrin through ankyrin and band 3 to the membrane protein, CD47 [73]. Mutations associated with hereditary spherocytosis are listed on the Human Gene Mutation Database [74].

Hereditary spherocytosis may be asymptomatic and only diagnosed incidentally or there may be symptomatic anaemia and intermittent jaundice. The spleen is sometimes enlarged. Because of the chronic haemolysis there is increased production of bilirubin and the incidence of gallstones is increased. Symptomatic anaemia may occur only when there is intercurrent bacterial infection, parvovirus B19 infection or folic acid deficiency. Hereditary spherocytosis may be ameliorated by co-inheritance of β thalassaemia trait [70].

Babies with hereditary spherocytosis usually have a normal Hb at birth. Neonatal jaundice is common and they may require phototherapy and, sometimes, exchange transfusion. Babies with hereditary spherocytosis are prone to develop a transient but severe anaemia around 20 days of age [75]. Blood transfusion is often needed at this stage. Spleno-megaly is common during the first year of life.

Blood film and count

Depending on the specific genetic abnormality, there may be either anaemia or compensated haemolysis. The blood film (Fig. 8.32) shows variable numbers of spherocytes and less easily recognized spherostom-atocytes. There are also some cells with normal central pallor. Scanning electron microscopy has shown that generally only a minority of the cells are spherical, the majority being discocytes, stomatocytes or spherostomatocytes [76]. In mild cases of hereditary spherocytosis it is sometimes very difficult to be certain, on examining the blood film, whether or not spherocytes are present and confirmatory tests are needed. In severe cases there is obvious spherocytosis, polychromasia and polychromatic macrocytes and sometimes the presence of other poikilocytes. The reticulocyte percentage and absolute count are elevated. After splenectomy the usual post-splenectomy features are seen but target cells are not a feature; spheroacanthocytes may be very numerous (Fig. 8.33). Ultrastructural studies show that splenectomy leads to disappearance of a minor

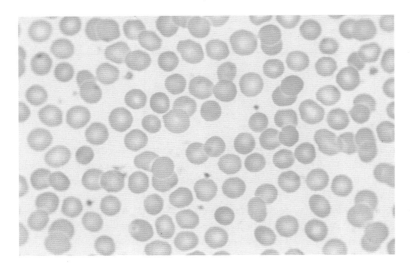

Fig. 8.32 The blood film of a patient with hereditary spherocytosis who had mild chronic haemolysis without anaemia showing moderately numerous spherocytes.

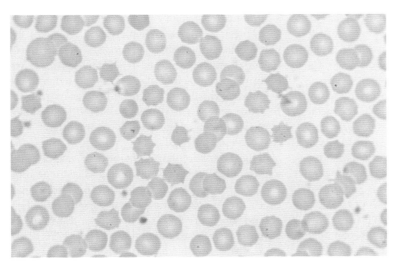

Fig. 8.33 The blood film of a patient with hereditary spherocytosis (the father of the patient shown in Fig. 8.32) who has been splenectomized, showing spheroacanthocytes.

population of microspherocytes [76]. Diagnosis can be difficult in the neonatal period with one-third of babies not showing a significant number of spherocytes [77].

Certain characteristic morphological features are associated with specific mutations [78–83]: the presence of both spherocytes and acanthocytes or spheroechinocytes has been associated with a mutant β spectrin with defective binding to protein 4.1 and with certain other mis-sense and null mutations of the β spectrin gene including a mutation leading to truncation of β spectrin [80] and a mutation of the initiation codon [82]; band 3 deficiency is associated with pincered or mushroom-shaped cells which are lost after splenectomy (see Fig. 3.51); band 4.2[Nippon] and band 4.2[Komatsu] can be associated with stomatocytes, ovalocytes and sphero-ovalocytes in homozygotes [72]; protein 4.2 deficiency is associated with ovalospherocytes and pincer cells [73]; severe spectrin and ankyrin deficiency has irregular spherocytes, some of which resemble the cells of hereditary pyropoikilocytosis. Heterozygosity for band 3[Coimbra] causes typical hereditary spherocytosis whereas the rare homozygous state is associated with a total absence of band 3 and very severe hereditary spherocytosis with spherocytosis and marked poikilocytosis, the poikilocytes including erythrocytes with stalk-like elongations [83].

The blood count in hereditary spherocytosis shows a normal or reduced Hb and a normal MCV and MCH, although the MCV is low if account is taken of the young age of the cells. With impedance counters, the MCHC is towards the upper limit of normal or somewhat increased. With Bayer H.1 series and Advia 120 instruments, the MCHC is increased in the majority of patients who also show an increased RDW and HDW and, on the histograms, a tail of microcytes and a tail of hyperchromic cells [84]. Red cell cytograms (Figs 8.34 and 8.35) show a characteristic increase of hyperchromic or hyperdense cells and, if there is significant macrocytosis, an increase of hypochromic macrocytes. An increased percentage of hyperdense cells is not specific for spherocytosis but examination of the blood film allows spherocytes to be distinguished from other hyperdense cells such as sickle cells and irregularly contracted

Fig. 8.34 Bayer H.2 scatter plots and histograms of a patient with hereditary spherocytosis. Both the red cell cytogram and the haemoglobin histogram show a large number of dense cells, which are the spherocytes.

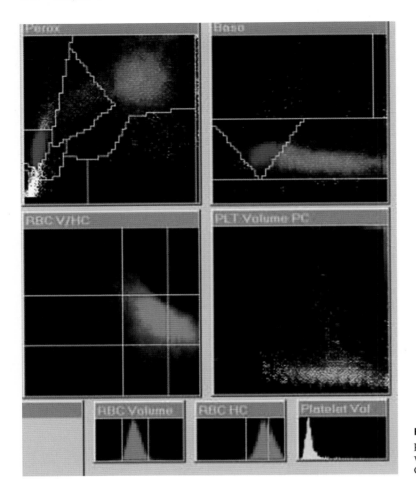

Fig. 8.35 Bayer Advia 120 scatter plots and histograms of a patient with hereditary spherocytosis. Courtesy of Ms Sue Mead.

cells. Post-splenectomy the Hb rises, usually to normal, and the RDW and HDW usually return to normal. Microcytes are less consistently present but increased numbers of hyperchromic cells are usually still present [84]. With the Beckman–Coulter LH750 instrument an MSCV (see p. 39) that is less than the MCV has been found to have a high sensitivity and reasonable specificity for hereditary spherocytosis [85].

Sudden worsening of anaemia in hereditary spherocytosis may be caused by: (i) megaloblastic anaemia consequent on folate deficiency; (ii) 'anaemia of chronic disease' developing during acute infection; or (iii) red cell aplasia induced by parvovirus B19 infection or, less often, resulting from infection by another virus (e.g. influenza virus) [86]. Because of the shortened red cell lifespan, the anaemia develops acutely. In megaloblastic anaemia, polychromasia is diminished in comparison with the stable state and some macrocytes, oval macrocytes and hypersegmented neutrophils are present (Fig. 8.36). In 'anaemia of chronic disease', e.g. in resulting from acute or chronic infection, polychromasia also diminishes and red cells become less spherocytic, some developing central pallor. The blood film may be dimorphic (Fig. 8.37). If the patient is not known to suffer from hereditary spherocytosis the diagnosis may be difficult to make at this stage. In pure red cell aplasia, cells remain spherocytic but polychromasia disappears and the reticulocyte count is close to zero. Previously undiagnosed hereditary spherocytosis may be unmasked by parvovirus infection and also by infectious mononucleosis, which aggravates the haemolysis. Diagnosis is more difficult

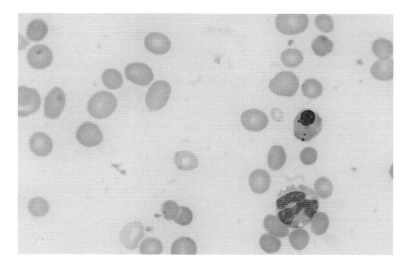

Fig. 8.36 The blood film of a patient with hereditary spherocytosis who has developed a megaloblastic anaemia consequent on inadequate dietary intake of folate in the face of increased requirements caused by chronic haemolysis. The film shows macrocytes, oval macrocytes, occasional spherocytes and a megaloblast containing Howell–Jolly bodies.

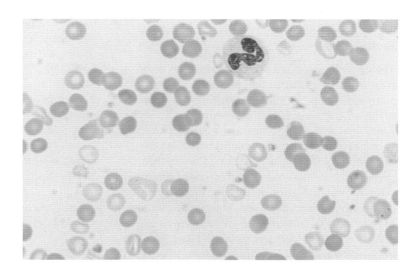

Fig. 8.37 The blood film of a patient with hereditary spherocytosis (the same patient as shown in Fig. 8.36) during an episode of 'anaemia of chronic disease' associated with intercurrent infection. Some cells have central pallor and are hypochromic and microcytic. The film is dimorphic.

during recovery from parvovirus-induced red cell aplasia as young red cells newly released from the bone marrow are not spherocytic. Haemolytic episodes can also be induced by exercise or precipitated by pregnancy. The predisposition to gallstones means that patients with hereditary spherocytosis have an increased likelihood of developing obstructive jaundice. When this occurs, more lipid is taken up into the red cell membrane and consequently spherocytosis and haemolysis lessen. Iron deficiency is also associated with a reduction of spherocytosis and sometimes a dimorphic blood film.

Differential diagnosis

The main differential diagnosis is warm autoimmune haemolytic anaemia (see p. 342). The blood films are often indistinguishable, and thus family history and a direct antiglobulin test are needed. Other causes of spherocytosis that may have to be considered in the differential diagnosis are shown in Table 3.3. Often the diagnosis is readily evident from the clinical history but laboratory features can help. In the mild, compensated haemolytic anaemia associated with the Rh deficiency syndrome (see

Table 8.4) there are some stomatocytes as well as spherocytes and there is reduced or absent expression of Rh antigens on red cell membranes. In Zieve's syndrome, an acute haemolytic anaemia associated with alcoholic liver disease, there are irregularly contracted cells as well as spherocytes. In *Clostridium perfringens* (previously known as *Clostridium welchii*) sepsis the red cell membrane may be so damaged that numerous ghosts are seen. Further lysis occurring in the blood specimen *in vitro* can cause artefactual elevation of the MCH and MCHC.

In the neonatal period, the differential diagnosis includes haemolytic disease of the newborn, particularly that due to ABO incompatibility (see p. 347). It should, however, be noted that clinically evident ABO incompatibility is commoner in babies who are subsequently found to have hereditary spherocytosis.

Further tests

The direct antiglobulin test is negative. An osmotic fragility test confirms the presence of osmotically fragile cells but does not distinguish between hereditary spherocytosis and warm autoimmune haemolytic anaemia or other causes of spherocytosis. In mild cases, an osmotic fragility test after the incubation of red cells at 37°C for 24 hours may be necessary to demonstrate the presence of abnormal cells. In very mild cases, the osmotic fragility may be normal, even after incubation. The osmotic fragility may be normal in hereditary spherocytosis in the presence of iron deficiency, obstructive jaundice or post-aplasia reticulocytosis. Post-splenectomy, the osmotic fragility test remains abnormal but a small population of very fragile cells may have disappeared; this population probably represents very abnormal cells resulting from damage within the spleen. When an automated counter that detects hyperdense cells is available, the need for an osmotic fragility test is much diminished and the detection of a MSCV/MCV discrepancy may play a similar role. If available, a flow cytometry test showing uptake of eosin-5-maleimide (which binds specifically to membrane band 3) obviates the need for an osmotic fragility test [86,87]: the majority of patients with hereditary spherocytosis show a reduction of mean fluorescence (whereas in autoimmune haemolytic anaemia results are normal); the exception is in

patient with hereditary spherocytosis with an isolated ankyrin deficiency in whom results are normal. Abnormal results are not specific for hereditary spherocytosis, being observed also in hereditary pyropoikilocytosis, South-East Asian ovalocytosis, congenital dyserythropoietic anaemia type II, cryohydrocytosis and in some patients with hereditary elliptocytosis [86,87]. However assessment of eosin-5-maleimide uptake together with the blood film features permits the correct diagnosis to be made. The glycerol lysis and cryohaemolysis tests are abnormal in hereditary spherocytosis. False positive results with a glycerol lysis test are seen in spherocytosis from other causes, hereditary persistence of fetal haemoglobin, pyruvate kinase deficiency and severe glucose-6-phosphate dehydrogenase (G6PD) deficiency and also in one-third of pregnant women and some patients with MDS or who are on dialysis for chronic renal failure [86]. False positive cryohaemolysis tests are seen in South-East Asian ovalocytosis and congenital dyserythropoietic anaemia type II [88]. The definitive test for hereditary spherocytosis, although not often needed, is quantification of spectrin and other proteins of the red cell membrane. Membrane spectrin is normal in autoimmune haemolytic anaemia. The most relevant genetic studies can be predicted from the defect demonstrated in membrane proteins:

spectrin and ankyrin deficient—investigate *ANK1* gene

spectrin deficient—investigate *SPTB* and *SPTA* genes

protein 3 deficient—investigate *AE1* gene.

Hereditary elliptocytosis and ovalocytosis

Hereditary elliptocytosis

The condition designated hereditary elliptocytosis is actually a heterogeneous group of inherited conditions characterized by elliptocytic red cells. The presence of at least 25% elliptocytes or ovalocytes has been suggested as a diagnostic criterion. However, subjects with mutations capable of leading to hereditary elliptocytosis can have from 0 to 100% elliptocytes so the selection of any cut-off point for diagnosis is arbitrary. Inheritance is usually autosomal dominant. Many ethnic groups are affected including individuals of African origin, northern European Caucasians, Chinese, Japanese and Indians.

The incidence is highest in West and Central Africa where the prevalence is at least six per 1000, and in Benin and some parts of central Africa is as high as 1% [77]. In Caucasians the prevalence is about one in 5000. Hereditary elliptocytosis results from a variety of genetic abnormalities that affect the integrity of the red cell cytoskeleton [67,78,79,89]. Most mutations leading to hereditary elliptocytosis affect the structure of α or β spectrin, causing either a truncated β spectrin chain or a defect in either the α or the β chain near the sites that are involved in the self-assembly of the spectrin heterodimers into tetramers, i.e. the NH_2-terminus of the α spectrin chain or the COOH-terminus of the β spectrin chain. As a result, the normal lattice of interconnected spectrin tetramers is disrupted. Overall, about 80% of cases of hereditary elliptocytosis are caused by a mutation in the a spectrin gene (*SPTA*), about 15% by a mutation in the protein 4.1 gene (*EPB41*) and about 5% by mutation in the β spectrin gene (*SPTB*) [68]. *SPTA* mutations predominate in Africans whereas *EPB41* mutations are common in Arabs [90]. Less commonly, there is a mutation in the glycophorin gene (*GYPC*), giving the rare Leach phenotype (lack of expression of Gerbich blood group antigens, glycophorin C and glycophorin D in association with elliptocytosis) [91]. Ovalocytosis in the Wosera region of Papua New Guinea has been associated with Gerbich negativity and a deletion in the *GPC* gene [92]. There is also a gene on the X chromosome, mutation of which can give rise to elliptocytosis associated with Alport's syndrome [68].

Mutations associated with hereditary elliptocytosis are listed on the Human Gene Mutation Database [74].

The majority of patients with hereditary elliptocytosis are asymptomatic and the diagnosis is made incidentally. In a minority there is symptomatic anaemia.

Blood film and count

The severity of hereditary elliptocytosis is very variable, ranging from a morphological abnormality without any shortening of the red cell lifespan, through mild or moderate compensated haemolysis to severe intermittent or severe chronic haemolytic anaemia. The majority of patients, however, are not anaemic. The blood film (Fig. 8.38) shows predominantly elliptocytes or, in some patients with the same genetic defect, ovalocytes [89]. Haemoglobinization of cells is normal. When there is anaemia, there is also polychromasia; more severe cases sometimes have a variety of other poikilocytes including fragments and spherocytes. A variant with sphero-elliptocytes has been associated with a β spectrin variant, spectrin Rouen [93]. Other cases of dominantly inherited spherocytic elliptocytosis (characterized by the presence of elliptocytes, spherocytes, micro-elliptocytes and microspherocytes) are of unknown molecular basis [90]. Spherocytes as well as elliptocytes can also be seen in patients with glycophorin C mutations [90]. Morphological abnormalities are greater in those who have inherited the low expression α spectrin allele, $α^{Lely}$, in *trans* to the

Fig. 8.38 The blood film of a patient with hereditary elliptocytosis showing elliptocytes and ovalocytes. The patient had a normal Hb and reticulocyte count.

hereditary elliptocytosis mutation [94]; such patients may have poikilocytes and fragments, in addition to elliptocytes, and sometimes have the clinicopathological features of hereditary pyropoikilocytosis (see below [95]). Conversely, the α^{Lely} mutation occurring in *cis* to a hereditary elliptocytosis mutation lessens the phenotypic abnormality.

The Hb and red cell indices are usually normal. The reticulocyte count is normal or increased. Cases with haemolytic anaemia have an increased RDW. Bayer H.1 series red cell cytograms are usually normal but, in cases with haemolysis, increased numbers of hyperdense and hypodense cells may be detected and the volume histograms may show two populations of red cells, normocytic and microcytic. The proportion of microcytes correlates with the severity of haemolysis [96].

In hereditary elliptocytosis, there is considerable variation in the severity of the defect between individuals who have the same genotype; the phenotype in heterozygotes for some defects varies from an asymptomatic state, with less than 2% elliptocytes, to mild or moderately severe hereditary elliptocytosis [78,79,89]. In subjects with the same genotype there is a correlation between the degree of abnormality of red cell shape and the severity of haemolysis. However, the genotypes that most often cause severe haemolysis are not those in which the cells are most elliptocytic or in which the percentage of elliptocytes is highest [89]. Despite the variable expression, some generalizations can be made with regard to the usual phenotypic expression of differ-

ent genetic abnormalities [78,79,89]. Glycophorin C deficiency causes no significant abnormality in heterozygotes while homozygotes have mild hereditary elliptocytosis. Protein 4.1 deficiency and several α spectrin variants cause a minimal or mild abnormality in heterozygotes and severe hereditary elliptocytosis in homozygotes [79,97,98]. The most severe elliptogenic mutations generally cause the phenotype of hereditary elliptocytosis in heterozygotes while homozygotes and certain compound heterozygotes have the phenotype of hereditary pyropoikilocytosis (see below).

Exacerbations of haemolysis are sometimes seen during infections, during pregnancy [99], in the postpartum period and when the microcirculation is compromised or there is reticuloendothelial hyperplasia, e.g. in disseminated intravascular coagulation, thrombotic thrombocytopenic purpura (TTP), malaria or infectious mononucleosis [78,89,90]. Patients with haemolysis severe enough to require splenectomy may thereafter have marked poikilocytosis, in addition to the usual post-splenectomy features; the poikilocytes include prominent spherocytes, microelliptocytes and fragments (Fig. 8.39). Patients with mild disease in whom splenectomy is carried out for other reasons, e.g. following trauma, may also have bizarre films post-splenectomy.

In general, subjects with hereditary elliptocytosis have very few elliptocytes at birth. However, some who in later life have typical hereditary elliptocytosis with only mild haemolysis may, in the neonatal period when haemoglobin F is high, have severe

Fig. 8.39 The blood film of a patient with severe hereditary elliptocytosis who required splenectomy for haemolysis, showing marked poikilocytosis with the poikilocytes including elliptocytes, ovalocytes and fragments. One ovalocyte contains a Howell–Jolly body. Courtesy of Dr Raina Liesner, London.

Fig. 8.40 The blood film of a neonate with hereditary elliptocytosis and neonatal poikilocytosis showing marked poikilocytosis with a mixture of elliptocytes and other poikilocytes. Courtesy of Dr Marilyn Treacy, London.

haemolysis and a blood film (Fig. 8.40) showing marked poikilocytosis with the presence not only of elliptocytes but also of fragments, irregularly contracted cells and microspherocytes [100,101]. The likely explanation of the more marked abnormality in the neonatal period is that haemoglobin F has a lower affinity for 2,3-diphosphoglycerate (2,3-DPG) than does haemoglobin A and the free 2,3-DPG destabilizes the spectrin–actin–protein 4.1 interaction, thus exacerbating the abnormality.

Differential diagnosis

When the blood film shows a high proportion of elliptocytes or ovalocytes the diagnosis of hereditary elliptocytosis is very probable. Rare patients with developing myelofibrosis [102] or myelodysplastic syndromes [103] have shown similar numbers of elliptocytes, and this may be attributable to an acquired deficiency of protein 4.1. The differential diagnosis of cases of hereditary elliptocytosis with marked neonatal poikilocytosis is hereditary pyropoikilocytosis. Follow-up beyond the neonatal period permits the two conditions to be distinguished; alteration of the phenotype can take from 4 months to 2 years [90].

Further tests

Osmotic fragility is normal except in those with severe haemolysis. Family studies are useful in confirming the inherited nature of the condition. A definitive diagnosis can be made by biochemical investigation of red cell membranes in a reference laboratory. Testing for Gerbich red cell antigens is useful in recognition of the Leach phenotype. Both normal [87] and abnormal [104] results for eosin-5-maleimide binding have been reported.

Hereditary pyropoikilocytosis

The condition designated hereditary pyropoikilocytosis is a heterogeneous group of inherited haemolytic anaemias characterized by recessive inheritance and bizarre poikilocytes including red cell fragments and microspherocytes. It has been described in Caucasian, Black and Arab populations. The condition is defined by enhanced red cell fragmentation on *in vitro* heating which occurs at a lower temperature than with normal red cells. This feature is indicated in the name 'pyropoikilocytosis'. Hereditary elliptocytosis shows a similar but milder defect on heat exposure. Red cell membranes often show two defects, a partial spectrin deficiency and a defect of self-assembly of spectrin dimers into tetramers, the latter as a result of an elliptogenic mutation. It may be the spectrin deficiency (absent in typical hereditary elliptocytosis) that leads to the presence of spherocytes as well as elliptocytes in patients with hereditary pyropoikilocytosis [90]. The underlying genetic defects are various [105]. There may be homozygosity or compound heterozygosity for a mutant spectrin that has a defect affecting dimer self-assembly and is also degraded rapidly. Alternatively, there may be compound heterozygosity for a mutant spectrin (α or β chain) and for a defect leading to a reduced rate of synthesis of α spectrin, α spectrin[Lely] occurring in *trans*. Parents of patients with hereditary pyropoikilocytosis may both have morphologically normal red cells or one or occasionally both parents may have typical hereditary elliptocytosis.

Patients with hereditary pyropoikilocytosis have a severe haemolytic anaemia. Anaemia tends to be more severe in the neonatal period since haemoglobin F binds 2,3-DPG less well than does haemoglobin A and the free 2,3-DPG weakens spectrin–actin interactions.

Blood film and count

There is anaemia and the blood film (Figs 8.41 & 8.42) shows gross anisocytosis and poikilocytosis with the poikilocytes including microspherocytes, cells with bud-like projections and fragments; elliptocytes may be a minor or a major component. Sometimes they are absent. The reticulocyte count is increased. The Hb is reduced. The MCV and MCH are markedly reduced. The MCV may be as low as 25 fl [77]. The RDW and HDW are increased.

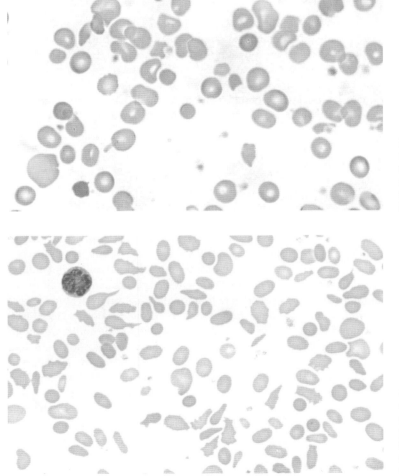

Fig. 8.41 The blood film of a patient with hereditary pyropoikilocytosis showing numerous spherocytes, other poikilocytes and polychromatic macrocytes. Courtesy of Professor Irene Roberts, London.

Fig. 8.42 The blood film of a patient with hereditary pyropoikilocytosis showing marked poikilocytosis and polychromatic macrocytes; among the poikilocytes, elliptocytes and spherocytes are prominent. Courtesy of Professor Irene Roberts.

Morphological abnormalities may be particularly marked in the neonatal period.

Differential diagnosis

In the neonatal period some cases of hereditary elliptocytosis have marked poikilocytosis (see above) and therefore resemble hereditary pyropoikilocytosis. Patients with homozygosity for protein 4.1 deficiency also have a severe anaemia and fragmenting elliptocytes but have normal thermal stability [90]. Haemoglobin H disease and the congenital dyserythropoietic anaemias also sometimes show a similar degree of poikilocytosis but they lack the microspherocytes and budding cells. Hereditary pyropoikilocytosis can be simulated by accidental *in vitro* heating of a blood specimen [106].

Further tests

Osmotic fragility and autohaemolysis are increased. The diagnosis is confirmed by demonstration of fragmentation on *in vitro* exposure to heat and by biochemical analysis of red cell membranes. Binding of eosin-5-maleimide, detected by flow cytometry, is abnormal.

South-East Asian ovalocytosis

South-East Asian ovalocytosis, also sometimes referred to as hereditary ovalocytosis of Melanesians, Melanesian elliptocytosis or stomatocytic elliptocytosis, is a distinct and homogeneous disorder that occurs in Melanesians in Papua and New Guinea, the Solomon and Torres Strait Islands, and in Malaysian aboriginals and the populations of Indonesia and the Philippines. The condition is recognized among the South African Cape Coloured population [107]. A single case has been described in a Mauritian Indian and single affected Afro-American and White families have has been reported [70]. Inheritance is autosomal dominant. In some of the affected ethnic groups, as many as 20–30% of the population are affected [108]. The underlying genetic defect is deletion of nine codons in the gene for band 3 (*SLC4A1* or *AE1*), which results in tight binding of band 3 to ankyrin, reduced lateral mobility and rigidity of the membrane. A polymorphic point mutation in the same gene, the Memphis polymorphism, usually occurs in *cis* to the deletion responsible for this condition.

Heterozygotes for South-East Asian ovalocytosis are usually completely asymptomatic but epidemiological studies suggest that homozygosity for this mutation is incompatible with fetal survival.

Blood film and count

In the vast majority of cases there is no anaemia. However a greater fall of Hb during intercurrent *Plasmodium falciparum* malaria has been observed in heterozygotes for this condition in comparison with subjects with normal red cell membranes [109]. Red cells are round or oval and include stomatocytes. There is a minor population of macro-ovalocytes, many of which are stomatocytic (Fig. 8.43). Stomas may be longitudinal, transverse, V-shaped or Y-shaped or there may be two stomas per cell. Some cases, diagnosed by molecular genetic analysis, have lacked ovalocytes but have shown stomatocytes or red cells with multiple irregular or linear pale areas [109]. The reticulocyte count is normal. The Hb, MCV, MCH and MCHC are normal.

Differential diagnosis

The blood film is so distinctive that as long as the characteristic features are known it is unlikely to be confused with any other condition.

Further tests

The blood film is pathognomonic so that further tests are unnecessary. However molecular genetic analysis is possible. There is reduced expression of many red cell antigens including Rh D so that subjects may type as D^U [110]. Binding of eosin-5-maleimide, detected by flow cytometry, is abnormal whereas it is generally normal in hereditary elliptocytosis [87]. Osmotic fragility is reduced [90].

Hereditary stomatocytosis and related conditions

Hereditary stomatocytosis and related disorders are a heterogeneous group of rare dominantly inherited

Fig. 8.43 The blood film of a patient with South-East Asian ovalocytosis showing several macro-ovalocytes one of which has a V-shaped stoma and the other an eccentric transverse stoma. Many of the smaller cells are either stomatocytes, ovalocytes or stomato-ovalocytes.

haemolytic anaemias and related conditions characterized by stomatocytes in blood films, an increased cation flux through red cell membranes or both. In the majority of cases there is increased intracellular sodium and decreased intracellular potassium. These disorders can be further categorized as shown in Table 8.3.

Hereditary stomatocytosis

The term hereditary stomatocytosis describes a heterogeneous group of rare inherited haemolytic anaemias characterized by a red cell membrane defect that leads to formation of overhydrated stomatocytic cells. An alternative designation is hereditary stomatocytosis, overhydrated variant, or 'hydrocytosis'. In some cases the erythrocyte membrane defect is in band 7.2 [111] while in others it is in band 4.2 [112] or in band 3, leading to impaired binding of band 3 to band 4.2 [113]. Observations in knock-out mice suggest that lack of the band 7.2 protein, stomatin, observed in some cases is not the cause of the abnormality [114]. There is a very marked increase in cation flux.

Haemolysis is often severe and patients are chronically jaundiced. When splenectomy has been performed, post-splenectomy thrombosis has sometimes been a problem. Intercurrent parvovirus B19 infection can lead to life-threatening and even fatal anaemia [116].

Blood film and count

Haemolysis may be compensated or there may be anaemia that is mild, moderate or severe. The blood film shows a variable number of stomatocytes,

Table 8.3 Hereditary stomatocytosis and related conditions [111–115].

Condition	Blood film	Other characteristics
Hereditary stomatocytosis, over-hydrated variant	Stomatocytes	Mild to severe haemolytic anaemia
Hereditary xerocytosis or hereditary stomatocytosis, dehydrated variant	Target cells and sometimes also stomatocytes	Haemolytic anaemia or compensated haemolysis
Familial pseudohyperkalaemia	Normal blood film	Fully compensated mild haemolytic anaemia; loss of potassium at room temperature
Cryohydrocytosis	Stomatocytes	Mild to moderate haemolytic anaemia with loss of potassium at low temperatures

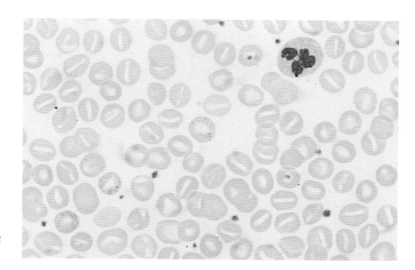

Fig. 8.44 The blood film of a patient with hereditary stomatocytosis showing basophilic stippling and numerous stomatocytes. Courtesy of Dr Carol Barton, Reading.

usually 10–30% (Fig. 8.44). In some variants there are also target cells [117].

There is an increased MCV and decreased MCHC. Red cell cytograms show increased normochromic and, in particular, hypochromic macrocytes. The HDW is increased. Typical red cell indices have been given as Hb 8–10 g/dl, MCV 120, MCHC 28 g/dl and reticulocyte count 10–30% [90].

Differential diagnosis

The differential diagnosis includes other inherited conditions characterized by stomatocytes and also the much more frequent cases of acquired stomatocytosis (see p. 84). Rh deficiency disease (see Table 8.4) has many characteristics in common with hereditary stomatocytosis. Blood films show similar numbers of stomatocytes together with a few spherocytes. Cation flux is abnormal. There is a mild haemolytic anaemia or well-compensated haemolysis. The demonstration of a total lack of Rh antigens allows the diagnosis to be made. Stomatocytes are also a feature of Mediterranean stomatocytosis/ macrothrombocytopaenia (see below) [118].

Further tests

Osmotic fragility is increased. There may be pseudohyperkalaemia consequent on leakage of potassium from cells if there is delay in processing blood specimens; this abnormality can be sought when stomato-cytosis is suspected. Blood grouping is indicated to exclude Rh null disease.

Hereditary xerocytosis

Hereditary xerocytosis, also referred to as the dehydrated variant of hereditary stomatocytosis, is a rare inherited haemolytic anaemia characterized by increased cation flux, normal or increased cellular cation content and loss of red cell water. Inheritance is autosomal dominant with variable penetrance. In some kindreds the gene responsible maps to 16q23-q24 [119]. Pseudohyperkalaemia may occur. Fetal ascites and neonatal ascites and peripheral oedema have been reported [120]. This condition is now recognized as being the same as that initially described under the designation 'high phosphatidyl choline haemolytic anaemia' [115,121]. It is both milder and more common than the overhydrated variant of hereditary stomatocytosis. When splenectomy has been performed, post-splenectomy thrombosis has sometimes occurred [115].

Blood film and count

Some patients are anaemic and some have compensated haemolysis. The blood film (Fig. 8.45) shows target cells, sometimes a small number of stomatocytes, echinocytes, irregularly contracted cells and cells with the haemoglobin apparently 'puddled' at the periphery or on one or two edges of the cell

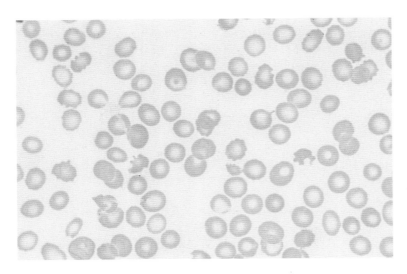

Fig. 8.45 The blood film of a patient with hereditary xerocytosis showing target cells, poikilocytes and several cells with haemoglobin distributed unevenly in the cell or 'puddled'. Courtesy of Dr J.L.L. Vives Corrons, Barcelona.

[122]. There is polychromasia and the reticulocyte count is increased. Stomatocytes may be more prominent on wet preparations.

The MCV is normal or low and the MCHC may be elevated. The RDW and HDW are increased. Typical red cell indices have been given as Hb 11–14 g/dl, MCV 110–120 fl, MCHC 36–37 g/dl and reticulocyte count 5–10% [90]. Red cell cytograms produced by the H.1 series of Bayer instruments may show a population of hyperdense cells.

Differential diagnosis

The differential diagnosis includes other causes of haemolytic anaemia, particularly those conditions that usually have some stomatocytes or target cells.

Further tests

The osmotic fragility is decreased although there may be a small tail of fragile cells. The demonstration of a population of cells with an increased MCHC is diagnostically useful. Patients may exhibit pseudohyperkalaemia if there is delay in measuring plasma potassium, as a result of leakage of potassium from the cell.

Familial pseudohyperkalaemia

This term refers to a heterogeneous group of inherited red cell membrane defects that lead to increased

cation flux with loss of potassium from red cells at room temperature [115,123]. Diagnosis of this condition usually follows observation of a falsely elevated plasma potassium concentration. In some kindreds the abnormality maps to 16q23-24, suggesting a close relationship to hereditary xerocytosis [67]. In cases it is probably a mild variant of hereditary cryohydrocytosis [90].

Blood film and count

There is fully compensated haemolysis so that the haemoglobin concentration is normal. The reticulocyte count may be slightly elevated. The blood film does not show any stomatocytes. There may be mild macrocytosis and the MCV may rise markedly on room temperature or cold storage [124].

Differential diagnosis

The differential diagnosis is hereditary stomatocytosis and other defects leading to pseudohyperkalaemia. The normal or near normal blood film and the mildness of the haemolysis distinguishes this condition from related disorders.

Cryohydrocytosis

This term refers to a very rare group of disorders with increased erythrocyte cation flux, loss of potassium from the red cell and red cell lysis at low temperatures

[125]. On storage in the cold, red cells swell so that the MCV rises and the MCHC falls. Band 7.2 protein, stomatin, was found to be missing from erythrocytes in one affected family but not in three other families [115,126]. Splenectomy is not of benefit but has not been reported to have any deleterious effects [126]. In a rare variant of stomatin-deficient cryohydrocytosis (two patients described) there is a congenital syndrome of mild or severe mental retardation, growth retardation, seizures, cataracts and massive hepatosplenomegaly [127].

Blood film and count

There is either haemolytic anaemia or compensated haemolysis. The blood film shows stomatocytes and macrospherocytes [126]. The MCHC is increased when measured without delay but decreases with storage, whereas the MCV rises with storage [115]. Storage effects are aggravated if storage is in the cold rather than at room temperature.

Differential diagnosis

The differential diagnosis is other types of hereditary stomatocytosis and other defects leading to pseudohyperkalaemia. Misdiagnosis as hereditary spherocytosis may occur because storage in the cold leads to the appearance of increased numbers of macrospherocytes and increasing osmotic fragility [126].

Mediterranean stomatocytosis/ macrothrombocytopaenia

Mediterranean stomatocytosis/macrothrombocytopaenia is now known to be the haematological manifestation of phytosterolaemia (also known as sitosterolaemia), an autosomal recessive disorder in which there is unselective and unrestricted absorption of dietary cholesterol and plant-derived cholesterol-like molecules (phytosterols) [128]. Serum phytosterols are increased and serum cholesterol may be increased. In addition to the haematological manifestations, the condition is characterized by short stature and xanthomas. Although initially described in Australians of Greek or Balkan origin, this condition is not confined to Mediterranean

populations. It has also been observed in northern Europeans and in an Indian family [118,128]. The underlying genetic defect is a mutation in either the *ABCG5* or the *ABCG8* gene at 2p21 [128].

Blood film and count

There is mild haemolysis with marked stomatocytosis. The platelet count is reduced and platelets are large.

Differential diagnosis

The differential diagnosis is other causes of stomatocytosis and others causes of thrombocytopenia with large platelets.

Other defects of the erythrocyte membrane

Other rare inherited defects of the red cell membrane leading to haemolytic anaemia are summarized in Table 8.4. In addition, familial hypercholesterolaemia is associated with a red cell membrane abnormality and a reduced red cell survival in the absence of any morphological abnormality [133]. When such patients are treated by plasmapheresis, haemolysis increases and iron deficiency anaemia subsequently develops.

Red cell enzyme abnormalities

The red cell contains many enzymes that are crucial for maintaining the integrity of the cell. The most important enzymatic pathways are the glycolytic pathway, which provides energy for the cell, and the pentose shunt, which protects the red cell from oxidant damage. These pathways are shown in Figs 8.46 and 8.47. Other enzymes are concerned with nucleotide metabolism. Deficiencies in any these pathways can lead to haemolytic anaemia. Individual mutations associated with non-spherocytic haemolytic anaemia are listed on the Human Gene Mutation Database [74].

Glucose-6-phosphate dehydrogenase (G6PD) deficiency

G6PD is an enzyme of the pentose shunt. G6PD deficiency is common in many ethnic groups including many African populations, Afro-Caribbeans and

Table 8.4 Other rare hereditary haemolytic anaemias caused by red cell membrane defects.

Defect	Antigenic or biochemical defect and genetic abnormality (when known)	Haematological features	Associated abnormalities
McLeod phenotype [129]	Lack of Kx antigen encoded by *KX* gene at Xp21; Kell antigens are generally reduced	Acanthocytosis, compensated haemolysis	Late onset of muscular and neurological abnormalities (neuropathy and choreiform movements), cardiomyopathy; when caused by a large deletion may occur in association with chronic granulomatous disease, Duchenne muscular dystrophy or retinitis pigmentosa
Neuroacanthocytosis [130]	Normal Kell and Kx antigens, mutation in *CHAC* gene or *JP3* gene (see p. 81)	Acanthocytosis	Dystonic and choreiform movements
Inherited CD59 deficiency [131]	Autosomal recessive inheritance of CD59 deficiency	Chronic haemolytic anaemia resembling acquired paroxysmal nocturnal haemoglobinuria	
Rh deficiency syndrome [132]	Rh_{null}. Lack of all Rh and LW antigens and also Fy5 antigen, reduced expression of CD47, Ss and U, caused either by homozygosity for a silent allele at the *RH* locus or homozygosity for an autosomal suppressor gene $X^o r$, an allele at the *RHAG* (Rh-associated glycoprotein) locus Rh_{mod} Reduced expression of Rh antigens caused by mutations in the *RHAG* gene	Chronic haemolytic anaemia or compensated haemolyis with spherocytes and stomatocytes; increased osmotic fragility	

Black Americans, populations around the Mediterranean basin, Middle-Eastern populations and those of the Indian subcontinent and in South-East Asia and Papua and New Guinea. The gene for G6PD is on the X chromosome so that most cases of G6PD deficiency are in hemizygous males. However, in populations with a high incidence of mutant genes, deficiency also occurs in homozygous females. In addition, because of random inactivation of one X chromosome, deficiency is sometimes seen in heterozygous females. In parts of Greece and the Middle-East the prevalence in males is as high as 35–40%. Depending on the severity of the defect, G6PD deficiency may present as neonatal jaundice, congenital non-spherocytic haemolytic anaemia or

intermittent haemolysis triggered by oxidant stress such as that caused by intercurrent infection, by eating broad beans (fava beans) or by exposure to naphthalene or oxidant drugs. Neonatal jaundice occurs in as many as one-third of affected males, being attributable to impaired liver function more than to haemolysis [134]. Haemolysis is acute and partly intravascular, leading to both haemoglobinuria and jaundice.

Blood film and count

When there is chronic haemolytic anaemia due to severe G6PD deficiency the blood film (Fig. 8.48) may show anisocytosis, poikilocytosis, basophilic

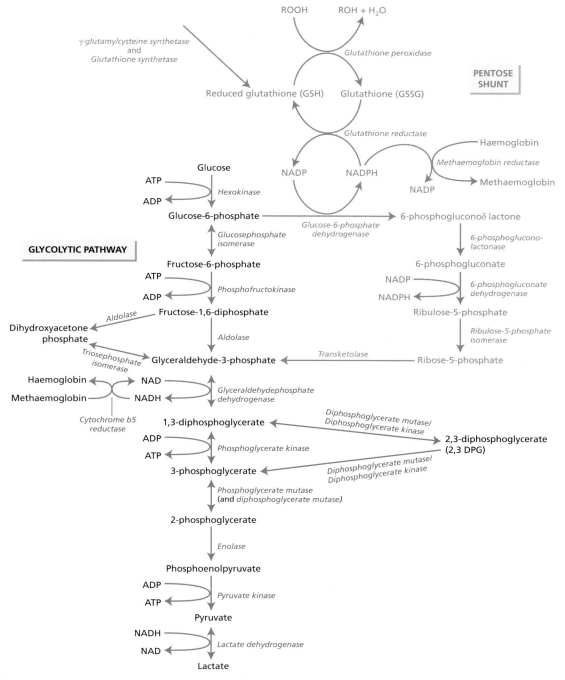

Fig. 8.46 The metabolites and enzymes of the red cell glycolytic pathway (Embden–Meyerhoff pathway).

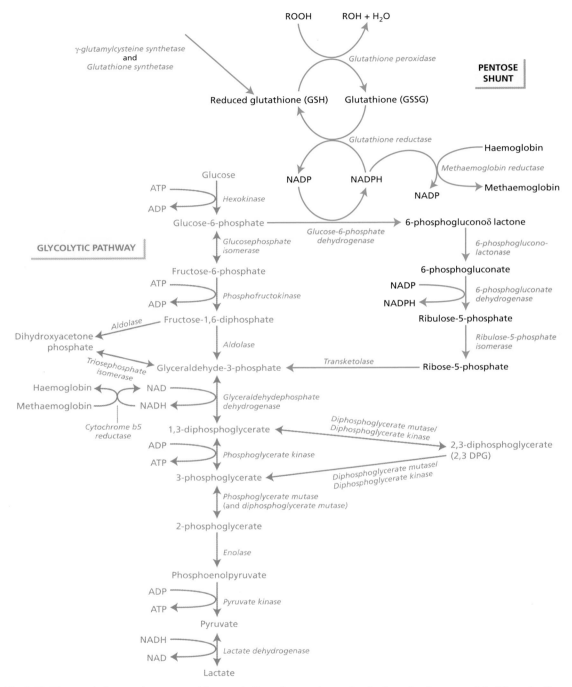

Fig. 8.47 The metabolites and enzymes of the metabolic pathways that maintain the reduction potential of the red cell (including the pentose shunt).

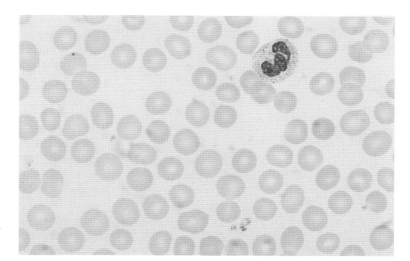

Fig. 8.48 The blood film of a patient with congenital non-spherocytic haemolytic anaemia caused by G6PD deficiency showing macrocytosis and slight polychromasia. Courtesy of Professor L. Luzzatto, Genoa.

Fig. 8.49 The blood film of an Afro-Caribbean child with G6PD deficiency who had suffered an episode of acute haemolysis, showing anaemia, irregularly contracted cells, a hemighost, a complete ghost, and a cell with a protrusion attributable to a Heinz body; the Heinz body preparation was positive.

stippling, macrocytosis and polychromasia without any specific diagnostic features. In less severe G6PD deficiency, the blood film is normal except during haemolytic episodes. When such an episode occurs, the morphological abnormalities are very characteristic (Figs 8.49 & 8.50). There are irregularly contracted cells, some of which have small protrusions caused by the presence of Heinz bodies. Keratocytes, often called 'bite cells', have an irregular gap in their outline, probably caused by removal of Heinz bodies by the spleen. In other cells, referred to as hemighosts or blister cells, the haemoglobin appears to have retracted to form a dense mass occupying half the cell while the rest of the cell appears empty. When haemolysis is very acute, a few complete ghosts may be present. At the height of a haemolytic episode there is a leucocytosis and neutrophilia and the features of hyposplenism can appear as a result of reticuloendothelial overload. In the few days following an episode of oxidant stress there may be a further fall in the Hb as damaged cells are cleared by the spleen. Subsequently, polychromatic macrocytes appear. Patients with chronic non-spherocytic haemolytic anaemia caused by G6PD deficiency can have their haemolysis exacerbated by infection or other oxidant stress.

Fig. 8.50 The blood film of a patient with acute haemolysis associated with G6PD deficiency showing a 'bite cell' and a cell with haemoglobin retracted from the cell margin.

G6PD deficient patients with chronic non-spherocytic haemolytic anaemia have a reduced Hb, RBC and Hct and an increased MCV and MCH. Those with episodic haemolysis have a reduced Hb, RBC and Hct during attacks together with an increased RDW, a population of cells with an increased haemoglobin concentration and, if haemolysis is very acute, an increased MCHC. When recovery starts, there is a further increase in the RDW and the MCV, MCH and HDW also increase.

Differential diagnosis

In the neonatal period, the differential diagnosis includes other causes of neonatal jaundice, particularly haemolytic disease of the newborn with an immune basis. In cases with chronic haemolysis, the differential diagnosis includes other causes of congenital non-spherocytic haemolytic anaemia (see below). In patients with intermittent haemolysis the differential diagnosis is other much less common defects of the pentose shunt and haemolytic anaemia due to exposure to oxidant drugs or chemicals in a patient with no underlying enzyme deficiency (see p. 353); when there is oxidant damage to red cells the blood films are indistinguishable whether or not

there is an underlying enzyme defect. To a lesser extent other causes of irregularly contracted cells, such as unstable haemoglobins, should be included in the differential diagnosis (see p. 310).

Further tests

There is haemoglobinuria and free haemoglobin may be present in the plasma during haemolytic episodes. Haptoglobin is greatly reduced or absent. Unconjugated bilirubin is increased. Diagnosis can be based on screening tests for G6PD deficiency or on an assay. Screening tests are very suitable for population surveys. During haemolytic episodes the high reticulocyte count can cause screening tests and sometimes even assays to be normal. This is particularly so in individuals of African ancestry who often have a G6PD mutation associated with relatively high enzyme levels in reticulocytes. It can also occur in female heterozygotes who haemolyse, since the deficient cells will be selectively lysed, leaving cells with a more normal G6PD content in the circulation [135]. If G6PD deficiency is suspected, on the basis of the clinical history and the blood count, and the assay is normal it should be repeated after the reticulocyte count has returned to normal.

In some countries with a high prevalence of G6PD deficiency, neonatal screening is performed on cord blood.

Pyruvate kinase deficiency

Pyruvate kinase deficiency is the most common of the congenital non-spherocytic haemolytic anaemias resulting from a glycolytic pathway enzyme deficiency. Its prevalence is about one in 20 000 [136], similar to that of non-spherocytic haemolytic anaemia due to G6PD deficiency. Pyruvate kinase deficiency is recessive so that affected individuals are either homozygotes or, more often, compound heterozygotes. This diagnosis should be suspected when there is either neonatal jaundice associated with haemolysis or chronic haemolysis in older children or adults without any specific morphological abnormality. Anaemia is very variable in severity with rare patients being transfusion dependent. Hydrops fetalis has occurred [136]. Extramedullary

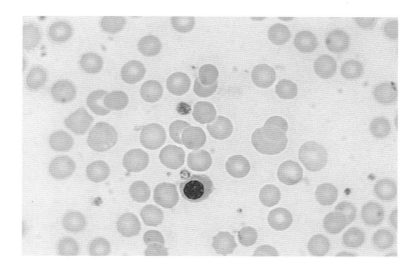

Fig. 8.51 The blood film of a patient with pyruvate kinase deficiency showing anisocytosis, macrocytosis, polychromasia and an NRBC.

haemopoiesis can lead to spinal cord compression [136]. Leg ulcers occasionally occur [137]. Anaemia may be aggravated by intercurrent infection, oxidant stress, pregnancy and possibly by administration of oral contraceptives [138]. Sudden worsening of anaemia may also result from pure red cell aplasia caused by parvovirus B19 infection. Iron overload sometimes occurs, particularly in individuals who are also heterozygous for familial haemochromatosis.

Pyruvate kinase deficiency is associated with increased levels of 2,3-DPG and therefore milder symptoms than would be expected for the degree of anaemia.

Blood film and count

There is chronic anaemia, varying from very severe to mild, or compensated haemolysis. The blood film (Fig. 8.51) usually shows only non-specific features such as anisocytosis, macrocytosis and polychromasia. There may be occasional ovalocytes and elliptocytes and small numbers of densely staining spiculated cells; in one study 3–30% of spiculated cells were seen in 15% of 61 patients [136]. It has been postulated that these spiculated cells are adenosine triphosphate (ATP)-depleted erythrocytes at the end of their lifespan. Elliptocytes have been attributes to associated dyserythropoiesis but the presence of appreciable numbers may indicate a coexisting membrane defect [139]. The reticulocyte count is increased but, because of the increased concentration of 2,3-DPG, less than might have been expected from the Hb. Some patients have leucopenia consequent on hypersplenism.

After splenectomy, the Hb usually rises by 1–3 g/dl and the MCV and MCH may rise. After splenectomy, some but not all cases have very frequent spiculated cells, resembling acanthocytes or abnormal echinocytes (Fig. 8.52) [140]; there may be a paradoxical rise in the reticulocyte count to 40–70% despite improvement in the haemolysis, the likely explanation being that prior to splenectomy some highly defective newly produced cells were removed rapidly by the spleen and also that reticulocytes are selectively sequestered in the spleen. When the spleen is removed these cells survive in the circulation.

Differential diagnosis

The differential diagnosis includes other causes of congenital non-spherocytic anaemia (see below).

Further tests

Pyruvate kinase deficiency is characterized by signs of haemolysis, such as increased non-conjugated bilirubin and increased lactate dehydrogenase (LDH). In some cases there is intravascular haemolysis, leading to reduced serum haptoglobin and the

Fig. 8.52 The blood film of a patient with pyruvate kinase deficiency who has been splenectomized showing macrocytosis and acanthocytosis.

presence of urinary haemosiderin. Osmotic fragility is normal in three-quarters and reduced in one-quarter of patients [136]. Increased autohaemolysis is seen in only about one-fifth of patients and is therefore not a useful test [136]. Definitive diagnosis requires a pyruvate kinase assay.

Congenital non-spherocytic haemolytic anaemia resulting from other red cell enzyme deficiencies

A variety of inherited congenital haemolytic anaemias consequent on a red cell enzyme deficiency have no characteristic abnormality of red cell shape and are grouped together under the designation 'congenital non-spherocytic haemolytic anaemia'. The two most common are pyruvate kinase deficiency and G6PD deficiency. All others are rare or very rare. They should be suspected when there is either neonatal jaundice associated with haemolysis or chronic haemolysis in older children or adults. Neonatal jaundice, which is in part hepatic in origin, is particularly a feature of G6PD deficiency. The underlying defect may be in enzymes of the: (i) glycolytic pathway; (ii) pentose shunt and glutathione synthesis and metabolism; or (iii) nucleotide metabolism. The inheritance and associated clinical features of these defects are summarized in Tables 8.5–8.7. In addition, an association of haemolytic anaemia with glyceraldehyde-3-phosphate dehydrogenase

deficiency has been suspected but not firmly established [137]. Deficiencies of a single enzyme are heterogeneous; the mutations differ and they occur in a variety of ethnic groups spread over a wide geographical area. Most enzyme deficiencies show an autosomal recessive inheritance with affected individuals being homozygotes or, more often, compound heterozygotes. Exceptions are phosphoglycerate kinase and G6PD deficiency, which have a sex-linked recessive inheritance, enolase deficiency, which is probably autosomal dominant, and the very rare haemolytic anaemia associated with adenosine deaminase excess, which is autosomal dominant. Heterozygotes do not suffer haemolysis with the exception of some female heterozygotes for phosphoglycerate kinase deficiency [142]. Anaemia may be aggravated by intercurrent infection or pregnancy. In defects in the pentose shunt or glutathione synthesis, haemolysis may be aggravated by infection, drugs or ingestion of fava beans [160]. Sudden worsening of anaemia can also result from pure red cell aplasia caused by parvovirus B19 infection. Iron overload sometimes occurs, particularly in individuals who are also heterozygous for familial haemochromatosis. In one kindred with pyrimidine 5' nucleotidase deficiency there was intravascular haemolysis leading to iron deficiency [157].

It should be noted that deficiencies of enzymes early in the glycolytic pathway lead to a reduced formation of 2,3-DPG which in turn causes a left

Table 8.5 Associated clinical features and inheritance of glycolytic pathway enzyme deficiencies, most of which cause congenital non-spherocytic anaemias [74,137,141–144].

Enzyme	Frequency	Inheritance-*	Associated features
Hexokinase [145,146]	Rare; 17 known families	AR* HK1 gene at 10q11.2; 7 known mutations	Multiple congenital abnormalities, latent diabetes mellitus or psychomotor retardation in some cases; intrauterine periventricular leucomalacia reported in a compound heterozygote and a homozygote with lethal haemolytic anaemia
Glucose phosphate isomerase [147]	Third most common enzyme deficiency causing haemolytic anaemia; 50 known cases in Caucasians, Afro-Americans, Turks, Japanese and Jews	AR GPI gene at 19q13.1; 29 known mutations	Five mutations have been associated with non-haematological abnormalities including myopathy, mental retardation and neurological dysfunction
Phosphofructokinase[†] [144,148]	Rare; 39 known families in Caucasians, Japanese and Jews	AR mutation in PFK-M gene at 12q13 (15 known) or in the PFK-L gene at 21q22.3	Myopathy (type VII glycogen storage disease) in about half; myopathy can also occur without haemolysis; some individuals with deficiency are asymptomatic
Aldolase [144,149,150]	Very rare, four cases in three kindreds	AR mutations in ALDOA gene at 16q22-23	Mental retardation, multiple congenital abnormalities, type VI glycogen storage disease in 1 of 3 kindreds; myopathy in two cases (rhabdomyolysis can occur)
Triose phosphate isomerase [144,151,152]	Rare; 35 known cases; however heterozygosity is unexpectedly common among Afro-Americans	AR 14 known mutations in TPI1 gene at 12p13	Progressive neuromuscular and cardiac dysfunction in the great majority of cases; sometimes mental retardation; increased susceptibility to infection; death in utero or early childhood
Phosphoglycerate kinase [144,148]	Rare; 28 known families	X-linked recessive PGK1 gene at Xq13.3; 17 known variants; female heterozygotes may have mild haemolytic anaemia	No associated defect or various combinations of myopathy with exercise-induced rhabdomyolysis, growth retardation, mental retardation and progressive neurological dysfunction; myopathy, neurological dysfunction or both can occur without haemolysis
2,3 diphosphoglycerate mutase [144][‡]	Rare; about 20 cases known	AR BPGM gene at 7q22-34	
Enolase [144]	Very rare 3 known families	? AD ENO1 gene at 1q36.13p-ter but no mutations identified	In these families enolase of about half normal is seen in individuals with hereditary spherocytosis with AD inheritance
Pyruvate kinase [144,153]	Similar frequency to G6PD deficiency as a cause of chronic haemolytic anaemia, more than 500 cases reported	AR PK-LR gene at 1q21; more than 130 known mutations	
Lactate dehydrogenase[§] [144]	Very rare	AR LDH-M gene at 11p15.4 or LDH-H gene at 12p12.2-12.2	

AD, autosomal dominant; AR autosomal recessive; G6PD, glucose-6-phosphate dehydrogenase.

* AD in two families with unusual morphological features.

[†] Can be associated with haemolytic anaemia, compensated haemolysis or mild polycythaemia.

[‡] Causes polycythaemia rather than anaemia because of decreased 2,3-DPG; compensated haemolysis has been described but a causal association has not been shown [137].

[§] Reduced enzyme level but no anaemia (although haemolysis is seen in deficient mice) [137].

Table 8.6 Clinical features and inheritance of deficiencies or excesses of enzymes involved in nucleotide metabolism, most of which cause congenital non-spherocytic anaemias [74,141–143,154].

Enzyme	Frequency	Inheritance	Associated features
Adenylate kinase* [144,154,155]	Rare	AR *AK1* gene at 9q34.1; at least 7 mutations known	Mental retardation in some patients
Pyrimidine 5′ nucleotidase[†] [19,156]	Rare; about 50 known cases in 35 families	AR Gene at 7p15-p14 [157]	Possible association with learning difficulties [157]
Adenosine deaminase excess[‡]	Rare	AD Gene on chromosome 20, over-expression is associated with an increase in mRNA	

AD, autosomal dominant; AR autosomal recessive.
* Association with anaemia is inconsistent [137].
[†] Correctly designated pyrimidine 5′ nucleotidase 1.
[‡] Deficiency causes immune deficiency but not anaemia.

Table 8.7 Clinical features and inheritance of deficiencies of enzymes of the hexose monophosphate shunt and enzymes concerned in glutathione synthesis and metabolism that can cause congenital non-spherocytic anaemias [74,141–144,158–161].

Enzyme	Frequency	Inheritance	Associated features
Glucose-6-phosphate dehydrogenase [158]	Similar frequency to pyruvate kinase deficiency as a cause of chronic haemolytic anaemia; occurs sporadically in many ethnic groups	X-linked, *G6PD* gene at Xq28	Neonatal jaundice
γ-glutamyl cysteine synthetase* [159]	Rare; Caucasian, Japanese and mixed Caucasian-American Indian	AR, mutations described in *GLCLC* gene at 6p12	Spinocerebellar disease and aminoaciduria in 2 brothers, but not in 6 other reported cases
Glutathione synthetase* [160]	Rare	AR *GSS* gene at 20q11.2	Mental retardation, ataxia and metabolic acidosis with 5-oxoprolinuria in some cases with generalized rather than red cell restricted deficiency; may have intermittent neutropenia [161]
Glutathione peroxidase [144]	Rare; Jewish and Mediterranean	Not known	
Glutathione reductase[†] [144]	Rare; 1 family	Probably AR gene on chromosome 8	

AR, autosomal recessive.
* Enzymes required for glutathione synthesis.
[†] Enzyme that favours maintaining glutathione in reduced state; acquired deficiency has been associated with haemolysis, panmyelopathy and a neurological disorder and is mainly caused by riboflavin deficiency.

shift of the oxygen dissociation curve, aggravates the symptoms of anaemia and provides a hypoxic drive to erythropoiesis. This may, paradoxically, lead to polycythaemia as has been observed for individuals with diphosphoglycerate mutase deficiency and some with phosphofructokinase deficiency. Conversely, deficiency of enzymes involved late in the glycolytic pathway is associated with increased levels of 2,3-DPG and milder symptoms than would be expected for the degree of anaemia.

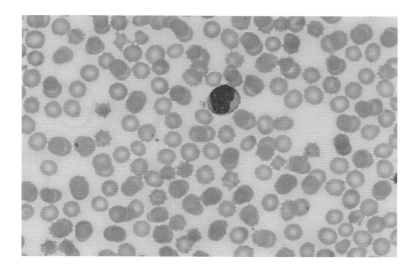

Fig. 8.53 The blood film of a patient with triose phosphate isomerase deficiency showing echinocytosis. Courtesy of Dr J.L.L. Vives Corrons.

Blood film and count

There is chronic anaemia, varying from very severe to mild, or compensated haemolysis. The blood film (see Fig. 8.51) usually shows non-specific features such as anisocytosis, macrocytosis, polychromasia and basophilic stippling. Sometimes there are echinocytes or other poikilocytes, usually in small numbers. Echinocytes have been noted in some cases of triose phosphate isomerase deficiency (Fig. 8.53) [162], aldolase deficiency [163] and phosphoglycerate kinase deficiency [164]. Small numbers of irregularly contracted cells have been noted in triose phosphate isomerase deficiency [165] and stomatocytes in glucose phosphate isomerase deficiency [166]. Irregularly contracted cells are also a feature of defects of glutathione biosynthesis. Adenylate kinase deficiency has been associated with small numbers of elliptocytes, spherocytes, schistocytes and stomatocytes [167,168]. Glutathione synthetase deficiency has been associated with teardrop poikilocytes [160]. One kindred with deficiency of 2,3-diphosphoglycerate mutase had occasional microspherocytes [169]. Enolase deficiency is unusual in that in the three reported kindreds it has been associated with the presence of spherocytes [142,144] but for convenience it is discussed here with other enzyme deficiencies. Only in pyrimidine 5'-nucleotidase deficiency is the blood film distinctive. In this condition there is very prominent basophilic

Fig. 8.54 The blood film of a patient with pyrimidine 5' nucleotidase deficiency showing prominent basophilic stippling. Courtesy of Dr J.L.L. Vives Corrons.

stippling (Fig. 8.54), best seen when the blood film is made from heparinized or non-anticoagulated blood rather than from ethylenediaminetetra-acetic acid (EDTA)-anticoagulated blood. Basophilic stippling disappears if EDTA-anticoagulated blood is stored for more than 4 hours [19]. In addition to basophilic stippling, it is common for there to be a low percentage of spherocytes or spiculated spherocytes (but with the osmotic fragility test usually being normal) [156]. The reticulocyte count is increased. Some cases have leucopenia consequent on hypersplenism.

After splenectomy, the Hb usually rises by 1–3 g/dl and the MCV and MCH may rise. If there is a poor response to splenectomy, thrombocytosis may be very marked. Splenectomy is not usually useful in pyrimidine 5′-nucleotidase deficiency [156].

Differential diagnosis

The differential diagnosis of pyruvate kinase deficiency and other enzyme deficiencies includes: (i) congenital haemolytic anaemias due to membrane abnormalities but with only minor morphological abnormalities such as congenital xerocytosis and some cases of congenital stomatocytosis; (ii) certain porphyrias; and (iii) lead poisoning. Congenital erythropoietic porphyria causes chronic haemolysis with or without anaemia. The blood film in this condition shows anisocytosis, poikilocytosis, basophilic stippling and polychromasia [170]; Howell–Jolly bodies are often present. Slender purple-violet crystals, often radially arranged, have been observed in erythrocytes (see Fig. 3.53); they are likely to represent crystallized porphyrins [171]. Hypersplenism is common with resultant leucopenia and thrombocytopenia [170]. One case of the very rare harderoporphyria showed basophilic stippling [172] but, in general, cases of porphyria with haemolysis have not shown any specific morphological features. Lead poisoning enters particularly into the differential diagnosis of pyrimidine 5′-nucleotidase deficiency, since it can cause a haemolytic anaemia with prominent basophilic stippling; the stippling is the result of an acquired deficiency of the same enzyme. In cases presenting beyond the neonatal period, the differential diagnosis also includes Wilson's disease, congenital erythropoietic porphyria and acquired haemolytic anaemias. Wilson's disease can cause acute haemolysis with minimal morphological abnormalities in advance of any obvious evidence of liver disease.

Further tests

Congenital non-spherocytic anaemia is characterized by signs of haemolysis, such as increased non-conjugated bilirubin. In some cases there is intravascular haemolysis, leading to reduced serum haptoglobin and the presence of urinary haemosiderin. The demonstration of normal osmotic fragility with or without increased autohaemolysis is consistent with a red cell enzyme deficiency. However, definitive diagnosis requires biochemical assays, which can generally only be performed in a reference laboratory. Congenital erythropoietic porphyria can be confirmed by demonstrating fluorescence in a proportion of erythrocytes and in the nuclei of any circulating erythroblasts when the blood is examined under ultraviolet light.

Acquired haemolytic anaemias

Acquired haemolytic anaemias with an immune mechanism

Warm autoimmune haemolytic anaemia

Most cases of autoimmune haemolytic anaemia are caused by warm-acting antibodies, usually IgG, which are directed at red cell membrane antigens. The phagocytic cells of the spleen, and to a lesser extent the liver, remove both whole cells and parts of the red cell membrane to which immunoglobulin and sometimes also complement have been bound. Removal of pieces of the red cell membrane leads to spherocyte formation. Autoimmune haemolytic anaemia may be primary, one feature of an autoimmune disease such as systemic lupus erythematosus or the autoimmune lymphoproliferative syndrome or secondary to other diseases such as chronic lymphocytic leukaemia (CLL), lymphoma or DiGeorge's syndrome; rarely, it may have been induced by a drug—in the past most often α-methyl dopa but occasionally levodopa, mefenamic acid, interferon alpha [173] or other drugs.

Blood film and count

The blood film (Fig. 8.55) shows spherocytosis and sometimes also polychromasia and polychromatic macrocytes. There may be phagocytosis of erythrocytes by neutrophils and monocytes but such phagocytic cells are sufficiently infrequent that they are only readily noted of a buffy coat preparation. In

Fig. 8.55 The blood film of a patient with autoimmune haemolytic anaemia showing spherocytes and polychromatic macrocytes.

severe cases, granulocyte precursors and NRBC are present and there may be features of hyposplenism consequent on reticuloendothelial overload. In occasional patients, teardrop poikilocytes have been prominent and have disappeared after splenectomy

[174]. Some patients have an associated immune thrombocytopenia, the combination being referred to as Evans' syndrome. More rare is immune pancytopenia in which there is also neutropenia. The blood film may show features of an underlying disease such as CLL, large granular lymphocyte leukaemia, non-Hodgkin's lymphoma or angio-immunoblastic lymphadenopathy.

The Hb, RBC and Hct are reduced. The MCH and MCV may be normal or elevated. The MCHC is elevated when measured by an instrument that is sensitive to changes in this variable. The RDW and HDW are increased. The reticulocyte count is increased. Bayer H.1 series instruments indicate the presence of hyperchromia. The red cell cytogram is not distinguishable from that of hereditary spherocytosis but, because haemolysis is often more severe, there may be a prominent population of hypochromic and normochromic macrocytes which represent reticulocytes and other young red cells (Fig. 8.56).

Differential diagnoses

The differential diagnosis includes hereditary spherocytosis and other causes of immune haemolytic

Fig. 8.56 Bayer H.2 red cell histograms and cytogram from a patient with autoimmune haemolytic anaemia showing dense cells, which are spherocytes, and hypochromic macrocytes, which are mainly reticulocytes. There is also eosinophilia evident in the peroxidase channel.

anaemia. Occasionally, there are specific blood film features suggestive of immune haemolysis, such as small red cell agglutinates, red cell phagocytosis by monocytes, rosetting of red cells around neutrophils [175] or thrombocytopenia. More often the peripheral blood features are indistinguishable from those of hereditary spherocytosis. Other immune haemolytic anaemias that can also be confused with autoimmune haemolytic anaemia if sufficient weight is not given to the clinical history are: (i) paroxysmal cold haemoglobinuria; (ii) drug-induced immune haemolytic anaemia; and (iii) alloimmune haemolytic anaemia (see below), including delayed transfusion reactions. In delayed transfusion reactions, examination of a blood film permits a diagnosis since only transfused cells are affected and the film is dimorphic (see Fig. 3.24). When ABO incompatible plasma or immunoglobulin is transfused, the spherocytosis is generalized so that the film appearances do not differ from those of autoimmune haemolytic anaemia. Spherocytosis may persist for weeks [176] so that confusion with autoimmune haemolytic anaemia is possible. Immediate transfusion reactions are unlikely to be confused with autoimmune haemolysis since most of the donor cells are destroyed and spherocytosis is not prominent.

Chronic haemolytic anaemia mediated by a cold agglutinin (see below) can usually be readily distinguished from warm autoimmune haemolytic anaemia on the blood film. The blood film of acute cold antibody haemolytic anaemia is more likely to cause confusion but, in comparison with warm autoimmune haemolytic anaemia, red cell agglutinates are more prominent and spherocytes are not so numerous.

Paroxysmal cold haemoglobinuria and drug-induced immune haemolytic anaemias (see below) can sometimes cause confusion since some spherocytes are present but consideration of the history should suggest the correct diagnosis.

Further tests

A positive direct antiglobulin test (Coombs' test) is critical in distinguishing autoimmune haemolytic anaemia from hereditary spherocytosis. There may also be free autoantibody in the plasma, detected by an indirect antiglobulin test. Some patients have other autoantibodies such as anti-DNA antibodies or antinuclear factor. An osmotic fragility test is positive in both hereditary spherocytosis and in autoimmune haemolytic anaemia so is not of use in distinguishing between these two conditions. In children, Evans' syndrome may be the initial presentation of the autoimmune lymphoproliferative syndrome; immunophenotyping to detect CD4-negative CD8-negative cells has therefore been advised [177].

Cold antibody-induced haemolytic anaemia

Haemolysis may be induced by autoantibodies that have maximal activity at low temperatures. Cold antibodies are often IgM antibodies that can cause both red cell agglutination and complement-mediated haemolysis. Clinical features may be mainly due to haemolysis or mainly due to red cell agglutination in small peripheral vessels following exposure to cold. Cold antibody production may be an acute phenomenon when polyclonal antibodies are produced following infections such as infectious mononucleosis or mycoplasma infection. In these cases acute haemolysis is the dominant clinical feature. Cold antibody production can also be chronic, when a clone of neoplastic lymphocytes produces a monoclonal cold agglutinin, the syndrome being known as cold haemagglutinin disease. The dominant clinical features are those of peripheral cyanosis (acrocyanosis) and ischaemia following cold exposure but there may also be some haemolysis and features, such as lymphadenopathy, suggestive of a lymphoproliferative disease.

Cold antibodies produced following infections such as measles and other viral infections can also cause a distinct clinical syndrome known as paroxysmal cold haemoglobinuria (see below).

Blood film and count

In acute cold antibody-induced haemolytic anaemia the peripheral blood (Fig. 8.57) shows red cell agglutinates, variable numbers of spherocytes and, subsequently, polychromasia and the presence of polychromatic macrocytes. Erythrophagocytosis is occasionally present. Variable numbers of atypical lymphocytes are present when haemolysis is caused

Fig. 8.57 The blood film of a patient with acute haemolytic anaemia caused by anti-i autoantibodies occurring as a complication of infectious mononucleosis. There are several spherocytes, a single small agglutinate and an atypical lymphocyte.

by infectious mononucleosis and, less often, when it is caused by other infections. In chronic cold agglutinin disease the dominant peripheral blood feature is red cell agglutination, which may be massive (see Fig. 3.2). Some cases also have lymphocytosis and plasmacytoid lymphocytes may be present. The presence of a cold agglutinin is often first suspected from the automated FBC as the red cell agglutinates cause a factitious elevation in the MCV, MCH and MCHC with impedance counters such as Coulter counters and, to a lesser extent, with light-scattering counters such as the Bayer H.1 series. Histograms and cytograms may show two populations of red cells, the apparent macrocytes being red cell agglutinates. The presence of a cold agglutinin is easily verified by warming the blood specimen and repeating the FBC.

Differential diagnosis

The differential diagnosis includes other causes of acute haemolysis, spherocytosis and red cell agglutination. The blood film in acute paroxysmal cold haemoglobinuria is easily confused with that of acute cold antibody-induced haemolytic anaemia.

Further tests

Confirmation that haemolysis or ischaemia is caused by a cold haemagglutinin is by a direct antiglobulin test which is positive for complement but not IgG and by the detection of a cold agglutinin. This is usually IgM. It most often has anti-I specificity and less often anti-i or other specificity. In mycoplasma infections anti-I specificity is usual and in infectious mononucleosis anti-i. Cold agglutinins are not uncommon in healthy subjects but in patients with relevant clinical features they are present at a high titre and/or have a wide thermal amplitude.

Paroxysmal cold haemoglobinuria

The term 'paroxysmal cold haemoglobinuria' (PCH) covers two distinct syndromes, both of which are caused by a biphasic antibody referred to as a Donath–Landsteiner antibody. A biphasic antibody is one that is bound to red cells at low temperature but causes potent complement activation on warming to 37°C. The antibody is usually IgG with anti-P specificity. In chronic PCH, there is episodic haemolysis, hence the designation 'paroxysmal'. In acute PCH, there is a single episode of haemolysis; the term 'paroxysmal cold haemoglobinuria' is therefore inappropriate but no more suitable alternative has been suggested. Chronic PCH may be idiopathic or secondary to syphilis or other infections. Rarely it is consequent on non-Hodgkin's lymphoma, the autoantibody being secreted by the lymphoma cells [178]. The clinical features are either of recurrent episodes of haemolysis or a

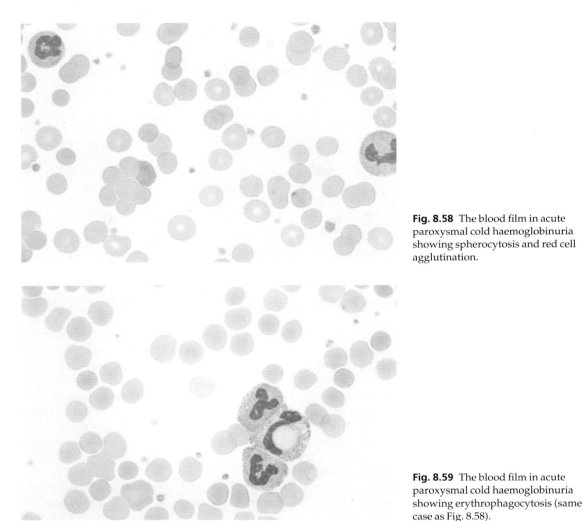

Fig. 8.58 The blood film in acute paroxysmal cold haemoglobinuria showing spherocytosis and red cell agglutination.

Fig. 8.59 The blood film in acute paroxysmal cold haemoglobinuria showing erythrophagocytosis (same case as Fig. 8.58).

single acute episode. Haemolysis is intravascular so that haemoglobinuria is a feature.

Blood film and count

The Hb, RBC and Hct are reduced and the reticulocyte count is increased. In acute PCH there are small red cell agglutinates and spherocytes (Fig. 8.58). Erythrophagocytosis by neutrophils is often prominent (Fig. 8.59). In chronic PCH there are no specific blood film features. Associated features sometimes present in PCH include leucopenia, neutropenia, eosinopenia, monocytopenia and a lesser degree of lymphopenia [179].

Further tests

The diagnosis of paroxysmal cold haemoglobinuria is confirmed by demonstration of the Donath–Landsteiner antibody, usually anti-P, which causes biphasic haemolysis, i.e. haemolysis on rewarming a previously chilled blood sample.

Immune haemolytic anaemia induced by drugs and other exogenous antigens

Drugs are now a rare but important cause of haemolytic anaemia. Antibodies are produced that damage red cells only in the presence of the drug.

Haemolysis is acute and severe when the red cell is an 'innocent bystander', damaged by drug–antibody complexes. When the antibody is directed at a drug bound to the red cell membrane ('hapten mechanism'), as in penicillin-induced haemolysis, haemolysis is usually less acute and less severe.

Immune haemolytic anaemia can be induced not only by drugs but also by exposure to other exogenous antigens such as pollens and plants containing flavonoids [180].

Blood film and count

In drug-induced haemolysis of the 'innocent bystander' type the blood film usually shows only the features of anaemia and spherocytes are rare.

In penicillin-induced haemolytic anaemia there may be moderate numbers of spherocytes.

Differential diagnosis

The differential diagnosis is with other causes of acute haemolysis and other causes of spherocytosis.

Further tests

Suspected drug-induced haemolysis can be confirmed serologically. With penicillin-induced haemolysis the direct antiglobulin test is positive in the absence of the drug and the patient's serum immunoglobulins bind to penicillin-coated cells. When there is haemolysis with an innocent-bystander mechanism the antiglobulin test is usually positive as complement is bound to the red cells. Serological tests using normal red cells, the patient's serum and the causative drug are positive.

Haemolytic disease of the newborn

IgG maternal alloantibodies cross the placenta and those with specificity for antigens on fetal red cells can cause hydrops fetalis and haemolytic disease of the newborn. The commonest form of haemolytic disease of the newborn is now that caused by anti-A or anti-B antibodies; clinically significant ABO haemolytic disease of the newborn occurs in one in 3000 pregnancies in the UK. Rh haemolytic disease of the newborn, caused by anti-D or other Rh antibodies, is now the second most common cause. Occasionally, haemolytic disease of the newborn is caused by antibodies of other systems such as Kell.

Blood film and count

Anaemia varies from mild to severe. The blood film in ABO haemolytic disease of the newborn shows prominent spherocytosis (Fig. 8.60) whereas in Rh haemolytic disease of the newborn the degree of spherocytosis is usually much less (Fig. 8.61). There is polychromasia and the number of NRBC is

Fig. 8.60 The blood film of a baby with ABO haemolytic disease of the newborn showing marked spherocytosis and an NRBC.

Fig. 8.61 The blood film of a baby with Rh haemolytic disease of the newborn showing that the degree of spherocytosis is much less than that which is seen in ABO haemolytic disease of the newborn (see Fig. 8.60).

increased. There may be associated neutropenia, lymphopenia, monocytopenia and thrombocytopenia [181,182]. The reticulocyte count is generally elevated.

In Kell haemolytic disease of the newborn the evidence of a bone marrow response to haemolysis (reticulocytosis and circulating NRBC) is not increased appropriately to the degree of anaemia as there is also an element of bone marrow suppression [183], attributable to suppression of proliferation of erythroid progenitors by antibodies to Kell group antigens [184]. Marked thrombocytopenia is also a particular feature of Kell haemolytic disease of the newborn and is attributable to inhibition of proliferation of megakaryocyte progenitors by antibodies to Kell group antigens [184].

Differential diagnosis

The main differential diagnosis is hereditary spherocytosis.

Further tests

The diagnosis is confirmed by a positive direct antiglobulin test in the baby and detection of an IgG antibody in maternal serum with specificity against a fetal red cell antigen. In the case of ABO

haemolytic disease of the newborn, a high titre IgG antibody will be demonstrated.

Other alloimmune haemolytic anaemias

Beyond the neonatal period, alloimmune haemolytic anaemia is uncommon. Delayed transfusion reactions following transfusion of incompatible red cells are alloimmune in nature as is immune haemolysis following transfusion of incompatible plasma, cryoprecipitate, high dose intravenous immunoglobulin or other blood products containing immunoglobulin such as some factor VIII or IX concentrates. Alloimmune haemolysis can result from administration of anti-D in the treatment of autoimmune thrombocytopenic purpura [185]; uncommonly there may be acute haemoglobinaemia and haemoglobinuria with a sudden marked fall in the Hb. Immune haemolysis can also follow transplantation of ABO-incompatible bone marrow. If peripheral blood is used as a source of stem cells, severe haemolysis can also follow a transplant showing minor ABO incompatibility (e.g. O donor with A or B recipient), presumably because of the greater content of lymphocytes with this type of transplantation [186].

Blood film and count

In delayed transfusion reactions, only a proportion of red cells are spherocytic, the patient's own cells either being normal or showing features of the underlying disease. In other types of alloimmune haemolytic anaemia spherocytosis is generalized.

Differential diagnosis

The differential diagnosis includes other causes of spherocytosis with a positive direct antiglobulin test, particularly autoimmune and immune drug-induced haemolytic anaemia.

Further tests

The direct antiglobulin test is positive, as are tests indicative of intravascular haemolysis—haemoglobinaemia and haemoglobinuria (when haemolysis is acute and severe), positive Schumm's test, low serum haptoglobin and presence of urinary haemosiderin. Otherwise the clinical history is of more importance than laboratory tests in elucidating the nature of the anaemia. Alloimmune haemolysis is sometimes severe enough to precipitate renal failure so that renal function should be monitored.

Haemolysis in familial autoimmune/lymphoproliferative syndrome

Haemolysis with either a positive or negative direct antiglobulin test, a poor reticulocyte response and associated dyserythropoiesis has been reported in the familial autoimmune/lymphoproliferative syndrome associated with mutations in the *FAS* gene and impaired Fas-mediated apoptosis [187].

Non-immune acquired haemolytic anaemias

Microangiopathic and related haemolytic anaemias

The term microangiopathic haemolytic anaemia refers to haemolytic anaemia caused by red cell fragmentation resulting from endothelial damage, fibrin deposition in capillaries or both. Causes are multiple (Table 8.8). In childhood the commonest cause is enteric infection, most often by a verocytotoxin-secreting *Escherichia coli*, resulting in haemolytic uraemic syndrome. In adults the commonest causes are probably idiopathic thrombotic thrombocytopenic purpura, pregnancy-associated hypertension and carcinoma. A similar haemolytic anaemia can occur with large vessel or valvular lesions and with prosthetic cardiac valves. In some of these instances there is thrombosis on an abnormal surface and in others there is red cell damage consequent on turbulent flow or on mechanical damage of red cells by components of a malfunctioning prosthetic valve.

Blood film and count

The blood film shows microspherocytes, keratocytes and other schistocytes and often polychromasia and polychromatic macrocytes. When there is associated platelet consumption, thrombocytopenia and large platelets are apparent. In the post-diarrhoeal haemolytic uraemia syndrome of childhood there is often leucocytosis and neutrophilia, the severity of which correlates with associated renal damage; the degree of elevation of the WBC and the duration of leucocytosis are both of prognostic

Table 8.8 Some causes of red cell fragmentation.

Microangiopathic haemolytic anaemia
Congenital, inherited and familial
  Familial thrombotic thrombocytopenic purpura resulting from deficiency of von Willebrand's factor-cleaving protease [188,189]
  Familial haemolytic uraemic syndrome (some caused by autosomal recessively inherited deficiency of complement factor H [190])
  Associated with congenital cobalamin C defect [191]
  Epidemic or sporadic haemolytic uraemic syndrome, thrombotic thrombocytopenic purpura and related thrombotic microangiopathies
  Following infection by Shigella, verotoxin-producing *E.coli*, *Campylobacter jejuni*, *Legionella pneumophila* [192], *Rickettsia rickettsii* [193], *Borrelia burgdorferi* [194], *Streptococcus pneumoniae* [195], *Aeromonas hydrophilia* [196], *Campylobacter upsaliensis* [196], *Campylobacter canimorsus* [196], other bacteria, *Mycoplasma pneumoniae*, viruses (including HIV, HTLV-I, CMV, varicella zoster, adenovirus and possibly human herpesvirus 6 [197]) or fungi [198–202] or following vaccination (influenza, polio, measles, smallpox, triple antigen or typhoid-paratyphoid) [203]
  Associated with pregnancy (including HELLP syndrome), oral contraceptive intake or the postpartum state
  Drug-toxicity [204]* including of mitomycin C, bleomycin, pentostatin [205], daunorubicin [206], gemcitabine [204], methyl-CCNU [207], tamoxifen [207], atorvastatin [207], penicillin, rifampicin [206], sulphonamides [206], quinolones [206], aciclovir [206], valaciclovir [206], penicillamine [199], ciclosporin, tacrolimus [208], sirolimus [207], simvastatin [209], ticlopidine [210], clopidogrel [206,211], risperidone [206], OKT3 [212], interferon β [196], interferon α therapy in CGL [213], heroin [196], traditional African medicine ('Pitocine') [214], quinine hypersensitivity [215], arsenic [207], iodine [207], 'crack' cocaine [207], anti-CD22 recombinant immunotoxin [216], treatment of acute promyelocytic leukaemia with all-*trans* retinoic acid [217]
  Associated with pancreatitis [218]

Continued p. 350

Table 8.8 *Continued*

Other pathological processes involving small vessels in the kidney (with or without extra-renal vascular lesions)
    Pregnancy-associated hypertension
    Malignant hypertension
    Renal cortical necrosis
    Microscopic polyarteritis nodosa
    Acute glomerulonephritis
    Renal involvement by systemic lupus erythematosus (may precede other manifestations of the disease) [219]
    Renal involvement by systemic sclerosis (scleroderma) [220]
    Wegener's granulomatosis
    Renal irradiation
    Rejection of transplanted kidney
    POEMS syndrome [212]
    Anti-phospholipid antibody syndrome [212]
    Dysfibrinogenaemia and other prothrombotic states [212]
Diabetic angiopathy [221]
Systemic amyloidosis
Disseminated intravascular coagulation (including that associated with malignant disease, aortic aneurysm and renal vein thrombosis)
Therapeutic defibrination (occasionally)
Atrial myxoma [222]
Disseminated carcinoma (particularly mucin-secreting carcinoma, particularly carcinoma of the stomach)
Following arteriography [223]
Reaction to bee sting [199]
Bone marrow transplantation
Thymoma-associated (1 case) [224]

Associated with vascular malformations and other large vessel and valvular lesions
Haemangioma
Haemangioendothelioma of the liver or spleen
Haemangioendotheliosarcoma
Plexiform pulmonary lesions of pulmonary hypertension
Plexiform pulmonary lesions of cirrhosis [225]
Giant cell arteritis [226]
Umbilical vein varix (in a fetus) [227]
Prosthetic valves (aortic more than mitral, much more common when there is regurgitation around a valve)
Homograft, xenograft (porcine) and fascia lata autograft valves (less likely than with prosthetic valves)
Acute rheumatic valvulitis [228]
Prosthetic patches, e.g. for ventricular septal defect
Endoluminal closure of patent ductus arteriosus [229]
Severe aortic stenosis (very uncommon)
Severe mitral valve disease and following valvuloplasty for mitral valve disease (rare)
Cardiac myxoma
Aortic coarctation (rare)
Use of subclavian dialysis catheters [230]

Associated with extracorporeal circulation (associated with thrombosis in the apparatus) [230] *and long-term extracorporeal membrane oxygenation in neonates* [231]

CGL, chronic granulocytic leukaemia; CMV, cytomegalovirus; HELLP syndrome, haemolysis, elevated liver enzymes, low platelet syndrome; HTLV-I, human T-cell lymphotropic virus type I; POEMS syndrome, polyneuropathy, organomegaly, endocrinopathy, M protein, skin changes syndrome.
* Drug-induced thrombotic microangiopathy may be either idiosyncratic (e.g. with quinine and ticlopidine) or dose-related (as with cytotoxic chemotherapeutic agents) [204].

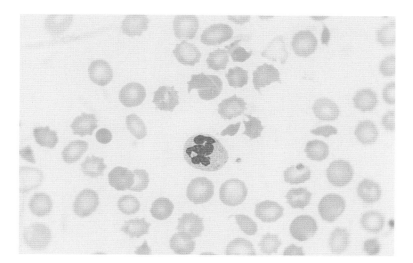

Fig. 8.62 The blood film of an adult patient at presentation with haemolytic uraemic syndrome, showing both fragments and echinocytes. Courtesy of Dr A. Eden, Southend-on-Sea.

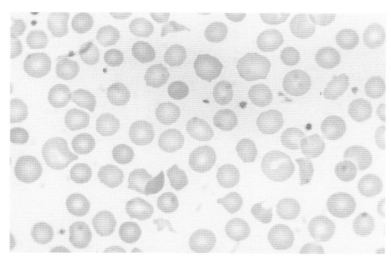

Fig. 8.63 The blood film of an adult with the haemolytic uraemic syndrome showing fragments, several spherocytes and several polychromatic macrocytes.

significance [232]. Prolonged thrombocytopenia is associated with long-term renal sequelae [196]. Occasionally, at presentation, there is also marked echinocytosis, probably indicative of damage to the red cell membrane by the toxin that is causing the haemolysis (Fig. 8.62). In microangiopathic haemolytic anaemia there is often associated thrombocytopenia but otherwise the blood films of microangiopathic haemolytic anaemia (Fig. 8.63) and of haemolytic anaemia caused by large vessel or valvular diseases or prostheses (Fig. 8.64) cannot be readily distinguished. Haemolysis in the microangiopathic and mechanical haemolytic anaemias is intravascular and when it is severe and chronic the resultant

haemoglobinuria can lead to complicating iron deficiency, the features of which are then apparent on the blood film (Fig. 8.65).

It should be noted that, although red cell fragmentation is often a feature of chronic disseminated intravascular coagulation (DIC), it is quite uncommon in acute DIC. Examination of a blood film is therefore not often a useful screening test if this diagnosis is suspected [233]. Conversely, blood film examination is very important if TTP or the haemolysis–elevated liver enzymes–low platelet count (HELLP) syndrome is suspected. It should, however, be noted that, in TTP, schistocytes are sometimes lacking in the first few days after presentation [234].

Fig. 8.64 The blood film of a patient with mechanical haemolytic anaemia, due to a defective prosthetic mitral valve, showing numerous fragments.

Fig. 8.65 The blood film of an Afro-Caribbean patient with iron deficiency as a complication of mechanical haemolysis from a defective prosthetic valve. The film shows fragments, hypochromia, microcytosis and one target cell. The patient also had haemoglobin C trait.

The FBC shows a reduced Hb, increased RDW and sometimes an increased MCV and HDW (consequent on reticulocytosis) or a low platelet count with an increased MPV. There may be 'flagging' indicating the presence of both microcytes and macrocytes. If there are large numbers of schistocytes there may be 'flagging' indicating poor separation of red cells and platelets and the possibility of factitious elevation of the platelet count. Red cell histograms and cytograms (Fig. 8.66) may show hyperchromic cells, normochromic and hyperchromic microcytes and hypochromic macrocytes.

Differential diagnosis

The blood film of microangiopathic and related haemolytic anaemias is distinctive and usually there is no diagnostic difficulty.

Further tests

The speedy recognition of haemolytic uraemic syndrome by the laboratory is of critical importance for optimal management. In addition to appropriate management of the renal failure, early stool culture is indicated and therapy that may aggravate the

```
SEQ#      0001156
TIME      16:38  01/06/94
SYS#      001
ID        000000108821
                CBC
      10.06    x10⁹/L    WBC
L     3.21     x10¹²/L   RBC
L     9.6      g/dL      HGB
L     .270               HCT
      84.3     fL        MCV
      29.8     pg        MCH
H     35.4     g/dL      MCHC
H     18.1     %         RDW
H     3.78     g/dL      HDW
L     33*      x10⁹/L    PLT
L     6.6*     fL        MPV
H     79.7*    %         PDW
L     .03*     %         PCT
RBC FLAGS                2311
      %       DIFF    x10⁹/L
      67.5     NEUT      6.79
      19.6     LYMP      1.98
      5.9      MONO H    .60
      1.7      EOS       .17
      .7       BASO      .07
H     4.6      LUC   H   .46
      LI                 2.12
      MPXI               -8.2
WBC FLAGS                4011
```

RBC

PEROX

HC

RBC VOLUME
(0–200 fL)

HGB CONC
(0–50 g/dL)

PLT VOLUME
(0–20 fL)

BASO

Fig. 8.66 Bayer H.2 red cell and platelet histograms and cytograms from a patient with microangiopathic haemolytic anaemia. There are many hyperchromatic cells (spherocytes and microspherocytes) and normochromic microcytic cells (other fragments). The platelet histogram illustrates that in this patient the platelet count was very low.

condition, e.g. antibiotics and agents to reduce gut motility, should be avoided [196]. Death associated with delay in diagnosis has been reported when a blood film was not examined [235]. Speedy diagnosis of TTP is likewise critical, but it must be remembered that initial absence of fragments does not exclude the diagnosis.

Bilirubin and LDH estimations and a reticulocyte count are useful in assessing the severity of the haemolysis. In cases with chronic mild haemolysis and few fragments the detection of haemosiderin in urinary sediment is useful in demonstrating that intravascular haemolysis has occurred.

Oxidant-induced haemolytic anaemia

Exposure to sufficiently potent oxidants, either drugs or chemicals, can cause haemolytic anaemia even in individuals in whom G6PD and other enzymes of the pentose shunt are normal. Neonates, especially premature neonates, are particularly susceptible to oxidant-induced haemolysis. Oxidants can cause

acquired methaemoglobinaemia, consequent on oxidation of haemoglobin, and acute or chronic haemolytic anaemia consequent on oxidation both of haemoglobin and of membrane components. When haemolysis is acute, oxidized haemoglobin precipitates as Heinz bodies, hence the name 'Heinz body-haemolytic anaemia'. Heinz bodies are cleared by the spleen but when haemolysis is acute they may be detected in circulating red cells.

Oxidant-induced haemolysis is most often caused by drugs, particularly dapsone and sulfasalazine. It can also result from nitrate contamination of drinking water or from accidental or deliberate exposure to agricultural and industrial chemicals.

It should be noted that, if patients have methaemoglobinaemia as well as oxidant-induced haemolysis, their symptoms are often more severe than would be expected from the degree of anaemia. This is because methaemoglobin does not function in oxygen transport and, in addition, causes a left shift of the oxygen dissociation curve, further reducing the capacity to deliver oxygen to tissues.

Fig. 8.67 The blood film of a patient taking dapsone for a skin condition showing macrocytosis, irregularly contracted cells and several bite cells.

Blood film and count

When the haemolysis is acute the blood film (Fig. 8.67) is similar to that of G6PD deficiency during acute haemolytic episodes. Heinz bodies may produce a visible protrusion of the surface of the red cell, the reason for this being apparent from electron microscopy [236]. Heinz bodies do not merely bind to the red cell membrane but protrude through it (Fig. 8.68). When haemolysis is milder and more chronic, there are variable numbers of irregularly contracted cells and sometimes also macrocytosis and polychromatic macrocytes.

Differential diagnosis

The differential diagnosis includes G6PD deficiency, unstable haemoglobins and other causes of irregularly contracted cells (see p. 74).

Further tests

The diagnosis can usually be made from the clinical history and the blood film. A Heinz body preparation is positive in acute cases. In some patients it may be necessary to confirm that the G6PD activity is normal after the episode of haemolysis has passed.

Neonatal glutathione peroxidase deficiency

Glutathione peroxidase deficiency can occur

Fig. 8.68 Scanning electron micrograph of an erythrocyte with a projecting Heinz body. Courtesy of Dr M. Amare and colleagues.

transiently in the neonatal period as a result of deficiency of selenium, an essential cofactor.

Blood film and count

The blood film shows irregularly contracted cells and other features similar to those of oxidant damage.

Renal disease

Red cell survival is usually reduced in acute renal failure. The features of a microangiopathic haemolytic anaemia are commonly present. Reduced red cell survival is one of the mechanisms, although not the principal one, in anaemia of chronic renal failure. Small numbers of keratocytes and other fragments may be present.

Liver disease

Liver disease is associated with several haemolytic syndromes. In Zieve's syndrome there is acute alcoholic liver disease associated with hyperlipidaemia and acute haemolysis. Zieve [237] and others [238] have described the abnormal cells as 'spherocytes' and in one case Zieve suspected an inherited haemolytic anaemia. However, illustrations have shown irregularly contracted cells [238] and these are sometimes prominent (Fig. 8.69). A distinct syndrome initially called 'spur cell haemolytic anaemia', which is characterized by numerous acanthocytes, (Fig. 8.70) is caused by liver failure of any aetiology.

Wilson's disease

Wilson's disease can cause both acute haemolytic anaemia with no morphological abnormality and an acute Heinz body haemolytic anaemia consequent on sudden release of copper from a gravely damaged liver [239] (Fig. 8.71). It is important to think of previously undiagnosed Wilson's disease when an acute haemolytic anaemia is unexplained since this may be the presenting feature of a condition that is fatal if left untreated.

Diabetes mellitus

Compensated haemolysis without anaemia or morphological abnormalities appears to be common in diabetes mellitus [240].

Vitamin E deficiency

Vitamin E deficiency can cause haemolysis, particularly in neonates and particularly when iron-supplemented milk is used for feeding. This may be the initial presentation of cystic fibrosis [241]. The blood film shows 'pyknocytes'—irregularly contracted spiculated cells, similar to the acanthocytes observed in other circumstances.

Phosphate depletion

Phosphate depletion, leading to reduced ATP, is a rare cause of haemolytic anaemia. This is the likely mechanism of haemolytic anaemia reported in association with hypophosphataemia during re-feeding of a patient with anorexia nervosa [242].

Fig. 8.69 The blood film of a patient with Zieve's syndrome as a complication of acute alcoholic liver disease showing irregularly contracted cells and polychromatic macrocytes.

Fig. 8.70 The blood film of a patient with terminal liver disease of unknown aetiology showing numerous acanthocytes ('spur cell' haemolytic anaemia).

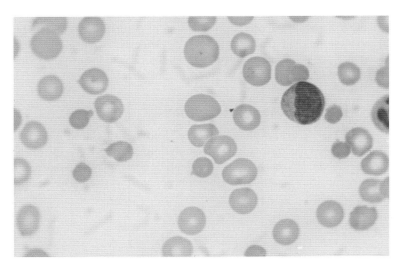

Fig. 8.71 The blood film in a patient with terminal liver failure as a complication of Wilson's disease showing irregularly contracted cells and polychromatic macrocytes.

Bacterial and parasitic infections

Bartonellosis, malaria and babesiosis characteristically cause haemolytic anaemia. Rarely this is also seen in patients with Whipple's disease who have been splenectomized. Bacterial and viral infections can be associated with microangiopathic haemolytic anaemia. Clostridial toxins can cause a severe spherocytic haemolytic anaemia. Bacterial infections can also alter red cell membrane antigens to cause T activation. Anti-T antibodies in the plasma can then bind to red cells causing spherocytosis and haemolysis. This has been observed with infection by *Staphylococcus aureus*, *Escherichia coli* and

pneumococcus and in necrotizing enteritis caused by *Clostridium perfringens* (previously known as *Clostridium welchii*). Acute haemolysis can follow transfusion of normal blood which contains anti-T antibodies and this type of haemolysis can therefore be confused with other types of haemolytic transfusion reaction [243].

Snake and insect bites

Bites of a number of snakes (Fig. 8.72) and insects can cause an acute spherocytic haemolytic anaemia, sometimes with associated disseminated intravascular coagulation and thrombocytopenia.

Fig. 8.72 The blood film of a Sri Lankan patient who had suffered a viper bite showing fragments and microspherocytes. Courtesy of Dr Sudharma Vidyatilake, Colombo.

Sometimes red cell fragments are the most prominent feature.

March haemoglobinuria

March haemoglobinuria describes haemolytic anaemia observed in soldiers on forced marches. Although haemolysis is mechanical, consequent on damage of red cells in blood vessels in the feet, it is rare for any fragments or other specific features to be observed. A similar type of haemolysis can be induced by jogging on hard surfaces, karate, drumming with the hands and even swimming. These conditions should be sought by specific questioning whenever there is mild unexplained anaemia in an apparently fit, usually young, person. (There may be factors other than haemolysis operating in some cases of exercise-induced anaemia, e.g. exercise-induced gastrointestinal haemorrhage.)

Haemolysis caused by infusion of hypotonic fluid

Acute intravascular haemolysis with no morphological abnormality can be caused by inadvertent intravenous infusion of hypotonic fluid.

Paroxysmal nocturnal haemoglobinuria

Paroxysmal nocturnal haemoglobinuria (PNH) is a clonal haemopoietic stem cell disorder in which red cells with a specific membrane defect are abnormally sensitive to complement-induced lysis. This results from an acquired somatic mutation in the phosphatidylinositol-glycan complementation class A (*PIG-A*) gene that leads to a deficiency of glycosylphosphatidylinositol (GPI) and therefore of the numerous membrane proteins that are anchored to GPI [244]. A tendency to bone marrow hypoplasia or aplasia must also be present so that the PNH clone is favoured. Some but not all patients give a history of nocturnal haemolysis, i.e. of the first urine specimen passed in the morning being red. A diagnosis of PNH should be considered when there is an unexplained haemolytic anaemia, particularly if associated with leucopenia or thrombocytopenia. Acute myeloid leukaemia (AML) and myelodysplastic syndromes (MDS) may develop during the course of PNH.

It should be noted that very rarely the phenotype of PNH results from an inherited deficiency of CD59 (membrane inhibitor of reactive lysis, MIRL) [245].

Blood film and count

There are no specific blood film features. Polychromatic macrocytes may be present (Fig. 8.73). Eighty per cent of patients have neutropenia or thrombocytopenia [244].

Differential diagnosis

The differential diagnosis includes other causes of normocytic anaemia and pancytopenia.

Fig. 8.73 The blood film of a patient with paroxysmal nocturnal haemoglobinuria (PNH) showing polychromatic macrocytes.

Further tests

A Ham test for lysis of red cells following exposure to acidified serum should be performed when this diagnosis is suspected. The diagnosis can also be confirmed by flow cytometry using monoclonal antibodies directed at GPI-anchored antigens such as CD55 and CD59 on red cells or neutrophils. The absence of such antigens can also be demonstrated by a modification of the gel technology used for blood grouping.

Miscellaneous causes of acquired haemolytic anaemia

Haemolytic anaemia with a negative direct and indirect antiglobulin test and with no specific morphological features has been described as a transient phenomenon, sometimes accompanied by thrombocytopenia, in patients with hepatitis C infection [246].

Dyserythropoietic anaemias

Congenital dyserythropoietic anaemias (CDA)

The congenital dyserythropoietic anaemias are inherited disorders characterized by ineffective and dysplastic erythropoiesis, shortened red cell lifespan and anaemia with marked poikilocytosis. There are three well-characterized types, the features of which are summarized in Tables 8.9 and 8.10. There are also cases that appear to conform to these types but have a different inheritance and therefore presumably a different underlying defect. There are autosomal dominant cases resembling type I and apparently autosomal recessive cases resembling type III. In addition there are individual cases or families with distinctive features. These include congenital megaloblastic anaemia independent of vitamin B_{12} or folate deficiency and cases with various red cell inclusions [247]. Variants have been described with microcytosis attributable to sideroblastic erythropoiesis [250] and with prominent ovalocytosis [251]. Two cases have been described with features resembling those of type II CDA but with spherocytosis and a negative acid lysis test [252]. Cases with X-linked inheritance and coexisting thrombocytopenia may be consequent on mutation in the *GATA1* gene [253,254]. Provisional categorization of some atypical forms as CDA, types IV–VII, has been proposed [247]. It has been suggested that cases of congenital ineffective erythropoiesis without significant erythroid dysplasia should also be included in the category of CDA [247].

In most cases of CDA the underlying abnormality is not understood although the genes that are mutated in the three major forms of CDA have been

Table 8.9 Inheritance pattern. Ethnic distribution and associated features in the congenital dyserythropoietic anaemias [247,248].

Type	Inheritance	Gene	Ethnic origin and associated features
Type I	AR	*CDAN1* at 15q15.1–15.3	Caucasians (including Russians), Israeli Bedouins, Lebanese, Japanese; associated constitutional abnormalities such as facial dysmorphism and abnormalities of distal limbs are common
Type II (HEMPAS)	AR	*CDNA2* at 20q11.2 in 90%, unknown in others	Caucasian, particularly Italian
Type III	AD	*CDNA3* at 20q21–25 in single Swedish family	Swedish, American and Argentinean families; Swedish family shows association with retinal abnormalities and plasma cell neoplasia

HEMPAS, hereditary erythroid multinuclearity with positive acidified-serum lysis test.

identified. Some cases, particularly of type I CDA, have other associated congenital abnormalities.

Patients typically present with anaemia, hepatomegaly, splenomegaly and intermittent jaundice. Cases of type III are typically milder than cases of types I and II. Coexisting β thalassaemia trait has been observed to aggravate type II.

Since interferon alpha has been found to be of considerable therapeutic benefit in type I CDA the laboratory diagnosis of these rare conditions is becoming increasingly important. Correct diagnosis may also lead to therapeutic measures to reduce iron overload and consequent organ damage.

Blood film and count

In a minority of cases the anaemia is severe. Usually it is mild or moderate. Some cases are macrocytic and others are normocytic. Cells show marked anisocytosis and striking poikilocytosis (Figs 8.74 and 8.75). Haemoglobinization is generally normal but some cells may be poorly haemoglobinized. The absolute reticulocyte count is normal. Some cases have had circulating NRBC, which become very numerous after splenectomy [255]. The RDW and HDW are increased, the RDW markedly so, and this is reflected in the red cell cytograms and histograms (Fig. 8.76).

In CDA resulting from mutation of the *GATA1* gene there is thrombocytopenia with large platelets. Acanthocytes, which are not often a feature of CDA, have been noted in this syndrome [253,254].

Differential diagnosis

The differential diagnosis includes haemolytic anaemias with marked morphological abnormalities,

Table 8.10 Peripheral blood features in the congenital dyserythropoietic anaemias [247,248].

Type	Red cell size	Other blood film features
Type I	Usually macrocytic	Round and oval macrocytes, marked anisocytosis, marked poikilocytosis including elliptocytes and teardrop poikilocytes, basophilic stippling, irregularly contracted cells, polychromasia
Type II (HEMPAS)	Normocytic	Moderate anisocytosis, variable anisochromasia, moderate poikilocytosis including 'pincer cells' [249], teardrop cells and irregularly contracted cells, basophilic stippling, some NRBC, polychromasia
Type III	Normocytic or slightly macrocytic	Marked anisocytosis with some large macrocytes, marked poikilocytosis including fragments and irregularly contracted cells, basophilic stippling, polychromasia; some patients have superimposed iron deficiency

HEMPAS, hereditary erythroid multinuclearity with positive acidified-serum lysis test. NRBC, nucleated red blood cells.

Fig. 8.74 The blood film of a patient with type I congenital dyserythropoietic anaemia showing marked anisocytosis, poikilocytosis and some macrocytes.

(a)

(b)

Fig. 8.75 (a,b) The blood film of a patient with type III congenital dyserythropoietic anaemia showing anisocytosis and poikilocytosis. Courtesy of Professor S.N. Wickramasinghe, London.

Fig. 8.76 Bayer H.2 red cell histograms and cytograms from a patient with type I congenital dyserythropoietic anaemia (same patient as in Fig. 8.74) showing a marked variation in red cell size (as reflected in the increased RDW) and a lesser degree of variation in red cell haemoglobinization (as reflected in the increased HDW).

particularly hereditary poikilocytosis and haemoglobin H disease. In both these conditions the reticulocyte count is elevated and in haemoglobin H disease there is hypochromia and microcytosis. Cases presenting beyond childhood need to be distinguished from the MDS and other conditions causing acquired dyserythropoiesis. Cases of CDA usually lack significant dysplastic features in non-erythroid lineages.

Further tests

A provisional diagnosis can be made from the blood film. Confirmation of the diagnosis requires bone marrow examination with ultrastructural examination being particularly useful. In type I CDA there may be an increased percentage of haemoglobin A_2 and a slight reduction in red cell membrane protein 4.1 [67]. In the case of suspected type II CDA, the demonstration of a positive acid lysis (Ham) test is useful; this may require testing with multiple fresh

sera. Type II CDA also shows increased expression of the i antigen and on SDS-polyacrylamide gel electrophoresis red cell membrane band 3, which is hypoglycosylated, shows an abnormal migration pattern. In type II CDA, binding of eosin-5-maleimide, detected by flow cytometry, is abnormal [87].

Bilirubin and LDH concentrations are generally increased and serum haptoglobin is decreased. In more severe cases there may be significant haemosiderinuria.

Acquired dyserythropoietic anaemias

Dyserythropoiesis as an acquired phenomenon can be secondary to severe protein–calorie malnutrition, acute severe illness, autoimmune disease, human immunodeficiency virus (HIV) infection or exposure to drugs (such as cytotoxic drugs) or to toxic substances (such as alcohol or arsenic). It can also be a manifestation of MDS (see p. 421) or of other haemopoietic neoplasms. Severe dyserythropoiesis has been observed in peripartum women with pregnancy-associated hypertension and parvovirus B19 infection [256].

Blood film and count

Red cells may show anisocytosis, poikilocytosis, macrocytosis or basophilic stippling and there may be a population of hypochromic microcytes. Neutrophils may show hypogranularity and defects of nuclear lobulation. The FBC may show anaemia, neutropenia or thrombocytopenia. Red cell histograms and cytograms may show an increased MCV, RDW and HDW.

Differential diagnosis

The differential diagnosis includes congenital dyserythropoietic anaemias and other causes of anaemia with or without other cytopenia.

Further tests

Which further tests are indicated is dependent on the clinical setting and the specific cytological abnormalities present.

Aplastic anaemias and pure red cell aplasia

Inherited aplastic anaemia

There are various inherited syndromes in which haemopoietic stem cells are abnormal, leading to the onset of aplastic anaemia during childhood or adolescence. The least uncommon of these is Fanconi's anaemia, a genetically diverse group of disorders in which there are often associated constitutional abnormalities; these may include mental retardation, abnormalities of skin pigmentation, urogenital abnormalities and abnormalities of limbs and digits. There appear to be at least eight different genes, designated *FANCA* to *FANCH*, mutation of which can lead to the phenotype of Fanconi's anaemia. Inheritance is autosomal recessive. Fanconi's anaemia may progress to MDS and AML. An even more rare inherited condition leading to aplastic anaemia is dyskeratosis congenita, some cases of which result

from mutation in the *DKC1* gene and others from mutation in the *TERC* gene; it is characterized by prominent abnormalities of skin and nails.

Blood film and count

There is thrombocytopenia, which is often the presenting feature. Anaemia is often macrocytic and is accompanied by reticulocytopenia. Sometimes anisocytosis and poikilocytosis are marked. With progression, there is pancytopenia.

Differential diagnosis

The differential diagnosis includes acquired aplastic anaemia and other causes of anaemia or pancytopenia.

Further tests

Diagnosis of aplastic anaemia requires bone marrow aspiration and a trephine biopsy. Diagnosis of Fanconi's anaemia is traditionally by demonstration of increased chromosomal breaks on exposure to clastogenic agents, but it should be noted that about 10% of patients do not show sensitivity to clastogenic agents [17].

A more economical screening test is measurement of serum alpha-fetoprotein; it is elevated in the majority of patients and is not elevated in other bone marrow failure syndromes [257].

Acquired aplastic anaemia

Aplastic anaemia may be: (i) a dose-related effect of irradiation or certain drugs or chemicals (e.g. chemotherapeutic agents or benzene); (ii) an idiosyncratic reaction to a drug (e.g. chloramphenicol or sulphonamides and related drugs including antithyroid drugs); (iii) the result of infection by certain viruses, possibly non-A, non-B non-C hepatitis or, in patients with defective immunity, the Epstein–Barr virus. In many cases the cause cannot be ascertained so that they are classified as idiopathic. Aplastic anaemia may lead to death from infection or haemorrhage. In patients who survive, e.g. following immunosuppressive treatment, PNH, MDS and AML may subsequently emerge.

Blood film and count

There is pancytopenia with a markedly reduced reticulocyte count. Red cells are normochromic and either normocytic or macrocytic. Poikilocytosis is sometimes marked. The neutrophils may show heavy granulation. Platelet size is normal on the blood film and MPV is not increased. In contrast to pancytopenia resulting from bone marrow infiltration, circulating granulocyte precursors and nucleated red blood cells are absent.

Differential diagnosis

The differential diagnosis included inherited causes of aplastic anaemia (particularly when there is a late onset and other constitutional abnormalities are minor or absent), an aplastic presentation of acute lymphoblastic leukaemia, hypoplastic AML and MDS, HIV infection and other causes of pancytopenia.

Further tests

Bone marrow aspiration and a trephine biopsy are required for diagnosis. Cytogenetic analysis is indicated, although the detection of an abnormal clone does not necessarily indicate that there will be rapid progression to a myelodysplastic syndrome or to acute myeloid leukaemia. Young patients, e.g. under the age of 35 years, should be tested for Fanconi's anaemia, even in the absence of evident constitutional abnormalities. This is particularly important if stem cell transplantation is being considered.

Inherited pure red cell aplasia

Diamond–Blackfan anaemia is a haemopoietic stem cell disorder of which the earliest manifestation is pure red cell aplasia. Later neutropenia and thrombocytopenia may also develop. Inheritance is usually autosomal dominant but in some families is autosomal recessive. About three-quarters of cases appear to be sporadic. In about one-quarter of familial cases, all autosomal dominant, the mutation responsible is in the ribosomal protein S19 (*RPS19*) gene at 19q13.2 [258]. Another gene implicated is at

8p23.3-23.1 [259]. Phenotypic expression of *RPS19* mutations is variable. In addition to red cell aplasia, there are some individuals in affected families in whom the gene is silent; in others it causes only macrocytosis, an elevated red cell adenosine deaminase activity or both. About 40% of patients have associated congenital abnormalities [259]. The incidence of AML is increased [17].

The prevalence is 5–7/100 000 live births [259].

Blood film and count

Initially there is anaemia and macrocytosis with a low reticulocyte count. The neutrophil count is normal or slightly reduced. The platelet count is normal or increased. With disease progression, there may be neutropenia or thrombocytopenia progressing to pancytopenia.

Differential diagnosis

The differential diagnosis includes transient erythroblastopenia of childhood and persistent parvovirus B19 infection.

Further tests

Serum soluble transferrin receptor is greatly reduced in all types of pure red cell aplasia. Erythrocyte adenosine deaminase activity is increased in about 40% of patients with Diamond–Blackfan syndrome whereas it is normal in transient erythroblastopenia of childhood [259]. Bone marrow examination usually shows reduction of proerythroblasts and marked reduction of later erythroblasts. In a minority, proerythroblast numbers are normal. Cells of other lineages are initially normal. In transient erythroblastopenia, the haemoglobin A_{1C} may be elevated, as a consequence of the increased mean age of the red cells, whereas in Diamond–Blackfan syndrome the haemoglobin A_{1c} would be expected to be normal as the decline in erythropoiesis has been very gradual [260].

Acquired pure red cell aplasia

Acquired pure red cell aplasia may be transient or persistent. Transient pure red cell aplasia is often caused by parvovirus B19 infection and, unless the patient has, coincidentally, a shortened red cell life-span, is so brief that it often goes undiagnosed. More prolonged pure red cell aplasia occurs in transient erythroblastopenia of childhood, which results, in some cases, from human herpesvirus 6 infection. Chronic pure red cell aplasia may result from persistent parvovirus B19 infection in patients with impaired immunity, e.g. in HIV infection or following immunosuppressive therapy. It may be immunological in origin, as when it is associated with thymoma, autoimmune disease, large granular lymphocyte leukaemia or chronic lymphocytic leukaemia. A significant proportion of cases represent the most prominent manifestation of MDS.

Blood film and count

There is a macrocytic or normocytic anaemia with marked reticulocytopenia. Depending on the aetiology, there may be dysplastic features in cells of other lineages or an increase in large granular lymphocytes. Transient erythroblastopenia of childhood is associated with a normal MCV, with a neutrophil count of less than $1 \times 10^9/l$ in up to one-fifth of patients and with thrombocytopenia in about 5% [261].

Differential diagnosis

The differential diagnosis includes other causes of a normocytic or macrocytic anaemia.

Further tests

Bone marrow examination is diagnostic. Depending on the clinical context, other indicated tests may include serological tests for herpesvirus 6 and parvovirus B19, tests for parvovirus DNA, screening for autoantibodies, chest radiology, immunophenotypic analysis of lymphocytes or cytogenetic analysis.

Polycythaemia

Polycythaemia refers to an increased RBC, Hb and PCV/Hct. It may be relative, resulting from a decreased plasma volume, or absolute, caused by an increase in the total volume of red cells in the circulation.

Relative polycythaemia

Relative or apparent or pseudo-polycythaemia may occur as a consequence of acute plasma loss, as in burns and dehydration. The explanation will be readily apparent from the clinical history and no further diagnostic tests are required. Relative polycythaemia also occurs as a chronic condition, which is sometimes attributable to cigarette smoking but is usually unexplained. The blood film appears 'packed' but is otherwise normal. The blood film cannot be distinguished from that in idiopathic erythrocytosis (see below), the distinction being made by radio-isotopic estimations of total plasma volume and total red cell volume (traditionally referred to as 'red cell mass'). Measurement of the Hb is not reliable in distinguishing a true from a relative polycythaemia. Even Hbs of over 20 g/dl may be observed in relative polycythaemia [262].

True polycythaemia

True polycythaemia refers to an increase in the total volume of circulating red cells ('red cell mass') above that which is predicted for the individual's height and weight. The total plasma volume is often increased but may be normal or decreased. True polycythaemia may result from:

1 chronic hypoxia such as that caused by living at altitude, cyanotic heart disease and chronic hypoxic lung disease;
2 increased secretion of erythropoietin as from renal cysts and tumours or other tumours;
3 idiopathic erythrocytosis (an unexplained condition);
4 polycythaemia rubra vera.

All these conditions cause a high RBC, Hb and PCV/Hct and the blood film appears 'packed'. With the exception of polycythaemia rubra vera (see below), the blood film and count are usually otherwise normal.

Polycythaemia rubra vera

Polycythaemia rubra vera (PRV), also known as polycythaemia vera and primary proliferative polycythaemia, is a myeloproliferative disorder in which there is increased production of red cells and sometimes also of granulocytes and platelets. PRV is largely a disease of the middle-aged and elderly, although occasional cases are seen in younger adults and very rare cases in children. Common clinical features are those resulting from the hyperviscosity of the polycythaemic blood, such as cerebrovascular accidents and peripheral gangrene, and those indicative of the myeloproliferative disorder, such as hepatomegaly, splenomegaly and pruritus.

PRV may eventually enter a 'burnt-out' phase or may be complicated by the development of myelofibrosis or AML.

Blood film and count

The peripheral blood film in polycythaemia of any aetiology shows a 'packed film' appearance since the viscosity of the blood means that the film of blood is not spread as thinly as normal (Fig. 8.77). The WBC, neutrophil and basophil counts are increased in the majority of cases. Monocyte and eosinophil counts are much less often increased. The platelet count is elevated in about two-thirds of cases and platelet size is increased. There may be circulating nucleated red blood cells or granulocyte precursors. Red cells may be normocytic and normochromic or, if hyperplastic erythropoiesis has led to exhaustion of iron stores, they may be hypochromic and microcytic. If complicating iron deficiency occurs there may be anaemia (Fig. 8.78) but the underlying polycythaemia is revealed if the patient is given iron. Less often PRV is masked by complicating vitamin B$_{12}$ or folate deficiency.

The FBC usually shows an elevated RBC, Hb and Hct and normal or reduced MCV and MCH. The platelet count may be increased. The MPV is raised in relation to the platelet count. In PRV complicated by iron deficiency the red cell indices are very similar to those of thalassaemia trait but the MCHC is reduced and the RDW is increased.

Differential diagnosis

The differential diagnosis includes other causes of polycythaemia (see Table 6.1). In particular, it is necessary to distinguish PRV from essential erythrocytosis. This term means that there is unexplained polycythaemia without clear clinical or laboratory evidence of a myeloproliferative disorder; some but not all of these patients subsequently develop features of PRV.

Neutrophilia, an increased basophil count, thrombocytosis, giant platelets and an elevated MPV favour a diagnosis of PRV. An increased basophilia count is particularly useful in the differential diagnosis since it is not seen in secondary polycythaemia or essential erythrocytosis.

Further tests

Polycythaemia should be confirmed by obtaining a repeat blood specimen, with minimal stasis, before

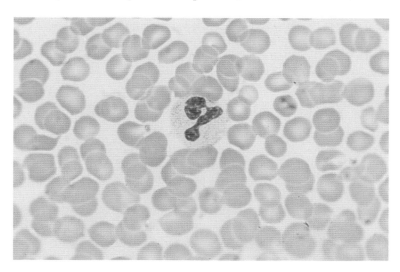

Fig. 8.77 A 'packed film' consequent on post-transplant polycythaemia. The Hb was 20 g/dl and the Hct 0.59. The MCV was increased to 114 fl as a consequence of azathioprine therapy.

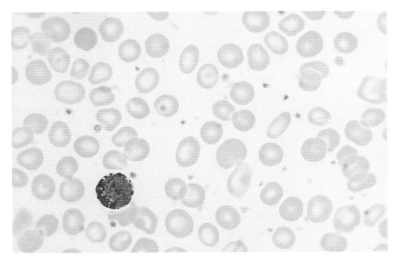

Fig. 8.78 The blood film of a patient with PRV complicated by iron deficiency, showing anaemia and thrombocytosis and some hypochromic and microcytic cells. There was an increased basophil count and there is one basophil in the field. FBC (Coulter S Plus IV) was: WBC $6.7 \times 10^9/l$, RBC $4.38 \times 10^{12}/l$, Hb 10.6 g/dl, Hct 0.33, MCV 75 fl, MCH 24.2 pg, MCHC 32.3 g/dl, RDW 24.9, platelet count $1056 \times 10^9/l$.

proceeding to further investigations. Determination of total red cell and plasma volume by radio-isotopic dilution studies excludes relative polycythaemia. The World Health Organization (WHO) classification of myeloproliferative disorders suggest that measurement of the red cell mass is unnecessary if the Hb is greater than 18.5 g/dl in a man or greater than 16.5 g/dl in a woman [263]. However in one comparison of true and relative polycythaemia the Hb exceeded these levels in 14% of men with relative polycythaemia and in 35% of women [262]. It therefore seems prudent to estimate the red cell mass and plasma volume whenever polycythaemia vera is suspected. The neutrophil alkaline phosphatase (NAP) score is often increased and is much less likely to be increased in secondary polycythaemia. The plasma erythropoietin concentration is often decreased whereas it is more likely to be normal in relative polycythaemia. A low serum erythropoietin has a high specificity but only moderate sensitivity [264]. However, it should also be noted that 30–50% of patients with essential thrombocythaemia show a reduced erythropoietin concentration [264,265] and this test therefore cannot be used to distinguish between these two conditions; a low level can also be seen in idiopathic erythrocytosis [266]. The serum ferritin is often low. Serum vitamin B_{12} is often elevated as a result of an increase of B_{12}-binding proteins in the plasma. Growth or erythropoietin-independent erythroid colonies from peripheral blood or bone marrow suggests polycythaemia vera although a significant proportion of cases of idiopathic erythrocytosis also show this phenomenon; this test is not widely used but a simplified method could make it more widely applicable [267]. A bone marrow aspirate and trephine biopsy are useful to confirm a myeloproliferative disorder and should be supplemented by cytogenetic analysis (since a clonal chromosomal abnormality is confirmatory of a haematological neoplasm). Analysis for a *JAK2* point mutation, which can be performed on the peripheral blood, also provides evidence that the process is neoplastic; such an abnormality is found in the majority of patients with PRV. An ultrasound examination of the abdomen is important, both to detect splenomegaly in patients with PRV and to exclude renal lesions as a cause of secondary polycythaemia. Arterial blood gas estimations are also relevant to exclude a pulmonary cause of secondary polycythaemia. Guidelines for the diagnosis of polycythaemia vera are available [266].

Secondary polycythaemia

A diagnosis of secondary polycythaemia can often be made by consideration of the blood count and film in the light of the clinical features. If it is not clear whether the patient has a secondary polycythaemia or PRV, investigations as above are indicated. Some patients with secondary polycythaemia have neutrophilia or thrombocytosis but an increased basophil count (confirmed on a blood film) and giant platelets are strongly suggestive of PRV. A raised serum erythropoietin has a high specificity but is observed in around 50% of patients; occasional patients even have a reduced concentration [264].

Relative polycythaemia

This condition is generally asymptomatic, the diagnosis being made incidentally.

Blood film and count

The RBC, Hb and Hct are increased. The white cell count and platelet count are normal. The blood film may appear 'packed', as a result of increased blood viscosity. Otherwise it is normal.

Differential diagnosis

The differential diagnosis is true polycythaemia, particularly essential erythrocytosis.

Further tests

Distinction from true polycythaemia is made by studies of total red cell and plasma volume. Bone marrow aspiration and trephine biopsy show no abnormality [268], although these tests are not necessary if blood volume studies are available. The serum erythropoietin concentration is usually normal but is occasionally low [264,268].

DISORDERS OF PLATELETS

Thrombocytopenia

Congenital thrombocytopenias

Congenital thrombocytopenia may be inherited or due to a pathological process, e.g. infection or exposure to an antibody or a toxic substance, occurring during intrauterine life. It may be caused by failure of production or increased consumption or destruction of platelets.

Congenital thrombocytopenia may be an isolated abnormality or may be associated with abnormalities of granulopoiesis or erythropoiesis or with constitutional abnormalities. In congenital amegakaryocytic thrombocytopenia resulting from a mutation in the *MPL* gene (the thrombopoietin receptor), there is slow progression to pancytopenia [269]. Patients with Fanconi's anaemia may also present with isolated thrombocytopenia, only later showing progression to pancytopenia. The rare syndrome of amegakaryocytic thrombocytopenia with radio-ulnar synostosis may show progression to hypoplastic anaemia or pancytopenia [270,271]. Inherited and other constitutional syndromes causing thrombocytopenia are summarized in Tables 8.11–8.13. It should be noted that the Bernard–Soulier syndrome is a severe bleeding disorder with giant platelets and abnormal platelet function as well as marked thrombocytopenia whereas heterozygosity for one of the Bernard–

Table 8.11 Inherited and other constitutional abnormalities leading to thrombocytopenia with small platelets [272].

Defect	Inheritance	Platelet functional defect	Associated abnormalities	Reference
Wiskott–Aldrich syndrome	Sex-linked recessive* (*WASP* gene at Xp11.22–23)	Yes (reduced dense granules and reduced expression of GpIIb/IIIa and IV)	Eczema and defective cell-mediated immunity	[273,274]
X-linked thrombocytopenia including intermittent X-linked thrombocytopenia with small platelets	Sex-linked recessive (*WASP* gene at Xp11.22–23)	Yes (reduced dense granules and reduced expression of GpIIb/IIIa and IV)	Isolated thrombocytopenia (although there is a mutation in the same gene as causes Wiskott–Aldrich syndrome)	[274,275]
Autosomal dominant with micro-thrombocytes	AD	Normal function		[276]

* Occasional cases occur in females, either because of extreme Lyonization or because of failure of the mechanism that usually ensures that in heterozygotes there is preferential proliferation/survival of cells expressing the paternal wild type *WASP* [273].

Table 8.12 Inherited and other constitutional abnormalities leading to thrombocytopenia with normal sized platelets [272].

Defect	Inheritance	Platelet functional defect	Associated abnormalities	Reference
Fanconi's anaemia	AR		Progression to pancytopenia; reduced stature, abnormal digits and other dysmorphic features	
Thrombocytopenia with absent radii	AR (rarely AD)		Absent radii, thrombocytopenia improves with age	
Amegakaryocytic thrombocytopenia	AR, mutation in *MPL* gene (encoding thrombopoietin receptor) at 1p34		Slow progression to pancytopenia	[270,271,277, 278]
Amegakaryocytic thrombocytopenia with radio-ulnar synostosis	AD, *HOXA11* gene		Radio-ulnar fusion (synostosis); progression to pancytopenia, possible sensorineural deafness	[270,271,277]
Autosomal dominant thrombocytopenia	AD, *FLJ14813* gene at 10p11.2–2			[279,280]
Familial platelet disorder with a propensity to develop AML	AD, *AML1* (*RUNX1*) mutation	Very abnormal platelet function, storage pool defect and greatly reduced aggregation with all agents	Propensity to develop AML	[281,282]
Quebec platelet disorder (previously known as factor V Quebec)	AD	Abnormal epinephrine-induced aggregation, delayed bleeding		[283]
Dysmega-karyopoietic thrombocytopenia	AR	Normal or increased numbers of small dysmorphic megakaryocytes		[284]

AD, autosomal dominant; AML, acute myeloid leukaemia; AR autosomal recessive.

Soulier mutations leads to a milder thrombocytopenia with giant but normally functioning platelets, resulting in either a mild bleeding tendency or no clinical abnormality. The four syndromes resulting from mutation in the *MHY9* gene, which encodes the heavy chain of non-muscle myosin IIA, differ in associated features and in the ultrastructure of any neutrophil inclusions [300]. There are other rare congenital syndromes in which thrombocytopenia has been described. The von Voss–Cherstvoy or DK-phocomelia syndrome is a syndrome of multiple congenital abnormalities, which may have associated thrombocytopenia and which is often fatal in the perinatal period [301]; bone marrow megakaryocytes are reduced. Congenital thrombocytopenia has also been associated with agenesis of the corpus callosum and distinctive facies [302]. Another autosomal dominant syndrome associates deformity of the upper limb, hearing loss, external ophthalmoplegia and thrombocytopenia [303].

Congenital thrombocytopenia may be immune in origin and transient, resulting from transplacental passage of maternal autoantibodies or alloantibodies (including anti-glycoprotein IV–anti-CD36).

Table 8.13 Inherited and other constitutional abnormalities leading to thrombocytopenia with large platelets.

Defect	Inheritance	Platelet functional defect	Associated abnormalities	Reference
Bernard–Soulier syndrome	AR, homozygosity or compound heterozygosity for mutations in the GpIbα gene (17pter-p12), GpIbβ gene (22q11.2) or Gp IX gene (3q21)	Abnormal glycoprotein Ib/IX/V complex with marked defect in von Willebrand factor-dependent aggregation	Nil	
Heterozygosity for Bernard–Soulier syndrome/ Mediterranean macrothrombo-cytopenia	AD, minimally expressed in heterozygotes; mutations as above	Normal	Nil	[278,285]
Mediterranean stomatocytosis/ macrothrombo-cytopaenia (phytosterolaemia)	AR, mutation in *ABCG5* or *ABCG8* gene	Abnormal with ristocetin; variable abnormalities with other agonists	Short stature, hyperphytosterolaemia, variable hypercholesterolaemia	[128]
Grey platelet syndrome	AR or AD	α granule defect with hypogranular platelets and mild functional defect; combined α and δ granule deficiency	Severely hypogranular neutrophils in some families	[286]
White platelet syndrome	AD	α granule defect, prominent Golgi complexes, defective aggregation with epinephrine and adenosine diphosphate		[287]
May–Hegglin anomaly	AD, non-muscle myosin heavy chain 9 gene (*MYH9/NMMHCIIA*) at 22q11–13	Reduced glycoprotein Ib/IX/V complex	Neutrophil inclusions	[288,289]
Fechtner syndrome	AD, non-muscle myosin heavy chain 9 gene (*MYH9* or *NMMHC-A*) at 22q11–13		Neutrophil inclusions, Alport-like syndrome—nephritis, sensorineural deafness, cataracts	[290,291]
Epstein syndrome	AD, muscle myosin heavy chain 9 gene (*MYH9/ NMMHCIIA*) 22q11–13		Alport-like syndrome—nephritis, sensorineural deafness, cataracts—but no neutrophil inclusions	[291]
Sebastian syndrome	AD, muscle myosin heavy chain 9 gene *MYH9* or *NMMHC-A* gene at 22q11–13	Reduced glycoprotein Ib/IX/V complex	Neutrophil inclusions	[288,290, 291]
Paris–Trousseau thrombocytopenia	Deletion of 11q23; a contiguous gene syndrome	Platelets have abnormally large α granules	Features of Jacobsen's syndrome; psychomotor retardation, facial dysmorphism and cardiac defects	[278,292]

Continued p. 370

Table 8.13 *Continued*

Defect	Inheritance	Platelet functional defect	Associated abnormalities	Reference
DiGeorge and velocardiofacial syndrome	AD, loss of function of *GP1BB* gene at 22q11; a contiguous gene syndrome		Cardiac, parathyroid and thymus abnormalities, cognitive impairment in velocardiofacial syndrome, also facial dysmorphism; autoimmune cytopenias	[278,293]
Homozygous Pelger–Huët anomaly	AD		Lack of lobulation in granulocytes and monocytes	[294]
X-linked thrombocytopenia, with abnormal erythropoiesis	X-linked, mutation in *GATA 1* at Xp11–12	Abnormal glycoproteins Ibβ and IX, abnormal ristocetin-induced aggregation, may have severe functional defect	Macrocytosis, dyserythropoiesis or dyserythropoietic anaemia in some families, β thalassaemia in some families	[253,254, 295]
Thrombocytopenia with neutropenia	Unknown but presumably inherited	Reduced glycoprotein Ib	Neutropenia with reduced sialyl-Lewis X on neutrophils	[296]
Down's syndrome	Trisomy 21		Other features of transient abnormal myelopoiesis	
Thrombocytopenia with large platelets in West Bengal	Unknown	Normal		[297]
Giant platelets with mitral valve insufficiency	Unknown	Reduced glycoproteins Ia, Ic and IIa, reduced aggregation with ADP and adrenaline	Mitral insufficiency	[298]
Giant platelets with ineffective thrombopoiesis	AD	Increased platelet glycoprotein Ib and IIb/IIIa	Nil	[299]
Montreal platelet syndrome	AD	Spontaneous platelet aggregation of resting or stirred platelets		
Macrothrombo-cytopenia with platelet expression of glycophorin A	AD	Defective aggregation with arachidonic acid		
Platelet-type von-Willebrand's disease	AD, GpIbα at 17p13	Increased aggregation with ristocetin		

AD, autosomal dominant; AR autosomal recessive.

Other congenital abnormalities may indicate either an inherited syndrome or exposure to a teratogenic substance *in utero*.

Blood film and count

The peripheral blood film may show platelets that are small, normal in size or large. Small platelets are uncommon but are seen in the Wiskott–Aldrich syndrome (see Fig. 3.135). Platelets of normal size are seen when there is bone marrow or megakaryocytic hypoplasia. Large platelets are common in various inherited causes of thrombocytopenia, e.g. Bernard–Soulier syndrome (Fig. 8.79) and May–Hegglin

anomaly (see Fig. 3.79) and a number of other more rare conditions. In Bernard–Soulier syndrome there is marked thrombocytopenia with giant platelets. In heterozygosity for the Bernard–Soulier syndrome the platelet count may be as low as $40–50 \times 10^9/l$ but in some individuals is normal; all have giant platelets [285]. In most disorders the platelets show normal granulation but in the rare grey platelet syndrome they appear agranular or hypogranular (Fig. 8.80) and in Paris–Trousseau thrombocytopenia (Jacobsen's syndrome) platelets have giant granules. Neutrophils should be examined for abnormal inclusions which are present in granulocytes not only in the May–Hegglin anomaly but also in Fechtner's

Fig. 8.79 The blood film of a patient with the Bernard–Soulier syndrome showing thrombocytopenia and three giant platelets.

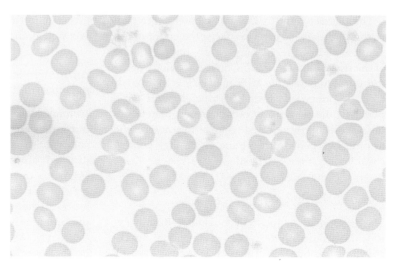

Fig. 8.80 The blood film of a patient with the grey platelet syndrome showing six agranular platelets.

syndrome and Sebastian's syndrome; in the May–Hegglin anomaly, inclusions tend to be spindle-shaped whereas in the other two syndromes they are more irregular [300]. These inclusions appear to result from abnormal localization of the non-muscle myosin IIA heavy chain in association with ribosomes [304]. At an ultrastructural level, May–Hegglin anomaly is characterized by granulocyte inclusions composed of clusters of ribosomes, segments of rough endoplasmic reticulum and parallel longitudinal filaments. The latter feature is not seen in either Sebastian's or Fechtner's syndrome [300]. A different ultrastructural feature, cross-striation of inclusions, in seen in Sebastian's syndrome [300]. Epstein's syndrome, also resulting from a mutation in the *MHY9* gene, lacks neutrophil inclusions [300]. In another rare congenital syndrome, the Upshaw–Schulman syndrome, there is episodic thrombocytopenia associated with microangiopathic haemolytic anaemia; this syndrome, which is responsive to plasma infusion, has been shown to result from a congenital deficiency of von Willebrand factor cleaving protease [305]. Red cells should be examined for anisocytosis, poikilocytosis and macrocytosis, which may be indicative of a mutation in the *GATA1* gene affecting both erythropoiesis and thrombopoiesis [254]. In babies with Down's syndrome, the blood film should be examined for features of transient abnormal myelopoiesis (see p. 421), which may cause thrombocytopenia. Rarely, in other thrombocytopenic babies, the blood film shows features of congenital leukaemia.

The platelet count is low but when a large proportion of platelets are very large the count on an automated instrument may be an underestimate of the true count. Depending on the aetiology of the thrombocytopenia, the MPV may be low, normal or high. In inherited thrombocytopenia with large platelets, the percentage of reticulated platelets is normal or slightly elevated whereas in autoimmune thrombocytopenic purpura the percentage is often considerably increased [306].

Differential diagnosis

The differential diagnosis of congenital thrombocytopenia includes all the causes of congenital thrombocytopenia listed in Tables 6.27 and 8.11–8.13.

A rare cause of thrombocytopenia that could be confused with the Bernard–Soulier syndrome is pseudo-Bernard–Soulier syndrome resulting from a drug-induced antiplatelet autoantibody [307].

Further tests

Whether further tests are needed and the choice of any further tests depends on the aetiology that is suspected on the basis of the clinical features and blood film and count. Useful tests may include study of platelet membrane antigens by immunological techniques, testing of the mother's serum for antibodies to Kell group antigens or specific antiplatelet antibodies, bone marrow examination, cytogenetic analysis (for the detection of a constitutional abnormality or a leukaemia-related clonal abnormality) and platelet function studies (e.g. showing aggregation only with ristocetin in Bernard–Soulier syndrome). Investigation of other family members may be useful. Ultrastructural examination of platelets or neutrophils is sometimes useful. If fetomaternal allo-immune thrombocytopenia is suspected the tests indicated are HPA typing on baby and mother and investigation of maternal serum for platelet allo-antibodies, most often anti-HPA-1a and less often anti-HPA-5b [308]. If Wiskott–Aldrich syndrome is suspected, assessment of immunological status is indicated. This diagnosis can also be confirmed by genetic analysis or by demonstration of absent or abnormal WAS protein [309]. Coagulation factors and von Willebrand factor multimer distribution require investigation if von Willebrand's disease or pseudo-von Willebrand's disease is suspected.

Autoimmune ('idiopathic') thrombocytopenic purpura (ITP)

Autoimmune or 'idiopathic' thrombocytopenic purpura is an acquired condition in which platelet survival is reduced by the presence of platelet-directed autoantibodies. Autoimmune thrombocytopenia can also occur as one feature of a more generalized autoimmune disease such as systemic lupus erythematosus or the rare autoimmune lymphoproliferative syndrome associated with Fas deficiency [187]. There is an increased incidence in DiGeorge's syndrome. Autoimmune thrombocytopenia is a common complication of chronic lymphocytic leukaemia and a less common complication of other lymphoproliferative disorders. Idiopathic autoimmune thrombocytopenic purpura has generally been regarded as particularly likely to occur in young women but in one population-based survey the incidence in adults was 1.6/10 000/year overall, was similar in men and women and was higher above the age of 60 years [310].

Blood film and count

The blood film shows thrombocytopenia and, unless the onset is very acute, increased platelet size (Fig. 8.81). Usually other cell lineages are normal but occasionally there is associated autoimmune haemolytic anaemia or evidence of an underlying causative condition such as CLL, lymphoma or large granular lymphocyte leukaemia.

The platelet count is reduced and, unless the onset is very acute, the MPV is increased. The percentage of reticulated platelets (see p. 54) is often considerably increased. Whether this is a useful variable for distinguishing increased platelet destruction from a failure of platelet production is not clear since conflicting results have been found in different studies [306,311].

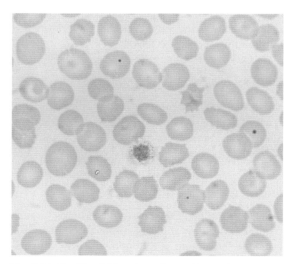

Fig. 8.81 The blood film of a patient with autoimmune thrombocytopenic purpura, post-splenectomy, showing thrombocytopenia, a single giant platelet and Howell–Jolly bodies.

Among childhood cases of ITP, less than one-fifth develop chronic disease [312]. Those with the lowest platelet counts are least likely to develop chronic ITP [312].

Differential diagnosis

The differential diagnosis includes thrombocytopenia following rubella and other viral infections, drug-induced thrombocytopenia and TTP. Cytomegalovirus infection, infectious mononucleosis and other viral infections can also present with severe thrombocytopenia as the major manifestation. Symptomatic thrombocytopenia may be the presenting feature of HIV infection. Hepatitis C infection is common in patients who would otherwise meet the diagnostic criteria for ITP, so testing for hepatitis C should be done in all patients; hepatitis C-related cases often have cryoglobulinaemia and anticardiolipin antibodies [313]. *Helicobacter pylori* infection has also been related to what would otherwise be categorized as ITP. Some cases have a rise in the platelet count in response to elimination of helicobacter, but how often this occurs is disputed.

Further tests

Before any other investigations are performed the blood film must be examined to confirm thrombocytopenia and, unless the patient has obvious petechiae or purpura, the thrombocytopenia must be confirmed on a second carefully taken blood specimen. The blood film should also be examined for spherocytes, red cell fragments, polychromasia, atypical lymphocytes, lymphoma cells and cryoglobulin deposits. Other tests that are indicated depend on the diagnosis suspected on the basis of the clinical features and the blood film examination. For example, if ITP seems the most likely diagnosis no further tests are usually required. However, in adults a bone marrow examination is considered indicated if: (i) there are atypical features; (ii) the patient is aged above 60 years; (iii) the patient has relapsed; or (iv) splenectomy is required [314]. Similarly, bone marrow aspiration is advised in children who: (i) have atypical features; (ii) relapse; or (iii) require corticosteroid therapy [314]. Tests for antinuclear antibodies and DNA binding should also be carried out since ITP may be the initial presentation of systemic lupus erythematosus. The presence of antiphospholipid antibodies also supports the diagnosis of immune-mediated thrombocytopenia. If atypical lymphocytes are detected, a Paul–Bunnell screening test for infectious mononucleosis and specific serology for Epstein–Barr virus (EBV) and cytomegalovirus may be useful and, if HIV infection appears clinically likely, a specific test for HIV infection should be considered. Serology for chronic hepatitis C infection is indicated, particularly in countries with a high prevalence of this virus [315], since this diagnosis has therapeutic implications. Investigation for *H. pylori* infection should be considered in countries with a high prevalence of this infection, e.g. Italy and Japan; however it is uncertain to what extent this is a worthwhile test since there are conflicting reports as to the likelihood of improvement following eradication of the bacterium [316,317]. The British Committee for Standards in Haematology (BCSH) recommends testing patients who relapse for *H. pylori* [314]. If red cell fragments are present, investigations relevant to TTP should be initiated as a matter of urgency.

Post-infection immune thrombocytopenic purpura

Immune thrombocytopenic purpura, in many ways resembling autoimmune thrombocytopenic purpura, can occur following various infections (e.g. rubella) or following vaccination, e.g. vaccination for rubella, influenza, measles, hepatitis B, poliomyelitis, mumps and triple vaccine for diphtheria, polio and tetanus (DPT) [318]. Post-infection thrombocytopenia is particularly common in children.

Thrombotic thrombocytopenic purpura (TTP)

TTP is a systemic disorder, usually of unknown cause, in which microthrombi in multiple organs lead to platelet consumption and renal and cerebral manifestations. The thrombocytopenia may lead to haemorrhage. A minority of cases follow identifiable infections such as *Escherichia coli* O157 : H7 [319] or Legionnaires' disease. TTP can occur during the course of HIV infection and can relapse following interruption of effective antiretroviral therapy [320].

Ticlopidine [321] and clopidogrel therapy can cause TTP and occasional cases have been linked to abuse of cocaine or Ecstasy [322] or to interferon therapy in chronic granulocytic leukaemia [323].

The incidence has been estimated at 1/1 000 000/ year [234]. The classic pentad of disease features is thrombocytopenia, microangiopathic haemolytic anaemia, renal impairment, neurological abnormalities and fever. However, since urgent treatment by plasma exchange is required it is recommended that a provisional diagnosis be made and treatment be started if a patient has thrombocytopenia and micro-angiopathic haemolytic anaemia for which there is no other apparent explanation [204].

Blood film and count

The blood film shows the features of a microangiopathic haemolytic anaemia (fragments and polychromasia) together with thrombocytopenia with platelet anisocytosis. Fragments comprising more than 1% of red cells have been found to be strongly suggestive of TTP [324]. However, red cell fragments may initially be quite infrequent [234] and if there is a strong clinical suspicion of this diagnosis blood films should be kept under very regular review. The RDW, MPV and PDW may be increased. The percentage of reticulated platelets is likely to be increased. Once treatment has commenced, the platelet count is the most important laboratory test for monitoring progress [204].

Differential diagnosis

The differential diagnosis includes other causes of red cell fragmentation, particularly those that can also cause thrombocytopenia. The possibility of familial TTP should be remembered.

Further tests

The LDH is often greatly elevated. A biopsy confirmation of capillary thrombi confirms the diagnosis but, since treatment is required urgently, a provisional diagnosis should be made on the basis of clinical and haematological features and treatment should be initiated. TTP is usually the result of an autoantibody to von Willebrand factor-cleaving protease, which is therefore the definitive test for this condition. HIV testing is important since TTP may be the initial presentation of HIV infection and patients require antiretroviral therapy in addition to plasma exchange.

Thrombocytosis

Familial thrombocytosis

Familial thrombocytosis is a rare condition with an autosomal dominant inheritance. It can result from a mutation in the promoter of *TPO,* the gene that encodes thrombopoietin, the mutation leading to an aberrantly stable messenger RNA. In another family it resulted from a dominant activating mutation in the *MPL* gene that encodes the thrombopoietin receptor [325].

Blood film and count

The platelet count is increased. Platelet size is normal and cells of other lineages are normal.

Differential diagnosis

The differential diagnosis is reactive thrombocytosis and essential thrombocythaemia. Familial thrombocytosis should be suspected and family studies should be performed when unexplained thrombocytosis is detected in a child or young adult.

Further tests

Genetic analysis is indicated, if available.

Essential thrombocythaemia

Essential thrombocythaemia is a myeloproliferative disorder characterized by increased platelet production. In the WHO classification it is defined as a Ph-negative, *BCR-ABL* negative condition. Essential thrombocythaemia is predominantly a disease of the middle-aged and elderly population but cases also occur in young adults and even in children. Clinical features are either caused directly by the thrombocytosis or reflect the abnormal proliferation of myeloid cells. They include microvascular obstruction, bleeding and, less often, splenomegaly and itch. However, the majority of patients are now diagnosed at a presymptomatic stage as a result of the increasing performance of blood counts for a variety of reasons. Since automated counters now generally in use include a platelet count in the FBC the incidental detection of thrombocytosis is not infrequent.

Essential thrombocythaemia terminates, uncommonly, in myelofibrosis and, rarely, in AML.

Blood film and count

Conventionally, the diagnosis is not usually made unless the platelet count is at least $600 \times 10^9/l$ and in many cases it is in excess of $1000 \times 10^9/l$. The blood film shows increased platelet anisocytosis and usually a large number of giant platelets (Fig. 8.82). Some of the platelets may be hypogranular. Neutrophilia is present in about one-third of patients. The basophil count is often elevated but does not usually exceed 3%. A basophil count of more than 5% suggests that the patient may be Philadelphia-positive. Occasional NRBC and immature granulocytes may be present. There may be features of iron deficiency as a consequence of bleeding. Rarely, there are features of hyposplenism following earlier splenic infarction.

The platelet count, MPV and PDW are elevated whereas in reactive thrombocytosis the MPV and PDW are not usually increased. Splenectomy or hyposplenism can, however, cause thrombocytosis with an increased MPV and PDW.

Differential diagnosis

The differential diagnosis includes many of the other causes of thrombocytosis (see Table 6.15), particularly those conditions that can cause reactive thrombocytosis without clear clinical features suggesting the underlying disease, e.g. occult neoplasms and connective tissue disorders. In iron deficient patients, uncomplicated iron deficiency should be included in the differential diagnosis since iron deficiency alone can cause a platelet count of $600 \times 10^9/l$ or even higher. Patients with iron deficiency may also have an occult neoplasm, occult haemorrhage or both as a cause of thrombocytosis. It can also be difficult or impossible to distinguish iron deficient PRV from

Fig. 8.82 The blood film of a patient with essential thrombocythaemia showing thrombocytosis with platelet anisocytosis and giant platelets. There is also red cell anisocytosis and poikilocytosis.

essential thrombocythaemia with iron deficiency but this distinction is not clinically important since satisfactory treatment does not require that the two conditions be distinguished.

Further tests

A bone marrow aspirate and trephine biopsy may provide evidence of a myeloproliferative disorder. Megakaryocytes are increased in number, large, well lobulated and clustered. It should be noted that iron deficiency alone can cause thrombocytosis, marked erythroid hyperplasia and quite a marked increase in megakaryocytes so that the diagnosis of essential thrombocythaemia should be made with caution in iron deficient patients. If histological features are not clear cut, a trial of iron therapy may be necessary to make the distinction. The NAP score is low in a minority of patients, elevated in some and normal in the majority; it is not useful in differentiating Philadelphia-positive and Philadelphia-negative cases. Cytogenetic analysis is indicated at least whenever it is not clear that the patient has a myeloproliferative disorder and if there are atypical disease characteristics—such as myelodysplastic features, blast cells or a markedly elevated basophil count—which suggest either Philadelphia-positivity or another unfavourable karyotype that would influence management. However, with the availability of imatinib, it is now reasonable to undertake cytogenetic or molecular genetic analysis (for the *BCR-ABL*

fusion gene) on all patients in order to identify any Ph-positive patients, who are likely to respond to this drug. Molecular analysis shows a *JAK2* mutation in a substantial proportion of patients, but this finding is less frequent than in polycythaemia vera. A low serum erythropoietin is seen in as many as one-third of patients so does not help to distinguish essential thrombocythaemia from masked polycythaemia rubra vera [264]. Plasma thrombopoietin may be normal or decreased but not elevated. Detection of splenomegaly on ultrasonography supports a diagnosis of essential thrombocythaemia and makes reactive thrombocytosis very unlikely [326]. Various laboratory tests, such as an elevated plasma fibrinogen, elevated C-reactive protein or an elevated ESR, can provide indirect evidence of an occult neoplasm or connective tissue disorder and thus support a diagnosis of reactive thrombocytosis rather than essential thrombocythaemia.

Ph-positive essential thrombocythaemia

Ph-positive essential thrombocythaemia is a rare myeloproliferative disorder in which there is thrombocytosis without the peripheral blood features of chronic myeloid leukaemia but with a Ph chromosome or a *BCR-ABL* fusion gene. In comparison with other cases of essential thrombocythaemia, there is an increased probability of development of myelodysplastic syndrome, myelofibrosis and blastic transformation. Ph-positive essential thrombocythaemia can transform into acute phase disease before there is any elevation of the white cell count. Because the condition is responsive to imatinib, making the distinction from Ph-negative essential thrombocythaemia is important.

Blood film and count

The blood film and count shows thrombocytosis without any significant increase of the total white cell count. There may be large platelets. Basophils may be increased.

Differential diagnosis

The differential diagnosis includes other causes of thrombocytosis, particularly Ph-negative essential thrombocythaemia.

Further tests

A bone marrow aspirate and trephine biopsy shows hypolobated rather small megakaryocytes, in contrast to the large clustered megakaryocytes of Ph-negative essential thrombocythemia, Cytogenetic or molecular genetic analysis is essential for the diagnosis.

Test your knowledge

Multiple choice questions (MCQs)

(1–5 answers may be correct)

MCQ 8.1 In anaemia secondary to chronic inflammatory disease
(a) Serum erythropoietin concentration is not elevated appropriately to the degree of anaemia
(b) Erythroid precursors are relatively resistant to the action of erythropoietin
(c) Serum ferritin is normal or elevated
(d) Serum iron may be markedly reduced despite normal bone marrow iron stores
(e) Serum iron-binding capacity is increased

MCQ 8.2 In relation to haemoglobin S (sickle cell haemoglobin)
(a) Paraproteins can cause a false-positive sickle solubility test
(b) In homozygosity for haemoglobin S there is 10–15% of haemoglobin A

(c) Haemoglobins D and G have the same mobility as haemoglobin S on cellulose acetate electrophoresis at alkaline pH
(d) A sickle solubility test is a reliable method for neonatal screening for sickle cell anaemia
(e) The presence of 95% of haemoglobin S with small amounts of haemoglobins F and A_2 is compatible with either sickle cell anaemia (homozygosity for haemoglobin S) or compound heterozygosity for haemoglobin S and β^0 thalassaemia

MCQ 8.3 An elevated haemoglobin concentration together with an elevated serum erythropoietin concentration is expected in
(a) Cyanotic congenital heart disease
(b) Pseudo or relative or 'stress' polycythaemia
(c) Renal artery stenosis
(d) Renal cell carcinoma
(e) Polycythaemia rubra vera

MCQ 8.4 Infection by parvovirus B19 may cause symptomatic anaemia or aggravation of pre-existing anaemia in patients
(a) With sickle cell anaemia
(b) With hereditary spherocytosis
(c) With polycythaemia rubra vera
(d) With acquired immune deficiency syndrome (AIDS)
(e) Having immunosuppressive therapy following renal transplantation

MCQ 8.5 An increased cold agglutinin titre is a recognized feature of
(a) Non-Hodgkin's lymphoma
(b) Paroxysmal nocturnal haemoglobinuria
(c) *Mycoplasma pneumoniae* infection
(d) Alpha-methyl dopa-induced haemolytic anaemia
(e) Infectious mononucleosis

MCQ 8.6 *Escherichia coli* O157 infection is a recognized cause of
(a) Crohn's disease
(b) Haemorrhagic colitis
(c) Haemolytic uraemic syndrome
(d) Tropical sprue
(e) A minority of cases of thrombotic thrombocytopenic purpura

MCQ 8.7 Glucose-6-phosphate dehydrogenase (G6PD) deficiency
(a) Occurs in Africans and Afro-Caribbeans
(b) May lead to haemolysis following dapsone therapy
(c) Causes clinical problems only in homozygotes
(d) Is not excluded by a normal G6PD assay during an acute haemolytic crisis
(e) Can result in haemosiderinuria

MCQ 8.8 A positive direct antiglobulin (Coombs') test is characteristic of
(a) Hereditary spherocytosis
(b) Hereditary elliptocytosis
(c) Haemolytic disease of the newborn
(d) Delayed haemolytic transfusion reaction
(e) Warm autoimmune haemolytic anaemia

MCQ 8.9 Thrombocytopenia with increased platelet size is characteristic of
(a) Essential thrombocythaemia
(b) Wiskott–Aldrich syndrome
(c) Bernard–Soulier syndrome
(d) May–Hegglin anomaly
(e) Grey platelet syndrome

MCQ 8.10 Glucose-6-phosphate dehydrogenase (G6PD) deficiency can cause
(a) Neonatal jaundice
(b) Chronic non-spherocytic haemolytic anaemia
(c) Aplastic anaemia
(d) Jaundice following ingestion of red kidney beans
(e) Heinz body haemolytic anaemia

Extended matching questions (EMQs)

Select the most accurate option for each of the stems. Each option may be used once, more than once or not at all. There is only one correct answer.

EMQ 8.1
Theme: anaemia and/or microcytosis
Options
A Iron deficiency anaemia
B Iron-deficient polycythaemia
C Iron deficiency resulting from coeliac disease
D Anaemia of chronic disease
E Congenital sideroblastic anaemia
F Acquired sideroblastic anaemia
G Lead poisoning
H β thalassaemia major
I β thalassaemia intermedia
J β thalassaemia trait
K $\delta\beta$ thalassaemia trait
L $\gamma\delta\beta$ thalassaemia trait
M Hereditary persistence of fetal haemoglobin
N α^+ thalassaemia trait
O α^0 thalassaemia trait
P Haemoglobin H disease

For each clinical history select the option that provides the most likely diagnosis—the diagnosis should be as precise as possible.

1 A 10-year-old Greek child is found to have a palpable spleen. Laboratory investigations show:
RBC 5.84×10^{12}/l
Hb 9.8 g/dl
Hct 0.36
MCV 62 fl
MCH 16.7 pg
MCHC 27.5 g/dl
Reticulocyte count 3.5%
Haemoglobins A, A_2, F and H detected—haemoglobin F 1.8%, haemoglobin H 5%
Answer:

2 A laboratory receives a request for a blood count on a 75-year-old northern European man on whom no clinical details are provided. The results of the FBC are:
WBC 25×10^9/l (neutrophils and basophils increased)
RBC 7.77×10^{12}/l
Hb 15.8 g/dl
Hct 0.518
MCV 67 fl
MCH 20.4 pg
MCHC 30.5 g/dl
RDW 18.7
Platelet count 512×10^9/l
Blood film: hypochromia, microcytosis, giant platelets
Answer:

3 A 50-year-old Indian woman had been unwell for 9 months. She had first experienced orthopnoea followed by loss of appetite, constant nausea and occasional vomiting. For the preceding 2 months she had suffered constant abdominal pain with inter-mittent superimposed colicky pain. For a few weeks she had noted ankle swelling and weakness of her arms and legs. Results of FBC were:
WBC 9.9×10^9/l
RBC 2.99×10^{12}/l
Hb 8.3 g/dl
Hct 0.25 l/l
MCV 84.8 fl
MCH 27.8 pg
MCHC 32.7 g/dl
Reticulocyte count 9.4% (281×10^9/l)
Blood film: polychromasia, stomatocytes, basophilic stippling, occasional NRBC
Bilirubin concentration was 32 µmol/l (normal range 3–20)
Answer:

4 A 45-year-old woman has recently suffered an exacerbation of her rheumatoid arthritis. At various times she has taken aspirin, non-steroidal anti-inflammatory drugs and corticosteroids. Results of laboratory investigations are:
WBC 12×10^9/l
Hb 8.5 g/dl
MCV 70 fl
Platelet count 450×10^9/l
Serum ferritin 103 µmol/l (normal range 15–200)
Serum iron 5 µmol/l (normal range 9–16)
Serum transferrin 20 µmol/l (normal range 23–38)
Erythrocyte sedimentation rate 53 mm/hr (normal range 1–20)
Answer:

5 A 35-year-old Irish woman presents with fatigue and a vague history of intermittent diarrhoea. Results of laboratory investigations are:
RBC 4.22×10^{12}/l
Hb 7 g/dl
Hct 0.39
MCV 67 fl
MCH 16.6 pg
MCHC 24.5 g/dl

Platelet count 450×10^9/l
Anti-endomysial antibodies: positive
Anti-gliadin antibodies: positive
Answer:

EMQ 8.2
Theme: thrombocytopenia
Options
A Idiopathic (autoimmune) thrombocytopenic purpura
B Immune thrombocytopenic purpura as a feature of systemic lupus erythematosus
C Alloimmune thrombocytopenia
D Haemolytic uraemic syndrome
E Thrombotic thrombocytopenic purpura
F Disseminated intravascular coagulation
G Factitious thrombocytopenia
H Bernard–Soulier syndrome
I Wiskott–Aldrich syndrome
J Fanconi's anaemia
K Heparin-induced thrombocytopenia
L Thrombocytopenia with absent radii

For each clinical history select the option that provides the most likely diagnosis—the diagnosis should be as precise as possible.

1 A 35-year-old HIV-positive man who has been poorly compliant with antiretroviral therapy presents with fever, mental confusion, jaundice and bruising. FBC shows:
WBC 10.2×10^9/l
Neutrophil count 9.0×10^9/l
Lymphocyte count 0.6×10^9/l
Hb 6.8 g/dl
MCV 106 fl
Platelet count 62×10^9/l
Reticulocyte count 250×10^9/l
Blood film: numerous fragments including micro-spherocytes, polychromatic macrocytes, thrombo-cytopenia, giant platelets
A coagulation screen shows only minor abnormalities
Serum creatinine is elevated to 150 µmol/l
Answer:

2 A 35-year old woman presents with the recent onset of bruising. For the preceding 3 months she

had noted a rash over her nose and both cheeks and had suffered from swelling and discomfort in various joints. She had been taking paracetamol but was on no other medications. A dipstick test done in the Accident and Emergency department was strongly positive for urinary protein. Laboratory tests show:
WBC $2.7 \times 10^9/l$
Neutrophil count $1.5 \times 10^9/l$
Lymphocyte count $1.0 \times 10^9/l$
Hb 12.5 g/dl
MCV 85 fl
Platelet count $10 \times 10^9/l$
Blood film: severe thrombocytopenia with occasional large platelets
Serum creatinine is elevated to 140 µmol/l
Antinuclear factor antibodies: positive
Answer:

3 A pregnant woman presents already in labour and shortly afterwards a full-term baby is delivered. Although the delivery was uneventful the baby shows severe bruising. He is afebrile and appears otherwise healthy. His blood count shows severe thrombocytopenia but no other abnormality. The blood film confirms severe thrombocytopenia with normal sized platelets and likewise shows no other abnormality. A coagulation screen is normal.

His mother has no history of thrombocytopenia and her platelet count is normal. This is her second pregnancy. She tells the obstetric staff that her first baby died *in utero* of an intracerebral haemorrhage and her second baby had Down's syndrome.
Answer:

4 A 65-year-old man suffers a myocardial infarction and is given an injection of abciximab, a monoclonal antibody directed at a platelet glycoprotein. Several hours later a routine blood count shows mild neutrophilia and a severely reduced platelet count. A blood film shows numerous large platelet aggregates.
Answer:

5 A 10-year-old boy presents with developmental delay. He is below the third percentile for height, his head appears smaller than normal and he has abnormal fingers and thumbs. His elder brother is said to also be short and to suffer from anaemia. His younger sister, mother and father are healthy. FBC shows:

WBC $7.0 \times 10^9/l$
Neutrophil count $1.3 \times 10^9/l$
Lymphocyte count $5.2 \times 10^9/l$
Hb 11.0 g/dl
MCV 98 fl
Platelet count $60 \times 10^9/l$
Answer:

EMQ 8.3
Theme: anaemia and macrocytosis
Options
A Vitamin B_{12} deficiency
B Pernicious anaemia
C Folic acid deficiency
D Folic acid deficiency resulting from coeliac disease
E Folic acid deficiency resulting from tropical sprue
F Myelodysplastic syndrome
G Refractory anaemia
H Refractory anaemia with ring sideroblasts
I Effects of excess alcohol
J Drug-induced macrocytosis
K Congenital dyserythropoietic anaemia
L Aplastic anaemia
M Fanconi's anaemia
N Chronic haemolytic anaemia

For each clinical history select the option which gives the most probable diagnosis—the diagnosis should be as precise as possible.

1 A 68-year-old English woman presents to her GP with a history of tiredness, lethargy, breathlessness and ankle swelling at the end of the day. On specific questioning she also complains of a sore tongue, numbness in her feet and tingling in her toes. She drinks 1–2 pints of beer a week and smokes 15 cigarettes a day. She has a good diet. She is found to be pale with slight jaundice and neurological examination shows reduced light touch, pain and proprioception in the feet. Tendon reflexes are reduced.
FBC shows:
WBC $3.1 \times 10^9/l$
Hb 5.8 g/dl
MCV 129 fl
RDW 17.2
Platelet count $129 \times 10^9/l$
Neutrophil count $1.7 \times 10^9/l$
Lymphocyte count $1.2 \times 10^9/l$

Blood film: anisocytosis ++, poikilocytosis +++, macrocytes, oval macrocytes, teardrop poikilocytes, occasional fragments, hypersegmented neutrophils
Answer:

2 A 30-year-old English woman presents with a history of weight loss and lethargy. She gives the history that, having been a blood donor for 5 years, the previous year she had been rejected as a donor because of anaemia and had been given a course of iron tablets. She does not smoke or drink, takes alcohol only rarely and has a good diet. She is on no medications. Laboratory investigations show:
WBC $5.2 \times 10^9/l$
RBC $2.67 \times 10^{12}/l$
Hb 9 g/dl
MCV 105 fl
MCH 33.7 pg
MCHC 32 g/dl
RDW 15.2
Platelet count $170 \times 10^9/l$
Serum ferritin 22 μmol/l (normal range 15–300)
Serum vitamin B_{12} 180 ng/l (normal range 212–1081)
Red cell folate 56 μg/l (normal range 146–528)
Antiendomysial antibodies: positive
Anti-gliadin antibodies: positive
Answer:

3 The laboratory received a blood sample from a 67-year-old man with a history of polycythaemia rubra vera. Initially he had been treated by venesection but his platelet count was persistently elevated so for the previous 5 months he had been receiving regular hydroxycarbamide (hydroxyurea). FBC was:
WBC $3.5 \times 10^9/l$
RBC $3.42 \times 10^{12}/l$
Hb 12.6 g/dl
MCV 115 fl
MCH 36.8 pg
MCHC 32 g/dl
Platelet count $520 \times 10^9/l$
Blood film: macrocytosis with some stomatocytes, platelet anisocytosis
Answer:

4 A 25-year-old Arab male whose parents are first cousins has splenomegaly and the following laboratory results:

WBC $7.8 \times 10^9/l$
RBC $3.10 \times 10^{12}/l$
Hb 9.8 g/dl
Hct 0.32
MCV 105 fl
MCH 31.9 pg
MCHC 30.6
RDW 27
Reticulocyte count 3%
Platelet count $370 \times 10^9/l$
Blood film: anisocytosis +++, poikilocytosis +++, macrocytes (some very large and some oval macrocytes), microcytes, fragments, irregularly contracted cells
Answer:

5 A 50-year-old northern European Caucasian presents with dysphagia and is found to have adenocarcinoma of the proximal stomach extending into the oesophagus. Laboratory tests show:
WBC $9.1 \times 10^9/l$
RBC $4.10 \times 10^{12}/l$
Hb 14.1 g/dl
Hct 0.427
MCV 104 fl
MCH 34.3 pg
MCHC 33.1 g/dl
RDW 14.2
Platelet count $269 \times 10^9/l$
Serum ferritin 250 μmol/l (normal range 15–300)
Serum vitamin B_{12} 145 ng/l (normal range 212–1081)
Red cell folate 223 μg/l (normal range 146–528)
Answer:

EMQ 8.4
Theme: disorders of globin chain synthesis
Options
A Sickle cell trait
B Sickle cell trait plus alpha thalassaemia trait
C Sickle cell anaemia (homozygosity for haemoglobin S)
D Sickle cell/β^0 thalassaemia compound heterozygosity
E Sickle cell/β^+ thalassaemia compound heterozygosity
F Sickle cell/haemoglobin C compound heterozygosity
G δβ thalassaemia trait

H β thalassaemia trait
I β thalassaemia major
J α thalassaemia trait
K Haemoglobin H disease
L Haemoglobin E heterozygosity
M Haemoglobin E homozygosity
N Hereditary persistence of fetal haemoglobin

For each patient choose the option that indicates the most likely diagnosis. Be as precise as possible.

1 An asymptomatic 18-year-old West African woman has the following laboratory results:
RBC $4.41 \times 10^{12}/l$
Hb 11.7 g/dl
Hct 0.36
MCV 83 fl
MCH 26.5 pg
MCHC 32.5 g/dl
Blood film: borderline hypochromia
Serum ferritin: normal
Haemoglobin electrophoresis: haemoglobin A 67%, haemoglobin S 30%
Answer:

2 A 34-year-old Burmese woman has the following laboratory results:
RBC $4.39 \times 10^{12}/l$
Hb 11 g/dl
Hct 0.32
MCV 74 fl
MCH 25.1 pg
MCHC 33.2 g/dl
Blood film: hypochromia, microcytosis, occasional target cells, occasional irregularly contracted cells
Serum ferritin: normal
Haemoglobin electrophoresis: haemoglobin A (64%) and an abnormal band (33%). The abnormal band has the mobility of $C/E/A_2$ on cellulose acetate at alkaline pH and the mobility of A on citrate agar at acid pH
Answer:

3 An 18-year-old Afro-Caribbean man who suffers from intermittent limb and chest pains has the following laboratory results:
RBC $3.68 \times 10^{12}/l$
Hb 7.0 g/dl

Hct 0.23
MCV 62 fl
MCH 19 pg
MCHC 30.4 g/dl
Blood film: hypochromia, microcytosis, sickle cells, boat-shaped cells, target cells, Howell–Jolly bodies, NRBC
Sickle solubility test: positive
High performance liquid chromatography: haemoglobin S 83%, haemoglobin A 7%, haemoglobin F 5%, haemoglobin A_2 5%
Answer:

4 A 23-year-old asymptomatic Spanish woman has the following laboratory results:
RBC $5.78 \times 10^{12}/l$
Hb 10.5 g/dl
Hct 0.32
MCV 56 fl
MCH 18.2 pg
MCHC 32.3 g/dl
Blood film: poikilocytosis, target cells, basophilic stippling
Haemoglobin electrophoresis: haemoglobin A 93%, haemoglobin A_2 7.3%
Answer:

5 A 33-year-old pregnant African woman has a normal full blood count and blood film. Haemoglobin electrophoresis done as part of an antenatal screening programme shows 69% haemoglobin A, 29% haemoglobin F and 1.8% haemoglobin A_2.
Answer:

EMQ 8.5
Theme: haemolytic anaemia
Options
A Hereditary spherocytosis
B Autoimmune haemolytic anaemia
C Paroxysmal nocturnal haemoglobinuria
D Paroxysmal cold haemoglobinuria
E Chronic cold haemagglutinin disease
F Oxidant-induced haemolysis
G Pyruvate kinase deficiency
H Microangiopathic haemolytic anaemia
I Haemolytic uraemic syndrome
J Thrombotic thrombocytopenic purpura
K March haemoglobinuria

L Sickle cell anaemia
M Sickle cell/haemoglobin C compound hetero-zygosity
N Haemoglobin C disease
O Haemoglobin H disease
P Glucose-6-phosphate dehydrogenase (G6PD) deficiency

For each clinical history select the option that gives the most likely diagnosis.

1 A 3-year-old child presented with fever and red urine that tested positively for blood. The FBC was:
WBC $17.0 \times 10^9/l$
RBC $3.42 \times 10^{12}/l$
Hb 7.5 g/dl (falling within days to 3.7 g/dl)
Hct 0.23
MCV 68 fl
MCH 22 pg
MCHC 32.4 g/dl
Platelet count $223 \times 10^9/l$
Blood film: neutrophilia, spherocytes, red cell agglutinates, erythrophagocytosis
Direct antiglobulin test positive: ++++ with poly-specific antisera; ++++ with anti-IgG antisera; ++++ with anti-C3d
Donath–Landsteiner test: positive
Serum ferritin: normal (the microcytosis remained unexplained)
Answer:

2 A 57-year-old builder had to give up work because of cold intolerance. If he worked outdoors he developed blueness and pain of his fingers, toes, nose and ears. He was jaundiced with no lym-phadenopathy, hepatomegaly or splenomegaly. Laboratory tests showed Hb 10.4 g/dl with MCV of 121 fl when measured on a Coulter counter and 94 fl when measured on a Bayer H.2 counter. Blood film showed very large red cell agglutinates and occa-sional plasmacytoid lymphocytes. Direct antiglobu-lin test was ++++ with polyspecific antisera, ++++ with anti-C3d and negative with anti-IgG. The bilirubin, LDH and transaminases were elevated. Immunophenotyping of peripheral blood lympho-cytes showed a monoclonal B-cell population, which was positive for CD23, CD79b and FMC7 and

showed moderately strong expression of λ (lambda) light chain.
Answer:

3 A 10-year-old girl is taken to her GP because her parents noted her to be jaundiced. She is otherwise well. Her father reports that he has been told that he also was intermittently jaundice during childhood. Results of laboratory investigations are:
WBC $5.9 \times 10^9/l$
RBC $4.07 \times 10^{12}/l$
Hb 10.5 g/dl
Hct 0.315
MCV 77.4 fl
MCH 25.7 pg
MCHC 33.2 g/dl
Blood film: spherocytes +++, polychromasia +
Direct antiglobulin: negative
Answer:

4 A 60-year-old Afro-Caribbean man is admitted for cholecystectomy and at surgery is found to have pigment gallstones. FBC shows:
WBC $4.9 \times 10^9/l$
RBC $4.59 \times 10^{12}/l$
Hb 13.5 g/dl
Hct 0.412
MCV 89.6 fl
MCH 29.4 pg
MCHC 32.8 g/dl
Platelet count $173 \times 10^9/l$
Blood film: irregularly contracted cells ++, target cells ++, polychromasia
Sickle solubility test: negative
Answer:

5 A 50-year-old Indian man is referred for assess-ment of chronic anaemia. He reports some episodes of passing red urine. Laboratory investigations show:
WBC $3.5 \times 10^9/l$
Hb 9.8 g/dl
MCV 104 fl
Platelet count $110 \times 10^9/l$
Reticulocyte count $180 \times 10^9/l$
Haemoglobin electrophoresis: normal
Serum haptoglobin: absent
Ham test: positive
Answer:

References

1 Jolobe OMP (2000) Prevalence of hypochromia (without microcytosis) vs microcytosis (without hypochromia) in iron deficiency. *Clin Lab Haematol*, **22**, 79–80.

2 Patton WN, Cave RJ and Harris RI (1991) A study of changes in red cell volume and haemoglobin concentration during phlebotomy induced iron deficiency and iron repletion using the Technicon H1. *Clin Lab Haematol*, **13**, 153–161.

3 Bessman JD, Gilmer PR and Gardner FH (1983) Improved classification of the anemias by MCV and RDW. *Am J Clin Pathol*, **80**, 322–326.

4 Schleper B and Stuerenburg HJ (2001) Copper deficiency-associated myelopathy in a 46-year-old woman. *J Neurol*, **248**, 705–706.

5 Intragumtornchai T, Rojnukkarin P, Swasdikul D and Israsena S (1998) The role of serum ferritin in the diagnosis of iron deficiency anemia in patients with liver cirrhosis. *J Intern Med*, **243**, 233–241.

6 Guyatt GH, Oxman AD, Ali M, Willan A, Mcilroy W and Patterson C (1992) Laboratory diagnosis of iron-deficiency anemia: an overview. *J Gen Intern Med*, **7**, 145–153.

7 Punnonen K, Irjala K and Rajamaki A (1997) Serum transferrin receptor and its ratio to serum ferritin in the diagnosis of iron deficiency. *Blood*, **89**, 1052–1057.

8 Cermak J and Brabec V (1998) Transferrin receptor-ferritin index: a useful parameter in differential diagnosis of iron deficiency and hyperplastic erythropoiesis. *Eur J Haematol*, **61**, 210–212.

9 Cook JD, Flowers CH and Skikne BS (2003) The quantitative assessment of body iron. *Blood*, **101**, 3359–3364.

10 Witte DL, Kraemer DF, Johnson GF, Dick FR and Hamilton H (1986) Prediction of bone marrow iron findings from tests performed on peripheral blood. *Am J Clin Pathol*, **85**, 202–206.

11 Howard MR, Morley P, Turnbull AJ, Hollier P, Webb R, Wilkinson H and Clarke A (2000) A prospective study of screening for coeliac disease in laboratory defined iron and folate deficiency. *Hematol J*, **1**, Suppl. 1, 41.

12 Weiss G and Goodnough LT (2005) Anemia of chronic disease. *N Engl J Med*, **353**, 1011–1023.

13 Marsh WL, Bishop JW and Darcy TP (1987) Evaluation of red cell volume distribution width (RDW). *Hematol Pathol*, **1**, 117–123.

14 Cazzola M, May A, Bergamaschi G, Cerani P, Rosti V and Bishop DF (2000) Familial-skewed X-chromosome inactivation as a predisposing factor for late-onset X-linked sideroblastic anemia in carrier females. *Blood*, **96**, 4363–4365.

15 Pagon RA, Bird TD, Detter JC and Pierce I (1985) Hereditary sideroblastic anaemia and ataxia: an X linked recessive disorder. *J Med Genet*, **22**, 267–273.

16 Maguire A, Hellier K, Hammans S and May A (2001) X-linked cerebellar ataxia and sideroblastic anaemia associated with a missense mutation in the *ABC7* gene predicting V411L. *Br J Haematol*, **315**, 910–917.

17 Sieff CA, Nisbet-Brown E and Nathan DG (2000) Congenital bone marrow failure syndromes. *Br J Haematol*, **111**, 30–37.

18 Borgna-Pignatti C, Marradi P, Pinelli L, Monetti N and Patrini C (1989) Thiamine-responsive anemia in DIDMOAD syndrome. *J Pediatr*, **114**, 405–410.

19 Vives i Corrons LJ-L (2000) Chronic non-spherocytic haemolytic anaemia due to congenital pyrimidine 5' nucleotidase deficiency: 25 years later. *Bailière's Clin Haematol*, **13**, 103–118.

20 Mazza U, Saglio G, Cappio FC, Camaschella C, Neretto G and Gallo E (1976) Clinical and haematological data in 254 cases of beta-thalassaemia trait in Italy. *Br J Haematol*, **33**, 91–99.

21 d'Onofrio G, Zini G, Ricerca BM, Mancini S and Mango G (1992) Automated measurement of red blood cell microcytosis and hypochromia in iron deficiency and β-thalassaemia trait. *Arch Pathol Lab Med*, **116**, 84–89.

22 Weatherall DJ and Clegg JB. *The Thalassaemia Syndromes*. Blackwell Scientific Publications, Oxford, 1981.

23 Mentzer WC (1973) Differentiation of iron deficiency from thalassaemia trait. *Lancet*, **i**, 882.

24 England JM and Fraser PM (1973) Differentiation of iron deficiency from thalassaemia trait by routine blood count. *Lancet*, **i**, 449–452.

25 England JM, Bain BJ and Fraser PM (1973) Differentiation of iron deficiency from thalassaemia trait. *Lancet*, **i**, 1514.

26 Srivastava PC (1973) Differentiation of thalassaemia minor from iron deficiency. *Lancet*, **ii**, 154–155.

27 Shine I and Lal S (1977) A strategy to detect β thalassaemia trait. *Lancet*, **I**, 692–694.

28 Green R and King R (1989) A new red cell discriminant incorporating volume dispersion for

differentiating iron deficiency anemia from thalassemia minor. *Blood Cells*, **15**, 481–495.

29 Jiminez CV, Minchinela J and Ros J (1995) New indices from H*2 analyzer improve differentiation between heterozygous β and δβ thalassaemia. *Clin Lab Haematol*, **17**, 151–155.

30 Bain BJ, *Haemoglobinopathy Diagnosis*, 2nd Edn. Blackwell Publishing, Oxford, 2006.

31 Bain BJ (1988) Screening of antenatal patients in a multiethnic community for β-thalassaemia trait. *J Clin Pathol*, **41**, 481–485.

32 Polliack A and Rachmilewitz EA (1983) Ultrastructural studies in β-thalassaemia major. *Br J Haematol*, **24**, 319–326.

33 Dozy AM, Kan YW, Embury SH, Mentzer WC, Wang WC, Lubin B *et al.* (1979) α-globin gene organization in blacks precludes the severe form of α-thalassaemia. *Nature*, **280**, 605–607.

34 Serjeant GR, Serjeant BE, Forbes M, Hages RJ, Higgs DR and Lehmann H (1986) Haemoglobin gene frequencies in the Jamaican population: a study of 100 000 newborns. *Br J Haematol*, **64**, 253–262.

35 Falusi AG, Esan GJF, Ayyub H and Higgs DR (1987) Alpha-thalassaemia in Nigeria: its interaction with sickle-cell disease. *Eur J Haematol*, **38**, 370–375.

36 Tzotzos S, Kavavakis E, Metaxotou-Mavromati A and Kattamis C (1986) The molecular basis of haemoglobin H disease in Greece. *Br J Haematol*, **63**, 263–271.

37 Serjeant GR. *The Clinical Features of Sickle Cell Disease*. North Holland Publishing Company, Amsterdam, 1974.

38 Wong W-Y, Zhou Y, Operskalski EA, Hassett J, Powars DR, Mosley JW, and the Transfusion Safety Study Group (1996) Hematologic profile and lymphocyte subpopulations in hemoglobin SC disease: comparison with hemoglobin SS and black controls. *Am J Hematol*, **52**, 150–154.

39 Davis LR (1976) Changing blood picture in sickle cell anaemia from shortly after birth to adolescence. *J Clin Pathol*, **29**, 898–901.

40 Serjeant GR, Grandison Y, Lowrie Y, Mason K, Phillips J, Serjeant BE and Vaidya S (1981) The development of haematological changes in homozygous sickle cell disease: a cohort study from birth to 6 years. *Br J Haematol*, **48**, 533–543.

41 Glader BE, Propper RD and Buchanan GR (1979) Microcytosis associated with sickle cell anemia. *Am J Clin Pathol*, **72**, 63–64.

42 Mohandas N, Kim YR, Tycko DH, Orlik J, Wyatt J and Groner W (1986) Accurate and independent measurement of volume and hemoglobin concentration of individual red cells by laser light scattering. *Blood*, **68**, 506–513.

43 Ballard SK and Smith ED (1992) Red blood cell changes during the evolution of the sickle cell painful crisis. *Blood*, **79**, 2154–2163.

44 Monplaisir N, Merault G, Poyart C, Rhoda MD, Craescu CT, Vidaud M *et al.* (1987) Hb-S-Antilles ($\alpha_2\beta_2$Glu Val, 23Va1 Ile): a new variant with lower solubility than Hb S and producing sickle cell disease in heterozygotes. *Acta Haematol*, **78**, 222.

45 Wilson CI, Hopkins PL, Cabello-Inchausti B, Melnick SJ and Robinson MJ (2000) The peripheral blood smear in patients with sickle cell trait: a morphologic observation. *Lab Med*, **31**, 445–447.

46 Mowafy N. Hematomorphology. XXXth Congress of the International Society of Hematology, Istanbul, 2005.

47 Sheehan RG and Frenkel EP (1983) Influence of hemoglobin phenotype on the mean erythrocyte volume. *Acta Haematol*, **69**, 260–265.

48 Mears JG, Lachman HM, Labie D and Nagel RL (1983) Alpha-thalassaemia trait is related to prolonged survival in sickle cell anemia. *Blood*, **62**, 286–290.

49 Beutler E and West C (2005) Hematologic differences between African-Americans and whites; the role of iron deficiency and α-thalassaemia on hemoglobin levels and mean corpuscular volume. *Blood*, **106**, 740–745.

50 Serjeant GR and Serjeant BE (1972) A comparison of erythrocyte characteristics in sickle cell syndromes in Jamaica. *Br J Haematol*, **23**, 205–213.

51 Serjeant GR, Sommereux A, Stevenson M, Mason K and Serjeant BE (1979) Comparison of sickle cell-β^0-thalassaemia with homozygous sickle cell disease. *Br J Haematol*, **41**, 83–93.

52 Bain BJ (1992) Blood film features of sickle cell–haemoglobin C disease. *Br J Haematol*, **83**, 516–518.

53 Diggs LW and Bell A (1965) Intraerythrocytic hemoglobin crystals in sickle cell-hemoglobin C disease. *Blood*, **25**, 218–223.

54 Lawrence C, Hirsch RE, Fataliev NA, Patel S, Fabry ME and Nagel RL (1997) Molecular interactions between Hb α-G Philadelphia, HbC and HbS: phenotypic implications for SC α-G Philadelphia disease. *Blood*, **90**, 2819–2825.

55 Ballas SK, Larner J, Smith ED, Surrey S, Schwartz E and Rappaport EF (1987) The xerocytosis of SC disease. *Blood*, **69**, 124–130.

56 Lachant NA (1987) Hemoglobin E: an emerging hemoglobinopathy in the United States. *Am J Hematol*, **25**, 449–462.

57 Bunyaratvej A, Sahaphong S, Bhamarapravati N and Wasi P (1985) Quantitative changes in red blood cell shapes in relation to clinical features in β-thalassemia/HbE disease. *Am J Clin Pathol*, **83**, 555–559.

58 Rieder RF and Bradley TB (1968) Hemoglobin Gun Hill: an unstable protein associated with chronic hemolysis. *Blood*, **32**, 355–369.

59 Whitehead VM, Rosenblatt DS and Cooper DA. Megaloblastic anemia. In: Nathan DG, Orkin SH, Ginsburg D and Look AT, *Nathan and Oski's Hematology of Infancy and Childhood*, 6th Edn. Saunders, Philadelphia, 2003.

60 van der Zee SP, Schretlen ED and Monnens LA (1968) Megaloblastic anaemia in the Lesch–Nyhan syndrome. *Lancet*, **i**, 1427.

61 Taylor C and Bain BJ (1991) Technicon H.1 automated white cell parameters in the diagnosis of megaloblastic erythropoiesis. *Eur J Haematol*, **46**, 248–249.

62 Bessman JD, Williams LJ and Gilmer PR (1982) Platelet size in health and hematologic disease. *Am J Clin Pathol*, **78**, 150–153.

63 Bain BJ and Taylor C. L'uso dei parametri leucocitari automatizzati nella diagnosi dell'anemia megaloblastica. Atti del V Incontro del Club Utilizzatori Sistemi Ematologici Bayer-Technicon, Montecatini Terme, Giugno, 1991.

64 Lindenbaum J, Savage DG, Stabler SP and Allen RH (1990) Diagnosis of cobalamin deficiency: II. Relative sensitivities of serum cobalamin, methylmalonic acid, and total homocysteine concentrations. *Am J Hematol*, **34**, 99–107.

65 Savage DG, Lindenbaum J, Stabler SP and Allen RH (1994) Sensitivity of serum methylmalonic acid and total homocysteine determinations for diagnosis of cobalamin and folate deficiencies. *Am J Med*, **96**, 239–246.

66 Muckerheide MM, Wolfman JA, Rohde DA and McManamy GE (1984) Studies on a radioassay for intrinsic factor antibody: comparison of methods and false positive results due to elevated serum B12 levels. *Am J Clin Pathol*, **82**, 300–304.

67 Delaunay J (2002) Molecular basis of red cell membrane disorders. *Acta Haematol*, **108**, 210–218.

68 Tse WT and Lux SE (1999) Red blood cell membrane disorders. *Br J Haematol*, **104**, 2–13.

69 Miraglia del Giudice E, Nobili B, Francese M, d'Urso L, Iolascon A, Eber S and Perrotta S (2001) Clinical and molecular evaluation of nondominant hereditary spherocytosis. *Br J Haematol*, **112**, 42–47.

70 Bruce LJ and Tanner MJA (2000) Erythroid band 3 variants and disease. *Baillière's Clin Haematol*, **12**, 637–654.

71 McMullin M (1999) The molecular basis of disorders of the red cell membrane. *J Clin Pathol*, **52**, 245–248.

72 Yawata Y (2001) Genotyping and phenotyping characteristics in hereditary red cell membrane disorders. *Gene Funct Dis*, **2**, 113–121.

73 Bruce LJ, Ghosh S, King MJ, Layton M, Mawby WJ, Stewart GJ *et al.* (2002) Absence of CD47 in protein 4.2-deficient hereditary spherocytosis in man: an interaction between the Rh complex and the band 3 complex. *Blood*, **100**, 1878–1885.

74 www.uwcm.ac.uk//uwcm/mg/hgmd01.html

75 Delhommeau F, Cynober T, Schischmanoff PO, Rohrlich P, Delaunay J, Mohandas N and Tchernia G (2000) Natural history of hereditary spherocytosis during the first year of life. *Blood*, **95**, 393–397.

76 Sugihara T, Miyashima K and Yawata Y (1984) Disappearance of microspherocytes in peripheral circulation and normalization of decreased lipids in plasma and in red cells of patients with hereditary spherocytosis after splenectomy. *Am J Hematol*, **17**, 129–139.

77 Gallagher PG and Lux SE, Disorders of the erythocyte membrane. In: Nathan DG, Orkin SH, Ginsburg D and Look AT, *Nathan and Oski's Hematology of Infancy and Childhood*, 6th Edn. Saunders, Philadelphia, 2003.

78 Palek J and Jarolim P (1993) Clinical expression and laboratory detection of red blood cell membrane protein mutations. *Semin Hematol*, **30**, 249–283.

79 Palek J and Sahr K (1992) Mutations of the red blood cell membrane proteins: from clinical evaluation to detection of the underlying genetic defect. *Blood*, **80**, 308–330.

80 Hassoun H, Vassiliadis JN, Murray J, Yi SJ, Hanspal M, Johnson CA and Palek J (1997) Hereditary spherocytosis with spectrin deficiency due to an unstable truncated β spectrin. *Blood*, **87**, 2538–2545.

81 Hassoun H, Vassiliadis JN, Murray J, Njolstad PR, Rogas JJ, Ballas SH *et al.* (1997) Characterisation of

the underlying molecular defect in hereditary spherocytosis associated with spectrin deficiency. *Blood*, **90**, 398–406.

82 Bassères DS, Vincentim DL, Costa FF and Saad STO (1998) β-spectrin Promissão: a translation initiation codon mutation of the β-spectrin gene (ATG→GTG) associated with hereditary spherocytosis and spectrin deficiency in a Brazilian family. *Blood*, **91**, 368–369.

83 Ribeiro ML, Alloisio N, Almeida H, Gomez C, Texier P, Lemos C et al. (2000) Severe hereditary spherocytosis and distal renal tubular acidosis associated with total absence of band 3. *Blood*, **96**, 1602–1604.

84 Pati AR, Patten WN and Harris RI (1989) The use of the Technicon H1 in the diagnosis of hereditary spherocytosis. *Clin Lab Haematol*, **11**, 27–30.

85 Chiron M, Cynober T, Mielot F, Tchernia G and Croisolle L (1999) The GEN-S: a fortuitous finding of a routine screening test for hereditary spherocytosis, *Hematol Cell Ther*, Spring 1999, 113–116.

86 Bolton-Maggs PH, Stevens RF, Dodd NJ, Lamont G, Tittensor P and King MJ; General Haematology Task Force of the British Committee for Standards in Haematology (2004) Guidelines for the diagnosis and management of hereditary spherocytosis. *Br J Haematol*, **126**, 455–474.

87 King M-J, Behrens J, Rogers C, Flynn C, Greenwood D and Chambers K (2000) Rapid flow cytometric test for the diagnosis of membrane cytoskeleton-associated haemolytic anaemia. *Br J Haematol*, **111**, 924–933.

88 King M-J (2000) Diagnosis of red cell membrane disorders. *CME Bull Haematol*, **3**, 39–41.

89 Lecomte MC, Garbarz M, Gautero H, Bournier A, Galand C, Boivin P and Dhermy D (1993) Molecular basis of clinical and morphological heterogeneity in hereditary elliptocytosis (HE) with spectrin I variants. *Br J Haematol*, **85**, 584–595.

90 Iolascon A, Perrotta S and Stewart GW (2003) Red blood cell membrane defects. *Rev Clin Exp Hematol*, **7**, 22–56.

91 Reid ME, Associations of red blood cell membrane abnormalities with blood group phenotype. In: Garratty G (ed.) *Immunobiology of Transfusion Medicine*, Marcel Dekker, New York, 1993.

92 Patel SS, Mehlotra RK, Kastens W, Mgone CS, Kazura JW and Zimmerman PA (2001) The association of the glycophorin C exon 3 deletion with ovalocytosis and malaria susceptibility in the Wosera, Papua New Guinea. *Blood*, **98**, 3489–3491.

93 Lecomte MC, Gautero H, Boumier O, Galand C, Lahary A et al. (1992) Elliptocytosis-associated spectrin Rouen (β$^{220/218}$) has a truncated but still phosphorylatable β chain. *Br J Haematol*, **80**, 242–250.

94 Bassères DS, Pranke PHL, Vincentim DL, Costa FF and Saad STO (1998b) Expression of spectrin αI/50 hereditary elliptocytosis and its association with the α^{LELY} allele. *Acta Haematol*, **100**, 32–38.

95 Bain BJ, Swirsky D, Bhavnani M, Layton M, Parker N, Makris M et al. (2001) British Society for Haematology Slide Session, Annual Scientific Meeting of BSH, Bournemouth, 2000. *Clin Lab Haematol*, **23**, 1–5.

96 Silveira P, Cynober T, Dhermy D, Mohandas N and Tchernia G (1997) Red blood cell abnormalities in hereditary elliptocytosis and their relevance to variable clinical expression. *Am J Clin Pathol*, **108**, 391–399.

97 Conboy JG, Mohandas N, Tchernia G and Kan YW (1986) Molecular basis of hereditary elliptocytosis due to protein 4.1 deficiency. *N Engl J Med*, **315**, 680–685.

98 Alloisio N, Morlé L, Pothier B, Roux A-F, Maréchal J, Ducluzeau M-T et al. (1988) Spectrin Oran (α$^{II/21}$), a new spectrin variant concerning the αII domain and causing severe elliptocytosis in the homozygous state. *Blood*, **71**, 1039–1047.

99 Pajor A and Lehozky D (1996) Hemolytic anemia precipitated by pregnancy in a patient with hereditary elliptocytosis. *Am J Hematol*, **52**, 240–241.

100 Austin RF and Desforges JF (1969) Hereditary elliptocytosis: an unusual presentation of hemolysis in the newborn associated with transient morphologic abnormalities. *Pediatrics*, **44**, 189–200.

101 Coetzer T, Lawler J, Prchal JT and Palek J (1987) Molecular determinants of clinical expression of hereditary elliptocytosis and pyropoikilocytosis. *Blood*, **70**, 766–772.

102 Djaldetti M, Cohen A and Hart J (1982) Elliptocytosis preceding myelofibrosis in a patient with polycythemia vera. *Acta Haematol*, **72**, 26–28.

103 Rummens IL, Verfaillie C, Criel A, Hidajat M, Vanhoof A, van den Berghe H and Louwagie A (1986) Elliptocytosis and schistocytosis in myelodysplasia: report of two cases. *Acta Haematol*, **75**, 174–177.

104 Kedar PS, Colah RB, Kulkarni S, Ghosh K and Mohanty D (2003) Experience with eosin-5′-maleimide as a diagnostic tool for red cell membrane cytoskeleton disorders. *Clin Lab Haematol*, **26**, 373–376.

105 Palek J and Lambert S (1990) Genetics of the red cell membrane skeleton. *Semin Hematol*, **27**, 290–332.

106 Bain BJ and Liesner R (1996) Pseudopyropoikilo-cytosis: a striking artefact. *J Clin Pathol*, **49**, 772–773.

107 Coetzer TL, Beeton L, van Zyl D, Field SP, Agherdien A, Smart E and Daniels GL (1996) Southeast Asian ovalocytosis in a South African kindred with hemolytic anemia. *Blood*, **87**, 1656–1657.

108 Liu S-C, Zhai S, Palek J, Golan DE, Amato D, Hassan K *et al.* (1990) Molecular defect of the band 3 protein in Southeast Asian ovalocytosis. *N Engl J Med*, **323**, 1530–1538.

109 O'Donnel A, Allen SJ, Mgone CS, Martinson JJ, Clegg JB and Weatherall DJ (1998) Red cell morphology and malaria anaemia in children with Southeast Asian ovalocytosis and band 3 in Papua and New Guinea. *Br J Haematol*, **101**, 407–412.

110 Booth PB, Serjeantson S, Woodfield DG and Amato D (1977) Selective depression of blood group antigens associated with hereditary ovalo-cytosis among Melanesians. *Vox Sang*, **32**, 99–110.

111 Stewart GW, Hepworth-Jones BE, Keen JN, Dash BCJ, Argent AC and Casimir CM (1992) Isolation of cDNA coding for a ubiquitous membrane protein deficient in high Na⁺, low K⁺ stomatocytic erythrocytes. *Blood*, **79**, 1593–1661.

112 Yawata Y, Kanzaki A, Sugihara T, Inoue T, Yawata A, Kaku M *et al.* (1996) Band 4.2 doublet Nagano: a trait with 72 kD and 74 kD peptides of red cell band 4.2 in equal amount and with increased red cell membrane cholesterol and phosphatidyl choline. *Br J Haematol*, **93**, Suppl. 2, 199.

113 Yawata Y, Kanzaki A, Inoue T, Yawata A, Kaku M, Takezono M *et al.* (1996b) Partial deficiency of band 4.2 due to its impaired binding to a mutated band 3 in a homozygote of band 3 Fukuoka (133 GGA→AGA:Gly→Arg). *Br J Haematol*, **93**, Suppl. 2, 199.

114 Mohandas N and Gascard P (2000) What do mouse gene knockouts tell us about the structure and function of the red cell membrane? *Baillière's Clin Haematol*, **12**, 605–20.

115 Stewart GW and Turner EJH (2000) The hereditary stomatocytoses and allied disorders of erythrocyte membrane permeability to Na and K. *Baillière's Clin Haematol*, **12**, 707–727.

116 Barton CJ, Chowdhury V and Marin D (2003) Hereditary haemolytic anaemias and parvovirus infections in Jehovah's witnesses. *Br J Haematol*, **121**, 675–676.

117 Otsuka A, Sugihara T and Yawata Y (1990) No beneficial effect of splenectomy in hereditary high red cell membrane phosphatidylcholine hemolytic anemia: clinical and membrane studies in 20 patients. *Am J Hematol*, **34**, 8–14.

118 Jackson JM, Stanley ML, Crawford IG, Barr AL and Hilton HB (1978) The problem of Mediterranean stomatocytosis. *Aust NZ J Med*, **8**, 216–217.

119 Grootenboer S, Schischmanhoff PO, Laurendeau I, Cynober T, Tchernia G, Dommergues JP *et al.* (2000) Pleiotropic syndrome of dehydrated hereditary stomatocytosis, pseudohyperkalemia, and perinatal edema maps to 16q23-q24. *Blood*, **96**, 2599–2605.

120 Grootenboer S, Schischmanhoff PO, Cynober T, Rodrigue J-C, Delaunay J, Tchernia G and Dommergues J-P (1998) A genetic syndrome associating dehydrated hereditary stomatocytosis, pseudohyperkalaemia and perinatal oedema. *Br J Haematol*, **103**, 383–386.

121 Yawata Y, Kanzaki A, Yawata A, Kaku M, Takezono M, Sugihara T *et al.* (1997) Hereditary xerocytosis is a phenotypically different entity from hereditary high red cell membrane phosphatidyl-choline hemolytic anemia. *Blood*, **90**, Suppl. 1, 5a.

122 Vives Corrons JL, Besson I, Merino A, Monteagudo J, Reverter JC, Aguilar JL and Enrich C (1991) Occurrence of hereditary leaky red cell syndrome and partial coagulation factor VII deficiency in a Spanish family. *Acta Haematol*, **86**, 194–199.

123 Stewart GW, Corrall RJM, Fyffe JA, Stockdill GM and Strong JA (1979) Familial pseudohyper-kalaemia: a new syndrome. *Lancet*, **ii**, 175–177.

124 Haines PG, Crawley C, Chetty MC, Jarvis H, Coles SE. Fisher J *et al.* (2001) Familial pseudo-hyperkalaemia Chiswick: a novel congenital thermotropic variant of K and Na transport across the human red cell membrane. *Br J Haematol*, **112**, 469–474.

125 Coles SE, Chetty MC, Ho MM, Nicolaou A, Kearney JW, Wright SD and Stewart GW (1999) Two British families with variants of the 'cryo-hydrocytosis' form of hereditary stomatocytosis. *Br J Haematol*, **105**, 1055–1065.

126 Haines PG, Jarvis HG, King S, Noormohamed FH, Chetty MC, Coles SE *et al.* (2001) Two further British families with the 'cryohydrocytosis' form of hereditary stomatocytosis. *Br J Haematol*, **113**, 932–937.

127 Fricke B, Jarvis HG, Reid CD, Aguilar-Martinez P, Robert A, Quitted P et al. (2004) Four new cases of stomatin-deficient hereditary stomatocytosis syndrome: association of the stomatin-deficient cryohydrocytosis variant with neurological dysfunction. *Br J Haematol*, **125**, 796–803.

128 Rees DC, Iolascon A, Carella M, O'Marcaigh AS, Kendra JR, Jowitt SN et al. (2005) Stomatocytic haemolysis and macrothrombocytopenia (Mediterranean stomatocytosis/macrothrombocytopenia) is the haematological presentation of phytosterolaemia. *Br J Haematol*, **130**, 297–309.

129 Redman CM, Russo D and Lee S (2000) Kell, Kx and the McLeod phenotype. *Baillière's Clin Haematol*, **12**, 621–635.

130 Hardie RJ (1989) Acanthocytosis and neurological impairment—a review. *Q J Med*, **71**, 291–306.

131 Yamashima M, Ueda E, Kinoshita T, Takami T, Ojima A, Ono H et al. (1990) Inherited complete deficiency of 20-kilodalton homologous restriction factor (CD59) as a cause of paroxysmal nocturnal hemoglobinuria. *N Engl J Med*, **328**, 1184–1189.

132 Cartron J-P (2000) *RH* blood group system and molecular basis of Rh-deficiency. *Baillière's Clin Haematol*, **12**, 655–689.

133 Wood L, Jacobs P, Byrne M, Marais D and Jackson G (1997) Iron deficiency as a consequence of serial plasma exchange for the management of familial hypercholesterolaemia. Proceedings of the 37th Annual Congress of the South African Societies of Pathology, 160.

134 Mehta A, Mason PJ and Vulliamy TJ (2000) Glucose-6-phosphate dehydrogenase deficiency. *Baillière's Clin Haematol*, **13**, 21–38.

135 Lim F, Vulliamy T and Abdalla SH (2005) An Ashenkenazi Jewish woman presenting with favism. *J Clin Pathol*, **58**, 317–319.

136 Zanella A, Fermo E, Bianchi P and Valentini G (2005) Red cell pyruvate kinase deficiency: molecular and clinical aspects. *Br J Haematol*, **130**, 11–25.

137 Mentzer WC. Pyruvate kinase deficiency and disorders of glycolysis. In: Nathan DG, Orkin SH, Ginsburg D and Look AT, *Nathan and Oski's Hematology of Infancy and Childhood*, 6th Edn. Saunders, Philadelphia, 2003.

138 Mainwaring CJ, James CM, Butcher J and Clarke S (2001) Haemolysis and the combined oral contraceptive pill. *Br J Haematol*, **115**, 710–714.

139 Branca R, Costa E, Rocha S, Coelho H, Quintanilha A, Cabeda JM et al. (2004) Coexistence of congenital red cell pyruvate kinase and band 3 deficiency. *Clin Lab Haematol*, **26**, 297–300.

140 Leblond PF, Lyonnais J and Delage J-M (1978) Erythrocyte populations in pyruvate kinase deficiency anaemias following splenectomy. *Br J Haematol*, **39**, 55–61.

141 Fujii H and Miwa S (1990) Recent progress in the molecular genetic analysis of erythroenzymopathy. *Am J Hematol*, **34**, 301–310.

142 Tanaka KR and Zerez CR (1990) Red cell enzymopathies of the glycolytic pathway. *Semin Hematol*, **27**, 165–185.

143 McMullin M (1999) The molecular basis of disorders of red cell enzymes. *J Clin Pathol*, **52**, 241–244.

144 Jacobasch G (2000) Biochemical and genetic basis of red cell enzyme deficiencies. *Baillière's Clin Haematol*, **13**, 1–20.

145 Kanno H (2000) Hekokinase: gene structure and mutations. *Baillière's Clin Haematol*, **13**, 83–88.

146 Kanno H, Murakami K, Hariyama Y, Ishikawa K, Miwa S and Fujii H (2002) Homozygous intragenic deletion of type I hexokinase gene causes lethal hemolytic anemia of the affected fetus. *Blood*, **100**, 1930.

147 Kugler W and Lakomek M (2000) Glucose-6-phosphate isomerase deficiency. *Baillière's Clin Haematol*, **13**, 89–102.

148 Fujii H and Miwa S (2000) Other erythrocyte enzyme deficiencies associated with non-haematological symptoms: phosphoglycerate kinase and phosphofructokinase deficiency. *Baillière's Clin Haematol*, **13**, 141–148.

149 Kreuder J, Borkhardt A, Repp R, Pekrun A, Gottsche B, Gottschalk U et al. (1996) Brief report: inherited metabolic myelopathy and hemolysis due to a mutation in aldolase A. *N Engl J Med*, **334**, 1100–1104.

150 Yao DC, Tolan DR, Murray MF, Harris DJ, Darras BT, Geva A and Neufeld EJ (2004) Hemolytic anemia and severe rhabdomyolysis caused by compound heterozygous mutations of the gene for erythrocyte/muscle isozyme of aldolase, ALDOA (Arg303X/Cys338Tyr). *Blood*, **103**, 2401–2403.

151 Schneider A (2000) Triosephosphate isomerase deficiency: historical perspectives and molecular aspects. *Baillière's Clin Haematol*, **13**, 119–140.

152 Valentin C, Pissard S, Martin J, Héron Labrune P, Livet M-O et al. (2000) Triose phosphate isomerase deficiency in 3 French families: two novel null alleles, a frameshift mutation (TPI Altfortville) and an

alteration in the initiation codon (TPI Paris) *Blood*, **96**, 1130–1135.

153 Zanella A and Bianchi P (2000) Red cell pyruvate kinase deficiency: from genetics to clinical manifestations. *Baillière's Clin Haematol*, **13**, 57–82.

154 Bianchi P, Zappa M, Bredi E, Vercellati C, Pelissero G, Barraco F and Zanella A (1999) A case of complete adenylate kinase deficiency due to a nonsense mutation in *AK-1* gene (Arg 107→Stop, CGA→TGA) associated with chronic haemolytic anaemia. *Br J Haematol*, **105**, 75–79.

155 Toren A, Brok-Simoni F, Ben-Bassat I, Holtzman F, Mandel M, Neumann Y *et al.* (1994) Congenital haemolytic anaemia associated with adenylate kinase deficiency. *Br J Haematol*, **87**, 376–380.

156 Bianchi P, Fermo E, Alfinito F, Vercellati C, Baserga M, Ferraro F *et al.* (2003) Molecular characterization of six unrelated Italian patients affected by pyrimidine 5'-nucleotidase deficiency. *Br J Haematol*, **122**, 847–851.

157 Rees DC, Duley DA and Marinaki AM (2003) Pyrimidine 5' nucleotidase deficiency. *Br J Haematol*, **120**, 375–383.

158 Fiorelli G, Martinez di Montmuros F and Cappellini MD (2000) Chronic non-spherocytic haemolytic disorders associated with glucose-6-phosphate dehydrogenase variants. *Baillière's Clin Haematol*, **13**, 39–55.

159 Ristoff E, Augustson C, Geissler J, de Rijk T, Carlsson K, Luo J-L *et al.* (2000) A missense mutation in the heavy subunit of γ-glutamylcysteine synthetase gene causes hemolytic anemia. *Blood*, **95**, 2193–2197.

160 Vives Corrons J-L, Alvarez R, Pujades A, Zarza R, Oliva E, Lasheras G *et al.* (2001) Hereditary non-spherocytic haemolytic anaemia due to red blood cell glutathione synthetase deficiency in four unrelated patients from Spain: clinical and molecular studies. *Br J Haematol*, **112**, 475–482.

161 Boxer LA, Oliver JM, Spielberg SP, Allen JM and Schulman JD (1979) Protection of granulocytes by vitamin E in glutathione synthetase deficiency. *N Engl J Med*, **310**, 901–905.

162 Schneider A, Westwood B, Yim C, Prchal J, Berkow R, Labotka R *et al.* (1995) Triosephosphate isomerase deficiency: repetitive occurrence of a point mutation in amino acid 104 in multiple apparently unrelated families. *Am J Hematol*, **50**, 263–268.

163 Miwa S, Fujii H, Tani K, Takahashi K, Takegawa S, Fujinami N *et al.* (1981) Two cases of red cell aldolase deficiency associated with hereditary hemolytic anemia in a Japanese family. *Am J Hematol*, **11**, 425–437.

164 Feo CJ, Tchernia G, Subtil E and Leblond PF (1978) Observations of echinocytosis in eight patients: a phase contrast and SEM study. *Br J Haematol*, **40**, 519–526.

165 Valentine WN, Schneider AS and Baughan MA (1966) Hereditary hemolytic anemia with triosephosphate isomerase deficiency. Studies in kindreds with coexisting sickle cell trait and erythrocyte glucose-6-phosphate dehydrogenase deficiency. *Am J Med*, **41**, 27–41.

166 Vives Corrons JL, Camera A, Triginer J, Kahn A and Rozman C (1974) Anemia hemolitica por déficit congénito en fosfohexosaisomerasa—descripcíon de una nueva variante (PHI Barcelon) con estomatocitosis y disminucíon de la resistencia osmotica eritrocitaria. *Sangre*, **20**, 197–206.

167 Qualtieri A, Pedoce V, Bisconte MG, Bria M, Gulino B, Andreoli V and Brancati C (1997) Severe erythrocyte adenylate kinase deficiency due to homozygous A→G substitution at codon 164 of human AK1 gene associated with chronic haemolytic anaemia. *Br J Haematol*, **99**, 770–776.

168 Fermo E, Bianchi P, Vercellati C, Micheli C, Marcello AP, Portaleone D and Zanella A (2004) A new variant of adenylate kinase (delG138) associated with severe hemolytic anemia. *Blood Cells Mol Dis*, **33**, 146–149.

169 Travis SF, Martinez J, Garvin J, Atwater J and Gillmer P (1978) Study of a kindred with partial deficiency of red cell 2,3-diphoshoglycerate mutase (2,3-DPGM) and compensated hemolysis. *Blood*, **51**, 1107–1116.

170 Desnick RJ and Astrin KH (2002) Congenital erythropoietic porphyria: advances in pathogenesis and treatment. *Br J Haematol*, **117**, 779–795.

171 Merino A, To-Figueras J and Herrero C (2006) Atypical red cell inclusions in congenital erythropoietic porphyria. *Br J Haematol*, **132**, 124.

172 Lamoril J, Puy H, Gouya L, Rosipal R, da Silva V, Grandchamp B *et al.* (1998) Neonatal hemolytic anemia due to inherited harderoporphyria: clinical characteristics and molecular basis. *Blood*, **91**, 1453–1457.

173 Stavroyianni N, Stamatopoulos K, Viniou M, Vaiopoulos G and Yataganas X (2001) Autoimmune haemolytic anemia during α-interferon treatment in a patient with chronic myelogenous leukemia. *Leuk Res*, **25**, 1097–1098.

174 Farolino DL, Rustagi PK, Currie MS, Doeblin TD and Logue GL (1986) Teardrop-shaped red cells in autoimmune hemolytic anemia. *Am J Hematol*, **21**, 415–418.

175 Pettit JE, Scott J and Hussein S (1976) EDTA dependent red cell neutrophil rosetting in autoimmune haemolytic anaemia. *J Clin Pathol*, **29**, 345–346.

176 Ervin DM, Christian RM and Young L (1950) Dangerous universal donors. *Blood*, **5**, 553–567.

177 Teachey DT, Manno CS, Axsom KM, Andrews T, Choi JK, Greenbaum BH *et al.* (2005) Unmasking Evans syndrome: T-cell phenotype and apoptotic response reveal autoimmune lymphoproliferative syndrome (ALPS). *Blood*, **105**, 2443–2448.

178 Sivakumaran M, Murphy PT, Booker DJ, Wood JK, Stampo R and Sohol RJ (1999) Paroxysmal cold haemoglobinuria caused by non-Hodgkin's lymphoma. *Br J Haematol*, **105**, 278–279.

179 Jordan WS, Prouty RL, Heinle RW and Dingle JH (1952) The mechanism of hemolysis in paroxysmal cold hemoglobinuria. *Blood*, **7**, 387–403.

180 Bauer P, Bellou A and El Kouch S (1998) Acute intravascular haemolysis after pollen ingestion. *Ann Intern Med*, **129**, 72–73.

181 Koenig JM and Christensen RD (1989) Neutropenia and thrombocytopenia in infants with Rh hemolytic disease. *J Pediatr*, **114**, 625–631.

182 Davies NP, Buggins AGS, Snijders AJM, Noble PN, Layton DM and Nicolaides KH (1992) Fetal leucocyte count in rhesus disease. *Arch Dis Child*, **67**, 404–406.

183 Vaughan JI, Manning M, Warwick RM, Letsky EA, Murray NA and Roberts IAG (1998) Inhibition of erythroid progenitor cells by anti-Kell antibodies in fetal alloimmune anemia. *N Engl J Med*, **338**, 798–803.

184 Wagner T, Bernaschek G and Geissler G (2000) Inhibition of megakaryopoiesis by Kell-related antibodies. *N Engl J Med*, **343**, 72.

185 Gaines AR (2000) Acute hemoglobinemia and/or hemoglobinuria and sequelae following $Rh_0(D)$ immune globulin intravenous administration in immune thrombocytopenic purpura patients. *Blood*, **95**, 2523–2529.

186 Bolan CD, Childs RW, Proctor JL, Barrett JA and Leitman SF (2001) Massive immune haemolysis after allogeneic peripheral blood stem cell transplantation with minor ABO incompatibility. *Br J Haematol*, **112**, 787–795.

187 Bader-Meunier B, Croisille L, Ledeist F, Rince P, Miélot F, Fabre M *et al.* (1997) Dyserythropoiesis and hemolytic anemia as initial presentation of Fas deficiency conditions. *Blood*, **90**, Suppl 1, 316a.

188 Schulman I, Pierce M, Lukens A and Currimbhoy Z (1960) Studies on thrombopoiesis I. A factor in normal human plasma required for platelet production, chronic thrombocytopenia due to its deficiency. *Blood*, **16**, 943–957.

189 Upshaw JD (1978) Congenital deficiency of a factor in normal plasma that reverses microangiopathic hemolysis and thrombocytopenia. *N Engl J Med*, **298**, 1350–1352.

190 Remuzzi G, Ruggenenti P, Codazzi D, Noris M, Cprioli J, Locatelli G and Gridelli B (2003) Combined kidney and liver transplantation for familial haemolytic uraemic syndrome. *Lancet*, **359**, 1671–1672.

191 Geraghty MT, Perlman EJ, Martin LS, Hayflick SJ, Casella JF, Rosenblatt DS and Valle D (1992) Cobalamin C defect associated with hemolytic-uremic syndrome. *J Pediatr*, **120**, 934–937.

192 Riggs SA, Wray NP, Waddell CC, Rossen RD and Gyorkey F (1982) Thrombotic thrombocytopenic purpura complicating Legionnaires' disease. *Arch Intern Med*, **142**, 2275–2280.

193 Case Records of the Massachusetts General Hospital (1997) A 43-year-old woman with rapidly changing pulmonary infiltrates and markedly increased intracranial pressure. *N Engl J Med*, **337**, 1149–1156.

194 Schröder St, Spyridopoulos I, König J, Jaschonek KG, Luft D and Seif FJ (1995) Thrombotic thrombocytopenic purpura (TTP) associated with a *Borrelia burgdorferi* infection. *Am J Hematol*, **50**, 72–73.

195 Communicable Disease Report (2000) Active surveillance for rare and serious diseases in children. *CDR Weekly*, **10**, 349 and 352.

196 Allford SL, Hunt BJ, Rose P and Machin SJ, on behalf of the Haemostasis and Thrombosis Task Force of the British Committee for Standards in Haematology (2003) Guidelines on the diagnosis and management of the thrombotic microangiopathic haemolytic anaemias. *Br J Haematol*, **120**, 556–573.

197 Matsuda Y, Hara J, Miyoshi H, Osugi Y, Fujisaki H, Takai K *et al.* (1999) Thrombotic microangiopathy associated with reactivation of human herpesvirus 6 following high-dose chemotherapy with autologous bone marrow transplantation in young children. *Bone Marrow Transplant*, **24**, 919–923.

198 Turner RC, Chaplinski TI and Adams HG (1986) Rocky Mountain spotted fever presenting as

thrombotic thrombocytopenic purpura. *Am J Med*, **81**, 153–157.

199 Kwaan HC (1987) Miscellaneous secondary thrombotic microangiopathy. *Semin Hematol*, **24**, 141–147.

200 Nishiura T, Miyazaki Y, Oritani K, Tominaga N, Tomiyama Y, Katagiri S *et al.* (1986) *Aspergillus* vegetative endocarditis complicated with schizocytic hemolytic anemia in a patient with acute lymphocytic leukemia. *Acta Haematol*, **76**, 60–62.

201 Meir BM, Amital H, Levy Y, Kneller A and Bar-Dayan Y (2000) *Mycoplasma-pneumoniae*-induced thrombotic thrombocytopenic purpura. *Acta Haematol*, **103**, 112–115.

202 Fassas AB-T, Buddharaju LN, Rapoport A, Cottler-Fox M, Drachenberg C, Meisenberg B and Tricot G (2001) Fatal disseminated adenoviral infection associated with thrombotic thrombocytopenic purpura after allogeneic bone marrow transplantation. *Leuk Lymphoma*, **42**, 801–804.

203 Brown RC, Blecher TE, French EA and Toghill PJ (1973) Thrombotic thrombocytopenic purpura after influenza vaccination. *BMJ*, **ii**, 303.

204 George JN (2000) How I treat patients with thrombotic thrombocytopenic purpura-hemolytic uremic syndrome. *Blood*, **96**, 1223–1229.

205 Leach JW, Pham T, Diamandidis D and Georg JN (1999) Thrombotic thrombocytopenia purpura—hemolytic uremic syndrome (TTP-HUS) following treatment with deoxycoformycin in a patient with cutaneous T-cell lymphoma (Sézary syndrome): a case report. *Am J Hematol*, **61**, 268–270.

206 Hankey GT (2000) Clopidogrel and thrombotic thrombocytopenic purpura. *Lancet*, **356**, 269–270.

207 Kwaan HC and Gordon LI (2001) Thrombotic microangiopathy in the cancer patient. *Acta Haematol*, **106**, 52–56.

208 Mach-Pascual S, Samii K and Beris P (1996) Microangiopathic hemolytic anemia complicating FK506 (tacrolimus) therapy. *Am J Hematol*, **52**, 310–312.

209 McCarthy LJ, Porcu P, Fausel CA, Sweeney CJ and Danielson CFM (1998) Thrombotic thombocytopenic purpura and simvastatin. *Lancet*, **352**, 1284–1285.

210 Kupfer Y and Tessler S (1997) Ticlopidine and thrombotic thrombocytopenic purpura. *N Engl J Med*, **337**, 1245.

211 Bennett CL, Connors JM, Carwile JM, Moake JL, Bell WR, Tarantolo SR, McCarthy LJ, Sarode R *et al.* (2000) Thrombotic thrombocytopenic purpura associated with clopidogrel. *N Engl J Med*, **342**, 1773–1777.

212 Case Records of the Massachusetts General Hospital (1999) A 54-year-old woman with acute renal failure and thrombocytopenia. *N Engl J Med*, **340**, 1900–1909.

213 Lipton JH and Minden M (1995) CML may not be part of HUS. *Am J Hematol*, **49**, 100–101.

214 Masokoane SI (2000) Dangers of uninformed use of 'African Pitocine'. 24th World Congress of Medical Technology, Vancouver, Canada.

215 Maguire RB, Stroncek DF and Campbell AC (1993) Recurrent pancytopenia, coagulopathy, and renal failure associated with multiple quinine-dependent antibodies. *Ann Intern Med*, **119**, 215–217.

216 Kreitman RJ, Wilson WH, Bergeron K, Raggio M, Stetler-Stevenson M, Fitzgerald DJ and Pastan I (2001) Efficacy of the anti-CD22 recombinant immunotoxin BL22 in chemotherapy-resistant hairy cell leukemia. *N Engl J Med*, **345**, 241–247.

217 Fujita H, Takemura S, Hyo R, Tanaka M, Koharazawa H, Fujisawa S *et al.* (2003) Pulmonary embolism and thrombotic thrombocytopenic purpura in acute promyelocytic leukemia treated with all-*trans* retinoic acid. *Leuk Lymphoma*, **44**, 1627–1629.

218 Silva VA (1995) Thrombotic thrombocytopenic purpura/hemolytic uremic syndrome secondary to pancreatitis. *Am J Clin Pathol*, **103**, 519.

219 Musa MA, Nounou R, Sahovic E, Seth P, Qadi A and Aljurf M (2000) Fulminant thrombotic thrombocytopenic purpura in two patients with systemic lupus erythematosus and phospholipid autoantibodies. *Eur J Haematol*, **64**, 433–435.

220 Salyer WR, Salyer DC and Heptinstall RH (1973) Scleroderma and microangiopathic hemolytic anemia. *Ann Intern Med*, **78**, 895–897.

221 Brunning RD, Jacob HS, Brenckman WD, Jimenez-Pasqau F and Goetz FC (1976) Fragmentation hemolysis in patients with severe diabetic angiopathy. *Br J Haematol*, **34**, 283–289.

222 Kaplon M, Karnad A, Mehata J and Krishnan J (1999) Left atrial myxoma complicated by microangiopathic haemolytic anemia (MAHA). *Blood*, **94**, Suppl. 1, Part 2, 6b.

223 Fairley S and Ihle BU (1986) Thrombotic microangiopathy and acute renal failure associated with arteriography. *BMJ*, **293**, 922–923.

224 Rauch AE, Tartaglia AP, Kaufman B and Kausel H (1984) RBC fragmentation and thymoma. *Arch Intern Med*, **144**, 1280–1282.

225 Paré PD, Chan-Yan C, Wass H, Hooper R and Hogg JC (1983) Portal and pulmonary hypertension with microangiopathic hemolytic anemia. *Am J Med*, **74**, 1093–1096.

226 Zauber NP and Echikson AB (1982) Giant cell arteritis and microangiopathic hemolytic anemia. *Am J Med*, **73**, 928–930.

227 Batton D, Amanullah A and Cornstock C (2000) Fetal schistocytic hemolytic anemia and umbilical vein varix. *J Pediatr Hematol Oncol*, **22**, 259–261.

228 Gudena M, Schmotzer J, Dopriak M, Novoa R and Morgan R (2004) Microangiopathic haemolytic anemia (MHA) associated with acute rheumatic valvulitis. *Blood*, **104**, 5b–6b.

229 Hayes AM, Redington AN and Rigby ML (1992) Severe haemolysis after transcatheter duct occlusion: a non-surgical remedy. *Br Heart J*, **67**, 321–322.

230 Nand S, Bansal VK, Kozeny G, Vertuno L, Remlinger KA and Jordan JV (1985) Red cell fragmentation syndrome with the use of subclavian hemodialysis catheters. *Arch Intern Med*, **145**, 1421–1423.

231 Steinhorn RH, Isham-Schopt B, Smith C and Green TP (1989) Hemolysis during long-term extracorporeal membrane oxygenation. *J Pediatr*, **115**, 625–630.

232 Green DA, Murphy WG and Uttley WS (2000) Haemolytic uraemic syndrome: prognostic factors. *Clin Lab Haematol*, **22**, 11–14.

233 Visudhiphan S, Piankijagum A, Sathayapraseart P and Mitrchai N (1983) Erythrocyte fragmentation in disseminated intravascular coagulation and other disease. *N Engl J Med*, **309**, 113.

234 Allford SA and Machin SJ (1999) Thrombotic thrombocytopenic purpura: current concepts. *CME Bull Haematol*, **2**, 80–84.

235 Casebook of the Medical Protection Society.

236 Amare M, Lawson B and Larsen WE (1972) Active extrusion of Heinz bodies in drug-induced haemolytic anaemia. *Br J Haematol*, **23**, 215–219.

237 Zieve L (1958) Jaundice, hyperlipidemia and hemolytic anemia: a heretofore unrecognized syndrome associated with alcoholic fatty liver and cirrhosis. *Ann Intern Med*, **48**, 471–496.

238 Melrose WD, Bell PA, Jupe DML and Baikie MJ (1990) Alcohol-associated haemolysis in Zieve's syndrome: a clinical and laboratory study of five cases. *Clin Lab Haematol*, **12**, 159–169.

239 Bain BJ (1999) Images in haematology: Heinz body haemolytic anaemia in Wilson's disease. *Br J Haematol*, **104**, 647.

240 Hudson PR, Tandy SC, Child DF, Williams CP and Cavill I (2001) Compensated haemolysis: a consistent feature of diabetes mellitus. *Br J Haematol*, **113**, Suppl. 1, 47.

241 Swann IL and Kendra JR (1998) Anaemia, vitamin E deficiency and failure to thrive in an infant. *Clin Lab Haematol*, **20**, 61–63.

242 Kaiser U and Barth N (2001) Haemolytic anaemia in a patient with anorexia nervosa. *Acta Haematol*, **106**, 133–135.

243 Placzek MM and Gorst DW (1987) T activation haemolysis and death after blood transfusion. *Arch Dis Child*, **62**, 743–744.

244 Hillmen P and Richards SJ (2000) Implications of recent insights into the pathophysiology of paroxysmal nocturnal haemoglobinuria. *Br J Haematol*, **108**, 470–479.

245 Yamashima M, Ueda E and Kinoshita T (1990) Inherited complete deficiency of 20-kilodalton homologous restriction factor (CD59) as a cause of paroxysmal nocturnal hemoglobinuria. *N Engl J Med*, **323**, 1184–1189.

246 Schreiber ZA (1999) Hemolytic anemia associated with hepatitis C infection. *Blood*, **94**, Suppl. 1, 7b.

247 Wickramasinghe SN (1997) Dyserythropoiesis and congenital dyserythropoietic anaemias. *Br J Haematol*, **98**, 788–787.

248 Delaunay J and Iolascon A (2000) The congenital dyserythropoietic anaemias. *Baillière's Clin Haematol*, **12**, 691–705.

249 McCann SR, Firth R, Murray N and Temperley IJ (1980) Congenital dyserythropoietic anaemia type II (HEMPAS): a family study. *J Clin Pathol*, **33**, 1197–1201.

250 Brien WF, Mant MJ and Etches WS (1985) Variant congenital dyserythropoietic anaemia with ringed sideroblasts. *Clin Lab Haematol*, **7**, 231–237.

251 Jankovic M, Sansone G, Comer V, Iolascon A and Masera G (1993) Atypical hereditary ovalocytosis associated with dyserythropoietic anemia. *Acta Haematol*, **89**, 35–37.

252 Bianchi P, Pelissero G, Bredi E, Zappa M, Vercellati C, Boscetti C *et al.* (1998) Two cases of atypical congenital dyserythropoietic anaemia (type II) presenting with laboratory features of hereditary spherocytosis. *Br J Haematol*, **102**, 300.

253 Nichols KE, Crispino JD, Poncz M, White JG, Orkin SH, Maris JM and Weiss MJ (2000) Familial dyserythropoietic anemia and thrombocytopenia due to an inherited mutation in *GATA1*. *Nat Genet*, **24**, 266–270.

254 Freson K, Devriendt K, Matthijs G, Van Hoof A, De Vos R, Thys C *et al.* (2001) Platelet characteristics in patients with X-linked macrothrombocytopenia because of a novel *GATA1* mutation. *Blood*, **98**, 85–92.

255 Bethlenfalvay NC, Hadnagy CS and Heimpel H (1985) Unclassified type of congenital dyserythropoietic anaemia (CDA) with prominent peripheral erythroblastosis. *Br J Haematol*, **60**, 541–550.

256 Yeh SP, Chiu CF, Lee CC, Peng CT, Kuan CY and Chow KC (2004) Evidence of parvovirus B19 infection in patients of pre-eclampsia and eclampsia with dyserythropoietic anaemia. *Br J Haematol*, **126**, 428–433.

257 Cassinat B, Guardiola P, Chevret S, Schlageter M-H, Tobert M-E, Rain J-D and Gluckman E (2000) Constitutive elevation of serum alpha-fetoprotein in Fanconi anemia. *Blood*, **96**, 859–863.

258 Willig T-N, Draptchinskaia N, Dianzani I, Ball S, Niemeyer C, Ramenghi U *et al.* (1999) Mutations in ribosomal protein S19 gene and Diamond–Blackfan anemia: wide variations in phenotypic expression. *Blood*, **94**, 4294–4306.

259 Freedman MH (2000) Diamond–Blackfan anaemia. *Baillière's Clin Haematol*, **13**, 591–606.

260 Karsten J, Anker AP and Odink RJ (1996) Glycosylated haemoglobin and transient erythroblastopenia of childhood. *Lancet*, **347**, 273.

261 Alter B. Inherited bone marrow failure syndromes. In: Nathan DG, Orkin SH, Ginsburg D and Look AT, *Nathan and Oski's Hematology of Infancy and Childhood*, 6th Edn. Saunders, Philadelphia, 2003.

262 Johansson PL, Safai-Kutti S and Kutti J (2005) An elevated venous haemoglobin concentration cannot be used as a surrogate marker for absolute erythrocytosis: a study of patients with polycythaemia vera and apparent polycythaemia. *Br J Haematol*, **129**, 701–705.

263 Pierre R, Imbert M, Thiele J, Vardiman JW, Brunning RD and Flandrin G, Polycythaemia vera, In Jaffe ES, Harris NL, Stein H and Vardiman JW, World Health Organization Classification of Tumours, Pathology and Genetics, Tumours of Haematopoietic and Lymphoid Tissues, IARC, Lyon, 2001, pp. 32–34.

264 Messinezy M, Westwood NB, El-Hemaidi I, Marsden JT, Sherwood RS and Pearson TC (2002) Serum erythropoietin values in erythrocytoses and in primary thrombocythaemia. *Br J Haematol*, **117**, 47–53.

265 Carneskog J, Kutti J, Wadenvik H, Lundberg P-A and Lindstedt G (1998) Plasma erythropoietin by high detectability immunoradiometric assay in untreated patients with polycythaemia rubra vera and essential thrombocythaemia. *Eur J Haematol*, **60**, 278–282.

266 McMullin MF, Bareford D, Campbell P, Green AR, Harrison C, Hunt B *et al.*, on behalf of the General Haematology Task Force of the British Committee for Standards in Haematology (2005) Guidelines for the diagnosis, investigation and management of polycythaemia/erythrocytosis. *Br J Haematol*, **130**, 166–173.

267 Tey S-K, Cobcroft R, Grimmett K, Marlton P, Gill D and Mills A (2004) A simplified endogenous erythroid colony assay for the investigation of polycythaemia. *Clin Lab Haematol*, **26**, 115–122.

268 Carneskog J, Safai-Kutti S, Suurküla M, Wadenvik H, Bake B, Lindstedt G and Kutti J (1998) The red cell mass, plasma erythropoietin and spleen size in apparent polycythaemia. *Eur J Haematol*, **62**, 43–48.

269 Germeshausen M, Ballmaier M and Welte K (2001) Implications of mutations in hematopoietic growth factor receptor genes in congenital cytopenias. *Ann N Y Acad Sci*, **938**, 305–320.

270 Thompson AA and Nguyen LT (2000) Amegakaryocytic thrombocytopenia and radio-ulnar synostosis are associated with *HOXA11* mutation. *Nat Genet*, **26**, 397–398.

271 Thompson AA, Woodruff K, Feig SA, Nguyen LT and Schanen NC (2001) Congenital thrombocytopenia and radio-ulnar synostosis: a new familial syndrome. *Br J Haematol*, **113**, 866–870.

272 Balduini CL, Cattaneo M, Fabris F, Gresele P, Iolascon A, Pulcinelli FM and Savoia A (2003) Inherited thrombocytopenias: a proposed diagnostic algorithm from the Italian Gruppo di Studio delle Piastrine. *Haematologica*, **89**, 325–329.

273 Lutskiy MI, Sasahara Y, Kenney DM, Rosen FS and Remold-O'Donnell E (2002) Wiskott–Aldrich syndrome in a female. *Blood*, **100**, 2763–2768.

274 Ho LL, Ayling J, Prosser I, Kronenberg H, Iland H and Joshua D (2001) Missense C168T in the Wiskott-Aldrich syndrome protein gene is a common mutation in X-linked thrombocytopenia. *Br J Haematol*, **112**, 76–80.

275 Notarangelo LD, Mazza C, Gilliani S, d'Aria C, Gandellini F, Locatelli MG *et al.* (2002) Missense mutations of the *WASP* gene cause intermittent X-linked thrombocytopenia. *Blood*, **99**, 2268–2269.

276 Jackson N, Mohammad S, Zainal N, Jamaluddin N, Hishamuddin M (1995) Autosomal dominant thrombocytopenia with microthrombocytes: a family study. *Med J Malaysia*, **50**, 421–424.

277 Ballmaier M, Germeshausen M, Schulze H, Cherkaoui K, Lang S, Gaudig A *et al.* (2001) c-*mpl* mutations are the cause of congenital amegakaryocytic thrombocytopenia. *Blood*, **97**, 139–146.

278 Drachman JG (2004) Inherited thrombocytopenia: when a low platelet count does not mean ITP. *Blood*, **103**, 390–398.

279 Savoia A, Del Vecchio M, Totaro A, Perrotta S, Amendola G, Moretti A *et al.* (1999) An autosomal dominant thrombocytopenia gene maps to chromosomal region 10p. *Am J Hum Genet*, **65**, 1401–1405.

280 Gandhi ML, Cummings CL and Drachman JG (2003) *FLJ14813*: a novel kinase mutated in autosomal dominant thrombocytopenia on human chromosome 10. *Blood*, **102**, 5a.

281 Song WJ, Sullivan MG, Legare RD, Hutchings S, Tan X, Kufrin D *et al.* (1999) Haploinsufficiency of CBFA2 causes familial thrombocytopenia with propensity to develop acute myelogenous leukaemia. *Nat Genet*, **23**, 166–175.

282 Buijs A, Poddighe P, van Wijk R, van Solinge W, Borst E, Verdonck L *et al.* (2001) A novel *CBFA2* single-nucleotide mutation in familial platelet disorder with propensity to develop myeloid malignancies. *Blood*, **98**, 2856–2858.

283 Hayward CP, Cramer EM, Kane WH, Zheng S, Bouchard M, Masse JM and Rivard GE (1997) Studies of a second family with the Quebec platelet disorder: evidence that the degradation of the alpha-granule membrane and its soluble contents are not secondary to a defect in targeting proteins to alpha-granules. *Blood*, **89**, 1243–1253.

284 van den Oudenrijn S, Bruin M, Folman CC, Bussel J, de Haas M, von dem Borne AEGK (2002) Three parameters, plasma thrombopoietin levels, plasma glycocalicin levels and megakaryocyte culture, distinguish between different causes of congenital thrombocytopenia. *Br J Haematol*, **117**, 390–398.

285 Savoia A, Balduini CL, Savino M, Noris P, del Vecchio M, Perrotta S *et al.* (2001) Autosomal dominant macrothrombocytopenia in Italy is most frequently a type of heterozygous Bernard–Soulier syndrome. *Blood*, **97**, 1330–1335.

286 Drouin A, Favier R, Massé J-M, Debili N, Schmitt A, Elbin C *et al.* (2001) Newly recognized cellular abnormalities in the gray platelet syndrome. *Blood*, **98**, 1382–1391.

287 White JG, Key N, King R and Vercellotti G (2003) The White platelet syndrome: an autosomal dominant platelet disorder. I. Structural defects. *Blood*, **102**, 12a.

288 Di Pumpo M, Noris P, Pecci A, Savoia A, Seri M, Ceresa IF and Balduini CL (2005) Defective expression of GPIb/IX/V complex in platelets from patients with May–Hegglin anomaly and Sebastian syndrome. *Haematologica*, **87**, 943–947.

289 Kunishima S, Kojima T, Matsushita T, Tanaka T, Tsurusawa M, Furukawa Y *et al.* (2001) Mutations in the NMMHC-A gene cause autosomal dominant macrothrombocytopenia with leukocyte inclusions (May–Hegglin anomaly/Sebastian syndrome). *Blood*, **97**, 1147–1149.

290 Bellucci S (1997) Megakaryocytes and inherited thrombocytopenias. *Baillière's Clin Haematol*, **10**, 149–162.

291 Toren A, Rozenfeld-Granot G, Rocca B, Epstein CJ, Amariglio N, Laghi F *et al.* (2000) Autosomal-dominant giant platelet syndromes: a hint of the same genetic defect as in Fechtner syndrome owing to a similar genetic linkage to chromosome 22q11–13. *Blood*, **96**, 3447–3451.

292 Favier R, Jondeau K, Boutard P, Grossfeld P, Reinert P, Jones C *et al.* (2003) Paris–Trousseau syndrome: clinical, hematological, molecular data of ten new cases. *Thromb Haemost*, **90**, 893–897.

293 Davies JK, Telfer P, Cavenagh JD, Foot N and Neat M (2003) Autoimmune cytopenias in the 22q11.2 deletion syndrome. *Clin Lab Haematol*, **25**, 195–197.

294 Erice JG, Perez JM and Pericas FS (1999) Homozygous form of the Pelger–Huet anomaly. *Haematologica*, **84**, 748.

295 Yu C, Niakan KK, Martsushita M, Stamatoyannopoulos G, Orkin SH and Raskind WH (2002) X-linked thrombocytopenia with thalassaemia from a mutation in the amino finger of GATA-1 affecting DNA binding rather than FOG-1 interaction. *Blood*, **100**, 2040–2045.

296 Willig T-N, Breton-Gorius J, Elbim C, Mignotte V, Kaplan C, Mollicone R *et al.* (2001) Macrothrombocytopenia with abnormal demarcation membranes in megakaryocytes and neutropenia with a complete lack of sialyl-Lewis-X antigens on leukocytes. *Blood*, **97**, 826–828.

297 Harris VK, Nair SC, Dolley D, Amelia SM and Chandy M (2002) Asymptomatic constitutional

macrothrombocytopenia among West Bengal blood donors. *Br J Haematol*, **117**, Suppl. 1, 88.

298 Becker PS, Clavell LA and Beardsley DS (1998) Giant platelets with abnormal surface glycoproteins: a new familial disorder associated with mitral valve insufficiency. *J Pediatr Hematol Oncol*, **20**, 69–73.

299 Fabris F, Fagioli F, Basso G and Girolami A (2002) Autosomal dominant macrothrombocytopenia with ineffective thrombopoiesis. *Haematologica*, **87**, ELT27.

300 Pujol-Moix N, Kelley MJ, Hernandez A, Muniz-Diaz E and Espanol I (2004) Ultrastructural analysis of granulocyte inclusions in genetically confirmed MYH9-related disorders. *Haematologica*, **89**, 330–337.

301 Lubinsky MS, Kahler SG, Speer IE, Hoyme HE, Kirillova IA and Lurie IW (1994) von Voss-Cherstvoy syndrome: a variable perinatally lethal syndrome of multiple congenital anomalies. *Am J Med Genet*, **52**, 272–278.

302 Braddock SR and Carey JC (1994) A new syndrome: congenital thrombocytopenia, Robin sequence, agenesis of the corpus callosum, distinctive facies and developmental delay. *Clin Dysmorphol*, **3**, 75–81.

303 Arias S, Penchaszadeh VB, Pinto-Cisternas J and Larrauri S (1980) The IVIC syndrome: a new autosomal dominant complex pleiotropic syndrome with radial ray hypoplasia, hearing impairment, external ophthalmoplegia, and thrombocytopenia. *Am J Med Genet*, **6**, 25–59.

304 Pecci A, Noris P, Invernizzi R, Savoia A, Seri M, Ghiggeri GM *et al.* (2002) Immunocytochemistry for the heavy chain of the non-muscle myosin IIA as a diagnostic tool for *MYH9*-related disorders. *Br J Haematol*, **117**, 164–157.

305 Yagi H, Matumoto M, Ishizashi H, Kinoshita S, Konno M, Matsui T *et al.* (2000) Plasmas with Upshaw–Schulman syndrome, a congenital deficiency of von Willebrand factor-cleaving protease, augment the aggregation of normal washed platelets under high-shear-stress. *Blood*, **96**, 630a.

306 Fabris F, Cordiano I, Steffan A, Ramon R, Scandellari R, Nichol JL and Girolami A (2000) Indirect study of thrombopoiesis (TPO, reticulated platelets, glycocalicin) in patients with hereditary macrothrombocytopenia. *Eur J Haematol*, **64**, 151–156.

307 Devine DV, Currie MS, Rosse WF and Greenberg CS (1987) Pseudo-Bernard–Soulier syndrome: thrombocytopenia caused by autoantibody to platelet glycoprotein Ib. *Blood*, **70**, 428–431.

308 Murphy MF and Williamson LM (2000) Antenatal screening for fetomaternal alloimmune thrombocytopenia: an evaluation using the criteria of the UK National Screening Committee. *Br J Haematol*, **111**, 726–732.

309 Qasim W, Gilmour KC, Heath S, Ashton E, Cranston T, Thomas A *et al.* (2001) Protein assays for diagnosis of Wiskott–Aldrich syndrome and X-linked thrombocytopenia. *Br J Haematol*, **113**, 861–863.

310 Neylon AJ, Saunders PWG, Howard MR, Proctor SJ and Taylor PRA on behalf of the Northern Region Haematology Group (2003) Clinically significant newly presenting autoimmune thrombocytopenic purpura in adults: a prospective study of a population-based cohort of 245 patients. *Br J Haematol*, **122**, 966–974.

311 Koh K-R, Yamane T, Ohta K, Hino M, Takubo T and Tatsumi N (1999) Pathophysiological significance of simultaneous measurement of reticulated platelets, large platelets and serum thrombopoietin in non-neoplastic thrombocytopenic disorders. *Eur J Haematol*, **63**, 295–301.

312 Rosthøj S, Hedlund-Treutiger I and Zeller B on behalf of the Nordic Society for Paediatric Haematology and Oncology Idiopathic Thrombocytopenic Purpura Working Group (2005) Factors predicting development of chronic disease in Nordic children with acute onset of idiopathic thrombocytopenic purpura. *Br J Haematol*, **130**, 148–149.

313 Rajan SK, Espina BM and Liebman HA (2005) Hepatitis C virus-related thrombocytopenia: clinical and laboratory characteristics compared with chronic immune thrombocytopenic purpura. *Br J Haematol*, **129**, 818–824.

314 British Committee for Standards in Haematology General Haematology Task Force (2003) Guidelines for the investigation and management of idiopathic thrombocytopenic purpura in adults, children and in pregnancy. *Br J Haematol*, **120**, 574–596.

315 Garcia-Suárez J, Burgaleta C, Hernanz N, Albarran F, Tobaruela P and Alvarez-Mon M (2000) HCV-associated thrombocytopenia: clinical characteristics and platelet response after recombinant α2b-interferon therapy. *Br J Haematol*, **110**, 98–103.

316 Kuga T, Kohda K, Koike K, Matsunaga T, Kogawa K, Kanisawa Y *et al.* (2001) Effect of *Helicobacter pylori* eradication on platelet recovery in chronic idiopathic thrombocytopenic purpura and secondary

autoimmune thrombocytopenic purpura. *Blood*, **98**, 520a.

317 Jarque I, Andrea R, Llopis I, de la Rubia J, Gomis F, Senent L *et al.* (2001) Absence of platelet response after eradication of *Helicobacter pylori* infection in patients with chronic idiopathic thrombocytopenic purpura. *Br J Haematol*, **115**, 1002–1003.

318 Petrov V, Vdovin V and Svirin P (2004) Vaccine-associated immune thrombocytopenic purpura in childhood. *Br J Haematol*, **125**, Suppl. 1, 50.

319 Su C and Brandt LJ (1995) *Escherichia coli* O157: H7 infection in humans. *Ann Intern Med*, **123**, 698–714.

320 Scully M, Miller R, Cohen H, Roedling S, Starke R, Edwards S *et al.* (2005) Treatment of HIV associated thrombotic thrombocytopenic purpura—importance of prompt diagnosis. *Br J Haematol*, **129**, Suppl. 1, 12.

321 Weinberg PD, Bennett CL, Rozenberg-Ben-Drot K, Kwaan HC and Green D (1997) Ticlopidine associated thrombotic thrombocytopenic purpura. *Blood*, **90**, Suppl. 1, 462a.

322 Schirron CA, Berghaus TM and Sackmann M (1999) Thrombotic thrombocytopenic purpura after Ecstasy-induced acute liver failure. *Ann Intern Med*, **130**, 163.

323 Rachmani R, Avigdor A, Youkla M, Raanani P, Zilber M, Ravid M and ben-Bassat I (1998) Thrombotic thrombocytopenic purpura complicating chronic myelogenous leukemia treated with interferon-α. *Acta Haematol*, **100**, 204–206.

324 Burns ER, Lou Y and Pathak A (2004) Morphologic diagnosis of thrombotic thrombocytopenic purpura. *Am J Hematol*, **75**, 18–21.

325 Ding J, Komatsu H, Wakita A, Kato-Uranishi M, Ito M, Satoh A *et al.* (2004) Familial essential thrombocythaemia associated with a dominant-positive activating mutation of the *c-MPL* gene, which encodes for the receptor for thrombopoietin. *Blood*, **103**, 4198–4200.

326 Picardi M, Martinelli V, Ciancia R, Soscia E, Morante R, Sodano A *et al.* (2002) Measurement of spleen volume by ultrasound scanning in patients with thrombocytosis: a prospective study. *Blood*, **99**, 4228–4230.

Answers to test questions

Multiple choice questions

MCQ 8.1	TTTTF
MCQ 8.2	TFTFT
MCQ 8.3	TFTTF
MCQ 8.4	TTFTT
MCQ 8.5	TFTFT
MCQ 8.6	FTTFT
MCQ 8.7	TTFTT
MCQ 8.8	FFTTT
MCQ 8.9	FFTTT
MCQ 8.10	TTFFT*

*Note: fava beans (broad beans) rather than red kidney beans cause haemolysis in G6PD deficiency.

Extended matching questions

EMQ 8.1
1 P
2 B
3 G
4 D
5 C

EMQ 8.2
1 E
2 B
3 C
4 G
5 J

EMQ 8.3
1 B
2 D
3 J
4 K
5 B

EMQ 8.4
1 B
2 L
3 E
4 H
5 N

EMQ 8.5
1 D
2 E
3 A
4 N
5 C

9 Disorders of white cells

Acquired disorders primarily involving white cells may be either reactive, to a primary usually non-haematological disease, or neoplastic. Neoplastic disorders result from the clonal proliferation of a haemopoietic stem cell, either myeloid or lymphoid, that has undergone mutation. Numerical changes in white cells are summarized in Chapter 6. Here the typical peripheral blood changes in reactive leucocyte disorders are described, followed by the characteristic features of haematological neoplasms.

Reactive changes in white cells

Bacterial infection

Acute and chronic bacterial infection

Blood film and count

In an adult, the usual response to a bacterial infection is a neutrophil leucocytosis with a left shift, toxic granulation, Döhle bodies and, when infection is severe, cytoplasmic vacuolation (Fig. 9.1). Occasionally, bacteria are seen within neutrophils (see p. 136). In severe infections there may be myelocytes, promyelocytes and even a few blast cells in the peripheral blood. The lymphocyte and eosinophil counts are reduced. A rise in the monocyte count occurs later than the rise in the neutrophil count. During recovery, there is a rise in the eosinophil count, sometimes to above normal. If infection persists, a normocytic normochromic anaemia develops and, if the infection becomes chronic, red cells may become hypochromic and microcytic. There is an increase in rouleaux formation and in background staining. The platelet count is often elevated during acute or severe chronic infection but is sometimes reduced. Sometimes bacterial infections are associated with pancytopenia as a consequence of haemophagocytosis.

In overwhelming sepsis, particularly in alcoholics and neonates, infection can be associated with

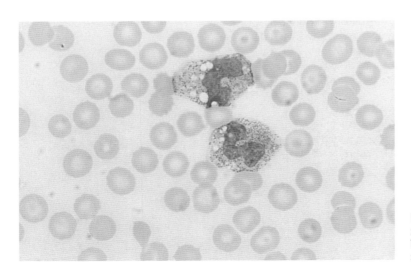

Fig. 9.1 Peripheral blood film in reactive neutrophilia; both cells are band forms showing vacuolation and marked toxic granulation.

paradoxical leucopenia and neutropenia. A left shift and toxic changes nevertheless occur. Neutropenia in bacteraemic patients is indicative of a worse prognosis [1]. Neutropenia in the course of infections that more often cause neutrophilia may be the result of increased margination of neutrophils, impaired granulopoiesis or migration of peripheral blood neutrophils to tissues at a faster rate than they can be replenished by a bone marrow with an inadequate reserve capacity. In some studies in neonates, an increased proportion of band cells has been found more useful than neutrophilia in identifying infected infants (see p. 91). However, others have found an increased band count to be no more sensitive in predicting a positive blood culture than an absolute neutrophil count [2].

Although neutrophilia is the characteristic response to bacterial infection, this is not invariable. Certain infections are characterized by either a normal white cell count (WBC) or even leucopenia and neutropenia, e.g. typhoid fever, brucellosis and rickettsial infections. Typhoid fever can also cause anaemia, isolated thrombocytopenia, bicytopenia or pancytopenia. Brucellosis occasionally causes isolated thrombocytopenia. Lymphocytosis is characteristic of pertussis (whooping cough). Infants and young children sometimes also respond to other bacterial infections with lymphocytosis rather than neutrophilia.

In addition to the elevated WBC, automated instruments may indicate a left shift, the presence of immature granulocytes or increased peroxidase activity of neutrophils.

Differential diagnosis

The differential diagnosis of neutrophil changes suggestive of infection includes other causes of neutrophilia (see p. 219). Toxic granulation and Döhle bodies are not specific for infection, being seen also in pregnancy, in inflammatory and autoimmune diseases, following administration of cytokines and when there is tissue damage or death, e.g. as a result of surgery, trauma or infarction. The presence of neutrophil vacuolation is more specific for infection, very commonly indicating septicaemia [3]. The observation of bacteria within neutrophils in a film made without delay (see p. 136) may indicate colonization of an indwelling venous line (if the blood specimen is obtained directly from the line) but otherwise is specific for bacteraemia. However, this finding is rare.

In the neonatal period, neutrophilia may be caused not only by infection but also by hypoxia or stressful labour, intrapartum oxytocin administration, maternal fever or seizures, neonatal hypoglycaemia and haemolytic disease of the newborn [4] (see p. 222). Even crying can cause an increase in WBC and the proportion of band cells [5].

Further tests

Characteristic peripheral blood features are often present in bacterial infection but, since they are neither specific nor invariably present, a definitive diagnosis necessitates consideration of clinical features and specific bacteriological tests. In patients with known bacterial infection the neutrophil count can be used to monitor the progress of the disease.

Tuberculosis

The haematological manifestations of tuberculosis are protean, although some of the abnormalities attributed to tuberculosis in the past are likely to have been caused by the coexistence of tuberculosis and a disease such as hairy cell leukaemia or idiopathic myelofibrosis.

Blood film and count

Pulmonary tuberculosis causes a normocytic normochromic anaemia with increased rouleaux formation and an increased erythrocyte sedimentation rate (ESR). When the disease is severe, leucocytosis and neutrophilia are common [6]. Lymphocytosis is present in about one-quarter of patients and lymphopenia in one-fifth. Although monocytosis has been regarded as characteristic of tuberculosis, it is present in only about one-quarter of patients while about half have monocytopenia. Thrombocytosis is common. Automated blood counts show a low haemoglobin concentration (Hb), normal or reduced mean cell volume (MCV) and increased red cell distribution width (RDW).

Patients with miliary tuberculosis [7] are usually anaemic. In contrast to acute pulmonary tuberculosis, leucocytosis is uncommon and leucopenia is common. Monocytosis occurs in about one-quarter of patients. Lymphopenia is usual. A minority of patients have pancytopenia (which is sometimes the result of haemophagocytosis).

Differential diagnosis

The haematological manifestations of tuberculosis are so variable that many infective, inflammatory and neoplastic conditions enter into the differential diagnoses.

Further tests

Bone marrow aspiration and trephine biopsy can be useful in the diagnosis of miliary tuberculosis. However blood cultures are also often positive so that bone marrow examination can be avoided.

Viral infections

Infectious mononucleosis

Infectious mononucleosis is an acute clinicopathological syndrome resulting from primary infection by the Epstein–Barr virus (EBV). It is predominantly a disease of adolescents and young adults. Common clinical features are fever, pharyngitis, lymphadenopathy (hence the common designation 'glandular fever'), splenomegaly and hepatitis. Haematologically, the disease is characterized by 'atypical mononuclear cells' or 'atypical lymphocytes' which are mainly activated T lymphocytes produced as part of the immunological response to EBV-infected B lymphocytes.

Blood film and count

There is often lymphocytosis and leucocytosis as a result of the presence of atypical lymphocytes. Suggested criteria alerting laboratory staff to the possibility of infectious mononucleosis are lymphocytes comprising at least 50% of peripheral blood leucocytes and atypical lymphocytes comprising at least 10% of circulating lymphocytes [8]; in one study the former observation had a sensitivity of 66% and the latter a sensitivity of 75% for

heterophile-positive disease among patients with suspected infectious mononucleosis [9]. Some patients are thrombocytopenic and a minority are anaemic. Atypical lymphocytes are highly pleomorphic (Fig. 9.2). Many are large, with diameters up to 15–30 µm, and have abundant strongly basophilic cytoplasm. Some have large central nucleoli and resemble immunoblasts (i.e. they have the same cytological features as lymphocytes stimulated *in vitro* by mitogens); others resemble the blasts of acute lymphoblastic leukaemia (ALL). Nuclei can be round, oval, reniform, lobulated or, occasionally, clover-leafed. In one study 15% of patients had cloverleaf nuclei, an observation of low sensitivity but high specificity in patients with suspected infectious mononucleosis [9]. In the same study 30% of patients had smear cells, also a highly specific observation in this group of patients [9]. The chromatin pattern may be diffuse or partly condensed. The cytoplasm may be vacuolated, foamy or (occasionally) granulated, and moderately or strongly basophilic. Cytoplasmic basophilia may be generalized or confined to the cytoplasmic margins. When the atypical cells have contact with other cells the cytoplasmic margins sometimes appear scalloped (see Fig. 9.2b). It should, however, be noted that both 'scalloping' and peripheral cytoplasmic basophilia can also be a features of lymphoma cells. Some cells have a hand-mirror conformation. Binucleate cells and mitotic figures may be seen. Apoptotic cells may be present, infectious mononucleosis being the most common cause of apoptosis in circulating lymphocytes [10]. Large granular lymphocytes may be increased and there may be some plasmacytoid lymphocytes and plasma cells. The abnormal cells can have cytochemical abnormalities such as block-positivity on a periodic acid–Schiff (PAS) stain—usually a feature of ALL—and tartrate-resistant acid phosphatase (TRAP) activity—usually a feature of hairy cell leukaemia. However, cytochemistry is not recommended in the diagnosis of infectious mononucleosis.

Changes in other cell lines are quite common although they tend to be overshadowed by the abnormalities in the lymphocytes. In one series 10% of patients had neutrophil counts of less than $1 \times 10^9/l$ [11]. Occasionally, neutropenia is very severe [12]. Neutrophilia can also occur. Neutrophils

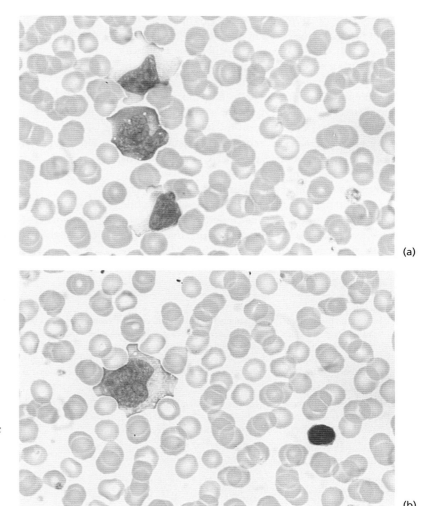

Fig. 9.2 Peripheral blood film in infectious mononucleosis showing atypical lymphocytes (atypical mononuclear cells): (a) pleomorphic cells, with plentiful cytoplasm; the largest cell has moderately basophilic vacuolated cytoplasm and a lobulated nucleus containing a nucleolus; and (b) a normal small lymphocyte and an atypical lymphocyte with voluminous cytoplasm and scalloped edges.

sometimes show toxic granulation, left shift and Döhle bodies; despite these changes, the neutrophil alkaline phosphatase (NAP) score is usually reduced. Reduction of the eosinophil count is usual; during recovery there is eosinophilia. Thrombocytopenia is not uncommon, the platelet count being less than $150 \times 10^9/l$ in about one-third of patients. Severe thrombocytopenia that sometimes occurs is likely to be due to immune destruction of platelets. Haemolytic anaemia due to a cold antibody can occur and the blood film then shows red cell agglutination, some spherocytes and, later, the development of polychromasia. A larger number of patients show some red cell agglutination without overt haemolysis.

Subjects with hereditary spherocytosis appear to be particularly prone to haemolysis during infectious mononucleosis. Some patients develop severe cytopenias consequent on virus-triggered haemophagocytosis. Aplastic anaemia is a rare complication, developing 1–6 weeks after presentation.

Not all patients with primary infection by EBV have the clinicopathological features of infectious mononucleosis. Young children have a greater degree of lymphocytosis and a lower percentage of atypical lymphocytes than older children but the absolute count of atypical lymphocytes is similar in children under and over 4 years of age [13]. In older patients the degree of lymphocytosis and the percentage of atypical lymphocytes may be less than is usually observed in adolescents and young adults [14]. Rare patients with infectious mononucleosis have severe lymphopenia [15]. This is associated with severe disease and a worse prognosis.

Automated counters usually 'flag' the presence of suspected blast cells, atypical (or 'variant') lymphocytes or both. Depending on the instrument, there may be an increase in 'monocytes', 'mononuclear cells' or large unstained cells (LUC) or a factitious increase in 'basophils'. In one study of patients with a clinical suspicion of infectious mononucleosis who had, or did not have, a positive test for a heterophile antibody a Coulter STKS instrument blast flag had a sensitivity of 41% for heterophile-positive disease while an atypical lymphocyte flag had a sensitivity

of 72%. For a Sysmex NE-8000, sensitivities were 43% and 16% respectively [9].

Differential diagnosis

The differential diagnosis of infectious mononucleosis includes other causes of atypical lymphocytes (Table 9.1) and, to a lesser extent, ALL and non-Hodgkin's lymphoma.

Further tests

The finding of a blood film suggestive of infectious mononucleosis is an indication to test for a heterophile antibody that agglutinates sheep or horse red cells and differs from heterophile antibodies in

Table 9.1 Some causes of atypical lymphocytes.

Viral infections
  Infectious mononucleosis (Epstein–Barr virus infection), cytomegalovirus infection*, infectious hepatitis (hepatitis A infection)*, measles (rubeola), German measles (rubella), echovirus infection, adenovirus infection*, chicken pox (varicella) and herpes zoster, herpes simplex infection, human herpesvirus 6 infection* [16], influenza, mumps, lymphocytic meningitis (lymphocytic choriomeningitis virus infection), human immunodeficiency virus (HIV) infection, human T-cell lymphotropic virus I (HTLV-I) infection, hantavirus pulmonary syndrome [17]

Bacterial infections
  Brucellosis, tuberculosis, syphilis, rickettsial infections* including tick typhus (*Rickettsia conorii*), scrub typhus (*Rickettsia tsutsugamushi*), murine typhus (*Rickettsia typhi*) [18,19], Ehrlichia infections (including Sennetsu fever (Japan) and ehrlichiosis (USA)) [20], *Mycoplasma pneumoniae* infection

Protozoan infections
  Toxoplasmosis*, malaria, babesiosis

Immunizations

Serum sickness (rarely)

Hypersensitivity to drugs*
  Hypersensitivity to para-aminosalicylic acid, sulfasalazine, sodium phenytoin, mesantoin, dapsone, phenothiazines, streptokinase [21]

Angioimmunoblastic lymphadenopathy [22]

Systemic lupus erythematosus [23]

Sarcoidosis [24]

Graft-versus-host disease

Graft rejection

Hodgkin's disease

Kawasaki's syndrome [25]

Familial haemophagocytic lymphohistiocytosis [26]

Transient idiopathic proliferation of monoclonal atypical lymphocytes [27]

* Conditions that can be associated with sufficiently large numbers of atypical lymphocytes to be confused with infectious mononucleosis.

other conditions in that it is adsorbed by ox red cells but not by guinea pig kidney. Rapid commercially available slide tests for heterophile antibodies are sensitive and very convenient with a false positive rate of 1–2%. At presentation, 60% of patients with infectious mononucleosis have a positive heterophile antibody test and up to 90% become positive if closely followed. In adolescents and adults, 'heterophile-negative infectious mononucleosis' most often represents either cytomegalovirus (CMV) or EBV infection. In one series of patients 70% of cases represented CMV infection and 16% EBV infection [28]. In another series, the percentages of patients with IgM antibodies to various viruses were 40% for EBV, 39% for CMV and 25% for human herpesvirus 6 [29], some patients having IgM antibodies to more than one virus; 3% of patients had toxoplasmosis. Well below half of infants with primary EBV infection have heterophile antibodies [13] so that in this age group EBV infection is the commonest cause of heterophile-negative infectious mononucleosis. Specific serological tests for IgM antibodies to EBV and CMV can clarify the diagnosis in heterophile-antibody negative cases. Serological tests for toxoplasmosis are also indicated and, in high-risk groups, testing for human immunodeficiency virus (HIV) should be considered (see below).

HIV infection and AIDS

HIV infection causes an acute illness at the time of seroconversion followed by a phase of latent infection before the manifestations of chronic infection appear. Chronic infection is associated with development of the acquired immune deficiency syndrome (AIDS). A transient expansion of CD8-positive large granular lymphocytes may occur as chronic HIV infection becomes clinically evident. Less often there is a persistent increase of large granular lymphocytes associated with a syndrome that clinically resembles Sjögren's syndrome, with lymphoid infiltration of salivary glands, lungs and kidneys [30].

Blood film and count

The acute illness can resemble infectious mononucleosis both clinically and haematologically but in general the number of atypical lymphocytes (Fig. 9.3)

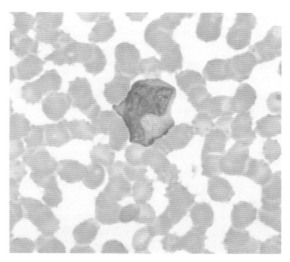

Fig. 9.3 Peripheral blood film showing an atypical lymphocyte during acute human immunodeficiency virus (HIV) infection.

is considerably less. Following recovery from the acute phase, the infected person is clinically and haematologically normal, often for many years. Isolated thrombocytopenia, resulting from immune destruction of platelets, can occur during this period of clinically latent infection.

Chronic infection is associated with a progressive decline in the number of CD4-positive lymphocytes and, usually, a decline in the total lymphocyte count. Reactive lymphocytosis consequent on an increase in CD8-positive lymphocytes (including CD8-positive CD57-positive large granular lymphocytes [30,31]) can initially mask the progressive decline in CD4-positive lymphocytes. The declining CD4-positive lymphocyte count is associated with a progressive decline in immune function, which eventually leads to infection or neoplasia. The development of certain specified infective or neoplastic conditions defines the patient as suffering from AIDS. Haematological features then include both the effects of HIV infection and the effects of intercurrent opportunistic infections. HIV infection itself causes a normocytic normochromic anaemia, thrombocytopenia and neutropenia with dysplastic neutrophils; one relatively specific neutrophil abnormality is the presence of detached nuclear fragments (see p. 97). Thrombotic thrombocytopenic purpura (TTP) may occur as a complication of HIV infection and the blood film then shows thrombocytopenia and red cell fragmentation. Recurrent infections contribute to the development of anaemia and are associated with increased rouleaux formation and increased background staining. Minor reactive changes in lymphocytes are common and may include cloverleaf forms. Bacterial infection can also be associated with toxic changes in neutrophils. Viral and mycobacterial infections can be associated with severe pancytopenia consequent on virus-associated haemophagocytosis. In the final stages of the disease there is a progressive pancytopenia.

Patients with HIV infection are also prone to iatrogenic haematological complications including macrocytosis and pancytopenia caused by zidovudine therapy, neutropenia caused by ganciclovir and oxidant-induced haemolytic anaemia caused by dapsone.

In patients with chronic HIV infection, the automated count with Bayer H.1 series counters can show increased peroxidase activity of neutrophils and a reduction of nuclear density seen as a reduced lobularity index. Both these features are indicative of dysplastic granulopoiesis.

Differential diagnosis

Depending on the stage of the disease and the specific haematological features, the differential diagnosis can include infectious mononucleosis and other viral infections, autoimmune ('idiopathic') thrombocytopenic purpura (ITP) and TTP. It is important to think of the possibility of HIV infection and consider performing specific serological tests in patients participating in high-risk activities who present with these haematological features. An expansion of large granular lymphocytes can be confused with large granular lymphocyte leukaemia, particularly as up to one-quarter of patients have evidence of a clonal expansion on T-cell receptor analysis [30]; the immunophenotype of the cells is CD8-positive, CD11a-positive, CD11c-positive and CD57-positive with strong expression of HLA-DR and negative reactions for CD16 and CD56. HIV infection is part of the differential diagnosis of chronic red cell aplasia since immune deficiency can lead to failure to eliminate parvovirus B19 so that virus-induced red cell aplasia is chronic rather than transient. Late in the disease, confusion with myelodysplastic syndromes (MDS) and other causes of bone marrow failure can occur.

Further tests

Diagnosis is customarily by serological detection of antibodies to HIV. If there is chronic red cell aplasia in an HIV-positive patient, serological tests for parvovirus should be supplemented by tests for parvovirus DNA since there may be a failure of specific antibody production.

Other viral infections

Viral infections may be acute or chronic. They cause a variety of effects on blood cells.

Blood film and count

Acute viral infections are associated with transient haematological abnormalities, most often lymphocytosis with reactive changes in lymphocytes. Large granular lymphocytes may be increased. With some viruses these changes can be sufficiently severe to simulate infectious mononucleosis (see Table 9.1). Other acute viral infections are associated with neutrophilia (see Table 6.4). The eosinophil count is reduced during acute infection and rises during recovery. Thrombocytopenia, as a consequence of platelet consumption, can occur during active viral infection. In the case of the viral haemorrhagic fevers, disseminated intravascular coagulation can cause severe thrombocytopenia. During recovery from some viral infections, e.g. rubella, there may be thrombocytopenia consequent on interaction of immune complexes with platelets. Acute haemolysis caused by the Donath–Landsteiner (anti-P) antibody can follow viral infections, e.g. measles, and acute haemolysis consequent on a cold agglutinin (anti-I or anti-i) can occur during other viral infections. Parvovirus infection in normal subjects causes acute, transient red cell aplasia associated with a slight fall in Hb and the disappearance of reticulocytes, and therefore a lack of polychromasia. In some patients there is associated neutropenia or thrombocytopenia. In patients with a shortened red cell lifespan, more severe but transient anaemia occurs. Some viruses, particularly herpesviruses, trigger a haemophagocytic syndrome, leading to pancytopenia. Infection by the Sin Nombre hantavirus has been observed to be associated with thrombocytopenia early in the illness with severe cardiopulmonary malfunction being predicted by a constellation of five peripheral blood features—thrombocytopenia, the presence of myelocytes, lack of marked toxic granulation (even if there was marked neutrophilia), increased haematocrit (attributable to a capillary leak syndrome) and the presence of more than 10% immunoblast-like cells or plasma cells [32].

The effects of chronic viral infection vary with the virus. There may be an increase of large granular lymphocytes. In chronic infection with human T-cell lymphotropic virus I (HTLV-I), there may be lymphocytosis with occasional atypical lymphocytes including some with cloverleaf nuclei (Fig. 9.4). Immunologically incompetent subjects, not only those with HIV infection but also those with congenital or iatrogenic immunosuppression, can develop chronic parvovirus infection with resultant chronic red cell aplasia. An apparent viral hepatitis, particularly non-A, non-B, non-C hepatitis [33], can be followed by aplastic anaemia. Patients with chronic infection by any of the hepatitis viruses can develop

Fig. 9.4 Peripheral blood film of a healthy carrier of the human T-cell lymphotropic virus I (HTLV-I virus) showing a lymphocyte with a flower-shaped nucleus.

haematological abnormalities resulting from chronic liver disease and hypersplenism and those with hepatitis C infection can develop cryoglobulinaemia.

Differential diagnosis

The differential diagnosis of the haematological effects of viral infection is complex, since the abnormalities caused are very variable. The differential diagnoses include the various conditions that can cause lymphocytosis, atypical lymphocytes and thrombocytopenia.

Further tests

Tests for heterophile antibodies and serological tests for specific viruses should be performed when clinically appropriate.

Persistent polyclonal B-cell lymphocytosis

Persistent polyclonal B-cell lymphocytosis is a rare condition occurring mainly in women and mainly in cigarette smokers. There is an association with the HLA-DR7 tissue type. Familial cases have been reported, both in several sets of siblings and in a parent and a child. An association with EBV infection has also been suspected. A minority of patients have hepatomegaly, splenomegaly or lymphadenopathy but most have only non-specific clinical features, such as fatigue. There is an association with chromosomal instability and acquired chromosomal abnormalities, particularly i(3)(q), trisomy 3 and dup(3)(q26q29) [34,35] which, remarkably, are present in both κ (kappa)-expressing and λ (lambda)-expressing lymphocytes and therefore cannot be taken as indicative of clonality.

Blood film and count

The abnormal lymphocytes include both large lymphocytes with increased cytoplasmic basophilia, resembling those seen in viral infections, and bilobed and binucleated lymphocytes (Fig. 9.5). The latter are strongly suggestive of this particular disorder. Some cells have nucleoli and among these there may also be some resembling prolymphocytes. The diagnosis can be made in patients without an absolute

Fig. 9.5 Peripheral blood film in a patient with persistent polyclonal B-cell lymphocytosis showing lobulated lymphocytes.

lymphocytosis if cytological and other features are typical. Such cases constituted 20% of patients in one series [36].

Differential diagnosis

The differential diagnosis includes reactive lymphocytosis and non-Hodgkin's lymphoma.

Further tests

Immunophenotyping is indicated to exclude a monoclonal proliferation of lymphocytes. The cells usually express IgM and IgD together with pan-B markers (such as CD19 and CD24), CD11c, CD21, CD25, CD27, CD95 and CD148 [37,38]. The proportion of B cells expressing CD5 and CD23 is lower than in normal controls, FMC7 is higher, and CD10 and CD38 are not usually expressed [37]. The abnormal cells appear to represent an expanded population of memory B cells [37], possibly analogous to marginal zone B cells [38]. Although the $\kappa : \lambda$ ratio may be abnormal, the atypical population includes both κ-expressing and λ-expressing cells. Polymerase chain reaction (PCR) shows that single or multiple *IGH-BCL2* fusion genes are often present. There is often a polyclonal increase in IgM. In addition to i(3q)

(leading to amplification of the *ATR* gene), del(6)(q), +8 and del(11)(q) have been observed [36].

Reactive eosinophilia

Reactive eosinophilia is common in a wide variety of allergic and parasitic conditions (see Chapter 6). Less often it represents a reaction to a neoplasm, e.g. carcinoma or sarcoma.

Blood film and count

Eosinophilia varies from mild to marked. Eosinophils may be cytologically normal or show a greater or lesser degree of degranulation or vacuolation. The blood film may also show lymphoma cells, blast cells or atypical lymphocytes. In reactive eosinophilia that occurs as a response to ALL, the leukaemic blasts may be very infrequent in the peripheral blood and the eosinophils very numerous.

Differential diagnosis

The differential diagnosis includes eosinophilic leukaemia and the idiopathic hypereosinophilic syndrome. The latter diagnosis (see below) requires that no evidence of an underlying cause can be found (see below).

Further tests

The most important initial step in investigating unexplained hypereosinophilia is a full history including a travel and drug history followed by a physical examination. These procedures may provide clues indicating the direction of further investigation. If parasitic infection appears likely, a considerable range of investigations may be necessary, the precise choice of test depending on the travel history and on any relevant features in the medical history or found on physical examination. Investigations that may be useful in patients with eosinophilia are shown in Table 9.2.

T-cell mediated hypereosinophilia

A proportion of patients with hypereosinophilia, often with cutaneous manifestations of the disease,

Table 9.2 Investigations that may be useful in unexplained eosinophilia.

If parasitic infection is suspected [39]

Examination of stools for parasites, cysts and ova

Examination of urine for *Schistosoma haematobium*

Rectal biopsy for *Schistosoma mansoni*

Serology—antibody tests for strongyloidiasis, toxocariasis, schistosomiasis, filariasis and a variety of other parasites (depending on the travel history) or antigen tests for cysticercosis, filariasis or a variety of other parasites

Examination of the blood for microfilariae

Duodenal aspiration

Assay of immunoglobulin E concentration

Chest radiology

Biopsy of skin or muscle

If neoplasia is suspected

Chest radiology

CT scan or other imaging of chest and abdomen

Bone marrow aspirate, trephine biopsy, cytogenetic analysis and molecular analysis (can be done on peripheral blood) for the *FIP1L1-PDGFRA* fusion gene

Biopsy of lymph node or other tissue

Immunophenotyping of peripheral blood lymphocytes or of any abnormal cell population in blood or bone marrow

T-cell receptor gene analysis to establish clonality of T lymphocytes

are found to have eosinophilia that is mediated by cytokines (e.g. interleukin 5) secreted by immunophenotypically aberrant T cells.

Blood film and count

There are no specific peripheral blood features. The lymphocyte count is usually normal and, if it is elevated, eosinophilia secondary to T-cell non-Hodgkin's lymphoma should be suspected.

Differential diagnosis

The differential diagnosis is the same as for reactive eosinophilia.

Further tests

Immunophenotyping shows a population of T cells with an aberrant phenotype, e.g. with failure to express CD3, with expression of CD3 but not CD4 or CD8 or with over- or under-expression of other T-cell associated antigens. Use of a panel of antibodies to variable domains of the T-cell receptor can provide evidence of clonality and clonal rearrangements of T-cell receptor genes can be demonstrated in about half of these patients. Cytogenetic abnormalities, e.g. 6q– or 10p–, can occur as secondary events.

Idiopathic hypereosinophilic syndrome

The term idiopathic hypereosinophilic syndrome (HES) is used to describe a heterogeneous group of conditions characterized by persistent unexplained eosinophilia and tissue damage (e.g. involving the heart and nervous system) attributable to the release of eosinophil granule contents. The condition is much more common in males. Cases are arbitrarily classified as idiopathic HES when the eosinophil count is in excess of 1.5×10^9/l, when unexplained eosinophilia persists for at least 6 months and when there is associated tissue damage [40]. Some cases appear to be attributable to an abnormality of T lymphocytes with eosinophilia provoked by lymphokines such as interleukin (IL) 2, IL3, IL5 and IL15 [41–43]. If the T lymphocytes can be shown to be clonal, the eosinophilia should probably be regarded as reactive to an overt or occult T-cell lymphoma but, if T cells are non-clonal, classification as 'idiopathic' remains appropriate. It is likely that certain other cases represent a myeloproliferative disorder with predominant eosinophilic differentiation, i.e. eosinophilic leukaemia, but if there is no proof of this, classification as 'idiopathic' is appropriate.

Blood film and count

The haematological features of idiopathic HES are currently ill-defined as previous series of patients included many who would now be recognized as having eosinophilic leukaemia. The description that follows should therefore be regarded as provisional.

There is a moderate or marked eosinophilia. Eosinophils often show marked degranulation and vacuolation including even completely agranular eosinophils (Fig. 9.6). Granules are often smaller than normal. Eosinophil nuclei may be hyperlobated, hypolobated or ring-shaped. Other haematological

Fig. 9.6 Peripheral blood film from a patient with the idiopathic hypereosinophilic syndrome (HES); the three eosinophils show various degrees of degranulation.

features can include anaemia, anisocytosis, poikilocytosis (including teardrop poikilocytes), a leucoerythroblastic blood film, basophilia, thrombocytopenia, thrombocytosis, neutrophilia and the presence of neutrophils with heavy rather basophilic granules (see Fig. 3.71). The latter abnormality may be so marked that the abnormal neutrophils are confused with basophils. A true increase in basophils can also occur [40]. The number of degranulated eosinophils is of prognostic significance. If they exceed $1 \times 10^9/l$ it is likely that cardiac damage is already present or will occur [44].

Differential diagnosis

Idiopathic HES is a diagnosis of exclusion. The diagnosis should not be made without excluding the presence of a *FIP1L1-PDGFRA* fusion gene, since many cases of what was previously classed as idiopathic HES are now know to represent eosinophilic leukaemia as a result of this fusion gene.

Many of the characteristic features are not specific. Tissue damage from the release of eosinophil granule contents can also occur both in reactive eosinophilia (see above) and in eosinophilic leukaemia. Degranulation and vacuolation of eosinophils can also be marked both in eosinophil leukaemia and in severe reactive eosinophilia. Peripheral blood features indis-

tinguishable from idiopathic HES can occur in some patients who are subsequently found to have systemic mastocytosis [45], ALL or lymphoma. Making a distinction between idiopathic HES and chronic eosinophilic leukaemia (see p. 432) at the onset of the disease can be difficult or even impossible.

Further tests

The patient should be appropriately investigated by history, physical examination and laboratory tests for known causes of eosinophilia. If no cause is identified, immunophenotypic analysis of peripheral blood lymphocytes should be performed to identify any population of lymphocytes expressing aberrant markers [42,43]. If an abnormal population is identified, T-cell receptor gene analysis should be performed to seek evidence that the abnormal population is clonal [42]. Bone marrow aspiration, a trephine biopsy and cytogenetic analysis are also indicated since detection of increased blast cells or a clonal cytogenetic abnormality permits the diagnosis of eosinophilic leukaemia. Systemic mastocytosis or a lymphoma may also be diagnosed on the bone marrow aspirate or trephine biopsy sections.

Although cases without evidence of an abnormal T-cell clone or specific features that identify them as 'leukaemia' are best classified as idiopathic HES some such patients subsequently show transformation of their disease to acute myeloid leukaemia (AML), providing evidence that the condition was neoplastic from the beginning. In others, an overt lymphoproliferative disorder subsequently becomes apparent. In some patients death occurs from the early or late effects of tissue damage without the true nature of the condition having become apparent.

Leukaemoid reactions

A leukaemoid reaction is a haematological abnormality that simulates leukaemia and thus may be confused with it, but that is, in fact, reactive to some other disease. In a leukaemoid reaction the abnormalities reverse when the underlying condition is corrected. In many of the early reports of leukaemoid reactions, the patient did not recover from the primary disease and correction of the haematological abnormality did not occur. In such cases, it is

Table 9.3 Some features that may be useful in distinguishing chronic granulocytic leukaemia from reactive neutrophilia.

Feature	Reactive neutrophilia	CGL
WBC	Rarely > $60 \times 10^9/l$	Usually $20–500 \times 10^9/l$ or higher
Left shift	May be moderate or marked; if slight in relation to neutrophilia supports reactive neutrophilia	Proportional to WBC; may be marked
White cell morphology	Toxic granulation, neutrophil vacuolation and Döhle bodies may be present	Toxic changes not present
Absolute eosinophil count	Usually reduced	Usually elevated; eosinophil myelocytes may be present
Absolute basophil count	Usually reduced	Almost invariably elevated; basophil myelocytes may be present
Absolute monocyte count	May be elevated	Usually moderately elevated
Erythropoiesis	Anaemia may be present; usually normocytic and normochromic but if hypochromic and microcytic supports a reactive neutrophilia; rouleaux may be present	Anaemia may be present; normocytic and normochromic
Platelet count	Thrombocytosis or thrombocytopenia may occur; if there is a reactive thrombocytosis the platelets are usually small	The platelet count is usually normal or high; giant platelets may be present; platelets are large, even in the presence of thrombocytosis; megakaryocytes may be present
NAP score	Usually elevated	Almost always reduced

NAP, neutrophil alkaline phosphatase; WBC, white blood cell count.

difficult to be sure that the patient did not have leukaemia coexisting with some other disease. This is so in many of the early reports of an apparent leukaemoid reaction with tuberculosis. Transient abnormal myelopoiesis in neonates with Down's syndrome (see p. 421) should not be described as a leukaemoid reaction. It is a neoplastic condition and is more correctly regarded as a spontaneously remitting leukaemia [46]. Leukaemoid reactions may be myeloid or lymphoid.

Myeloid leukaemoid reactions

Leukaemoid reactions rarely simulate chronic granulocytic leukaemia (CGL) since the characteristic spectrum of changes (see p. 425) is virtually never seen in reactive conditions. The differences are summarized in Table 9.3. The myeloid leukaemias that are most likely to be simulated by a leukaemoid reaction are AML, atypical Philadelphia-negative chronic myeloid leukaemia (aCML), chronic myelomonocytic leukaemia (CMML), juvenile myelomo-

nocytic leukaemia (JMML), neutrophilic leukaemia and eosinophilic leukaemia. Causes of myeloid leukaemoid reactions (Fig. 9.7) include any strong stimulus to bone marrow activity such as severe bacterial infection (particularly if complicated by megaloblastic anaemia, alcohol-induced bone marrow damage or prior agranulocytosis), tuberculosis, certain viral infections, haemorrhage and carcinoma or other malignant disease (with or without bone marrow metastases). Leukaemoid reactions in carcinoma may precede other manifestations of the carcinoma, sometimes by a number of years [47]. Myeloid leukaemoid reactions have been recognized in ALL [48]. The diagnosis of such reactions in AML is more problematical, often requiring cytogenetic and molecular genetic studies; the administration of growth factors or of high dose chemotherapy can lead to pseudo-relapse, with circulating immature but non-leukaemic cells, but growth factors can also lead to the appearance of leukaemic cells in the blood. Leukaemoid reactions in neonates may result from congenital syphilis [49] and in infants may be

Fig. 9.7 Peripheral blood film of a patient with a leukaemoid reaction consequent on severe postoperative sepsis due to a Gram-negative organism. WBC was $92 \times 10^9/l$ with a neutrophil count of $74 \times 10^9/l$ and a monocyte count of $16 \times 10^9/l$; the film shows a band form, a macropolycyte and monocytes with increased cytoplasmic basophilia.

consequent on the syndrome of thrombocytopenia with absent radii, particularly if complicated by haemorrhage [50]. Although it has been considered that there is an association between multiple myeloma, and other plasma cell neoplasms, and neutrophilic leukaemia it appears more likely that the neutrophilia in these patients represents a leukaemoid reaction [51,52], mediated by granulo-cyte colony-stimulating factor (G-CSF) secreted by the myeloma cells [53]; however in one such patient AML developed only 1.5 years after presentation [54] (rather too short an interval for an alkylating agent-related leukaemia) and the exact nature of this condition remains uncertain. Ectopic G-CSF secretion by other tumours can cause a neutrophilic leukaemoid reaction similar to that seen in multiple myeloma; this has been observed in sarcoma and in carcinomas of the lung, thyroid, stomach, gall bladder and urinary bladder [53,55,56]. Leukaemoid reaction can result from administration of growth factors such as G-CSF, granulocyte macrophage colony-stimulating factor (GM-CSF) and IL3. If the clinical history is not known to the laboratory staff, CMML, aCML or eosinophilic leukaemia may be suspected. Cases may have up to 30% circulating myeloblasts so can also simulate AML [57]. Various infections in children can lead to a leukaemoid reaction that simulates JMML. These include histo-plasmosis, toxoplasmosis, mycobacterial infection [58] and infection by *Mycoplasma pneumoniae* [59],

EBV [60], CMV [61], human herpesvirus 6 infection [62] and parvovirus B19 [63]. The blood film in osteopetrosis may simulate JMML [64] (Fig. 9.8).

Useful features in making the distinction between leukaemia and a leukaemoid reaction include toxic changes, such as toxic granulation and vacuolation, and a preponderance of more mature cells (in a leukaemoid reaction) and hypogranular neutrophils and the presence of a disproportionate number of myeloblasts (in many leukaemias). A low NAP score is strongly in favour of a diagnosis of leukaemia since it is almost invariably raised in leukaemoid reactions. If Auer rods are seen in blast cells, a con-fident diagnosis of leukaemia or MDS can be made.

If clinical and haematological features do not per-mit the distinction between leukaemia and a leukae-moid reaction then bone marrow aspiration with cytogenetic analysis and microscopy and culture for *Mycobacterium tuberculosis* is indicated.

'Pseudo-relapse' resulting from growth factor administration can be distinguished from relapse of leukaemia by cytogenetic or molecular genetic analysis, which shows that a leukaemia-associated abnormality is no longer present.

Lymphoid leukaemoid reactions

The blood film of whooping cough (Fig. 9.9) and of infectious lymphocytosis may simulate chronic lymphocytic leukaemia (CLL) but, since the clinical

Fig. 9.8 Peripheral blood film of a child with a leukaemoid reaction as a result of early onset osteopetrosis.

Fig. 9.9 Peripheral blood film of a child with whooping cough showing a cleft lymphocyte, a lymphocyte of normal morphology and a smear cell.

features and the age range of the two diseases are totally different, no problem occurs in practice. CLL has also been misdiagnosed in patients with post-splenectomy lymphocytosis. Knowledge of the high levels that the lymphocyte count can reach post-splenectomy, and careful examination of the peripheral blood film for post-splenectomy features will avoid this problem. Post-splenectomy lymphocytosis can also simulate large granular lymphocyte leukaemia since the dominant cell can be a large granular lymphocyte (Fig. 9.10). Considerable numbers of

large granular lymphocytes have also been reported in association with rituximab-induced autoimmune neutropenia [65]. Persistent polyclonal B-cell lymphocytosis can also be confused with CLL or non-Hodgkin's lymphoma, occasionally even leading to inappropriate chemotherapy. Knowledge of this syndrome and detection of the characteristic cytological features (see above) allows a distinction to be made. Hyper-reactive malarial splenomegaly can be associated with lymphocytosis with numerous villous lymphocytes and can thus simulate splenic

Fig. 9.10 Peripheral blood film following splenectomy for hereditary spherocytosis. The white blood cell count (WBC) was $29.3 \times 10^9/l$ and the lymphocyte count $24 \times 10^9/l$. The lymphocytes were predominantly large granular lymphocytes. Courtesy of Dr J. Houghton, Salford.

Fig. 9.11 Peripheral blood film from a child with severe burns showing blast cells as part of a leukaemoid reaction. By courtesy of Dr T. Corbett, London.

lymphoma with villous lymphocytes (SLVL) [66]; however immunophenotyping is essential to be certain that the patient does not in fact have SLVL since this lymphoma occurs in the same geographical area and may represent a neoplasm arising, as a result of chronic antigenic stimulation, in a patient with prior hyper-reactive malarial splenomegaly. A peripheral blood picture resembling Sézary cell leukaemia has been observed as part of a drug reaction [67]. Circulating plasma cells sufficient to simulate plasma cell leukaemia have been reported in a patient with bone marrow aplasia preceding ALL [68].

ALL can be simulated by infectious mononucleosis and other viral infections that cause atypical lymphocytes to appear in the blood, by reactions to stress in children (Fig. 9.11) and by mycoplasma infection [59], tuberculosis and congenital syphilis. Lymphocytosis with immature lymphoid cells of T lineage has been described in acute HTLV-I infection [69] and in ehrlichiosis [70]. When there is diagnostic uncertainty immunophenotyping is required. However, it should be noted that phenotypically abnormal lymphoid cells can appear in the blood during lymphoid leukaemoid reactions, e.g. CD10-

positive B-cell precursors or T-cells co-expressing CD4 and CD8 [59].

Haematological neoplasms

Acute myeloid leukaemia

AML is a disease resulting from proliferation of a clone of myeloid stem cells that show defective or absent maturation. Disease manifestations are those resulting from cell proliferation, such as hepatomegaly and splenomegaly, and those resulting from replacement of normal bone marrow, such as anaemia and bleeding. The neoplastic clone is usually derived from a multipotent myeloid stem cell but in some cases it may be derived either from a lineage-committed progenitor or a pluripotent lymphoid–myeloid stem cell.

Blood film and count

The majority of patients have leukaemic blast cells in the peripheral blood. These may be myeloblasts, monoblasts, megakaryoblasts, early erythroblasts or a mixed population. There may be some maturing cells, most often promyelocytes. In some patients an abnormal promyelocyte is the dominant cell. Most patients are neutropenic but in some types of AML there is maturation of the leukaemic clone with consequent neutrophilia or, less often, eosinophilia. Rarely, there is an increase in basophils. Most patients have a normocytic normochromic anaemia or, if there has been preceding MDS (see below), a macrocytic anaemia. Most patients are thrombocytopenic but in a minority there is a normal platelet count or even thrombocytosis. Peripheral blood cells may show dysplastic features similar to those of MDS. In a minority of patients, there is cytopenia, usually pancytopenia, without any circulating immature cells.

AML is further classified on the basis of peripheral blood and bone marrow features. Until now the most generally accepted classification is that of the French–American–British (FAB) cooperative group [71–75] but the World Health Organization (WHO) classification is being increasingly adopted [76]. Because application of the WHO classification requires knowledge of cytogenetic and molecular genetic abnormalities there is necessarily some delay in making a definitive diagnosis. A preliminary morphological diagnosis based on the FAB classification therefore remains appropriate. The FAB classification also remains important in parts of the world where cytogenetic analysis is not available. The most important difference between these two classifications is that, in the FAB classification, the bone marrow blast cell percentage must be at least 30% for a diagnosis of AML whereas, in the WHO classification, the defining criterion is a bone marrow blast cell count of at least 20%. These classifications are summarized in Tables 9.4 and 9.5. Different FAB subtypes of acute leukaemia are illustrated in Figs 9.12–9.21. It should be noted that the WHO classification is hierarchical with cases first being assigned to the category of therapy-related AML, if appropriate, and then to other categories, in the order shown in Table 9.5.

Differential diagnosis

The differential diagnosis is mainly ALL, transformation of CGL and other myeloproliferative disorders, MDS and other causes of bone marrow failure such as aplastic anaemia. Occasionally, it is necessary to distinguish between acute leukaemia and a leukaemoid reaction (see p. 408).

Further tests

When AML is suspected, a bone marrow aspiration is indicated, together with cytochemical stains to confirm granulocytic or monocytic differentiation and cytogenetic analysis, both for further classification and to give information on prognosis. Trephine biopsy is of use in some patients in whom the bone marrow is hypocellular or a poor aspirate is obtained because of fibrosis. Immunophenotyping (Table 9.6) can also be useful but is not essential in all patients unless it is intended to subsequently use immunophenotyping for monitoring of minimal residual disease. The most useful cytochemical reactions are myeloperoxidase (MPO) or Sudan black B (SBB), to confirm granulocyte differentiation, and a 'nonspecific' esterase reaction, such as α-naphthyl acetate esterase (ANAE), to confirm monocytic differentiation. A positive chloroacetate esterase (CAE) reaction confirms neutrophilic differentiation and can be combined with ANAE, as a combined esterase

Table 9.4 The French–American–British (FAB) classification of acute myeloid leukaemia (AML) [71–75].

M1 (*AML without maturation*)
Blasts ≥ 90% of NEC; ≥ 3% of blasts positive for peroxidase or SBB; monocytic component ≤ 10% of NEC; granulocytic component ≤ 10% of NEC

M2 (*AML with granulocytic maturation*)
Blasts 30–89% of NEC; granulocytic component > 10% of NEC; monocytic component < 20% of NEC

M3 and M3 variant
Characteristic morphology

M4 (*Acute myelomonocytic leukaemia*)
Blasts ≥ 30% of NEC; granulocytic component (including myeloblasts) ≥ 20% of NEC

AND

EITHER	OR
BM monocytic component ≥ 20% of NEC and PB monocyte count ≥ 5 × 10^9/l	BM resembling M2 but PB monocyte count ≥ 5 × 10^9/l and lysozyme elevated*
OR	OR
BM monocytic component ≥ 20% of NEC and lysozyme elevated	BM resembling M2 but PB monocyte count ≥ 5 × 10^9/l and cytochemical demonstration of monocytic component in BM
OR	
BM monocytic component ≥ 20% of NEC and cytochemical confirmation of monocyte component in BM†	

M5 (*acute monocytic/monoblastic leukaemia*)

M5a (*without maturation or acute monoblastic leukaemia*)
Monocytic component ≥ 80% of NEC; monoblasts ≥ 80% of monocytic component

M5b (*with maturation or acute monocytic leukaemia*)
Monocytic component ≥ 80% of NEC; monoblasts < 80% of monocytic component

M6 (*erythroleukaemia*)
Erythroblasts ≥ 50%; blasts ≥ 30% of NEC

M7 (*megakaryoblastic leukaemia*)
Blasts demonstrated to be megakaryoblasts, for example by ultrastructural cytochemistry showing the presence of platelet peroxidase or by immunological cell marker studies showing the presence of platelet antigens

M0 (*AML with minimal evidence of myeloid differentiation*)
Peroxidase and SBB positive in < 3% of blasts but blasts demonstrated to be myeloid by immunophenotyping

BM, bone marrow; NEC, non-erythroid cells; PB, peripheral blood; SBB, Sudan black B.
* Lysozyme in serum or urine elevated threefold compared with normal.
† Positive for naphthol AS acetate esterase activity, with activity being inhibited by fluoride.

Table 9.5 The World Health Organization (WHO) classification of acute myeloid leukaemia (AML) [76].

AML and myelodysplastic syndromes, therapy-related
Alkylating agent-related
Epipodophyllotoxin-related
Other types

AML with recurrent cytogenetic/genetic abnormalities
AML with t(8;21)(q22;q22), *AML1(CBFA)-ETO* fusion gene
Acute promyelocytic leukaemia (AML with t(15;17)(q22;q11–12) and *PML-RARA* fusion gene or variants with *RARA* rearrangement)
AML with abnormal bone marrow eosinophils (inv(16)(p13q22) or t(16;16)(p13;q11), *CBFB-MYH11* fusion gene)
AML with 11q23 (*MLL*) rearrangement

*AML with multilineage myelodysplasia**
With prior myelodysplastic or myelodysplastic/myeloproliferative syndrome
Without prior myelodysplastic syndrome

AML not otherwise categorized
AML minimally differentiated
AML without maturation
AML with maturation
Acute myelomonocytic leukaemia
Acute monocytic leukaemia
Acute erythroid leukaemia
Acute megakaryocytic leukaemia
Acute basophilic leukaemia
Acute panmyelosis with myelofibrosis

* Defined as dysplastic features in more than 50% of cells in two or more cell lines.

Fig. 9.12 Peripheral blood film in acute myeloid leukaemia (AML) without maturation (FAB type M1 AML). The blast cells have a fine chromatin pattern; they resemble lymphoblasts in having small nucleoli and a high nucleocytoplasmic ratio; in this patient only occasional blast cells had fine azurophilic granules but myeloperoxidase, Sudan black B (SBB) and chloroacetate esterase (CAE) were positive in a high percentage of cells.

Fig. 9.13 Peripheral blood film in acute myeloid leukaemia with maturation (FAB type M2 AML) showing leukaemic cells that are maturing beyond the blast stage. Both cells are promyelocytes, one with a nucleus of abnormal shape. Differentiation in M2 AML can be neutrophilic, eosinophilic, basophilic or any combination of these.

Fig. 9.14 Peripheral blood films of two patients with acute hypergranular promyelocytic leukaemia (FAB type M3 AML) showing: (a) hypergranular promyelocytes, one of which has a giant granule. *Continued p. 416*

(a)

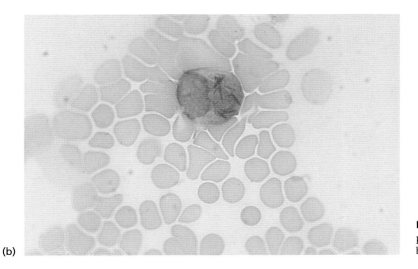

(b)

Fig. 9.14 *Continued* (b) a promyelocyte with few granules but stacks of Auer rods.

Fig. 9.15 Peripheral blood film in the hypogranular or microgranular variant of acute promyelocytic leukaemia (M3 variant AML) showing cells with characteristic bilobed nuclei; only occasional cells have granules visible by light microscopy but despite this there was strong cytoplasmic positivity with Sudan black B (SBB), myeloperoxidase and chloroacetate esterase (CAE).

Fig. 9.16 Peripheral blood film of a patient with acute myelomonocytic leukaemia (FAB type M4 AML) showing one myeloblast and two monoblasts; the monoblasts are large cells with lobulated nuclei, a fine lacy chromatin pattern, several nucleoli per nucleus and voluminous finely granulated cytoplasm whereas the myeloblast is smaller with a higher nucleocytoplasmic ratio. In M4 AML the granulocytic differentiation may be neutrophilic, eosinophilic (see Fig. 9.17) or basophilic.

Fig. 9.17 Peripheral blood film in acute myelomonocytic leukaemia with eosinophilia (FAB type M4 Eo AML) showing a myeloblast, a monocyte and an eosinophil myelocyte in which some granules have basophilic staining characteristics. Courtesy of Dr D. Swirsky, Leeds.

Fig. 9.18 Peripheral blood film in acute monoblastic leukaemia (FAB type M5a AML) showing a monoblast with a non-lobulated nucleus and a vesicular nucleolus. Monoblasts are usually strongly positive for non-specific esterase reactions, such as α-naphthyl acetate esterase (ANAE), and may have a few myeloperoxidase and Sudan black B (SBB)-positive granules.

Fig. 9.19 Peripheral blood film in acute monocytic leukaemia (FAB type M5b AML) showing one promonocyte and one monocyte; the promonocyte has moderately basophilic cytoplasm which is granulated and vacuolated; promonocytes are positive with Sudan black B (SBB), myeloperoxidase and non-specific esterase reactions.

stain, for the easy identification of acute myelomonocytic (M4) leukaemia. When there is no cytological or cytochemical evidence of myeloid differentiation, immunophenotypic analysis is essential to distinguish AML with minimal evidence of myeloid differentiation (M0 AML) from ALL [74]. Whenever resources permit, all cases of suspected AML should have cytogenetic analysis performed. Selective molecular genetic analysis is indicated to detect all good prognosis genetic abnormalities (*AML1-ETO*, *PML-RARA* and *MYH11-CBFB* fusion genes) and to detect poor prognosis genetic abnormalities that might need to be considered in planning treatment (e.g. *BCR-ABL* fusion). The accurate diagnosis of acute

Fig. 9.20 Peripheral blood film in acute erythroleukaemia (FAB type M6 AML) showing a circulating nucleated red blood cell (NRBC), which is megaloblastic.

Fig. 9.21 Peripheral blood film in acute megakaryoblastic leukaemia (FAB type M7 AML) showing a neutrophil and two blast cells; the blasts have no cytological features that permit their identification as megakaryoblasts but they expressed platelet-associated antigens detectable on immunophenotyping; the giant hypogranular platelet adjacent to the neutrophil is the only clue that this leukaemia may be of megakaryocyte lineage.

promyelocytic leukaemia is required urgently since specific treatment (all-*trans* retinoic acid) is needed. This is often possible on the basis of cytology but, if there is any doubt, fluorescence *in situ* hybridization (FISH) or analysis of the distribution of PML protein within the nucleus is needed [75].

Acute basophil leukaemia

Acute basophil leukaemia is a rare type of AML that is recognized as a specific category in the WHO but not in the FAB classification.

Blood film and count

There may be blast cells or mature basophils of blast cells alone. Some cases can be recognized cytologically because of characteristic basophil granules (Fig. 9.22). Others need ultrastructural examination.

Differential diagnosis

The differential diagnosis includes other AML in which blast cells have large granules with basophilic staining characteristics, particularly mast cell leukaemia and to a lesser extent acute hypergranular promyelocytic leukaemia. The granules in the latter condition are often reddish-purple rather than being deep purple.

Other tests

Cytochemical stains are useful. Cytogenetic and molecular genetic analysis are indicated. If t(9;22) or a *BCR-ABL* fusion gene is found, the possibility that the case represents transformation of CGL should be considered.

Table 9.6 Typical immunophenotypic findings in acute myeloid leukaemia, according to French–American–British (FAB) category (expression is on the surface membrane unless otherwise specified).

Type of leukaemia	Immunophenotype	
M0	Expression of some or all of CD13, CD33, CD65, CD117 and MPO*; variable expression of HLA-DR and CD34; expression of TdT† and CD7 in a minority of cases; CD56 may be expressed	Often express CD34, TdT, HLA-DR and CD7
M1		
M2		Expression of CD15
M3		CD34, HLA-DR and TdT usually negative; CD2 is expressed in a minority
M4		Expression of CD15 and CD11b; frequent expression of CD4, CD14, CD16, CD24 and CD64
M5		
M6		Expression of CD71, glycophorin and spectrin
M7		Expression of CD41, CD42a, CD42b and CD61

* Myeloperoxidase (cytoplasmic expression).
† Terminal deoxynucleotidyl transferase (nuclear expression).

Fig. 9.22 Peripheral blood film from a patient with acute basophilic leukaemia. Courtesy of Robyn Wells, Brisbane.

Mast cell leukaemia

Mast cell leukaemia is a rare disease which may occur *de novo* or as a complication of systemic mastocytosis. A mast cell leukaemia or mixed mast cell/basophil leukaemia can also occur as a terminal phase of CGL [77]. Since the mast cell is derived from a haemopoietic stem cell, mast cell leukaemia should be regarded as a variant of AML. It should be noted, however, that the majority of cases of acute leukaemia supervening in systemic mastocytosis are not mast cell leukaemia but other types of AML.

Blood film and count

Normal mast cells have a small oval nucleus that is not obscured by the purple granules that pack the cytoplasm (see Fig. 3.132). In mast cell leukaemia (Fig. 9.23), some neoplastic cells may resemble normal mast cells, while others have larger nuclei or nuclei that are bilobed or multilobed. Granules vary in colour from red to dark purple and may or may not obscure the nucleus. They may fuse into homogeneous masses. Less mature cells may have scanty granules and a nucleus that is oval or kidney-shaped with nucleoli [78,79].

Differential diagnosis

The differential diagnosis includes other leukaemias

Fig. 9.23 Peripheral blood film of a patient with acute mast cell leukaemia showing two mast cells. Courtesy of Miss Desley Scott and Dr I. Bunce, Brisbane.

Table 9.7 Some cytochemical tests useful in distinguishing between basophils, mast cells and hypergranular promyelocytes.

Cell type	Basophiloblast	Basophil	Mast cell	Hypergranular promyelocyte
Myeloperoxidase	–	– or +*	–	+++
Sudan black B	–	– or +	– or +	+++
Chloroacetate esterase	–	–†	+++	+++
Toluidine blue (metachromatic staining)	– or +	+++	+++	–

– Negative; + weakly positive; +++ strongly positive.
* Positive in basophil promyelocytes to metamyelocytes.
† Positive in basophil promyelocytes to metamyelocytes and may be positive in leukaemic basophils [80].

with hypergranular neoplastic cells, specifically hypergranular promyelocytic leukaemia (M3 AML) and basophilic leukaemia. The presence of Auer rods suggests a diagnosis of acute hypergranular promyelocytic leukaemia.

Further tests

Bone marrow aspiration and cytochemistry (Table 9.7) are useful in confirming the diagnosis. Mast cells can also be distinguished from basophils by electron microscopy which shows basophils to have granules that are either of a uniform consistency or finely particulate whereas mast cell granules are heterogeneous and contain whorled, scrolled, lamellate and

crystalline structures. Serum tryptase is expected to be elevated but it can also be elevated in other types of acute myeloid leukaemia.

Acute myelofibrosis

Acute myelofibrosis is a specific clinicopathological presentation of AML, mainly acute megakaryoblastic leukaemia (M7 AML), consequent on bone marrow fibrosis, which is reactive to the leukaemic infiltration. In the WHO classification, cases of acute leukaemia with bone marrow fibrosis in which differentiation is not largely megakaryocytic are designated acute panmyelosis with myelofibrosis [76]. Acute megakaryoblastic leukaemia is also a recognized WHO category. Clinical features result from anaemia and cytopenia. There is no splenomegaly.

Blood film and count

The blood film shows pancytopenia and sometimes occasional blast cells. There is little poikilocytosis.

Differential diagnosis

The differential diagnosis includes aplastic anaemia, acute panmyelosis with myelofibrosis and other causes of pancytopenia and bone marrow fibrosis.

Further tests

Bone marrow aspiration is often unsuccessful or yields an undiagnostic specimen so that bone marrow trephine biopsy is essential for diagnosis.

Transient abnormal myelopoiesis of Down's syndrome

Transient abnormal myelopoiesis or transient myeloproliferative disorder of Down's syndrome occurs in neonates (and during intrauterine life). Cytogenetic and molecular evidence indicate that this disorder is actually spontaneously remitting AML, often acute megakaryoblastic leukaemia [81,82]. Remission occurs within a few weeks but, in a significant percentage of affected infants, AML develops at 1–2 years of age.

Blood film and count

The blood film cannot be distinguished from that of AML. The WBC may be moderately to greatly elevated with a high percentage of blast cells. There may be anaemia and thrombocytopenia.

Differential diagnosis

The differential diagnosis is congenital leukaemia of other types.

Further tests

Cytogenetic analysis is indicated in order to both confirm Down's syndrome by demonstration of trisomy 21 and to exclude cytogenetic abnormalities that may be associated with other cases of congenital leukaemias. Molecular genetic analysis is indicated since a mutation in the *GATA1* gene is uniformly present [82]. Otherwise there are no laboratory investigations that will distinguish transient abnormal myelopoiesis from other forms of AML. In the absence of molecular analysis, this is achieved only by being aware of this disorder and observing its clinical course.

The myelodysplastic syndromes and myelodysplastic/myeloproliferative disorders

The MDS are a morphologically heterogeneous group of conditions that result from the proliferation of a clone of neoplastic haemopoietic cells showing abnormalities of proliferation and maturation. Haemopoiesis is functionally ineffective and morphologically dysplastic. MDS is potentially preleukaemic although some patients die from complications of cytopenia without evolution to AML. MDS may arise *de novo* or follow exposure to mutagenic agents such as ionizing radiation, benzene and anti-cancer agents including alkylating agents. The FAB group have categorized MDS as shown in Table 9.8 and the WHO group as shown in Table 9.9. The WHO classification of MDS is hierarchical with cases first being assigned, if appropriate, to the category of MDS with isolated 5q– and then subsequently to other categories, as shown in Table 9.9. Therapy-related cases should be specifically noted. The WHO classification also includes a category designated myelodysplastic/myeloproliferative disorders (Table 9.10), with CMML being assigned to this category rather than to MDS.

Blood count and film

The peripheral blood film usually shows features suggesting the diagnosis (Figs 9.24–9.26). Most patients are anaemic with red cells being normochromic and either normocytic or macrocytic. In patients with sideroblastic erythropoiesis, there is a minor population of hypochromic microcytes and Pappenheimer bodies are present. Red cells may also show anisocytosis, poikilocytosis and basophilic stippling. There may be leucocytosis or leucopenia. Leucocytosis is

Table 9.8 The French–American–British (FAB) classification of the myelodysplastic syndromes [71,75].

Category	Peripheral blood		Bone marrow
Refractory anaemia or refractory cytopenia*	Anaemia, *blasts $\leq$ 1%, monocytes $\leq 1 \times 10^9/l$	AND	Blasts < 5%, ringed sideroblasts $\leq$ 15% of erythroblasts
Refractory anaemia with ringed sideroblasts	Anaemia, blasts $\leq$ 1%, monocytes $\leq 1 \times 10^9/l$	AND	Blasts < 5%, ringed sideroblasts > 15% of erythroblasts
Refractory anaemia with excess of blasts (RAEB)	Anaemia, monocytes $\leq 1 \times 10^9/l$ — Blasts > 1% BUT Blasts < 5%	OR / AND	Blasts $\geq$ 5% / Blasts $\leq$ 20%
Chronic myelomonocytic leukaemia (CMML)	Monocyte count $> 1 \times 10^9/l$, granulocytes often increased, blasts < 5%		Blasts up to 20%, promonocytes often increased
Refractory anaemia with excess of blasts in transformation (RAEB-T)	Blasts $\geq$ 5%	OR Auer rods in blasts in blood or marrow / OR	Blasts > 20% BUT Blasts < 30%

* Or in the case of refractory cytopenia either neutropenia or thrombocytopenia.

Table 9.9 The World Health Organization (WHO) classification of the myelodysplastic syndromes [83].

Disease	Peripheral blood findings	Bone marrow findings
MDS associated with isolated del(5q)	Anaemia, platelet count usually normal or elevated, < 5% blasts	Megakaryocytes in normal or increased numbers but with hypolobated nuclei, < 5% blasts, no Auer rods, 5q– as sole cytogenetic abnormality
Refractory anaemia (RA)*	Anaemia, blasts rarely seen and always less than 1%	Dysplasia[†] confined to erythroid lineage, < 5% blasts, < 15% ringed sideroblasts
Refractory anaemia with ringed sideroblasts (RARS)*	Anaemia, no blasts	Dysplasia confined to erythroid lineage, < 5% blasts, $\geq$ 15% ringed sideroblasts
Refractory cytopenia with multilineage dysplasia (RCMD)[‡]	Cytopenias (bicytopenia or pancytopenia), no or rare blasts, no Auer rods, $< 1 \times 10^9/l$ monocytes	Dysplasia in $\geq$ 10% of the cells of two or more myeloid cell lineages, < 5% blasts, < 15% ringed sideroblasts, no Auer rods
Refractory cytopenia with multilineage dysplasia and ringed sideroblasts (RCMD-RS)[‡]	Cytopenias (bicytopenia or pancytopenia), no or rare blasts, no Auer rods, $< 1 \times 10^9/l$ monocytes	Dysplasia in $\geq$ 10% of the cells of two or more myeloid cell lineages, < 5% blasts, $\geq$ 15% ringed sideroblasts, no Auer rods
Refractory anaemia with excess blasts-1 (RAEB-1)[‡]	Cytopenias, < 5% blasts, no Auer rods, $< 1 \times 10^9/l$ monocytes	Unilineage or multilineage dysplasia, 5–9% blasts, no Auer rods
Refractory anaemia with excess blasts-2 (RAEB-2)[‡]	Cytopenias, 5–19% blasts, Auer rods sometimes present, $< 1 \times 10^9/l$ monocytes	Unilineage or multilineage dysplasia, 10–19% blasts, Auer rods sometimes present
Myelodysplastic syndrome-unclassified (MDS-U)[‡]	Cytopenias, no or rare blasts, no Auer rods	Unilineage dysplasia, < 5% blasts No Auer rods

* By definition, an isolated 5q– is not present.
[†] A lineage is regarded as dysplastic if at least 10% of cells of that lineage show dysplastic features.
[‡] If cases are therapy-related, this should be specified and it should be further specified whether cases are alkylating agent-related (the majority) or topoisomerase II-interactive-drug-related (a small minority); therapy-related cases are categorized with therapy-related AML.

Table 9.10 The World Health Organization (WHO) classification of the myeloproliferative and myelodysplastic/myeloproliferative disorders [84].

Myeloproliferative diseases
Chronic myelogenous leukaemia, Philadelphia chromosome positive (t(9;22)(q34;q11), *BCR-ABL*)
Chronic neutrophilic leukaemia
Chronic eosinophilic leukaemia/hypereosinophilic syndrome*
Chronic idiopathic myelofibrosis
Polycythaemia vera
Essential thrombocythaemia
Myeloproliferative disorders, unclassifiable

Myelodysplastic/myeloproliferative disorders
Chronic myelomonocytic leukaemia
Atypical chronic myelogenous leukaemia
Juvenile myelomonocytic leukaemia
Other myelodysplastic/myeloproliferative disorder, unclassifiable

* Cases with an increase in blast cells or demonstrable clonality of myeloid cells should be classified as eosinophilic leukaemia rather than as idiopathic hypereosinophilic syndrome; a hypereosinophilic syndrome should not be classified as eosinophilic leukaemia unless there is some evidence that it is leukaemic in nature.

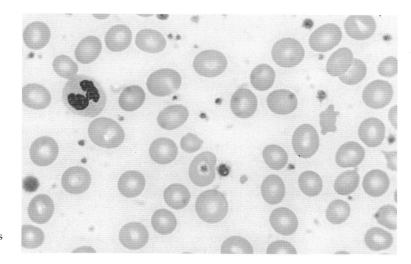

Fig. 9.24 Peripheral blood film of a patient with a myelodysplastic syndrome (MDS)—refractory anaemia (FAB classification), showing anisocytosis, macrocytosis and one poikilocyte; the neutrophil is hypogranular.

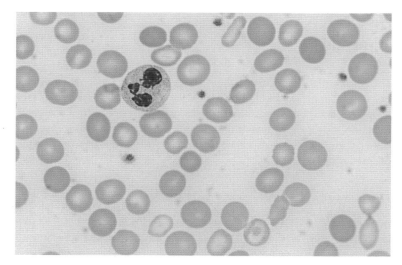

Fig. 9.25 Peripheral blood film of a patient with myelodysplastic syndrome (MDS)—refractory anaemia with ring sideroblasts (FAB classification), showing one target cell and several hypochromic microcytes; the remainder of the erythrocytes are normochromic cells which are either normocytic or macrocytic; MCV was 103 fl.

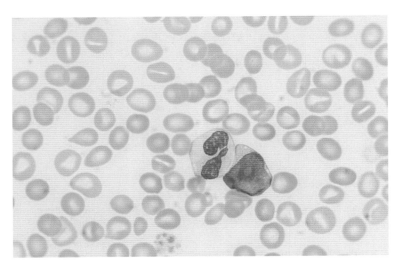

Fig. 9.26 Peripheral blood film of a patient with a myelodysplastic syndrome (MDS)—refractory anaemia with excess of blasts (FAB classification), showing a myeloblast and a hypogranular neutrophil; the red cells show anisocytosis and poikilocytosis including teardrop cells and stomatocytes.

usually attributable to monocytosis, sometimes with associated neutrophilia. An increase of eosinophils or basophils is very uncommon. Blast cells may be present and they may contain Auer rods. There may be occasional promyelocytes, myelocytes or nucleated red blood cells (NRBC).

Neutrophils commonly show dysplastic features, particularly hypogranularity (see Fig. 9.26) and the acquired Pelger–Huët anomaly (see Fig. 3.64). Detection of neutrophil hypogranularity requires that the blood film be correctly stained; a useful check is that at least some of the platelets are pale blue with lilac granules. The platelet count is often reduced but in a minority of patients it is increased. Platelets may show dysplastic features such as large size and hypogranularity.

Differential diagnosis

The differential diagnosis includes other causes of macrocytic anaemia and cytopenia, AML and non-neoplastic conditions causing dysplasia such as HIV infection, exposure to heavy metals and the direct rather than long-term effects of the administration of anti-cancer drugs.

Further tests

Bone marrow aspiration with cytochemical stains is often necessary for diagnosis and is always neces-sary for further classification (see Tables 9.8–9.10) and for determining prognosis. Either an MPO or a SBB stain is necessary for the reliable detection of Auer rods and a Perls' stain is essential for identification of ring sideroblasts. When cytological evidence is insufficient for a firm diagnosis, cytogenetic analysis or other investigations to establish clonality of haemopoietic cells may be essential for diagnosis. Cytogenetic analysis is important for determining prognosis and is essential for applying the WHO classification. Trephine biopsy can be useful, particularly if the bone marrow is hypocellular or if a poor aspirate is obtained because of fibrosis.

Chronic myeloid leukaemias

The chronic myeloid leukaemias differ from AML in that there is effective maturation with production of granulocytes. The majority of cases of chronic myeloid leukaemia represent the specific entity, variously referred to as chronic granulocytic leukaemia (CGL), chronic myelogenous leukaemia or chronic myeloid leukaemia, that is associated with a translocation giving rise to the Philadelphia (Ph) chromosome. The term 'chronic granulocytic leukaemia' has the advantage that it is unambiguous whereas the term 'chronic myeloid leukaemia' (CML) is sometimes used to refer to this specific Ph-positive entity and is sometimes used more generally. Although the term 'chronic granulocytic leukaemia' is currently falling out of favour it is used in this book to avoid ambiguity. Other categories of chronic myeloid leukaemia include chronic neutrophilic leukaemia and chronic eosinophilic leukaemia. All these are classified as myeloproliferative disorders in the WHO classification. Other chronic myeloid leukaemias—specifically aCML, CMML and JMML—are assigned by the WHO group to the myelodysplastic/myeloproliferative group of disorders (see above).

Chronic granulocytic leukaemia

CGL is mainly a disease of adults characterized clinically by anaemia, splenomegaly and hepatomegaly.

Blood film and count

The WBC is elevated, often markedly so. The differential count (Fig. 9.27) [85] and blood film (Fig. 9.28) are very characteristic with myelocytes and neutrophils being the most frequent cells. In patients with a very high WBC, the blast cells may be as high

Fig. 9.27 A diagrammatic representation of the typical differential count in chronic granulocytic leukaemia (CGL) based on 1500 cell differential counts in 50 patients with Philadelphia-positive CGL [85]. BL, blasts; P, promyelocytes; MY, myelocytes; ME, metamyelocytes; N, neutrophils; B, basophils; E, eosinophils; L, lymphocytes; MO, monocytes.

as 15% but nevertheless blasts remain less frequent than promyelocytes; similarly, promyelocytes are less frequent than myelocytes. There is an increase in the absolute basophil count in almost every case and an increase in the absolute eosinophil count in more than 90% of cases. Some eosinophils may have a proportion of granules with basophilic staining characteristics. Monocytes are increased, but not in proportion to neutrophils. Some NRBC are present. Dysplastic features are minor. The platelet count is usually normal or increased but in a minority of cases it is decreased. Platelet size is increased. Circulating megakaryocytes, mainly almost bare nuclei, are sometimes present.

Occasional patients with CGL have striking cyclical changes in WBC with a periodicity of 50–70 days, and with the WBC varying from frankly leukaemic levels to almost normal. All myeloid cells participate in the cycles.

A minority of patients have bone marrow fibrosis at presentation and the typical peripheral blood features of myelofibrosis are then superimposed on the features of CGL.

Most patients with CGL present with symptoms and well-established disease. However, an increasingly large proportion of patients are diagnosed incidentally while still asymptomatic. Occasional patients who have developed the disease while being monitored haematologically have allowed the early stages of the disease to be defined. The first detectable peripheral blood features are an increase in the basophil count, thrombocytosis and a low NAP score. Following this, the neutrophil count and the WBC rise and small numbers of immature cells appear. With the progressive rise of WBC that follows, the percentage of immature cells steadily increases.

CGL terminates in myelofibrosis or in blast transformation (see below), often preceded by an accelerated phase.

Differential diagnosis

The differential diagnosis includes reactive neutrophilia, other types of chronic myeloid leukaemia and the early stages of polycythaemia vera and essential thrombocythaemia. Features useful in distinguishing CGL from reactive neutrophilia are

(a)

(b)

Fig. 9.28 Peripheral blood film in Philadelphia-positive chronic granulocytic leukaemia (CGL) showing: (a) a promyelocyte, an eosinophil myelocyte, three basophils and a number of neutrophils and band forms; and (b) a promyelocyte, several myelocytes, neutrophil band forms and neutrophils; the presence of a binucleate neutrophil is relatively uncommon.

shown in Table 9.3 but, in practice, diagnostic difficulty only rises in early cases of CGL.

Further tests

Cytogenetic analysis is indicated to confirm the diagnosis. The great majority of cases of CGL are associated with the presence of the Philadelphia chromosome, an abbreviated chromosome 22 resulting from a t(9;22)(q34;q11) translocation. A minority of cases of CGL that are Philadelphia-negative and lack the classical microscopically detectable translocation nevertheless have a related DNA rearrangement (a

BCR-ABL fusion gene). Such cases, which are clinically and haematologically indistinguishable from the Philadelphia-positive cases, should be classified as Philadelphia-negative CGL. When facilities permit, molecular analysis for *BCR-ABL* should also be performed in patients with t(9;22) detected by cytogenetic analysis since identification of the specific breakpoints facilitates later monitoring of minimal residual disease. FISH analysis using *BCR* and *ABL* probes is also a useful technique, particularly during follow-up.

The NAP score is reduced in more than 90% of cases of chronic phase CGL but its importance in

Table 9.11 Some haematological abnormalities that may be detected during the accelerated phase of chronic granulocytic leukaemia.

Red cells and precursors
Anaemia (including that due to red cell aplasia in which reticulocytes are very infrequent or absent), macrocytosis, marked poikilocytosis (may be consequent on bone marrow fibrosis), vacuolated erythroblasts (PAS-positive), hypochromia and microcytosis

White cells and precursors
Refractory leucocytosis, increasing basophil count, disappearance of eosinophilia, increasing monocytosis, acquired Pelger–Huët anomaly of neutrophils or eosinophils, hypogranular neutrophils, vacuolated neutrophils, pseudo-Chédiak–Higashi anomaly (giant granules) of neutrophils and precursors, binuclearity and other dysplastic features of neutrophil precursors, increasing blast cell percentage with decreasing percentage of more mature cells, Auer rods in blast cells

Platelets and megakaryocytes
Thrombocytopenia, thrombocytosis, micromegakaryocytes, bare megakaryocyte nuclei

General
Pancytopenia (may be consequent on refractory splenomegaly or, rarely, bone marrow necrosis)

PAS, periodic acid–Schiff.

diagnosis has decreased with the more ready availability of cytogenetic and molecular analysis.

Chronic granulocytic leukaemia in accelerated phase and acute transformation

In the majority of patients with CGL a chronic phase, which lasts for weeks, months or years, is followed by blast transformation. This is sometimes preceded by an accelerated phase. Clinical features of disease evolution are pallor and bruising, increasing hepatomegaly and splenomegaly, lymphadenopathy or, less often, soft tissue tumours, bone pain and refractoriness to treatment.

Blood film and count

During the accelerated phase there may be anaemia, leucocytosis, thrombocytopenia, thrombocytosis, a rising basophil count, an increasing blast cell percentage and the appearance of dysplastic features (Table 9.11). Blast transformation may occur without any warning or be preceded by an accelerated phase. Blast transformation is lymphoblastic in about one-quarter of cases and myeloid or mixed lymphoblastic and myeloid in the remainder (Table 9.12). Myeloid transformation is often megakaryoblastic or mixed myeloblastic/megakaryoblastic. A patient who remits from one blast crisis (e.g. lymphoblastic)

Table 9.12 Types of transformation that can occur in chronic granulocytic leukaemia.

Myeloblastic transformation
Lymphoblastic transformation
Megakaryocytic transformation (with micromegakaryocytes and thrombocytosis)
Megakaryoblastic transformation
Erythroblastic transformation [86] and acquired sideroblastic erythropoiesis
Monoblastic transformation [87]
Basophil blast transformation [88]
Mast cell and mixed basophil/mast cell transformation [77]
Eosinophil blast transformation [89] including M4Eo type of transformation
Hypergranular promyelocytic transformation [90]
Transformations with various mixtures of cell types
Acute myelofibrosis

may subsequently suffer a second blast crisis with cells of different lineage (e.g. megakaryoblastic).

Differential diagnosis

Patients may present already in blast transformation in which case the differential diagnosis is acute leukaemia. Patients presenting in accelerated phase can also simulate atypical chronic myeloid leukaemia or other myeloid neoplasms. In patients presenting in chronic phase, the likely diagnosis is usually readily evident from the clinical and haematological features.

Further tests

Bone marrow aspiration is indicated unless there are large numbers of blasts in the peripheral blood. Cytogenetic analysis is indicated since cytogenetic evolution often precedes or occurs simultaneously with the development of acceleration or acute transformation. Immunophenotyping of blast cells may be useful since there is more likelihood of a response to treatment in lymphoblastic transformation.

Atypical chronic myeloid leukaemia

Atypical CML (aCML) is a myeloproliferative/myelodysplastic condition, designated as such in the WHO classification. It is a disease of adults. The clinical features are similar to those of CGL.

Blood film and count

Patients are anaemic and have a moderate to marked elevation in the WBC. On average, patients with aCML present with a lower Hb and a lower WBC than patients with CGL. Peripheral blood features (Fig. 9.29) differ from those of CGL in that monocytosis and thrombocytopenia are more common while basophilia and eosinophilia are less common. Granulocyte precursors are present. Dysplastic features are common. In comparison with CMML, there are more granulocyte precursors in the peripheral

(a)

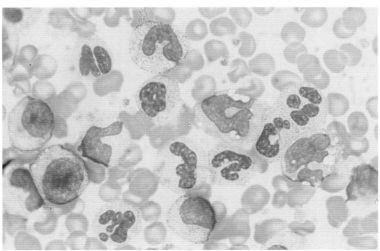

(b)

Fig. 9.29 Peripheral blood film in atypical chronic myeloid leukaemia (aCML) showing: (a) a normal neutrophil, a macropolycyte, a monocyte and a somewhat immature monocyte; there is one large platelet (b) numerous neutrophils, band forms, monocytes and hypogranular myelocytes.

Table 9.13 World Health Organization (WHO) criteria for diagnosing atypical chronic myeloid leukaemia (aCML) and chronic myelomonocytic leukaemia (CMML) and for distinguishing between them [91,92].

	aCML*	CMML*
Peripheral blood monocytes	Less than 10% of leucocytes	Greater than $1 \times 10^9/l$, almost always greater than 10% of leucocytes
Peripheral blood immature granulocytes (promyelocytes, myelocytes and metamyelocytes)	At least 10% of leucocytes	Usually less than 10% of leucocytes
Dysplasia	Granulocytic dysplasia	Dysplasia in at least one myeloid lineage or alternative supporting criteria must be met[†]

* In both conditions t(9;22) and *BCR-ABL* are absent and in both peripheral blood blast cells plus promonocytes are less than 20%.
[†] If there is not dysplasia in at least one lineage either a clonal cytogenetic abnormality must be present **or** the monocytosis must persist for at least 3 months **and** all other causes of monocytosis must be excluded.

blood, monocytes are less prominent and dysplasia is more prominent. The WHO diagnostic criteria are shown, in comparison with those of CMML, in Table 9.13.

Atypical CML may terminate in blast transformation.

Differential diagnosis

The differential diagnosis includes leukaemoid reactions and other types of CML.

Further tests

Bone marrow aspiration and cytogenetic analysis may be useful in diagnosis, e.g. for assessing erythroid and megakaryocytic hyperplasia and to exclude a diagnosis of AML. However, generally the peripheral blood features are more important than the bone marrow in categorizing the myelodysplastic/myeloproliferative syndromes. The Philadelphia chromosome is not detected but other clonal cytogenetic abnormalities may be present. The *BCR-ABL* fusion gene is absent. The NAP score is low in the majority of patients but elevated in a minority.

Chronic myelomonocytic leukaemia

CMML is classified by the FAB group as MDS and by the WHO group as a myeloproliferative/myelodysplastic disorder. It is a disease of the elderly, characterized by anaemia, hepatospleno-

megaly and, occasionally, significant tissue infiltration by leukaemic monocytes.

Blood film and count

The blood film (Fig. 9.30) shows monocytosis and most patients also have anaemia and neutrophilia. As defined by the FAB group (see Table 9.8), the monocyte count must be greater than $1 \times 10^9/l$. The monocytes may be somewhat immature with cytoplasmic basophilia or nucleoli. Granulocyte precursors may be present but they are usually less than 5% of white cells whereas in aCML there are significant numbers of immature granulocytes, often over 15% and almost always over 5%; the FAB group have suggested, as one of the criteria for CMML, that immature granulocytes be less than 10% of circulating leucocytes. Basophilia and eosinophilia are quite uncommon, except in association with certain specific cytogenetic abnormalities. Bone marrow blast cells are less than 20%. Dysplastic features in other lineages are often but not invariably present. The WHO diagnostic criteria are shown, in comparison with those of aCML, in Table 9.13.

CMML may terminate by evolving into AML.

Differential diagnosis

The differential diagnosis includes reactive conditions, other chronic myeloid leukaemias, MDS and MPD. The response to administration of G-CSF can simulate CMML.

Fig. 9.30 Peripheral blood film in chronic myelomonocytic leukaemia (CMML) showing a hypogranular neutrophil and three abnormal monocytes.

Further tests

Bone marrow aspiration, trephine biopsy and cytogenetic analysis are useful in diagnosis. The Philadelphia chromosome and the *BCR-ABL* fusion gene are not detected but other clonal cytogenetic abnormalities may be present. Patients with the clinical picture of CMML with eosinophilia may be found to have t(5;12)(q33;p13).

Juvenile myelomonocytic leukaemia

Children may develop typical Philadelphia-positive CGL although it is rare before adolescence. Children below the age of 5 years may also develop a distinctive, Philadelphia-negative condition previously known as juvenile CML and now usually designated juvenile myelomonocytic leukaemia (JMML). JMML encompasses also the childhood monosomy 7 syndrome. Usual clinical features are anaemia, splenomegaly, sometimes hepatomegaly, lymphadenopathy and a rash. JMML is more prevalent among children with neurofibromatosis or Noonan's syndrome.

Blood film and count

The blood count shows anaemia, neutrophilia and monocytosis. In comparison with CGL, the WBC is usually lower and myelocytes are less frequent, while monocytosis, thrombocytopenia and circulating NRBC are common features. Monocytosis is

particularly important in diagnosis since it is almost always present. Dysplastic features are present (Fig. 9.31). Diagnostic criteria proposed by the WHO are shown in Table 9.14. A high blast count, large numbers of NRBC and a low platelet count are indicative of a worse prognosis [94].

The disease may terminate in acute transformation but slow progression and death without transformation is more usual.

Differential diagnosis

The differential diagnosis includes reactive conditions that can cause monocytosis and dysplasia in infants and young children, particularly viral and bacterial infections (see p. 409). It should be noted that children with Noonan's syndrome may develop a spontaneously remitting condition that resembles JMML as well as having an increased incidence of JMML.

Further tests

Bone marrow aspiration and cytogenetic analysis are indicated. Cytogenetic analysis is often normal at presentation but monosomy 7, trisomy 8 or other clonal cytogenetic abnormality may be present or may appear during disease evolution. The NAP score may be high, normal or low. Commonly associated abnormalities include features associated with fetal haemopoiesis, specifically high haemoglobin F, low

Fig. 9.31 Peripheral blood film in juvenile myelomonocytic leukaemia (JMML) showing several neutrophils, a blast, a promyelocyte and several very dysplastic cells, which may be of monocyte lineage. Courtesy of Dr O. Oakhill and Dr G.R. Standen, Bristol. The patient was a child of 6 months with hepatosplenomegaly, WBC $94 \times 10^9/l$, Hb 10.2 g/dl, platelet count $28 \times 10^9/l$, NAP score 10 and haemoglobin F concentration 11%.

Table 9.14 World Health Organization (WHO) criteria for diagnosing juvenile myelomonocytic leukaemia (JMML) [93].

1. Monocyte count greater than $1 \times 10^9/l$
2. Blasts plus promonocytes less than 20% in peripheral blood and bone marrow
3. No Ph chromosome or *BCR-ABL* fusion gene
4. Two or more of the following:
    Haemoglobin F percentage increased for age
    Immature granulocytes in the peripheral blood
    White cell count greater than $10 \times 10^9/l$
    Clonal chromosomal abnormality present
    Myeloid progenitors hypersensitive to GM-CSF *in vitro*

Ph, Philadelphia chromosome; GM-CSF, granulocyte monocyte colony-stimulating factor.

haemoglobin A_2, low red cell carbonic anhydrase, reduced expression of the red cell I antigen and increased expression of the red cell i antigen. Serum immunoglobulin concentration may be increased. Molecular analysis is indicated if there is any difficulty in diagnosis since mutations are often present in either the *NF1* gene or the *PTP11* gene. *RAS* mutations are also present in 20–30% of children.

Neutrophilic leukaemia

Neutrophilic leukaemia is a rare condition characterized clinically by anaemia, splenomegaly and sometimes hepatomegaly.

Blood film

There is anaemia and a marked neutrophilia with very few circulating immature cells (Fig. 9.32). The WBC is usually of the order of $40–70 \times 10^9/l$. There is no basophilia, eosinophilia or monocytosis. Neutrophils may have both toxic granulation and Döhle bodies [95]. Ring neutrophils are relatively common [96]. Some cases have also had marked dysplastic features [97] although it should be noted that the WHO definition of this condition excludes cases with dysplasia [98]. The disease may terminate in acute transformation.

Differential diagnosis

The differential diagnosis includes reactive neutrophilia (including neutrophilic leukaemoid reaction associated with multiple myeloma or monoclonal gammopathy of undetermined significance) and other chronic leukaemias and myeloproliferative disorders.

Further tests

Bone marrow aspiration and cytogenetic analysis are indicated. The NAP score is usually high. When no clonal cytogenetic abnormality is present, a period of observation may be necessary to make the distinction from reactive neutrophilia.

Fig. 9.32 Peripheral blood film in chronic neutrophilic leukaemia. The neutrophils show 'toxic' granulation and vacuolation. One giant platelet is present. Other neutrophils showed Döhle bodies and macropolycytes were present.

Chronic eosinophilic leukaemia

Eosinophilia, which is sometimes very marked, can be a feature of AML. AML with eosinophilia falls into the FAB M2 or M4 categories and is often referred to as M2Eo or M4Eo AML. There are also cases of leukaemia in which the leukaemic cells are almost exclusively mature eosinophils or both mature and immature cells of eosinophil lineage but with there being fewer than 20% bone marrow blast cells. These cases are referred to either as eosinophilic leukaemia or as chronic eosinophilic leukaemia. The prognosis is variable and is related to the percentage of blast cells and to the extent of tissue damage consequent on the release of eosinophil granule contents. The WHO classification requires that the eosinophil count is greater than $1.5 \times 10^9/l$ and that **either** blast cells are greater than 2% in the blood or greater than 5% in the bone marrow **or** that there is cytogenetic or molecular genetic evidence of clonality [99]. The diagnosis of eosinophilic leukaemia in a significant proportion of cases that could previously only be categorized as having the idiopathic hypereosinophilic syndrome has been made possible by the discovery of the occurrence of a clonal molecular genetic abnormality, a *FIP1L1-PDGFRA* fusion gene, in a significant proportion of such cases [100]. Because of the therapeutic implications of correct diagnosis, eosinophilic leukaemia is dealt with here at greater length than a condition of this rarity would otherwise warrant;

cases with *FIP1L1-PDGFRA* fusion or *PDGFRB* rearrangement are imatinib responsive.

Blood film and count

The blood film (Fig. 9.33) shows mature eosinophils and sometimes also blast cells, promyelocytes and eosinophil myelocytes. The mature eosinophils often show hypogranularity, vacuolation and hypolobulation (Fig. 9.34) but sometimes they are cytologically normal. Eosinophils and eosinophil myelocytes may contain some granules with basophilic staining characteristics. In acute eosinophilic leukaemia, the blast cells and, occasionally, maturing cells may contain Auer rods but these are not seen in chronic eosinophilic leukaemia. Anaemia and thrombocytopenia are common. Neutrophils may be increased in number and often show heavy granulation. The monocyte count may be increased.

Differential diagnosis

The differential diagnosis includes reactive eosinophilia (see p. 406), aCML with eosinophilia, CMML with eosinophilia and idiopathic HES. Idiopathic HES (see p. 407) is only diagnosed if all other causes of eosinophilia are excluded after appropriate investigation. Reactive eosinophilia that can be confused with eosinophilic leukaemia includes that which occasionally occurs in ALL (Fig. 9.35) and non-Hodgkin's lymphoma.

Fig. 9.33 Peripheral blood film in eosinophilic leukaemia showing a blast cell and two vacuolated and partly degranulated eosinophils.

Fig. 9.34 Peripheral blood film in a patient with eosinophilic leukaemia associated with a *FIP1L1-PDGFRA* fusion gene showing eosinophils with varying degrees of degranulation, one of which is non-lobulated.

Fig. 9.35 Peripheral blood film of a patient with acute lymphoblastic leukaemia (ALL) with reactive eosinophilia showing a lymphoblast and a partially degranulated hypolobulated eosinophil.

Further tests

Bone marrow aspiration, cytogenetic analysis and molecular genetic analysis are indicated. The bone marrow should be specifically examined for increased blast cells (either myeloblasts or lymphoblasts), lymphoma cells and abnormal mast cells. If there is doubt as to the diagnosis, a trephine biopsy should also be performed since the features of lymphoma or systemic mastocytosis may be revealed. Cytogenetic analysis has revealed a variety of clonal chromosomal abnormalities, including trisomy 8, 20q–, an isochromosome of 17q and rearrangements involving the long arm of chromosome 5. The recurring cytogenetic abnormality, t(5;12)(q33;p13) leading to a *ETV6-PDGFRB* fusion gene, has been associated both with chronic eosinophilic leukaemia and with aCML with eosinophilia. A number of translocations involving 8p11–12, of which the most common is t(8;13)(p11;q12), are indicative of a pluripotent stem cell disorder presenting as chronic eosinophilic leukaemia, AML or T-lineage lymphoblastic lymphoma. Molecular genetic analysis, either FISH or reverse transcriptase PCR (RT-PCR), should be performed to detect the *FIP1L1-PDGFRA* fusion gene.

It can be useful to perform immunophenotyping of peripheral blood lymphocytes and T-cell receptor analysis, to establish T-cell clonality, in patients in whom there is neither evidence of an underlying cause of reactive eosinophilia nor conclusive morphological or cytogenetic evidence that the eosinophilia represents eosinophilic leukaemia. Many otherwise 'idiopathic' cases represent a response to an aberrant T-cell clone, rather than an eosinophilic leukaemia.

The diagnosis of eosinophilic leukaemia is readily established in those cases in which there is a significant increase in blast cells and other immature cells, dysplasia of other lineages, a clonal cytogenetic abnormality or other evidence of clonality of myeloid cells. A history of preceding myelodysplastic syndrome or the presence of soft tissue tumours composed of immature granulocytic cells also confirms the diagnosis. In cases with predominantly mature eosinophils, the diagnosis can be difficult to establish. The presence of marked morphological abnormalities confined to eosinophils is *not* useful in diagnosis since such abnormalities can be seen also in reactive eosinophilia and in systemic mastocytosis. In some cases, which cannot initially be distinguished from idiopathic HES, only subsequent evolution of the disease confirms the leukaemic nature.

Cases that are found to have the Philadelphia chromosome, a rare occurrence, are best classified as variants of CGL and treated accordingly.

Other chronic myeloproliferative disorders

The major diseases classified as chronic myeloproliferative disorders are the chronic myeloid leukaemia (see above), polycythaemia rubra vera (see p. 364), essential thrombocythaemia (see p. 375), chronic idiopathic myelofibrosis and systemic mastocytosis.

Chronic idiopathic myelofibrosis

Chronic idiopathic myelofibrosis or myelofibrosis with myeloid metaplasia is a haematological neoplasm characterized by extramedullary haemopoiesis together with bone marrow fibrosis that is reactive to the underlying proliferation of myeloid cells.

Blood film and count

The blood film is leucoerythroblastic and shows anisocytosis and poikilocytosis, particularly the presence of teardrop poikilocytes (Fig. 9.36). In the early stages of the disease there may be leucocytosis and thrombocytosis. Later in the course there is pancytopenia. Often there are some giant platelets and occasional circulating micromegakaryocytes or megakaryocyte nuclei. In multivariate analysis, the severity of the anaemia and the degree of elevation of the WBC are of independent prognostic significance [101].

Therapy with cytoreductive agents such as hydroxycarbamide leads to macrocytosis, stomatocytosis and reduction of the WBC and platelet count. Treatment with thalidomide may increase the WBC, Hb and platelet count [102].

Differential diagnosis

The differential diagnosis includes other causes of a leucoerythroblastic blood film and other causes of pancytopenia (see Tables 6.19 and 6.30).

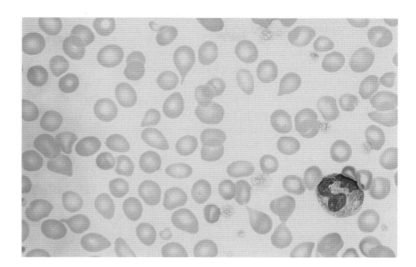

Fig. 9.36 Peripheral blood film in chronic idiopathic myelofibrosis showing anisocytosis and poikilocytosis with prominent teardrop poikilocytes.

Further tests

A bone marrow trephine biopsy is required for diagnosis. Cytogenetic analysis can be useful, particularly to exclude the presence of the Philadelphia chromosome. A clonal cytogenetic abnormality is sometimes demonstrated. Molecular genetic analysis shows a mutation in *JAK2* is present in a significant minority of patients.

Systemic mastocytosis

Since the mast cell is derived from a multipotent myeloid stem cell it is appropriate that systemic mastocytosis be classified with the chronic myeloproliferative disorders although it should be noted that the WHO group classifies it with other mast cell disorders rather than with the myeloproliferative disorders. Systemic mastocytosis is usually an indolent disorder, characterized by systemic symptoms resulting from the release of mast cell granule contents. Patients with lymphadenopathy and eosinophilia, associated myelodysplastic features or associated myeloproliferative disorder involving other lineages have a more aggressive course. A minority of patients have urticaria pigmentosa, resulting from skin infiltration by mast cells. The disease may terminate by transformation to AML, which is more often of lineages other than mast cell.

Blood film and count

The blood film and count may show proliferative or dysplastic features such as eosinophilia, monocytosis and thrombocytosis or anaemia and thrombocytopenia. There may be small numbers of circulating mast cells.

Differential diagnosis

The differential diagnosis includes other myeloproliferative disorders and MDS. Chronic eosinophilic leukaemia or aCML with eosinophilia associated with a *FIP1L1-PDGFRA* fusion gene is important in the differential diagnosis since this condition is often associated with increased bone marrow mast cells and increased serum tryptase.

Further tests

A bone marrow aspirate for cytogenetic and molecular genetic analysis and a trephine biopsy are required for diagnosis. Cytogenetic analysis may show a clonal abnormality and molecular genetic analysis shows a *KIT* mutation in the majority of patients. Because of the therapeutic implications, exclusion of a *FIP1L1-PDGFRA* fusion gene is necessary. Measurement of serum mast cell tryptase is useful.

Acute lymphoblastic leukaemia

Acute lymphoblastic leukaemia (ALL) is most common in children under 10 years of age but continues throughout childhood, adolescence and adult life. Clinical features are those due to leukaemic cell proliferation, such as bone pain, hepatosplenomegaly and lymphadenopathy, and those that are an indirect consequence of bone marrow infiltration, such as pallor and bruising. ALL may be of T or B lineage. The FAB classification of ALL includes cases with blastic cytology but the immunophenotype of a mature lymphocyte, these having the cytological features designated L3 ALL. In the WHO classification these cases are categorized as lymphoma rather than as acute leukaemia; this more accurately reflects the nature of the disease and the therapeutic implications.

Blood film and count

Some cases present with anaemia and thrombocytopenia without any circulating leukaemic cells. Others have variable numbers of lymphoblasts in the peripheral blood with the WBC sometimes being greatly elevated. There is usually anaemia, neutropenia and thrombocytopenia but occasionally there are normal numbers of neutrophils, platelets or both. Occasional patients have an increased platelet count [103]. Reactive eosinophilia is present in a minority of patients. ALL has been categorized by the FAB group [71] as L1, L2 and L3. In L1 ALL (Fig. 9.37) the blast cells are small to medium in size and are fairly uniform in appearance. Larger cells have diffuse chromatin and sometimes small nucleoli whereas the smaller blasts have no visible nucleolus and show some chromatin condensation. Cytoplasm is scanty and weakly to moderately basophilic. There may be a few cytoplasmic vacuoles. In L2 ALL (Fig. 9.38) the blasts are larger and more pleomorphic with more irregular nuclei, more prominent nucleoli and more abundant cytoplasm. Cytoplasm is weakly to strongly basophilic and may contain some vacuoles. L3 ALL (Fig. 9.39) is characterized by moderately intense cytoplasmic basophilia and variable but usually heavy cytoplasmic vacuolation.

Differential diagnosis

The differential diagnosis is mainly AML and reactive lymphocytosis.

Some cases of ALL have a few azurophilic granules and some cases of AML lack any granules or other light microscopy signs of myeloid differentiation so that reliable differentiation of the two conditions requires further tests. L2 ALL is most readily confused with AML. L1 ALL can usually be distinguished from AML on cytological features. There are

Fig. 9.37 Peripheral blood film in L1 acute lymphoblastic leukaemia (ALL) showing lymphoblasts and one nucleated red blood cell (NRBC). The lymphoblasts vary in size but are relatively uniform in morphology. The smaller blast cells show some chromatin condensation, which can be a feature of lymphoblasts but not of myeloblasts. This case was shown on immunophenotyping to be of B lineage.

Fig. 9.38 Peripheral blood film in L2 acute lymphoblastic leukaemia (ALL). The blast cells are larger and more pleomorphic than in LI ALL and in this case have a more diffuse chromatin pattern; one of the blasts has a hand-mirror conformation. This case was shown on immunophenotyping to be of T lineage.

Fig. 9.39 Peripheral blood film in L3 acute lymphoblastic leukaemia (ALL). The blast cells are medium sized with strongly basophilic vacuolated cytoplasm. This case was shown to have a mature B-cell immunophenotype.

usually some quite small blast cells, barely any bigger than a normal lymphocyte, and these cells show some chromatin condensation whereas the blasts of AML are rarely this small and usually have a diffuse chromatin pattern. L3 ALL is so distinctive that a diagnosis based on cytology alone is rarely wrong. However, it should be noted that B- and T-lineage ALL and even non-haemopoietic tumours sometimes have these cytological features. Cases of small cell tumours of childhood with circulating neoplastic cells are sometimes also confused with other types of ALL. Immunophenotyping may be necessary to make the distinction.

In cases of ALL with only small numbers of circulating blasts it is sometimes necessary to do further tests, e.g. a bone marrow aspiration, to distinguish ALL from lymphocytosis with atypical lymphocytes resulting from infection.

In cases with no circulating leukaemic cells the differential diagnosis includes aplastic anaemia and other causes of bone marrow failure. Concern is often expressed as to whether children with severe

Table 9.15 Typical immunophenotypic findings in acute lymphoblastic leukaemia (expression is on the surface membrane unless otherwise specified).

B-lineage

Expression of CD19, CD22, CD24, CD79a* and HLA-DR; TdT[†‡] and CD45 usually expressed; variable expression of CD34, CD10, CD20, CD79b and cytoplasmic μ chain; FMC7 not expressed; surface membrane immunoglobulin is generally not expressed and cases showing expression are better classified as non-Hodgkin's lymphoma rather than acute lymphoblastic leukaemia

T-lineage

Expression of CD7, CD45, cytoplasmic CD3 and nuclear TdT[†‡]; variable expression of CD1a, CD2, membrane CD3[§], CD5, CD4, CD8, CD10 (weaker than in B-lineage ALL) and T-cell receptor αβ or γδ; HLA more often not expressed

* Monoclonal antibodies in use detect a cytoplasmic epitope.
[†] Terminal deoxynucleotidyl transferase.
[‡] Nuclear expression.
[§] Expression may be cytoplasmic only.

thrombocytopenia, consistent with autoimmune thrombocytopenic purpura, are actually suffering from ALL. When there are no atypical lymphoid cells and no anaemia this is possible but is quite uncommon and unless there are atypical features or corticosteroid therapy is to be given, bone marrow aspiration is not usually considered necessary.

Further tests

Bone marrow aspiration and immunophenotyping of either peripheral blood or bone marrow blast cells are essential to confirm the diagnosis of ALL (Table 9.15). Cytogenetic analysis to identify prognostically important subgroups is also strongly recommended. Molecular analysis is becoming increasingly important, both to identify good prognosis cases, in which stem cell transplantation in first remission is inappropriate, and to identify poor prognosis cases, in which intensive and innovative forms of therapy are justified; among the poor prognosis groups, detection of the 25–30% of adult patients with the Ph chromosome and *BCR-ABL* fusion is important. Cases of L1 and L2 ALL may be of either B or T lineage. Cases of L3 ALL are almost always of B lineage with the blasts being mature B cells expressing surface membrane immunoglobulin.

Chronic lymphoid leukaemias and lymphomas

Both chronic lymphoid leukaemias and lymphomas are lymphoid neoplasms. By definition, in chronic lymphoid leukaemias there are circulating leukaemic cells whereas lymphomas primarily involve lymph nodes and other tissues. Lymphomas may, however, have a leukaemic phase, either at presentation or with disease progression. The term 'lymphoproliferative disorder' includes both leukaemias and lymphomas. Cytology is very useful in the differential diagnosis of these disorders [104] but it is not always possible to arrive at a definitive diagnosis on the basis of cytological features alone. Diagnosis should be based on clinical features, blood count, cytology and immunophenotype supplemented when necessary by cytogenetic and molecular genetic analysis. In some patients, histological examination of the bone marrow or lymph nodes is also necessary. Only peripheral blood features will be discussed in any detail here. For further information on immunophenotype and histology the reader is referred to Tables 9.16 and 9.17 and references [75] and [104–106].

B-lineage lymphoproliferative disorders

Chronic lymphocytic leukaemia

Chronic lymphocytic leukaemia (CLL) is a chronic condition characterized by accumulation of mature small B cells with consequent development of lymphadenopathy, hepatomegaly and splenomegaly. In early cases there may be no abnormal physical findings and the diagnosis is made incidentally on a routine blood count. The peripheral blood and bone marrow are always involved.

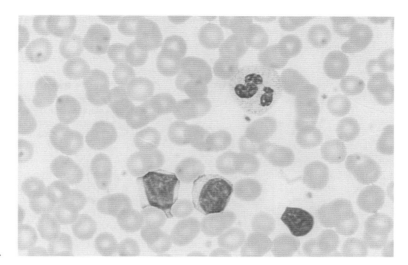

Fig. 9.40 Peripheral blood film in chronic lymphocytic leukaemia (CLL) showing a neutrophil, two mature lymphocytes and a smear cell.

Blood film and count

The WBC and lymphocyte count range from just above normal to greatly elevated. The Hb and platelet count may be normal or reduced. In the untreated patient, the neutrophil count is rarely reduced. The lymphocytes are similar in size to normal lymphocytes but are more uniform in appearance (Fig. 9.40). The chromatin is usually clumped and nucleoli are small and inconspicuous. Cytoplasm is scanty and weakly basophilic. In some cases there are cytoplasmic crystals (Fig. 9.41) or globular inclusions. Vermiform inclusions representing immunoglobulin in dilated cisternae of the endoplasmic reticulum have also been described [107]. Because CLL cells have increased mechanical fragility, there are increased numbers of smear cells. There may be a small number of larger cells with prominent nucleoli resembling the cells of prolymphocytic leukaemia (PLL). If there are more than 10% of prolymphocytes or the degree of pleomorphism is greater than usual, the diagnosis of CLL of mixed cell type (CLL/PL) is preferred [105]. Anaemia is usually normocytic and normochromic. If there is complicating auto-immune haemolytic anaemia there are spherocytes and polychromasia.

Differential diagnosis

The differential diagnosis includes other chronic lymphoproliferative disorders, particularly follicular

Fig. 9.41 Peripheral blood film in chronic lymphocytic leukaemia (CLL) showing two lymphocytes, one of which contains two crystals. Courtesy of Professor D. Catovsky, London.

lymphoma, SLVL, mantle cell lymphoma and the small cell variant of T-lineage PLL. Benign conditions that can be confused with CLL include post-splenectomy lymphocytosis and lymphocytosis induced by acute stress. If the blood film is examined in isolation without reference to the age and clinical features then whooping cough and infectious lymphocytosis can also be confused with CLL.

Table 9.16 Typical immunophenotypic findings in chronic lymphoid leukaemias and non-Hodgkin's lymphoma of B-lineage*.

Condition		Immunophenotype	
Chronic lymphocytic leukaemia		Weak expression of SmIg; expression of CD5 and CD23; lack of expression or weak expression of CD20, CD22 and CD79b; CD35 and FMC7 not expressed	
Prolymphocytic leukaemia, hairy cell leukaemia and non-Hodgkin's lymphoma	Prolymphocytic leukaemia	Moderate or strong expression of SmIg; lack of expression of CD23; expression of FMC7, CD20, CD22, CD35 and CD79b; variable expression of CD5 and CD10	
	Hairy cell leukaemia		Expression of CD11c, CD25, CD103 and CD123; CD22 strongly expressed
	Follicular lymphoma		CD10 most often expressed in this subtype
	Mantle cell lymphoma		Expression of CD5 and nuclear cyclin D1
	Splenic lymphoma with villous lymphocytes		CD11c and CD103 sometimes expressed
	Large cell lymphoma		Variable expression of CD5 and CD10
Plasma cell leukaemia		Expression of monotypic (κ or λ) cytoplasmic immunoglobulin (but not SmIg); expression of CD38 and CD138	

SmIg, surface membrane immunoglobulin.
* All this group of disorders are likely to express surface membrane immunoglobulin (SmIg), CD19 and CD79a (cytoplasmic epitope detected); they express CD37 strongly whereas it is expressed weakly by T cells; they express CD40, which is expressed by some myeloid cells but not by T cells; terminal deoxynucleotidyl transferase is not expressed.

Further tests

The diagnosis should be confirmed by immunophenotyping (Table 9.16), which may be supplemented by cytogenetic analysis (particularly FISH) and trephine biopsy of the bone marrow.

Monoclonal B-cell lymphocytosis

Monoclonal B-cell lymphocytosis or monoclonal lymphocytosis of undetermined significance is an asymptomatic condition that is sometimes detected in apparently healthy people. The clonal B-cells may have the immunophenotype of CLL or of non-Hodgkin's lymphoma. The probability of this condition evolving into an overt lymphoproliferative disorder is not yet known although it is known that in the short term the condition may regress, be stable or progress.

Blood film and count

The blood count may be normal or there may be a mild increase in the total lymphocyte count. A few smear cells may be seen. This condition has been detected as the result of observation of crystalline inclusions in lymphocytes, leading to immunophenotyping [108].

Differential diagnosis

The differential diagnosis is with overt lymphoproliferative disorders. Criteria have been proposed to help make this distinction [109].

Further tests

The diagnosis will only be made if immunophenotyping is carried out either in individuals with a mild lymphocytosis or, as part of a research project, in individuals who are apparently haematologically normal. A paraprotein is sometimes present at a low concentration. No further tests are indicated.

B-lineage prolymphocytic leukaemia

B-lineage prolymphocytic leukaemia (B-PLL or PLL) is characterized clinically by marked splenomegaly with trivial lymphadenopathy. The peripheral blood and bone marrow are always involved. There may be anaemia and other cytopenias. The disease is more rapidly progressive than CLL.

Blood film and count

The WBC is usually greatly elevated. The neoplastic cells are larger than those of CLL and often show more variation in size. They are predominantly round with round nuclei and weakly basophilic cytoplasm, which is more abundant than in CLL (Fig. 9.42). Many cells, particularly the larger ones, have large and prominent nucleoli. There is moderate chromatin condensation, which is enhanced around the large nucleolus, giving it a 'vesicular' appearance. If blood films are dried too slowly, cell shrinkage can lead to artefactual hairy projections and a less conspicuous nucleolus [110].

Differential diagnosis

The differential diagnosis includes other chronic lymphoproliferative disorders, particularly CLL/PL and T-lineage PLL. The best criterion to separate PLL from CLL/PL is that in PLL prolymphocytes are at least 55% of circulating lymphoid cells [111]. In T-lineage PLL, the cells are more irregular in shape, more pleomorphic and often smaller than in B-lineage PLL. Occasionally, the leukaemic phase of large cell lymphoma resembles PLL but generally the degree of pleomorphism is much greater in large cell lymphoma. Plasma cell leukaemia can also occasionally be difficult to distinguish but usually there are some cells with more evident plasma cell features such as an eccentric nucleus and cytoplasmic basophilia with a paranuclear Golgi zone.

Further tests

Immunophenotyping (see Table 9.16) supports a provisional diagnosis of PLL and permits a distinction from plasma cell leukaemia. Cytogenetic analysis

Fig. 9.42 Peripheral blood film in B-lineage prolymphocytic leukaemia (PLL) showing a neutrophil and three prolymphocytes with characteristic vesicular nucleoli.

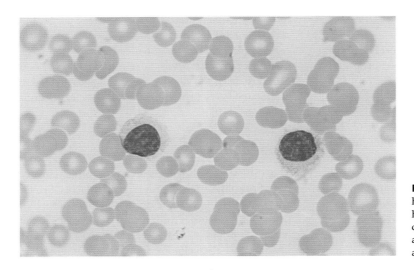

Fig. 9.43 Peripheral blood film in hairy cell leukaemia showing two hairy cells; both have plentiful cytoplasm with irregular margins and in one fine hair-like projections are present.

may show clonal cytogenetic abnormalities including trisomy 3, t(11;14)(q13;q32) and other rearrangements with a 14q32 breakpoint. The nature of cases with t(11;14) is disputed; they may be better regarded as a variant of mantle cell lymphoma.

Hairy cell leukaemia

Hairy cell leukaemia is a chronic disorder characterized by splenomegaly without lymphadenopathy. Early cases may have no abnormal physical findings and diagnosis may then be made incidentally because of cytopenia.

Blood film and count

The WBC is usually not elevated and hairy cells (Fig. 9.43) are infrequent in the peripheral blood. When they are very infrequent making a buffy coat preparation can be useful.

There is usually normocytic anaemia and marked monocytopenia. In more advanced disease there is also neutropenia and thrombocytopenia. Hairy cells are larger than normal lymphocytes. They have abundant weakly basophilic cytoplasm with irregular 'hairy' margins. Occasionally, there are cytoplasmic inclusions, which represent the ribosomal–lamellar complex that has been identified on electron microscopy; on light microscopy these inclusions appear

as two indistinct parallel lines (Fig. 9.44). The nucleus may be round, oval, dumbbell-shaped or bilobed. It has a bland appearance with little chromatin condensation and sometimes an indistinct nucleolus.

Differential diagnosis

The differential diagnosis includes other lymphoproliferative disorders, particularly the variant form of hairy cell leukaemia, and SLVL. Hairy cells do not have the prominent nucleolus of the neoplastic cells in the variant form of hairy cell leukaemia and have more plentiful cytoplasm than the cells of SLVL. Since there may be pancytopenia with very infrequent leukaemic cells, hairy leukaemia can also be confused with aplastic anaemia. The disproportionate reduction of the monocyte count is a useful indicator of the correct diagnosis. A condition similar to hairy cell leukaemia but with a higher WBC and a different immunophenotype has been reported from Japan [112]. In addition, rare cases of polyclonal hairy B lymphocyte proliferation have been reported in Japanese people [112].

Further tests

The diagnosis is confirmed by immunophenotyping [104] (see Table 9.16), TRAP activity and a highly

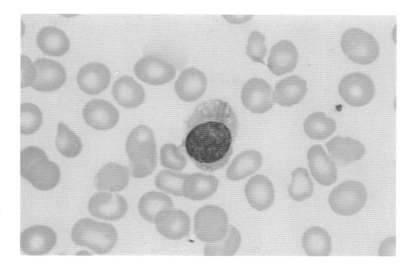

Fig. 9.44 Peripheral blood film in hairy cell leukaemia showing a hairy cell containing a ribosomal–lamellar complex. These structures are more readily observed by ultrastructural examination but can occasionally be identified by light microscopy as two parallel basophilic lines. Courtesy of Dr Laura Sainati, Padua, and Professor D. Catovsky.

characteristic trephine biopsy in which neoplastic cells are spaced apart. There may be clonal cytogenetic abnormalities but no specific rearrangement has been identified.

Hairy cell leukaemia variant

A variant form of hairy cell leukaemia has been recognized. It has similar clinical features to hairy cell leukaemia but some of the haematological, cytological and immunophenotypic features differ.

Blood film and count

In hairy cell leukaemia variant, the WBC is often elevated and neoplastic cells are numerous. Severe monocytopenia is not a feature. Otherwise haematological features are similar to those of hairy cell leukaemia. The neoplastic cells have similar cytoplasmic characteristics to hairy cells but have a prominent vesicular nucleolus, resembling that of the prolymphocyte (Fig. 9.45).

Fig. 9.45 Peripheral blood film in the variant form of hairy cell leukaemia showing cells with the cytoplasmic characteristics of hairy cells but with a prominent nucleolus. There is one binucleate cell. Courtesy of Professor D. Catovsky.

Fig. 9.46 Peripheral blood film in splenic lymphoma with villous lymphocytes (SLVL).

Differential diagnosis

The differential diagnosis is hairy cell leukaemia and SLVL. In SLVL the neoplastic cells have less abundant cytoplasm and the nucleolus, if visible, is less prominent than in hairy cell leukaemia variant.

Further tests

Immunophenotyping, cytochemistry and a trephine biopsy are useful in confirming the diagnosis. The immunophenotype of hairy cell variant differs from that of hairy cell leukaemia and TRAP activity is generally negative. The trephine biopsy usually does not show the spaced cells that are almost invariable in hairy cell leukaemia. SLVL has a similar immunophenotype to hairy cell leukaemia variant so that distinction is mainly on cytological features.

Splenic lymphoma with villous lymphocytes (splenic marginal zone lymphoma)

The clinical features of SLVL are prominent splenomegaly with only minor lymphadenopathy. In the WHO classification, SLVL is regarded as a variant of splenic marginal zone lymphoma.

Blood film and count

The WBC varies from normal to moderately ele-

vated. The blood film (Fig. 9.46) shows variable numbers of mature small lymphocytes, which are not as uniform in appearance as those of CLL. The nucleus is round with chromatin clumping and sometimes an inconspicuous nucleolus. Cytoplasm is scanty to moderate in amount and weakly to moderately basophilic. Some of the neoplastic cells have irregular or 'villous' margins, sometimes at one pole of the cell. Some neoplastic cells show plasmacytoid differentiation. Some cases show increased rouleaux formation indicating the presence of a paraprotein.

Differential diagnosis

The differential diagnosis is CLL and the variant form of hairy cell leukaemia.

Further tests

The immunophenotype is useful in making the distinction from CLL (see Table 9.16). Analysis of serum immunoglobulins may demonstrate a paraprotein.

Lymphoplasmacytic lymphoma

Lymphoplasmacytic lymphoma, as defined by the WHO group, is a lymphoma in which some cells show differentiation to plasma cells. This condition has previously often been referred to as

Fig. 9.47 Peripheral blood film in lymphoplasmacytic lymphoma.

lymphoplasmacytoid lymphoma. Lymphoplasma-cytic lymphoma is usually a disease of lymph nodes and sometimes of the spleen and other lymphoid organs. A proportion of cases have involvement of the peripheral blood and bone marrow. There is often secretion of a paraprotein, most often but not always IgM. Sometimes the paraprotein is a cryoglobulin or shows cold agglutinin activity. The term 'Waldenström's macroglobulinaemia', as described by Waldenström, refers to a lymphoplasma-cytic lymphoma with a marked increase in plasma IgM concentration leading to hyperviscosity and it would be preferable if use of this term were restricted to cases with these features.

Blood film and count

When the bone marrow is infiltrated, a normocytic normochromic anaemia is common and other cytopenias can also occur. The blood film may show only rouleaux and increased background staining, reflecting the presence of a paraprotein, or there may be circulating lymphoma cells (Fig. 9.47). In a minority of cases, there is red cell agglutination or cryoglobulin deposition. Circulating lymphoma cells resemble small lymphocytes but show some plasmacytoid features such as cytoplasmic basophilia or an eccentric nucleus. A few mature plasma cells must also be present (in peripheral blood or other tissues) to meet the WHO criteria for this diagnosis.

Sometimes cells have cytoplasmic crystals or globular inclusions.

Differential diagnosis

The differential diagnosis includes CLL and SLVL. Waldenström's macroglobulinaemia and chronic cold haemagglutinin disease represent subsets of lymphoplasmacytic lymphoma in which the dominant clinical and haematological features are caused by hyperviscosity and cold-induced red cell agglutination respectively. In chronic cold haemagglutinin disease the lymphoma itself is often very low grade and sometimes clinically inapparent. Type I and type II cryoglobulinaemia also are lymphoid neoplasms in which a paraprotein is either a cryoglobulin (type I) or has rheumatoid factor activity, complexing with polyclonal immunoglobulin to form a cryoglobulin (type II). Many patients with type II cryoglobulinaemia have chronic hepatitis C infection. The neoplastic clone may be occult in cryoglobulinaemia, sometimes becoming clinically apparent during the course of the illness. Diagnosis of these three conditions rests on assessment of all disease features rather than just the peripheral blood abnormalities.

Further tests

Bone marrow aspiration and trephine biopsy, immunophenotyping and investigations for a serum paraprotein and for urinary Bence-Jones protein (free monoclonal immunoglobulin light chains) are indicated. The immunophenotype is similar to that of other non-Hodgkin's lymphomas but there may be, in addition, cytoplasmic immunoglobulin and expression of CD38.

Follicular lymphoma

Follicular or centroblastic/centrocytic lymphoma is mainly a disease of the lymph nodes although in advanced disease the liver and spleen are also involved. Circulating neoplastic cells may be pre-

sent at diagnosis or a leukaemic phase may develop with disease progression.

Blood film and count

The WBC varies from normal to greatly elevated. The Hb and platelet count may be normal but, in advanced disease, anaemia and thrombocytopenia can develop. Circulating lymphoma cells may be rare or present in large numbers. Lymphoma cells (Fig. 9.48) are often very small with scanty, almost inapparent, weakly basophilic cytoplasm. Some nuclei show notches or deep narrow clefts. These

(a)

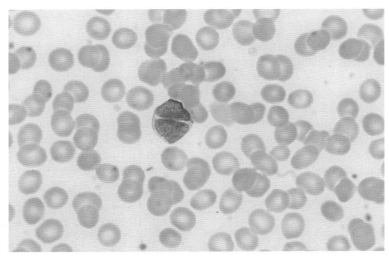

(b)

Fig. 9.48 Peripheral blood film in follicular lymphoma showing: (a) a neutrophil and a cleft lymphocyte; and (b) a cleft lymphocyte.

cytological features are particularly typical of cases with a high WBC. Other cases have larger, more pleomorphic cells, some of which have small but distinct nucleoli. Again there are notches or clefts in a proportion of cells. Smear cells are not a feature. Rarely the cells contain crystals [113].

Differential diagnosis

The differential diagnosis includes CLL and other non-Hodgkin's lymphomas, particularly mantle cell lymphoma.

Further tests

Immunophenotyping is very useful in making the distinction between follicular lymphoma and CLL. The immunophenotypes of follicular lymphoma and mantle cell lymphoma are more similar but mantle cell lymphoma is characteristically CD5-positive whereas follicular lymphoma is CD5-negative (see Table 9.16). When cytological features are insufficient to make a diagnosis, lymph node biopsy or cytogenetic/molecular genetic analysis may be needed.

Mantle cell lymphoma

Mantle cell lymphoma, previously known as diffuse centrocytic lymphoma and lymphoma of intermediate differentiation, is mainly a lymph node disease but the peripheral blood is involved in one-fifth to one-quarter of cases.

Blood film and count

Lymphoma cells vary from small to medium in size (Fig. 9.49). Some cases have been confused with CLL but, in general, the cells are more pleomorphic. Cells are variable in shape and nucleocytoplasmic ratio. Some have cleft or irregular nuclei. Chromatin condensation is less than in CLL and some cells appear blastic. Some cells are nucleolated. In the blastoid variant, most cells resemble blast cells.

Differential diagnosis

The differential diagnosis includes other non-Hodgkin's lymphomas and CLL and CLL/PL. In the blastoid variant a diagnosis of ALL may also have to be considered.

Further tests

The immunophenotype is quite distinct from that of CLL and shows subtle differences from that of other non-Hodgkin's lymphomas (see Table 9.16). In general, cytological and immunophenotypic features are not sufficiently distinctive for a definite diagnosis and either lymph node histology or cytogenetic/molecular genetic analysis is needed for confirmation.

Fig. 9.49 Peripheral blood film of a patient with mantle cell lymphoma showing a neutrophil and three highly pleomorphic lymphocytes. Courtesy of Dr Estella Matutes, London.

Fig. 9.50 Peripheral blood film of a patient with large cell lymphoma (centroblastic) showing large pleomorphic lymphoma cells with cleft nuclei.

This lymphoma is characterized by t(11;14)(q13;q32) (detectable by FISH analysis), rearrangement of the *BCL1* oncogene and expression of cyclin D1 (detectable immunohistochemically and by flow cytometry).

Other B-lineage lymphomas

Burkitt's lymphoma may involve the peripheral blood. In endemic Burkitt's lymphoma, leukaemia usually occurs only in advanced disease. In non-endemic and AIDS-associated Burkitt's lymphoma peripheral blood involvement is much more common. When a leukaemic phase occurs, the cells have the cytological features described by the FAB group as 'L3 ALL'.

A leukaemic phase is much less common in B-lineage large cell lymphomas than in the low grade lymphoproliferative disorders described above. When it occurs, the cells have a diameter about three times that of a red cell (Fig 9.50). They are usually pleomorphic with abundant moderately basophilic cytoplasm [114]. Nuclei are often lobulated and there may be prominent nucleoli. In some cases the cells resemble monoblasts. A single case of angiotropic large B-cell lymphoma has been reported in which diagnosis followed observation of clumps of lymphoma cells in a blood film [115].

Certain low-grade lymphomas, e.g. mucosa-associated lymphoid tissue (MALT) type lymphoma and monocytoid B-cell lymphoma, rarely have a leukaemic phase although occasional cases have shown peripheral blood dissemination. In monocytoid B cell lymphoma, the circulating neoplastic cells may have voluminous cytoplasm and somewhat irregular nuclei [17].

Multiple myeloma and plasma cell leukaemia

Multiple myeloma and plasma cell leukaemia are disseminated plasma cell neoplasms. Multiple myeloma is characterized by proliferation of abnormal plasma cells (myeloma cells) in the bone marrow and, in the great majority of patients, secretion of a monoclonal immunoglobulin or immunoglobulin light chain, which is referred to as a paraprotein. The monoclonal immunoglobulin is detectable in the serum. The monoclonal light chain, being of low molecular weight, is excreted in the urine where it is referred to as Bence-Jones protein. In multiple myeloma there may be some 'spillover' of neoplastic cells into the peripheral blood.

The term 'plasma cell leukaemia' indicates that significant numbers of neoplastic plasma cells are circulating in the blood. Plasma cell leukaemia may occur *de novo* or as the terminal phase of multiple myeloma. The FAB group [105] have suggested that this term be restricted to a *de novo* presentation in leukaemic phase but others, including the WHO

Fig. 9.51 Peripheral blood film in multiple myeloma.

expert group, have used it more generally [116,117]. Plasma cell leukaemia has been arbitrarily defined as an absolute plasma cell count of more than $2 \times 10^9/l$ with the plasma cells also being more than 20% of peripheral blood cells [116]. In the WHO classification, either of these criteria is considered sufficient for the diagnosis [117]. Plasma cell leukaemia is particularly common in IgD myeloma.

The picture of plasma cell leukaemia can also occur transiently when infection occurs in a patient with multiple myeloma, probably as a consequence of stimulation of plasma cells by IL6 [118].

The most typical clinical features of multiple myeloma are anaemia, bone pain, hypercalcaemia and renal failure.

Blood film and count

The blood film in multiple myeloma usually shows normocytic normochromic anaemia but sometimes there is macrocytosis. In the majority of cases in which there is a serum paraprotein there is also increased background staining and increased rouleaux formation (Fig. 9.51). Cases with Bence-Jones protein but no serum paraprotein do not have increased rouleaux or increased background staining so the absence of these features does not exclude the diagnosis. The WBC and platelet count are usually

not elevated and may be reduced. There may be occasional NRBC and immature granulocytes. Circulating myeloma cells may be absent, infrequent or numerous. Circulating myeloma cells may be cytologically normal but often they show abnormalities such as nuclear immaturity (a diffuse chromatin pattern and a nucleolus), high nucleocytoplasmic ratio, reduction of cytoplasmic basophilia and poorly developed Golgi zone, mitotic figures, binuclearity and dissociation of maturation of the nucleus and the cytoplasm. The number of circulating myeloma cells has been found to be of prognostic significance with 4% or more plasma cells being indicative of a worse prognosis [119].

In plasma cell leukaemia (Fig. 9.52), the neoplastic cells may resemble mature plasma cells or, particularly in the cases with a *de novo* presentation, may be highly abnormal with an immature chromatin pattern, nucleoli and minimal features of plasma cell differentiation.

In some patients with multiple myeloma, the paraprotein is a cryoglobulin or has cold agglutinin activity. In such cases, precipitated cryoglobulin or red cell agglutinates may be noted in blood films.

When paraproteins are cold agglutinins or cryoglobulins they may cause factitious results with automated blood cell counters (see Chapter 4).

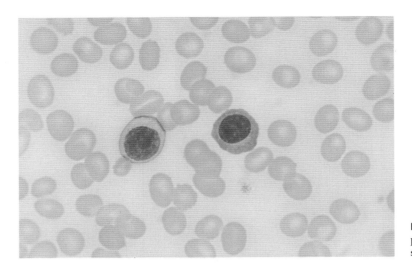

Fig. 9.52 Peripheral blood film of a patient with plasma cell leukaemia showing two neoplastic plasma cells.

Differential diagnosis

In patients with circulating myeloma cells the differential diagnosis is reactive plasmacytosis. Both conditions may have increased rouleaux formation and background staining. These abnormalities are usually, but not always, much more striking in multiple myeloma. Neutrophilia, monocytosis, thrombocytosis and reactive changes in neutrophils are often present in patients with reactive plasmacytosis but they are quite uncommon in multiple myeloma. However, rarely, there is a neutrophilic leukaemoid reaction in myeloma. Marked cytological abnormalities in plasma cells are indicative of a neoplastic condition.

The differential diagnosis in cases without circulating plasma cells includes other causes of normocytic normochromic anaemia (see p. 232), particularly conditions, such as AIDS, chronic inflammation and cirrhosis of the liver, in which an increased concentration of plasma proteins leads to increased rouleaux formation.

When the neoplastic cells are cytologically very atypical the differential diagnosis includes prolymphocytic leukaemia and non-Hodgkin's lymphoma.

Further tests

The ESR is commonly markedly elevated in multiple myeloma and is often used as a screening test for this condition. However, it should be noted that, if there is marked hyperviscosity, the ESR may be normal and in cases without a serum paraprotein the ESR may not show much elevation. When multiple myeloma is suspected, tests indicated to confirm the diagnosis are bone marrow aspiration, a radiological survey of the skeleton, serum calcium and creatinine estimation and investigation for serum and urinary paraproteins. Suitable tests include serum protein electrophoresis and immunofixation, immunofixation of a concentrated urine sample and nephelometry for assessment of the ratio of free κ chain to free λ chains in the serum. The latter technique will detect an abnormality in patients with Bence-Jones myeloma and in the majority of patients with non-secretory myeloma [120]. Immunophenotyping is not needed unless there is any reason to doubt that the plasma cells are neoplastic in which case use of anti-κ and anti-λ reagents will give evidence of clonality. Immunophenotyping is also useful when there is doubt as to whether highly abnormal circulating cells are neoplastic or when their lineage is not apparent. The immunophenotype of the terminally differentiated plasma cell differs from that of non-Hodgkin's lymphoma cells (see Table 9.16).

T-lineage lymphoproliferative disorders

T-lineage lymphoproliferative disorders are less common than B-lineage disorders. Precise diagnosis

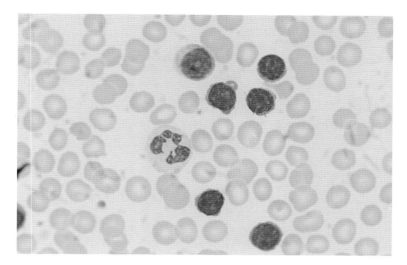

Fig. 9.53 Peripheral blood film of a patient with T-lineage prolymphocytic leukaemia (T-PLL) showing lymphocytes with irregular hyperchromatic nuclei, inconspicuous nucleoli and scanty moderately basophilic cytoplasm, which in one cell is forming blebs. Only one of the cells resembles those of B-lineage PLL, being larger with a moderate amount of cytoplasm and a more prominent nucleolus.

requires immunophenotyping and, sometimes, cytogenetic analysis or histological examination of lymph nodes, skin or other tissues.

T-lineage prolymphocytic leukaemia

T-lineage prolymphocytic leukaemia (T-PLL) is most often a disease of elderly people. Splenomegaly is the commonest clinical feature. A rash, indicative of skin infiltration, is sometimes present.

Blood count and film

The WBC is moderately to greatly elevated. T-lineage prolymphocytes (Fig. 9.53) are smaller and more pleomorphic than B-lineage prolymphocytes. Nuclei are irregular or lobulated. Cytoplasm is often scanty and may be moderately basophilic. Some cases cells have protruding cytoplasmic 'blebs'. Nucleoli may be inapparent or prominent but are rarely as large or as prominent as in B-lineage PLL.

Differential diagnosis

The differential diagnosis is mainly B-lineage CLL and PLL.

Further tests

Immunophenotyping is essential to confirm a diagnosis. Cells characteristically express CD7, which is usually negative in other T-lineage lymphoproliferative disorders (Table 9.17).

Cutaneous T-cell lymphomas

Mycosis fungoides and Sézary's syndrome are T-cell lymphomas that characteristically infiltrate the skin. The presence of circulating lymphoma cells is essential for the diagnosis of Sézary's syndrome, in which there is widespread disease dissemination at diagnosis, whereas in mycosis fungoides circulating lymphoma cells are seen only in patients with advanced stage disease. The cytological features do not differ between Sézary's syndrome and mycosis fungoides although they differ greatly between cases.

Blood count and film

The blood count may be normal, apart from sometimes showing lymphocytosis. Sometimes there is also eosinophilia. Lymphoma cells, known as Sézary cells, may be predominantly either small (Fig. 9.54) or large (Fig. 9.55) or a case may show a mixture of large and small cells. The most characteristic feature of the Sézary cell is a convoluted or cerebriform nucleus with tightly intertwined nuclear lobes. The cytoplasm is weakly basophilic and may contain a ring of vacuoles, which has been likened to rosary beads. In the small Sézary cell, there is scanty cytoplasm and a compact nucleus, the surface of which appears grooved. In large Sézary cells, there is more

Table 9.17 Typical immunophenotypic findings in chronic T-lineage and natural killer (NK)-lineage lymphoproliferative disorders.

Condition	Immunophenotype	
Prolymphocytic leukaemia	Variable expression of CD2, CD3, CD5 and CD7; CD1 and TdT not expressed; expression of T-cell receptor αβ or γδ	CD4 and CD7 usually expressed
Sézary syndrome/mycosis fungoides		CD4 usually expressed
Adult T-cell leukaemia/lymphoma		CD4 and CD25 usually expressed; HLA-DR expressed in half and CD38 in two-thirds of patients
Large cell lymphoma		
Large granular lymphocyte leukaemia—T-cell		Most often expression of CD2, CD3, CD8, CD57 and T-cell receptor αβ; CD4 and CD16 usually not expressed
Large granular lymphocyte leukaemia—natural killer cell	CD3 and T-cell receptors not expressed; CD1a and TdT not expressed	Variable expression of CD2 and CD8; CD4 usually not expressed; expression of CD11b, CD16, CD56 and sometimes CD57; expression of CD158a, CD158b or CD158e or failure to express any CD158 epitope

TdT, terminal deoxynucleotidyl transferase.

Fig. 9.54 Peripheral blood film of a patient with Sézary's syndrome showing small Sézary cells with hyperchromatic convoluted or cerebriform nuclei.

plentiful cytoplasm and a larger nucleus with more obvious nuclear lobes.

Differential diagnosis

The differential diagnosis includes other lymphomas and benign dermatological conditions, in which cells resembling Sézary cells are sometimes seen [121].

'Sézary cell leukaemia', in which skin infiltration is absent, is now thought to be a variant of T-PLL.

Further tests

Skin biopsy and immunophenotyping (see Table 9.17) are useful in diagnosis. Intra-epidermal lymphocyte accumulations (Pautrier's micro-abscesses)

(a)

(b)

Fig. 9.55 Peripheral blood film of a patient with Sézary's syndrome showing large Sézary cells.

are characteristic. It is sometimes difficult to recognize small Sézary cells by light microscopy. Ultrastructural examination can be useful in such cases since the complex nuclear form is then readily apparent (see Fig. 7.17).

Adult T-cell leukaemia/lymphoma

ATLL is a disease that develops in a minority of adults who are long-term carriers of the HTLV-I retrovirus. Such carriers mainly live in, or originate from, Japan and the Caribbean but the disease is also found in Taiwan, the Middle-East, Central and West Africa, South America, south-eastern USA and in Native Americans in North America. In the majority of cases the disease manifests itself as leukaemia and in a minority as a lymphoma. In those who present with leukaemia there is usually lymphadenopathy and sometimes hepatomegaly and splenomegaly. Skin infiltration and hypercalcaemia are common. Patients with ATLL are also prone to opportunistic infections.

Blood count and film

The WBC is often greatly elevated. Leukaemic cells are generally large and very pleomorphic. Nuclei are often polylobated, their shape resembling a flower or a cloverleaf (Fig. 9.56). Some nuclei have condensed chromatin while others have a diffuse chromatin pattern. Some cells are nucleolated. There is a variable amount of cytoplasm, which may be basophilic. A minority of cells resemble those of Sézary's syndrome. Some patients have associated eosinophilia. Anaemia and thrombocytopenia may be minimal at diagnosis.

Differential diagnosis

The differential diagnosis is cutaneous T-cell lymphoma and other lymphomas of mature T cells. The degree of pleomorphism and the presence of at least a minority of cells with flower-shaped nuclei are useful in the differential diagnosis. The typical acute form of ATLL should also be distinguished from smouldering or chronic ATLL, which generally lacks organomegaly, cytopenia and biochemical abnormalities. It also needs to be distinguished from the carrier state for HTLV-I in which there may be small numbers of polyclonal atypical lymphocytes in the peripheral blood, including some lymphocytes with polylobated nuclei.

Other tests

Serological tests for HTLV-I are indicated (not forgetting that a patient who is seropositive for HTLV-I may develop another type of lymphoma or lymphoid leukaemia). Immunophenotyping is also useful in

Fig. 9.56 Peripheral blood film of a patient with adult T-cell leukaemia/lymphoma (ATLL) showing four pleomorphic lymphocytes and a smear cell; one of the lymphoma cells has a flower-shaped nucleus and two others have convoluted nuclei.

the differential diagnosis since CD25 is commonly positive whereas it is usually negative in other leukaemias and lymphomas of phenotypically mature T cells (see Table 9.17).

Large granular lymphocyte leukaemia

Large granular lymphocyte leukaemia is a heterogeneous group of disorders in which the neoplastic cells have the cytological features of large granular lymphocytes and the immunophenotypic features of either cytotoxic T cells or natural killer cells. The clinical course is variable. Some patients have little organomegaly and a slowly progressive disease, but the course may be complicated by the effects of cytopenia, most often neutropenia. Other patients, particularly those whose cells have the phenotype of natural killer cells, have more typical features of lymphoma and a more rapid clinical course.

Blood count and film

In most cases the leukaemic cells are cytologically very similar to normal large granular lymphocytes (Fig. 9.57) with a small nucleus with condensed chromatin, plentiful weakly basophilic cytoplasm and

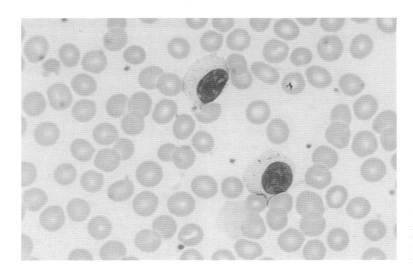

Fig. 9.57 Peripheral blood film of a patient with large granular lymphocyte leukaemia showing two large granular lymphocytes.

prominent azurophilic granules in at least some of the cells. Sometimes cells are larger with some nuclear irregularity and cytoplasmic basophilia. Sometimes there is neutropenia or, less often, anaemia or thrombocytopenia. Cytopenias may be profound, being the result of abnormal immune responses rather than bone marrow infiltration.

Differential diagnosis

The differential diagnosis is a reactive increase of large granular lymphocytes, e.g. that caused by a chronic viral infection, occurring post-splenectomy or associated with rituximab-induced autoimmune neutropenia.

Other tests

When the diagnosis is in doubt, immunophenotyping and tests to demonstrate clonality can be of use. Cells usually express CD2 and CD8 and do not express CD4 (see Table 9.17). In T-lineage cases, they express CD3, T-cell receptor antigens and usually CD57. Natural killer (NK)-lineage cases do not express CD3 or T-cell receptor antigens; they may express CD11b, CD16 and CD56 and, less often, CD57. A very uniform immunophenotype is suggestive of clonality and therefore of neoplasia. Clonality can be demonstrated in CD3-positive cases by molecular genetic analysis to demonstrate rearrangement of T-cell

receptor genes. In CD3-negative cases, cytogenetic analysis demonstrates an abnormal clone in some cases. In a larger group, analysis of CD158a, CD158b and CD158e (Killer Inhibitory Receptor) expression provides indirect evidence of clonality [122]. Polyclonal NK cells express all three antigens whereas monoclonal NK cells express one or none.

Other T-cell lymphomas

T-cell lymphomas are less common than B-cell lymphomas and less often have a leukaemic phase.

Blood count and film

Circulating lymphoma cells are often medium sized or large and quite pleomorphic (Figs 9.58 and 9.59).

Differential diagnosis

T-cell lymphomas cannot be reliably distinguished from certain B-cell lymphomas, particularly mantle cell lymphoma and B-lineage large cell lymphomas. Occasionally, they can also be confused with AML, particularly acute monoblastic leukaemia.

Other tests

Immunophenotyping is indicated and confirms the diagnosis. Cells express T-cell markers but the

Fig. 9.58 Peripheral blood film of a patient with large cell lymphoma of T lineage showing two large lymphoma cells.

Fig. 9.59 Peripheral blood film of a patient with large cell anaplastic lymphoma of T lineage showing very large pleomorphic lymphoma cells. By courtesy of Dr D. Clark, Grantham.

immunophenotype is often aberrant. Molecular analysis shows rearrangement of T-cell receptor genes.

Hodgkin's disease

Hodgkin's disease (Hodgkin lymphoma) is of B-lymphocyte origin. The disease is now divided into two major categories, nodular lymphocyte-predominant Hodgkin's disease and classical Hodgkin's disease. The former is clearly of B-cell origin whereas in the latter the neoplastic cells (Reed–Sternberg cells and mononuclear Hodgkin's cells) are defective B-cells that fail to express many B-lineage associated surface antigens. Classical Hodgkin's disease is further divided into nodular sclerosing Hodgkin's disease, mixed cellularity Hodgkin's disease, lymphocyte-depleted Hodgkin's disease and lymphocyte-rich classical Hodgkin's disease. The usual clinical presentation is with lymphadenopathy, with or without systemic symptoms.

Blood count and film

Hodgkin's disease can cause anaemia, leucocytosis, neutrophilia, eosinophilia, lymphopenia and thrombocytosis. The anaemia may be normocytic and normochromic or microcytic and hypochromic, with the characteristics of anaemia of chronic disease. There may also be increased background staining and increase rouleaux formation. When there is bone marrow infiltration there may be anaemia, leucopenia or pancytopenia. On multivariate analysis, an elevated WBC and a reduced lymphocyte count correlate with worse prognosis [123].

Differential diagnosis

The differential diagnosis includes non-Hodgkin's lymphoma and a variety of infective and inflammatory conditions. There are no specific peripheral blood features to point to a diagnosis of Hodgkin's disease.

Other tests

The ESR is increased, serum iron and transferrin concentration are reduced and serum ferritin is normal or elevated. Diagnosis usually requires a lymph node biopsy although occasionally a bone marrow aspirate and trephine biopsy give the diagnosis.

Test your knowledge

Multiple choice questions (MCQs)

(1–5 answers may be correct)

MCQ 9.1 A middle-aged man presents with an Hb of 8 g/dl and splenomegaly. A likely diagnosis is
(a) Chronic granulocytic (myeloid) leukaemia
(b) Autoimmune haemolytic anaemia
(c) β thalassaemia major
(d) Acute lymphoblastic leukaemia
(e) Sickle cell anaemia

MCQ 9.2 Recognized features of juvenile myelomonocytic leukaemia include
(a) Rash
(b) Lymphadenopathy
(c) High haemoglobin F percentage
(d) High haemoglobin A_2 percentage
(e) The Philadelphia chromosome

MCQ 9.3 HIV infection may cause
(a) Lymphocytosis
(b) Lymphopenia

(c) Atypical lymphocytes

(d) Detached nuclear fragments in neutrophils

(e) Auer rods in neutrophil precursors

MCQ 9.4 The translocation t(9;22)(q34;q11) is recognized in association with a significant proportion of cases of

(a) Acute lymphoblastic leukaemia

(b) Acute myeloid leukaemia

(c) Myelodysplastic syndromes

(d) Chronic myelomonocytic leukaemia

(e) Chronic neutrophilic leukaemia

MCQ 9.5 Auer rods may occur in

(a) M0 AML

(b) M3 AML

(c) M6 AML

(d) T-lineage ALL

(e) Biphenotypic acute leukaemia

MCQ 9.6 A myeloid leukaemoid reaction in children can result from infection by

(a) Human immunodeficiency virus (HIV)

(b) Epstein–Barr virus (EBV)

(c) Cytomegalovirus (CMV)

(d) Human herpesvirus 6 (HHV6)

(e) Human T-cell lymphotropic virus (HTLV-I or II)

Extended matching questions (EMQs)

Select the most accurate term from the options listed for each of the stems. Each option may be used once, more than once or not at all. Only one answer is correct.

EMQ 9.1

Theme: lymphadenopathy

Options

A Tuberculous lymphadenopathy

B Streptococcal pharyngitis with reactive lymphadenopathy

C Infection by human lymphotropic virus I (HTLV-I)

D Hodgkin's disease with iron deficiency

E Hodgkin's disease with anaemia of chronic disease

F Infectious mononucleosis caused by primary EBV infection

G Castleman's disease

H Toxoplasmosis

I Chronic lymphocytic leukaemia

J Chronic lymphocytic leukaemia with complicating autoimmune haemolytic anaemia

K Primary human immunodeficiency virus (HIV) infection

L Mantle cell lymphoma

M Splenic lymphoma with villous lymphocytes

N Infectious mononucleosis-like illness cause by primary cytomegalovirus (CMV) infection

O Follicular lymphoma

P Acute lymphoblastic leukaemia

For each clinical history select the option that provides the most likely diagnosis—your answer should be as complete as possible.

1 A 22-year-old university student presents with acute pharyngitis, high fever and cervical lymphadenopathy. She reports a prodromal illness of chills, sweats and malaise. On examination, she has palatal petechiae, marked tonsillar enlargement with pseudomembrane formation, faint jaundice and cervical lymphadenopathy. Her spleen can be tipped on inspiration. FBC shows:

WBC $11.0 \times 10^9/l$

Neutrophil count $3.7 \times 10^9/l$

Lymphocyte count $6.8 \times 10^9/l$

Platelet count $345 \times 10^9/l$

Blood film: numerous atypical mononuclear cells; these are large with either uniformly basophilic cytoplasm or basophilia at the cytoplasmic margins; cytoplasm is sometimes 'scalloped' around erythrocytes; some nuclei are irregular, some are nucleolated and some have an immature chromatin pattern; apoptotic cells are increased.

Answer:

2 A 67-year-old Caucasian male presents with breathlessness, fatigue, jaundice, generalized lymphadenopathy, hepatomegaly and splenomegaly. FBC shows:

WBC $82 \times 10^9/l$

Neutrophil count $3.2 \times 10^9/l$

Lymphocyte count $77 \times 10^9/l$

Hb 6.5 g/dl

MCV 102 fl

Platelet count $250 \times 10^9/l$

Blood film: lymphocytosis with increased mature small lymphocytes, smear cells, marked spherocytosis, polychromasia.
Answer:

3 A 24-year-old northern European woman presents with bilateral cervical lymphadenopathy (posterior triangle). She has also had a dry cough for the previous 2 months and has noticed lethargy, easy fatigability and increased sweating. Lymph nodes are firm and non-tender. Chest X-ray shows considerable widening of the upper mediastinum. Laboratory investigations show:
WBC 14.2
Neutrophil count $10.2 \times 10^9/l$
Lymphocyte count $1.0 \times 10^9/l$
Eosinophil count $2.7 \times 10^9/l$
Hb 10.5 g/dl
MCV 75 fl
Platelet count $470 \times 10^9/l$
ESR 43 mm/hr
Blood film: mild hypochromia and microcytosis, neutrophilia, eosinophilia, increased rouleaux formation
Answer:

4 A 67-year-old man presents with generalized lymphadenopathy, splenomegaly and low grade fever. FBC shows:
WBC $65.7 \times 10^9/l$
Neutrophil count $2.7 \times 10^9/l$
Lymphocyte count $62.5 \times 10^9/l$
Hb 12.8 g/dl
MCV 96 fl
Platelet count $138 \times 10^9/l$
Blood film: normocytic, normochromic; lymphocytes are small and mature with evenly condensed chromatin and, in some cells, cleft or notched nuclei or an indefinite nucleolus
Immunophenotyping shows lymphocytes to be CD19-positive, CD5-negative, CD10-positive, CD23-negative, CD79a-positive, CD79b-positive, FMC7-positive, κ-positive (strong), λ-negative
Answer:

5 A 24-year-old bisexual male presents with the acute onset of fever, arthralgia, myalgia, lethargy, non-exudative pharyngitis, mouth ulcers and a generalized rash. FBC shows:
WBC $6.0 \times 10^9/l$

Neutrophil count $1.5 \times 10^9/l$
Lymphocyte count $4.0 \times 10^9/l$
Hb 13.3 g/dl
Platelet count $140 \times 10^9/l$
A blood film shows small numbers of atypical lymphocytes
A mononucleosis screening test is negative. IgG antibodies to Epstein–Barr virus (EBV) and cytomegalovirus (CMV) are detected but not IgM antibodies
Answer:

EMQ 9.2
Theme: suspected acute leukaemia and myelodysplastic syndrome
Options
A M0 AML
B M1 AML
C M3 AML
D M4 AML
E M5 AML
F M6 AML
G M7 AML
H Refractory anaemia
I Refractory anaemia with ring sideroblasts
J Refractory anaemia with excess of blasts
K Refractory anaemia with excess of blasts in transformation
L B-lineage acute lymphoblastic leukaemia
M T-lineage acute lymphoblastic leukaemia
N Acute biphenotypic leukaemia

For each clinical description choose the option that provides the most likely diagnosis, according to the FAB classification.

1 A ten-year-old Indian child presents with respiratory distress, distended neck veins and generalized lymphadenopathy. His FBC is:
WBC $180 \times 10^9/l$
Hb 9.3 g/dl
MCV 73 fl
Platelet count $43 \times 10^9/l$
Blood film: numerous blast cells lacking granules or Auer rods. Myeloperoxidase and Sudan black B stains negative
Immunophenotype: CD19 6%, CD10 1%, CD2 96%, mCD3 78%, CD4 91%, CD5 93%, CD7 88%, CD8 79%, CD11b 8% CD16 1%, CD56 4%, CD57 6%
Answer:

2 A 75-year-old Caucasian man presents with recurrent infections. Other than pallor, there is no abnormality on physical examination. FBC shows:

WBC $3.4 \times 10^9/l$
Neutrophil count $0.6 \times 10^9/l$
Lymphocyte count $2.3 \times 10^9/l$
Monocyte count $0.5 \times 10^9/l$
Hb 10 g/dl
MCV 106 fl
Platelet count $70 \times 10^9/l$

Blood film: dimorphic with many hypogranular and hypolobated neutrophils
Bone marrow: hypercellular, M : E ratio 1 : 1, blast cells 5%, moderate erythroid dysplasia, 18% ring sideroblasts
Answer:

3 A 65-year-old Pakistani man with a history of diabetes mellitus, tuberculosis and coronary heart disease presents with fever, pallor and bruising. FBC shows:

WBC $33.6 \times 10^9/l$
Hb 10.4 g/dl
MCV 96 fl
Platelet count $90 \times 10^9/l$

The blood film shows 99% blast cells. These are large cells with a high nucleocytoplasmic ratio; they lack granules and Auer rods and are negative for Sudan black B, chloroacetate esterase and α-naphthyl acetate esterase
Immunophenotype: CD2 12%, CD7 12%, CD10 1%, CD13 71%, CD14 9%, CD15 2%, CD19 0%, CD22 0%, CD33 13%, CD34 61%, CD79a 2%, cytoplasmic μ chain 1%, terminal deoxynucleotidyl transferase 48%
Answer:

4 A 5-year-old child presents with bone pain and pallor. There is a minor degree of lymphadenopathy. FBC shows:

WBC $5.1 \times 10^9/l$
Hb 5.9 g/dl
MCV 86 fl
Platelet count $136 \times 10^9/l$

The blood film shows lymphocytes and moderate numbers of blast cells; the latter are small cells with a high nucleocytoplasmic ratio and an indistinct nucleolus
Immunophenotyping shows: CD10 21%, CD19 20%, cytoplasmic μ chain 7%, mCD3 36%, terminal deoxy-

nucleotidyl transferase 24%. Results are negative for CD13, CD33, CD117 and anti-myeloperoxidase
Answer:

5 A 33-year-old Welsh male presents with fever, pallor, bruising and skin infiltration. FBC shows:

WBC $92 \times 10^9/l$
Hb 8.6 g/dl
MCV 88 fl
Platelet count $25 \times 10^9/l$

The blood films shows that the predominant cell is a blast cell; these are very large with voluminous cytoplasm, round or oval nuclei and large nucleoli. The bone marrow is largely replaced by similar cells Sudan black B and peroxidase stains show small numbers of fine positively-staining granules; α-naphthyl acetate esterase is positive
Answer:

EMQ 9.3

Theme: suspected acute leukaemia or myelodysplastic or myelodysplastic/myeloproliferative syndrome
Options
A Refractory anaemia
B Refractory anaemia with ring sideroblasts
C Refractory cytopenia with multilineage dysplasia
D Refractory cytopenia with multilineage dysplasia and ring sideroblasts
E Refractory anaemia with excess of blasts
F 5q– syndrome
G Atypical chronic myeloid leukaemia
H Chronic myelomonocytic leukaemia
I Juvenile chronic myelomonocytic leukaemia
J Acute myeloid leukaemia

For each clinical description choose the option that provides the most likely diagnosis, according to the WHO classification.

1 A 35-year-old Australian woman presents with lethargy and fatigue. She is pale with no other abnormal physical findings. Her FBC shows: WBC $5.4 \times 10^9/l$ with normal differential count, Hb 5.6 g/dl, MCV 115 fl, platelet count $430 \times 10^9/l$. Her blood film shows only macrocytosis. Assays of vitamin B_{12} and folic acid are normal. Bone marrow aspirate is hypercellular with erythroid hyperplasia and 4% blast cells. There are 3% ring sideroblasts. Karyotype is: 46,XX, del(5)(q13q33) [18], 46,XX [2].
Answer:

2 A 75-year-old Caucasian man presents with recurrent infections. Other than pallor, there is no abnormality on physical examination. FBC shows:
WBC 3.4×10^9/l
Neutrophil count 0.6×10^9/l
Lymphocyte count 2.3×10^9/l
Monocyte count 0.5×10^9/l
Hb 10 g/dl
MCV 106 fl
Platelet count 70×10^9/l
Blood film: dimorphic with many hypogranular and hypolobated neutrophils
Bone marrow: hypercellular, M : E ratio 1 : 1, blast cells 5%, moderate erythroid dysplasia, 18% ring sideroblasts
Answer:

3 A 65-year-old Afro-Caribbean woman with a past history of carcinoma of the breast treated by 'lumpectomy' followed by chemotherapy is found at routine follow-up to have the following FBC: WBC 5.8×10^9/l, Hb 8.6 g/dl, MCV 105 fl, platelet count 60×10^9/l. There are 2% blast cells and many of the neutrophils are hypogranular with a pseudo-Pelger–Huët anomaly. Bone marrow aspirate shows micromegakaryocytes and 28% blast cells.

4 A 69-year-old Scottish engineer presents with bruising and is found to have a spleen enlarged 5 cm below the costal margin. FBC shows: WBC 35×10^9/l, Hb 8.7 g/dl, MCV 93 fl and platelet count 105×10^9/l. The differential count shows 2% blast cells, 4% pro-myelocytes, 14% myelocytes and 2% monocytes, 77% neutrophils, 1% eosinophils and rare basophils.
Answer:

5 A 78-year-old English housewife who has never previously sought medical care presents with recurrent skin and respiratory infections. Her FBC is: WBC 3.0×10^9/l, Hb 9.0 g/dl, MCV 95 fl and platelet count 62×10^9/l. The neutrophil count is 0.8×10^9/l and neutrophils are dysplastic. Bone marrow aspirate shows 15% blast cells and cytogenetic analysis shows monosomy 7.
Answer:

EMQ 9.4
Theme: leucocytosis

Options
A Chronic granulocytic leukaemia (Ph-positive chronic myeloid leukaemia)
B Chronic granulocytic leukaemia in blast transformation
C Chronic myelomonocytic leukaemia
D Atypical (Ph-negative) chronic myeloid leukaemia
E Chronic neutrophilic leukaemia
F Refractory anaemia with ring sideroblasts
G Reactive neutrophilia
H Reactive eosinophilia
I Chronic eosinophilic leukaemia
J Juvenile myelomonocytic leukaemia (juvenile chronic myeloid leukaemia)
K Idiopathic hypereosinophilic syndrome
L Refractory anaemia with excess of blasts

For each clinical history choose the option that gives the most likely diagnosis.

1 A 25-year-old man presents with a rash and slight splenomegaly. His FBC shows:
WBC 15.0×10^9/l
Neutrophil count 7.8×10^9/l
Eosinophil count 6.3×10^9/l
Hb 12.5 g/dl
MCV 103 fl
Platelet count 112×10^9/l
The blood film shows anisocytosis and moderate poikilocytosis. Some of the eosinophils are degranulated and vacuolated. There are occasional eosinophil myelocytes.
The bone marrow shows an increased of both mature eosinophils and their precursors. There are 12% blast cells. Cytogenetic analysis yields no metaphases.
Answer:

2 A 35-year old woman presents with a 9-month history of amenorrhoea, abdominal swelling and weight loss. On examination, she has gross hepatomegaly and splenomegaly. Her FBC shows:
WBC 68.6×10^9/l
Neutrophil count 24.4×10^9/l
Eosinophil count 2.3×10^9/l
Basophil count 2.0×10^9/l
Lymphocyte count 1.1×10^9/l
Monocyte count 0.4×10^9/l
Myelocytes 14.0×10^9/l
Promyelocytes 4.3×10^9/l

Blasts cells $20 \times 10^9/l$
Hb 9.4 g/dl
MCV 89 fl
Platelet count $500 \times 10^9/l$
Cytogenetic analysis showed 46,XX [2], t(9:22)(q34;q11)[6], t(9:22)(q34;q11),+22q–[3]
Answer:

3 A 70-year-old man presents with pleuritic chest pain and fever. There is no hepatomegaly or spleno-megaly. He appears very ill. His FBC shows:
WBC $26.6 \times 10^9/l$
Hb 13.3 g/dl
Platelet count $410 \times 10^9/l$
The blood film shows neutrophilia, left shift, toxic granulation, neutrophil vacuolation and Döhle bod-ies. Myelocytes and promyelocytes are present. The basophil count is not increased and eosinophil and lymphocyte counts are reduced.
Answer:

4 A 23-year-old man presents with a vasculitic skin rash. Several toes are cold and blue. He has a cardiac murmur indicative of mitral regurgitation and is in heart failure. FBC shows:
WBC $15.2 \times 10^9/l$
Neutrophil count $7.2 \times 10^9/l$
Eosinophil count $3.0 \times 10^9/l$
Hb 12.7 g/dl
MCV 87 fl
Platelet count $170 \times 10^9/l$
The blood film shows both hypersegmented and non-lobed eosinophils, many of which are vacuo-lated and degranulated.
Extensive investigation shows no evidence of para-sitic, allergic or connective tissue disease. Peripheral blood analysis shows no immunophenotypic abnor-mality and no rearrangements of T-cell receptor genes. A bone marrow aspirate shows increased eosinophils and precursors. Bone marrow blast cells are 3%. Cytogenetic analysis of the bone marrow shows 46, XY[20]. FISH analysis shows a *FIP1L1-PDGFRA* fusion gene.
Answer:

5 A 71-year-old man presents with lethargy and fatigue. On examination, he is pale with the spleen being enlarged 4 cm below the costal margin. FBC shows:

WBC $15.3 \times 10^9/l$
Neutrophil count $12.8 \times 10^9/l$
Monocyte count $1.8 \times 10^9/l$
Hb 10.6 g/dl
MCV 110 fl
Platelet count $60 \times 10^9/l$
The blood film shows macrocytosis, occasional hypo-chromic microcytes and hypogranular neutrophils. There are occasional blast cells.
The bone marrow aspirate is hypercellular with granulocytic and erythroid hyperplasia and dysery-thropoiesis. Megakaryocytes are normal in number but many are small and hypolobated. There are 15% blast cells and 22% ring sideroblasts.
Answer:

EMQ 9.5
Theme: lymphocytosis
Options
A Whooping cough (pertussis)
B Acute infectious lymphocytosis
C Infection by human T-cell lymphotropic virus I (HTLV-I)
D Persistent polyclonal B-cell lymphocytosis
E Post-splenectomy lymphocytosis
F Infectious mononucleosis caused by primary Epstein–Barr (EBV) infection
G Follicular lymphoma
H Follicular lymphoma plus post-splenectomy lymphocytosis
I Chronic lymphocytic leukaemia
J Mantle cell lymphoma
K Primary human immunodeficiency virus (HIV) infection
L Stress-induced lymphocytosis
M Dermatopathic lymphadenopathy
N Infectious mononucleosis-like illness cause by primary cytomegalovirus (CMV) infection
O Large granular lymphocyte leukaemia
P Adult T-cell leukaemia/lymphoma

For each clinical history, choose the option that is most likely to indicate the correct diagnosis—be as precise as possible.

1 A 42-year old man with a strong family history of coronary artery disease is admitted to an Accident and Emergency Department with a severe crushing central chest pain radiating to the neck and the left arm. He appears shocked. Myocardial infarction is suspected. FBC shows:

WBC $13.4 \times 10^9/l$

Neutrophil count $5.6 \times 10^9/l$

Lymphocyte count $7.3 \times 10^9/l$

Platelet count $421 \times 10^9/l$

Blood film: somewhat pleomorphic lymphocytes including small mature lymphocytes and large granular lymphocytes

Answer:

2 A 32-year-old female cigarette smoker presents with weight loss, fever, sweats and malaise. FBC shows:

WBC $11.4 \times 10^9/l$

Lymphocyte count $6.3 \times 10^9/l$

Hb 13.5 g/dl

Platelet count $304 \times 10^9/l$

The blood film shows pleomorphic lymphocytes including lobulated and binucleated lymphocytes and lymphocytes with increased cytoplasmic basophilia

Immunophenotype: CD2 42%, CD19 40%, CD5 45%, CD20 52%, CD22 53%, CD23 25%, CD79b 52%, FMC7 43%, κ 22% (strong), λ 24% (strong).

Answer:

3 A 67-year-old English woman presents with cervical lymphadenopathy. FBC shows:

WBC $49.5 \times 10^9/l$

Lymphocyte count $42 \times 10^9/l$

Hb 12.7 g/dl

Platelet count $142 \times 10^9/l$

The blood film shows mature lymphocytes and occasional smear cells

Immunophenotyping shows CD2 35%, CD19 65%, CD5 87%, CD23 58%, CD79b 20% +/−, FMC7 8%+, κ 58% (weak), λ negative

Answer:

4 A 44-year-old Afro-Caribbean man, who came to the UK at the age of 4 years, presents with the slow onset of spastic paraparesis. A routine blood count shows neutropenia (interpreted as ethnic neutropenia) and mild lymphocytosis with some atypical lymphocytes. The atypical lymphocytes include some with highly lobulated nuclei.

Answer:

5 A 52-year-old man presents with generalized lymphadenopathy with nodes measuring up to 3 cm in diameter. He suffers from psoriasis. Ten years before presentation he had required splenectomy following a road traffic accident. FBC shows:

WBC $19.4 \times 10^9/l$

Lymphocyte count $10.3 \times 10^9/l$

Hb 13 g/dl

Platelet count $368 \times 10^9/l$

The blood film shows features of hyposplenism. There are both increased numbers of large granular lymphocytes and a population of small lymphocytes with densely condensed chromatin, a high nucleo-cytoplasmic ratio and nuclear clefting.

Immunophenotyping shows CD3 51% ++, CD4 40% +++, CD5 30% +++, CD8 55% +++, CD10 16% +, CD19 34% +++, CD22 9% +/−, CD79b 18% +++, CD56 27% ++, CD57 26% +++, FMC7 11% ++, κ 1% +/−, λ 17% +++

Answer:

References

1 Leibovici L, Drucker M, Samra Z, Konisberger H and Pitlik SD (1995) Prognostic significance of the neutrophil count in immunocompetent patients with bacteraemia. *Q J Med*, **88**, 181–189.

2 Gombos MM, Bienkowski RS, Gochman RF and Billett HH (1998) The absolute neutrophil count: is it the best indicator of bacteremia in infants? *Am J Clin Pathol*, **109**, 221–225.

3 Lascari AD. *Hematologic Manifestations of Childhood Diseases*. Theme-Stratton, New York, 1984.

4 Manroe BL, Weinberg AG, Rosenfeld CR and Browne R (1979) The neonatal blood count in health and disease. I. Reference values for neutrophilic cells. *J Pediatr*, **95**, 89–98.

5 Christensen RD and Rothstein G (1978) Pitfalls in the interpretation of leukocyte counts in newborn infants. *Am J Clin Pathol*, **72**, 609–611.

6 Morris CDW, Bird AR and Nell H (1989) The haematological and biochemical changes in severe pulmonary tuberculosis. *Q J Med*, **73**, 1151–1159.

7 Glasser RM, Walker RI and Herion JC (1990) The significance of hematologic abnormalities in patients with tuberculosis. *Arch Intern Med*, **125**, 691–695.

8 Hoagland RJ (1960) The clinical manifestations of infectious mononucleosis: a report of two hundred cases. *Am J Med*, **240**, 21–29.

9 Brigden ML, Au S, Thompson S, Brigden S, Doyle P and Tsaparas Y (1999) Infectious mononucleosis in an outpatient population: diagnostic utility of 2 automated hematology analyzers and the sensitivity and specificity of Hoagland's criteria in heterophile-positive patients. *Arch Pathol Lab Med*, **123**, 875–881.

10 Lach-Szyrma V and Brito-Babapulle F (1999) The clinical significance of apoptotic cells in peripheral blood smears. *Clin Lab Haematol*, **21**, 277–280.

11 Cantow EF and Kostinas JE (1966) Studies on infectious mononucleosis. IV. Changes in the granulocytic series. *Am J Clin Pathol*, **46**, 43–47.

12 Habib MA, Babka JC and Burningham RA (1973) Profound granulocytopenia associated with infectious mononucleosis. *Am J Med Sci*, **265**, 339–346.

13 Sumaya CV and Ench Y (1985) Epstein–Barr virus infectious mononucleosis in children. I. Clinical and general laboratory findings. *Pediatrics*, **75**, 1003–1010.

14 Carter JW, Edson RS and Kennedy CC (1978) Infectious mononucleosis in the older patient. *Mayo Clin Proc*, **53**, 146–150.

15 Bar RS, Adlard J and Thomas FB (1975) Lymphopenic infectious mononucleosis. *Arch Intern Med*, **135**, 334–337.

16 Akashi K, Eizuru Y, Sumiyoshi Y, Minematsu T, Hara S, Harada M *et al.* (1993) Severe infectious mononucleosis-like syndrome and primary human herpesvirus 6 infection in an adult. *N Engl J Med*, **329**, 168–171.

17 Foucar K, *Bone Marrow Pathology*, 2nd Edn. ASCP Press, Chicago, 2001.

18 McDonald JC, MacLean JD and McDade JE (1988) Imported rickettsial disease: clinical and epidemiologic features. *Am J Med*, **85**, 799–805.

19 Wilson ME, Brush AD and Meany MC (1989) Murine typhus acquired during short-term urban travel. *Am J Med*, **57**, 233–234.

20 McDade JE (1990) Ehrlichiosis—a disease of animals and humans. *J Infect Dis*, **161**, 609–617.

21 Chesterman CN (1992) Late adverse effects of streptokinase. *Aust NZ J Med*, **22**, 106–108.

22 Cullen MH, Stansfeld AG, Oliver RTD, Lister TA and Malpas JS (1979) Angio-immunoblastic lymphadenopathy: report of ten cases and review of the literature. *Q J Med*, **48**, 151–177.

23 Delbarre F, Le Go A and Kahan A (1975) Hyperbasophilic immunoblasts in the circulating blood in chronic inflammatory rheumatic and collagen diseases. *Ann Rheum Dis*, **34**, 422–430.

24 Daniele R and Rowlands DT (1976) Lymphocyte subpopulations in sarcoidosis: correlation with disease activity and duration. *Ann Intern Med*, **85**, 593–600.

25 Craig J and Isaacs D (1993) Kawasaki syndrome in a Sydney hospital. *Aust NZ J Med*, **23**, 440.

26 Karandikar NJ, Kroft SH, Yegappan S, Rogers BB, Aquino VM, Lee KM *et al.* (2004) Unusual immunophenotype of CD8+ T cells in familial hemophagocytic lymphohistiocytosis. *Blood*, **104**, 2007–2009.

27 Nakahara K, Utsunomiya A, Hanada S, Takeshita T, Uozumi K, Yamamoto K *et al.* (1998) Transient appearance of CD3+CD8+ T lymphocytes with monoclonal gene rearrangement of T-cell receptor beta locus. *Br J Haematol*, **100**, 411–414.

28 Horwitz CA, Henle W, Henle G, Polesky H, Balfour HH, Siem RA *et al.* (1977) Heterophile-negative infectious mononucleosis and mononucleosis-like illnesses. *Am J Med*, **63**, 947–957.

29 Tsaparas YF, Brigden M, Mathias R, Thomas E, Raboud J and Doyle PW (2000) Proportion positive for Epstein–Barr virus, cytomegalovirus, human herpesvirus 6, *Toxoplasma*, and human immunodeficiency virus types 1 and 2 in heterophile-negative patients with an absolute lymphocytosis and an instrument-generated atypical lymphocyte flag. *Arch Pathol Lab Med*, **124**, 1324–1330.

30 Smith PR, Cavenagh JD, Milne T, Howe D, Wilkes SJ, Sinnott P, Forster GE and Helbert M (2000) Benign monoclonal expansion of CD8+ lymphocytes in HIV infection. *J Clin Pathol*, **53**, 177–181.

31 Milne TM, Cavenagh JD, Macey MG, Dale C, Howes D, Wilkes S and Newland AC (1998) Large granular lymphocyte (LGL) expansion in 20 HIV infected patients; analysis of immunophenotype and clonality. *Br J Haematol*, **101**, Suppl. 1, 107.

32 Koster F, Foucar K, Hjelle B, Scott A, Chong Y-Y, Larson R and McCabe M (2001) Rapid presumptive diagnosis of hantavirus cardiopulmonary syndrome by peripheral blood smear review. *Am J Clin Pathol*, **116**, 665–672.

33 Pol S, Thiers V, Driss F, Devergie A, Berthelot P and Bréchot C (1993) Lack of evidence for a role of HCV in hepatitis-associated aplastic anaemia. *Br J Haematol*, **85**, 808–810.

34 Mossafa H, Malaure H, Maynadie M, Valensi F, Schillinger F, Garand G *et al.* (1999) Persistent polyclonal B lymphocytosis with binucleated lymphocytes: a study of 25 cases. Groupe Français

d'Hématologie Cellulaire. *Br J Haematol*, **104**, 486–493.

35 Callet-Bauchu E, Gazzo S, Poncet C, Pages J, Morel D, Alliot C *et al.* (2000) Distinct chromosome 3 abnormalities in persistent polyclonal B-cell lymphocytosis. *Genes Chromosomes Cancer*, **26**, 221–228.

36 Mossafa H, Tapia S, Flandrin G, Troussard X and the Groupe Français d'Hématologie Cellulaire (GFHC) (2004) Chromosomal instability and the ATR amplification gene in patients with persistent and polyclonal B-cell lymphocytosis (PPBL). *Leuk Lymphoma*, **45**, 1401–1406.

37 Himmelmann A, Gautsschi O, Nawrath M, Bolliger U, Fehr J and Stahel RA (2001) Persistent polyclonal B-cell lymphocytosis is an expansion of functional IGD+CD27+ memory B cells. *Br J Haematol*, **114**, 400–405.

38 Salcedo I, Campos-Caro A, Sampalo A, Reales E and Brieva JA (2002) Persistent polyclonal B lymphocytosis: an expansion of cells showing IgVH gene mutations and phenotypic features of normal lymphocytes with the CD27+ marginal zone B-cell compartment. *Br J Haematol*, **116**, 662–666.

39 Leder K and Weller PF (2000) Eosinophilia and helminth infections. *Baillière's Clin Haematol*, **13**, 301–317.

40 Chusid ML, Dale DC, West BC and Wolff SM (1975) The hypereosinophilic syndrome. *Medicine*, **54**, 1–27.

41 Cogan E, Schandené L, Crusiaux A, Cochaux P, Velu T and Goldman M (1994) Clonal proliferation of type 2 helper T cells in a man with the hypereosinophilic syndrome. *N Engl J Med*, **330**, 535–538.

42 Simon H-U, Plotz SG, Dummer R and Blaser K (1999) Abnormal clones of T cells producing interleukin-5 in idiopathic eosinophilia. *N Engl J Med*, **341**, 1112–1120.

43 Means-Markwell M, Burgess T. de Keratry D, O'Neil K, Mascola J, Fleisher T and Lucey D (2000) Eosinophilia with aberrant T cells and elevated serum levels of interleukin-2 and interleukin-15. *N Engl J Med*, **342**, 1568–1571.

44 Spry C. Discussion: Management of the idiopathic hypereosinophilic syndrome. In: Mahmoud AAF, Austere KP, Simon AS (eds), *The Eosinophil in Health and Disease*, Grune & Stratton, New York, 1980: 341.

45 Parker RI (1991) Hematologic aspects of mastocytosis. II. Management of hematologic disorders in association with systemic mast cell disease. *J Invest Dermatol*, **96**, 52S–53S.

46 Bain B (1991) Down's syndrome—transient abnormal myelopoiesis and acute leukaemia. *Leuk Lymphoma*, **3**, 309–317.

47 Ferrer A, Cervantes F, Hernández-Boluda JC, Alvarez A and Montserrat E (1999) Leukemoid reaction preceding the diagnosis of colorectal carcinoma by four years. *Haematologica*, **84**, 671–672.

48 Olipitz E, Strunk D, Beham-Schmid C and Sill H (2004) Neutrophilic leukaemoid reactions as the presenting feature of de novo and therapy-related acute leukemias. *Acta Haematologica*, **111**, 233–234.

49 Stevens MCG, Darbyshire PJ and Brown SM (1987) Early congenital syphilis and severe haematological disturbance. *Arch Dis Child*, **62**, 1073–1075.

50 Willoughby MLN. *Paediatric Haematology*. Churchill Livingstone, Edinburgh, 1977.

51 Standen GA, Steers FJ and Jones L (1998) Clonality of chronic neutrophilic leukaemia associated with myeloma: analysis using the X-linked probe M27β. *J Clin Pathol*, **46**, 297–298.

52 Nagai M, Oda S, Iwamoto M, Marumoto K, Fujita M and Takahara J (1996) Granulocyte-colony stimulating factor concentrations in a patient with plasma cell dyscrasia and clinical features of chronic neutrophilic leukaemia. *J Clin Pathol*, **49**, 858–860.

53 Kohmura K, Miyakawa Y, Kameyama K, Kizaki M and Ikeda Y (2004) Granulocyte colony stimulating factor-producing multiple myeloma associated with neutrophilia. *Leuk Lymphoma*, **45**, 1475–1479.

54 Dinçol G, Nalçaci M, Dogan O, Aktan M, Küçükkaya R, Agan M and Dinçol K (2002) Coexistence of chronic neutrophilic leukemia with multiple myeloma. *Leuk Lymphoma*, **43**, 649–651.

55 Marui T, Yamamoto T, Akisue T, Hitora T, Yoshiya S and Kurosaka M (2003) Granulocyte colony-stimulating factor–producing undifferentiated sarcoma occurring in previously fractured femur. *Arch Pathol Lab Med*, **127**, e186–e189.

56 Sonobe H, Ohtsuki Y, Ido E, Furihata M, Iwata J, Enzan H *et al.* (1997) Epithelioid sarcoma producing granulocyte colony-stimulating factor. *Hum Pathol*, **28**, 1433–1435.

57 Reykdal S, Sham R, Phatak P and Kouides P (1995) Pseudoleukemia following the use of G-CSF. *Am J Hematol*, **49**, 258–259.

58 Pinkel D (1998) Differentiating juvenile myelomonocytic leukemia from infectious disease. *Blood*, **91**, 365–367.

59 Beigelman A, Moser AM, Shubinsky G, Ben-Harosh M, Alon H, Benjamin G and Kapelushnik J (2003)

The leukemoid reaction – clinical and molecular characterization in the pediatric population. *Blood*, **102**, 53b.

60 Herrod HG, Dow LW and Sullivan JL (1983) Persistent Epstein–Barr virus infection mimicking juvenile chronic myelogenous leukemia: immunologic and hematologic studies. *Blood*, **61**, 1098–1104.

61 Kirby MA, Weitzman S and Freedman MH (1990) Juvenile chronic myelogenous leukemia: differentiation from infantile cytomegalovirus infection. *Am J Pediatr Hematol Oncol*, **12**, 292–296.

62 Lorenzana A, Lyons H, Sawal H, Higgins M, Carrigan D and Emanuel P (1997) Human herpes virus-6 (HHV-6) infection in an infant mimicking juvenile chronic myelogenous leukemia (JCML). *J Pediatr Hematol Oncol*, **19**, 370.

63 Yetgin S, Çetin M, Yenicesu I, Özaltin F and Uçkan D (2000) Acute parvovirus B19 infection mimicking juvenile myelomonocytic leukemia. *Eur J Haematol*, **65**, 276–278.

64 Toren A, Neumann Y, Meyer JJ, Mandel M, Schiby G, Kende G *et al.* (1993) Malignant osteopetrosis manifested as juvenile chronic myeloid leukemia. *Pediatr Hematol Oncol*, **10**, 187–189.

65 Papadaki T, Stamatopoulos K, Stavroyianni N, Paterakis G, Phisphis M and Stefanoudaki-Sofianatou K (2002) Evidence for T-large granular lymphocyte-mediated neutropenia in Rituximab-treated lymphoma patients: report of two cases. *Leuk Res*, **26**, 597–600.

66 Bates I, Bedu-Addo G, Rutherford TR and Bevan DH (1997) Circulating villous lymphocytes—a link between hyperreactive malarial splenomegaly and splenic lymphoma. *Trans R Soc Trop Med Hyg*, **91**, 171–174.

67 Jabbar A and Siddique T (1998) A case of pseudo-lymphoma leukaemia syndrome following cefixime. *Br J Haematol*, **101**, 209.

68 Kikuchi M, Ohsaka A, Chiba Y, Sato M, Muraosa Y and Hoshino H (1999) Bone marrow aplasia with prominent atypical plasmacytic proliferation preceding acute lymphoblastic leukemia. *Leuk Lymphoma*, **35**, 213–217.

69 Ehrlich GD, Han T, Bettigole R, Merl SA, Lehr B, Tomar RH and Poiesz BJ (1988) Human T lymphotropic virus type I-associated benign transient immature T-cell lymphocytosis. *Am J Hematol*, **27**, 49–55.

70 Caldwell CW, Poje E and Cooperstock M (1991) Expansion of immature thymic precursor cells in peripheral blood after acute bone marrow suppression. *Am J Clin Pathol*, **95**, 824–827.

71 Bennett JM, Catovsky D, Daniel M-T, Flandrin G, Galton DAG, Gralnick H and Sultan C (1976) Proposals for the classification of the acute leukaemias (FAB cooperative group). *Br J Haematol*, **33**, 451–459.

72 Bennett JM, Catovsky D, Daniel MT, Flandrin G, Galton DAG, Gralnick H and Sultan C (1985) Proposed revised criteria for the classification of acute myeloid leukemia. *Ann Intern Med*, **103**, 620–625.

73 Bennett JM, Catovsky D, Daniel M-T, Flandrin G, Galton DAG, Gralnick H and Sultan C (1985) Criteria for the diagnosis of acute leukemia of megakaryocyte lineage (M7): a report of the French–American–British Cooperative Group. *Ann Intern Med*, **103**, 460–462.

74 Bennett JM, Catovsky D, Daniel M-T, Flandrin G, Galton DAG, Gralnick H and Sultan C (1991) Proposal for the recognition of minimally differentiated acute myeloid leukaemia (AML M0). *Br J Haematol*, **78**, 325–329.

75 Bain BJ. *Leukaemia Diagnosis: a Guide to the FAB Classification*, 3rd Edn. Blackwell Publishing, Oxford, 2003.

76 Brunning RD, Matutes E, Harris NL, Flandrin G, Vardiman J, Bennett J and Head D, Acute myeloid leukaemia: introduction. In: Jaffe ES, Harris NL, Stein H and Vardiman JW (eds), *World Health Organization Classification of Tumours: Pathology and Genetics of Tumours of Haematopoietic and Lymphoid Tissues*, IARC Press, Lyon, 2001, pp. 77–80.

77 Soler J, O'Brien M, Tavaras de CJ, San Miguel JF, Kearney L, Goldman JM and Catovsky D (1985) Blast crisis of chronic granulocytic leukemia with mast cell and basophil precursors. *Am J Clin Pathol*, **83**, 254–259.

78 Coser P, Quaglino D, de Pasquale A, Colombetti V and Prinoth O (1980) Cytobiological and clinical aspects of tissue mast cell leukaemia. *Br J Haematol*, **45**, 5–12.

79 Efrati P, Klajman A and Spitz H (1957) Mast cell leukemia? Malignant mastocytosis with leukemia-like manifestations. *Blood*, **12**, 869–882.

80 Parwaresch MR. *The Human Blood Basophil. Morphology, Origin, Kinetics, Function and Pathology*. Springer-Verlag, Berlin, 1976.

81 Bain BJ (1994) Transient leukaemia in newborn infants with Down's syndrome. *Leuk Res*, **18**, 723–724.

82 Hitzler JK, Cheung J, Yue LI, Scherer SW and Zipursky A (2003) GATA1 mutations in transient leukemia and acute megakaryoblastic leukemia of Down syndrome. *Blood*, **101**, 4301–4304.

83 Brunning RD, Bennett JM, Flandrin G, Matutes E, Head D, Vardiman JW and Harris NL, Myelodysplastic syndromes: introduction. In: Jaffe ES, Harris NL, Stein H and Vardiman JW (eds), *World Health Organization Classification of Tumours: Pathology and Genetics of Tumours of Haematopoietic and Lymphoid Tissues*, IARC Press, Lyon, 2001.

84 Vardiman JW, Myelodysplastic/myeloproliferative disease: introduction. In: Jaffe ES, Harris NL, Stein H and Vardiman JW (eds), *World Health Organization Classification of Tumours: Pathology and Genetics of Tumours of Haematopoietic and Lymphoid Tissues*, IARC Press, Lyon, 2001.

85 Spiers ASD, Bain BJ and Turner JE (1977) The peripheral blood in chronic granulocytic leukaemia. Study of 50 untreated Philadelphia chromosome-positive cases. *Scand J Haematol*, **18**, 25–38.

86 Srodes CH, Hyde EH and Boggs DR (1973) Autonomous erythropoiesis during erythroblastic crisis of chronic myelocytic leukaemia. *J Clin Invest*, **52**, 512–515.

87 Ondreyco SM, Kjeldsberg CR, Fineman RM, Vaninetti S and Kushner JP (1981) Monoblastic transformation in chronic myelogenous leukemia. *Cancer*, **48**, 957–963.

88 Rosenthal S, Schwartz JKH and Canellos GP (1977) Basophilic chronic granulocytic leukaemia with hyperhistaminaemia. *Br J Haematol*, **36**, 367–372.

89 Marinone G, Rossi G and Verzura P (1983) Eosinophilic blast crisis in a case of chronic myeloid leukaemia. *Br J Haematol*, **55**, 251–256.

90 Hogge DE, Misawa S, Schiffer CA and Testa JR (1984) Promyelocytic blast crisis in chronic granulocytic leukaemia with 15;17 translocation. *Leuk Res*, **8**, 1019–1023.

91 Vardiman JW, Pierre R, Bain B, Bennett JM, Imbert M, Brunning RD and Flandrin G. Chronic myelomonocytic leukaemia. In: Jaffe ES, Harris NL, Stein H and Vardiman JW (eds), *World Health Organization Classification of Tumours: Pathology and Genetics of Tumours of Haematopoietic and Lymphoid Tissues*, IARC Press, Lyon, 2001.

92 Vardiman JW, Imbert M, Pierre R, Bain B, Bennett JM, Brunning RD and Flandrin G. Atypical chronic myeloid leukaemia. In: Jaffe ES, Harris NL, Stein H and Vardiman JW (eds), *World Health Organization Classification of Tumours: Pathology and Genetics of Tumours of Haematopoietic and Lymphoid Tissues*, IARC Press, Lyon, 2001.

93 Vardiman JW, Pierre R, Imbert M, Bain B, Bennett JM, Brunning RD and Flandrin G. Juvenile myelomonocytic leukaemia. In: Jaffe ES, Harris NL, Stein H and Vardiman JW (eds), *World Health Organization Classification of Tumours: Pathology and Genetics of Tumours of Haematopoietic and Lymphoid Tissues*, IARC Press, Lyon, 2001.

94 Castro-Malaspina H, Schaison G, Passe S, Pasquier A, Bergen R, Bayle-Weisgerber C *et al.* (1984) Subacute and chronic myelomonocytic leukemia in children (juvenile CML). *Cancer*, **54**, 675–686.

95 You W and Weisbrot IM (1984) Chronic neutrophilic leukemia, report of two cases and review of the literature. *Am J Clin Pathol*, **72**, 233–242.

96 Kanoh T, Saigo K and Yamagishi M (1986) Neutrophils with ring-shaped nuclei in chronic neutrophilic leukemia. *Am J Clin Pathol*, **86**, 748–751.

97 Zoumbos NC, Symeonidis A and Kourakli-Symeonidis A (1989) Chronic neutrophilic leukemia with dysplastic features: a new variant of myelodysplastic syndromes? *Acta Haematol*, **82**, 156–160.

98 Imbert M, Bain B, Pierre R, Vardiman JW, Brunning RD and Flandrin G. Chronic neutrophilic leukaemia. In: Jaffe ES, Harris NL, Stein H and Vardiman JW (eds), *The World Health Organization Classification of Tumours: Pathology and Genetics of Tumours of Haemopoietic and Lymphoid Tissues*, IARC Press, Lyon, 2001.

99 Bain BJ, Pierre R, Imbert M, Vardiman JW, Brunning RD and Flandrin G. Chronic eosinophilic leukaemia and the idiopathic hypereosinophilic syndrome. In: Jaffe ES, Harris NL, Stein H and Vardiman JW (eds), *The World Health Organization Classification of Tumours: Pathology and Genetics of Tumours of Haemopoietic and Lymphoid Tissues*, IARC Press, Lyon, 2001.

100 Cools J, DeAngelo DJ, Gotlib J, Stover EH, Legare RD, Cortes J *et al.* (2003) A tyrosine kinase created by the fusion of the PDGFRA and FIP1L1 genes as a therapeutic target of imatinib in idiopathic hypereosinophilic syndrome. *N Engl J Med*, **348**, 1201–1214.

101 Arora B, Sirhan S, Hoyer JD, Mesa RA and Tefferi A (2005) Peripheral blood CD34 count in myelofibrosis with myeloid metaplasia: a prospective evaluation of prognostic value in 94 patients. *Br J Haematol*, **128**, 42–48.

102 Tefferi A and Elliott MA (2000) Serious myelo-proliferative reactions associated with the use of thalidomide in myelofibrosis with myeloid metaplasia. *Blood*, **96**, 4007.

103 Blatt J, Penchansky L and Horn M (1989) Thrombocytosis as a presenting feature in acute lymphoblastic leukemia of childhood. *Am J Hematol*, **31**, 46–49.

104 Bain BJ and Catovsky D (1994) The leukaemic phase of non-Hodgkin's lymphoma. *J Clin Pathol*, **48**, 189–193.

105 Bennett JM, Catovsky D, Daniel M-T, Flandrin G, Galton DAG and Gralnick H and Sultan C (1989) Proposals for the classification of chronic (mature) B and T lymphoid Leukaemias *J Clin Pathol*, **42**, 567–584.

106 Bain BJ, Clark D, Lampert IA and Wilkins BS, *Bone Marrow Pathology*, 3rd Edn. Blackwell Science, Oxford, 2000.

107 Dorion RP and Shaw JH (2003) Intracytoplasmic filamentous inclusions in the peripheral blood of a patient with chronic lymphocytic leukemia: a bright-field, electron microscopic, immunofluorescent, and flow cytometric study. *Arch Pathol Lab Med*, **127**, 618–620.

108 Girodon F, Poillot N, Martin I, Carli PM and Maynadie M (2004) Crystalline inclusions in B monoclonal lymphocytes. *Haematologica*, **89**, ECR40.

109 Marti GE, Rawstron AC, Ghia P, Hillmen P, Houlston RS, Kay N *et al.* on behalf of The International Familial CLL Consortium (2005) Diagnostic criteria for monoclonal B-cell lymphocytosis. *Br J Haematol*, **130**, 325–332.

110 Nguyen D and Diamond L, *Diagnostic Hematology: a Pattern Approach*. Butterworth-Heinemann, Oxford, 2000.

111 Melo JV, Catovsky D and Galton DAG (1986) The relationship between chronic lymphocytic leukaemia and prolymphocytic leukaemia. I. Clinical and laboratory features of 300 patients and characterisation of an intermediate group. *Br J Haematol*, **63**, 377–387.

112 Machii T, Yamaguchi M, Inoue R, Tokumine Y, Kuratsune H, Nagai H *et al.* (1997) Polyclonal B-cell lymphocytosis with features resembling hairy cell leukemia-Japanese variant. *Blood*, **15**, 2008–2014.

113 Groom DA, Wong D, Brynes RK and Macaulay LK (1991) Auer rod-like inclusions in circulating lymphoma cells. *Am J Clin Pathol*, **96**, 111–115.

114 Bain BJ, Matutes E, Robinson D, Lampert IA, BritoBabapulle V, Morilla R and Catovsky D (1991) Leukaemia as a manifestation of large cell lymphoma. *Br J Haematol*, **77**, 301–310.

115 Cobcroft R (1999) Images in haematology: diagnosis of angiotropic large B-cell lymphoma from a peripheral blood film. *Br J Haematol*, **104**, 429.

116 Kyle RA, Maldonado JE and Bayrd ED (1974) Plasma cell leukaemia. Report on 17 cases. *Arch Intern Med*, **133**, 813–818.

117 Grogan TM, van Camp B, Kyle RA, Müller-Hermelink HK and Harris NL (2001) Plasma cell neoplasms. In: Jaffe ES, Harris NL, Stein H and Vardiman JW (eds), *World Health Organization Classification of Tumours: Pathology and Genetics of Tumours of Haematopoietic and Lymphoid Tissues*, IARC Press, Lyon, 2001.

118 Murayama K, Sawamura M and Tamura K (1993) Transient plasmacytosis with acute infection in myeloma. *Br J Haematol*, **82**, 475.

119 Witzig TE, Gertz MA, Lust JA, Kyle RA, O'Fallon WM and Greipp PR (1996) Peripheral blood monoclonal plasma cells as a predictor of survival in patients with multiple myeloma. *Blood*, **88**, 1780–1787.

120 Drayson M, Tang LX, Drew R, Mead GP, Carr-Smith H and Bradwell AR (2001) Serum free light-chains measurements for identifying and monitoring patients with nonsecretory multiple myeloma. *Blood*, **97**, 2900–2903.

121 Duncan SC and Winkelman RK (1978) Circulating Sézary cells in hospitalized dermatology patients. *Br J Dermatol*, **99**, 171–178.

122 Morice WG, Kurtin PJ, Leibson PJ, Tefferi A and Hanson CA (2003) Demonstration of aberrant T-cell and natural killer-cell antigen expression in all cases of granular lymphocytic leukaemia. *Br J Haematol*, **120**, 1026–1036.

123 Portlock CS, Donnelly GB, Qin J, Straus D, Yahalom J, Zelenetz A *et al.* (2004) Adverse prognostic significance of CD20 positive Reed–Sternberg cells in classical Hodgkin's disease. *Br J Haematol*, **125**, 701–708.

Answers to questions

MCQs

MCQ 9.1	TTFFF
MCQ 9.2	TTTFF

MCQ 9.3   TTTTF   **EMQ 9.3**
MCQ 9.4   TTFFF   1 F
MCQ 9.5   FTTFT   2 D
MCQ 9.6   FTTTF   3 J
                                           4 G
                                           5 E

EMQs

EMQ 9.1   **EMQ 9.4**
1 F   1 I
2 J   2 B
3 E   3 G
4 O   4 I
5 K   5 C

EMQ 9.2   **EMQ 9.5**
1 M   1 L
2 I   2 D
3 A   3 I
4 L   4 C
5 E   5 H

Index

Page numbers in *italics* represent figures, those in **bold** represent tables